PATHOLOGY ILLUSTRATED

PATHOLOGY ILLUSTRATED

ALASDAIR D T GOVAN PhD FRCP(Glas) FRCP(Edin) FRCOG FRCPath

Formerly Consultant Pathologist, Glasgow Royal Maternity Hospital

PETER S MACFARLANE MBChB FRCP(Glas) FRCP(Edin) FRCPath

Formerly Consultant Pathologist and Honorary Clinical Lecturer,
University of Glasgow at the Western Infirmary

ROBIN CALLANDER FFPh FMAA AIMBI

Formerly Director, Medical Illustration Unit,
University of Glasgow

THIRD EDITION

CHURCHILL LIVINGSTONE
EDINBURGH LONDON MELBOURNE AND NEW YORK 1991

CHURCHILL LIVINGSTONE
Medical Division of Longman Group UK Limited

Distributed in the United States of America by Churchill
Livingstone Inc., 1560 Broadway, New York, N.Y.
10036, and by associated companies, branches and
representatives throughout the world.

First published/edition 1981
Second edition 1986
  Reprinted 1986, 1988, 1989
Third edition 1991

ISBN 0-443-04167-9

British Library Cataloguing in Publication Data
Govan, Alexander D.T. (Alexander David Telford) *1913-*
    Pathology illustrated. – 3rd ed.
    1. Medicine. Pathology
    I. Title   II. Macfarlane, Peter S.   III. Callander, Robin
    1922-
    616.07
Library of Congress Cataloging in Publication Data
Govan, Alasdair D.T.
    Pathology illustrated/Alasdair D.T. Govan, Peter S. Macfarlane,
    Robin Callander. – 3rd ed.
    p. cm.
    Includes index.
    1. Pathology.   I. Macfarlane, Peter S.   II. Callander, Robin.
    III. Title.
    [DNLM: 1. Pathology.]
    RB111.G68 1991
    616.07 – dc20

Produced by Longman Group (FE) Ltd
Printed in Hong Kong

PREFACE

In the preface to the first edition we stated our motive as follows: "We believe that communication by verbal and written methods is the fundamental basis for study and learning. Nevertheless, in the modern setting where knowledge is increasing so rapidly and in a subject such as pathology where morphological changes are a major component, we consider that the visual image has an important facilitating role. We therefore offer this book as a companion to its predecessors in the Illustrated Series on medical subjects."

In this third edition the general layout and style have been retained: we have attempted, with no little difficulty, to accommodate, but at the same time keep in perspective, the important advances arising from the continuing explosive growth of knowledge of cellular and subcellular activities.

Glasgow, 1991

A.D.T. Govan
P.S. Macfarlane
R. Callander

CONTENTS

INTRODUCTION
 1. Cell and Tissue Damage   1
 2. Inflammation   29
 3. Infection   47
 4. Healing   75
 5. Immunity   93
 6. Circulatory Disturbances   119
 7. Neoplasia   159
 8. Cardiovascular System   207
 9. Respiratory System   287
10. Alimentary System   365
11. Liver, Gall Bladder and Pancreas   439
12. Haemopoietic and Lympho-Reticular Tissues   499
13. Genitourinary System   611
14. Nervous System   709
15. Musculo-Skeletal System   779
16. Endocrine System   823
Index   847

INTRODUCTION

INTRODUCTION

Students of pathology have already studied anatomy and physiology which represent the scientific study of the structure and function of the body in the process of normal living. At every level of measurement a range is established within which normal structure and function are defined. They have learned the relationship between form and function and must now enter the world of clinical medicine and the concept of disease.

Disease occurs when there are variations of structure and/or function outside the normal range.

PATHOLOGY is the scientific study of DISEASE. It is concerned with the causes and mechanisms by which disease is produced, with the descriptions of the manifestations of disease and with its progress and sequels. It is therefore one of the important sciences on which the practice of clinical medicine and surgery is based.

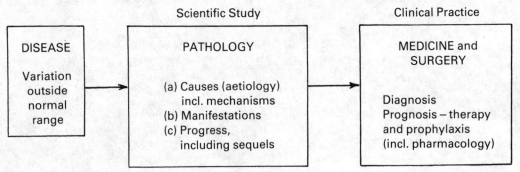

Because of the close relationship between the subjects, anatomical and physiological resumés are given throughout the book.

MANIFESTATIONS of DISEASE are essentially a summation of the damage done by a harmful agent and the body's response to it.

DAMAGE done by *HARMFUL AGENT* + *BODY'S REACTION* = *DISEASE*.

The components of this simple equation are themselves so very diverse and subject to modification by many factors that the spectrum of disease processes is very broad. Nonetheless scientific study demands analysis followed by resynthesis in the form of CLASSIFICATION.

The important broad groups of disease are:-

INFLAMMATORY   **DEGENERATIVE**   **NEOPLASTIC**
(incl. infections)   (excl. ageing)   (tumours)

Streptococcal sore throat is an example of a disease process caused by a single harmful agent.

- Streptococcal infection of throat
- General body reactions e.g. fever, malaise

1. 'Poisons' damage cells locally.
2. Local inflammatory response
3. Immune response

(a) *Usual* or (b) *Abnormal*

- Cure of infection
- Local abscess formation
- Rheumatic fever
- Nephritis

However in many diseases the harmful agents are multiple and the manifestations and progress of the disease very complex.

Age and disease

In young subjects a single harmful agent may cause disease leading to death if a vital organ is affected. With increasing age the chances of several harmful agents each causing separate diseases are enhanced and death is often due to the cumulative effect of such independant disease processes.

Physiological ageing implies a gradual loss of cellular and body vitality usually associated with atrophy of tissues and organs. This process is accentuated and mimicked by the degenerative diseases of old age (particularly arterial disease) so that the physiological and pathological states tend to merge. Nevertheless the student should try to identify the distinctions between ageing and disease although in some instances they may prove difficult to define.

Causes of disease

There are 2 broad groups.

1. Genetically determined disease

- Abnormalities of the chromosomes and component genes cause many diseases. The chromosomal changes are called mutations: the majority occur spontaneously (or without known cause): in some cases radiations, chemical or infective agents can be incriminated. The diseases produced range from serious defects incompatible with life to mild disorder presenting in adulthood. An important subdivision is the group of hereditary diseases in which family studies are particularly informative.

- Susceptibility to some diseases has long been linked with particular genetic types. The susceptibility of fair skin to damage caused by the ultraviolet rays in sunlight is well known and the mechanism — lack of the protective pigment mechanism — is obvious.
  More recently, associations between *particular normal genetic types* and *particular disease processes* have been discovered:

(i)   The blood group A is associated with an increased incidence of gastric cancer and pernicious anaemia and the blood group B with duodenal ulcer.

(ii) Another example is the ability of subjects who have inherited a particular blood group (Duffy negative) to resist infection by Plasmodium Vivax (a type of malaria).

(iii) The Human Leucocyte Antigen (HLA) system recently has been shown to have important associations with diseases, particularly infections and autoimmune processes. The system consists of protein substances on the surface of all cells (discovered first on leucocytes). The genetic control of the protein is on chromosome 6.

Chromosome 6   D   B   C   A   — genes on 4 loci,
                                                 each with many alleles.

The important rôles so far discovered are

(a) a close connection with graft rejection (the better the HLA match between subjects the better the chances of graft survival), and

(b) associations with disease processes of many types. The most striking association is of HLA B27 with ankylosing spondylitis (90 per cent of AS subjects are HLA B27).
   The mechanisms by which these associations are effected are currently the subject of intensive study.

Chromosome 6   D   B   C   A

Locus concerned with the
immune response –
particularly lymphocyte function:
implicated in auto-immune disease.

Loci concerned with infection
and graft rejection – important
implications in carcinogenesis
and transplant surgery.

2. Acquired Disease   The many causes can be classified under the following general headings:-

- **Physical agents** Among these are trauma, radiations, extremes of heat and cold, electrical power, i.e. the application to the body of an excess of physical energy in any form.
- **Chemical poisons** These are increasing in number particularly with the advances in industrial processing. Some act in a general manner, such as cyanide which is toxic to all cells. Others act locally, for example strong acids and caustics. Another group exhibit a predilection for certain organs — paraquat affects the lungs, phosphorus and organic solvents cause damage especially in the liver and kidneys.

  Iatrogenic disease is an important subgroup, not uncommon in present times due to the development of powerful drugs, many of which have undesirable side-effects.
- **Nutritional deficiencies** These may arise as a result of poor supply, interference with absorption, inefficient transport within the body or defective utilisation. In addition, the effects may be of a general nature as in starvation or lack of oxygen or they cause specific damage, for example, in vitamin deficiencies.
- **Infections and infestations** Viruses, bacteria, fungi, protozoa and metazoa all cause disease. They may do so by causing cell destruction directly as in certain virus infections, for example poliomyelitis, or protozoal infections, for example malaria. In many cases, however the damage is done by toxins elaborated by the infecting agent as in diphtheria and tetanus. As with poisons they may have a general effect or show a predilection for certain tissues.
- **Abnormal immunological reactions** The immune process is normally protective but in certain circumstances the reaction may become deranged. Hypersensitivity to various substances can lead to alarming shock-like conditions — anaphylaxis or to more localised lesions such as asthma. In other circumstances the immune process may act against the body cells — autoimmunity. This can be seen in certain endocrine diseases such as thyroiditis.
- **Psychological factors** cause and influence disease processes in several ways: (a) psychological stress may lead to mental illness; (b) their influence on the individual's symptoms and reaction to established somatic disease is apparent; (c) they are important components in disease caused by addiction, for example alcohol, tobacco; (d) finally it is thought that psychogenetic factors, by as yet ill-defined mechanisms, may be causally related to such diseases as hypertension, peptic ulcer, coronary arterial thrombosis and ulcerative colitis.

Although the causes of disease are divided into these two main groups, (i) genetically determined (ii) acquired, causes from both groups are operative in most disease processes.

The new technologies, particularly the use of genetic probes, which allow the identification of individual genes and their specific functions have increased our knowledge of the genetic component in many acquired diseases, for example where there is a high familial incidence of a particular disease it is now possible in some to identify the abnormal genes which may be contributing to the disorder. Another example is the discovery of acquired specific genetic abnormalities in stem cells, which potentiate the development of malignant tumours. The genes involved are proto-oncogenes (and virus oncogenes) which control cell proliferation and antioncogenes which control differentiation. The agents causing the abnormalities include chemicals, radiations and viruses.

Congenital disease is present at birth. It can either be genetically determined or acquired. An example of the latter type are the deformities caused by thalidomide taken by the mother during early pregnancy and it is becoming clear that environmental factors, for example nutritional factors and smoking, are very important environmental causes of congenital disease.

Investigation of disease

In medical practice the objective of the study of disease is twofold.
1. To determine the nature of the disease process and if possible its causation i.e. to establish a diagnosis.
2. To monitor the extent and progress of the disease and provide an indication of prognosis.

Historically the study of disease was based on morphological observations, first at a gross level and from the nineteenth century at cellular level and morbid anatomy and histology remain the corner stones of pathological study. The emergence of subspecialities, for example biochemistry and haematology has led to greater understanding in depth. But it is important that such knowledge should not be compartmentalised and one of the tasks of the modern student is to integrate information about disease from various sources and thus acquire a breadth of pathological knowledge.

Methods in pathology

The traditional methods of careful naked eye and light microscopic examination of organs and tissues at autopsy have been supplemented by the much wider use in clinical practice of *biopsy* which is the removal of tissue during life for diagnostic purposes. With the development of modern instrumentation biopsies are obtained from many parts of the body.

In addition, numerous technological advances have been applied to pathological methods at various levels with advantage. The following is a brief outline of these levels:

Level A. Morbid anatomy reveals the gross changes in diseased organs and indicates the secondary effects in other parts of the body.

Level B. Histology: diseases generally have a distinct pattern which can be recognised using the light microscope. Extensions of the method are histochemistry and immunohistochemistry by which the presence of various chemicals can be revealed.

Level C. Cytology: the study of cellular detail is of course a part of histology but the study of individual cells in detail is now important particularly in the diagnosis of cancer.

Level D. Electron-microscopy (EM) reveals the cellular organelles and various patterns of change found in disease.

Level E. The ultimate level, which is as yet beyond the scope of pathology in most cases, is in the field of molecular biology where form and function become one. At this level important advances in pathological knowledge have been made for example in the understanding of the roles of many chemical messengers and receptors.

These increasingly sophisticated methods tend to influence the student to focus on detailed mechanisms occurring at microscopic level. Without discouraging such an approach to the subject it must not be forgotton that the observations obtained over many years using the relatively simple methods of naked eye examination and histological assessment of routinely stained specimens are fundamental.

The following descriptions therefore begin with gross pathology and proceed stepwise to the detailed cellular changes where these are known. The students will find that such an approach is the basis of their learning and progress in clinical practice.

CHAPTER I

CELL AND TISSUE DAMAGE
Degenerations and Depositions

CELL DAMAGE

Visible changes occur in cells as a result of noxious agents, the degree of change varying with the severity of the damaging process.

CAUSES OF CELL DAMAGE

These are innumerable but are grouped as follows (the individual diseases mentioned are illustrative examples):

1. **Reduced oxygen supply** — respiratory disease, cardiovascular disease, anaemia
2. **Physical agents** — mechanical trauma, excessive heat or cold, radiations
3. **Chemical agents** — these continue to increase enormously with the complexity of industrial processes
4. **Toxins** — bacteria, plants, animals e.g. snakes
5. **Viruses**
6. **Abnormal immunological reaction** — hypersensitivity states, glomerulonephritis
7. **Nutritional deficiencies** — vitamin deficiency, malabsorption
8. **Genetic abnormalities** — Down's syndrome

NECROSIS

When, as a result of damage by the various agents mentioned above, cells or groups of cells die while still part of the living body the term **necrosis** is used. Death of the cell is associated with rapid depletion of intracellular energy systems. Initially there are no morphological changes. What we describe as necrosis is the result of the liberation of intracellular enzymes following upon the disruption of cytoplasmic organelles, disintegration of the nucleus and changes in the plasma membrane.

Group of necrotic cells

Passage into cell of Ca^{++} and Na^+

Passage out of cell of K^+ and ENZYMES

Loss of PLASMA MEMBRANE BARRIER FUNCTION

Blood vessel

Concentration of enzymes increases in blood — used in diagnostic tests.

Necrosis is associated with visible changes:

1. **Coagulative necrosis** is the classical appearance.
2. Several other descriptive forms where the appearances are modified by additional local factors, particularly the action of released enzymes.

NECROSIS

COAGULATIVE NECROSIS

This type of necrosis is frequently caused by lack of blood supply and is exemplified well in infarcts of solid organs, e.g. heart, spleen and kidney.

Naked eye appearance of kidney

Microscopic appearance

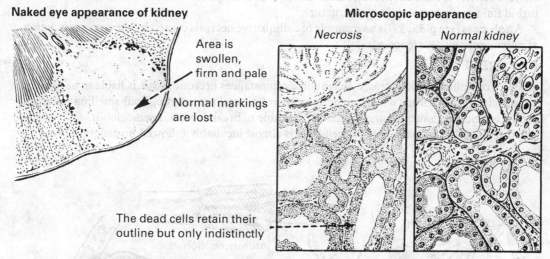

Area is swollen, firm and pale

Normal markings are lost

Necrosis

Normal kidney

The dead cells retain their outline but only indistinctly

At *light microscopic level* the following changes in the cell are seen:

1. The nucleus shows one of two changes (a) Karyolysis (b) Karyorrhexis.
2. The cytoplasm becomes opaque and strongly eosinophilic (affinity for the red dye, eosin).

Normal cell

Translucent granular cytoplasm

Nucleus with vesicular chromatin

damaging agent

Necrosis

(a)

or

(b)

Nucleus fades and dissolves = KARYOLYSIS

Cytoplasm opaque

Nucleus shrinks and becomes dense = PYKNOSIS

Nucleus fragments = KARYORRHEXIS

At *electron microscope (E.M.) level*, in addition to the above nuclear changes, disorganisation and disintegration of the cytoplasmic organelles and severe damage to the plasma membrane are seen.

NECROSIS

COLLIQUATIVE NECROSIS

In the brain consistently, and in other tissues when they contain a large amount of fluid and enzyme activity is marked, necrotic areas undergo softening and are filled with pigmented or turbid fluid, with complete loss of structure.

An **abscess** (see p.38, 39) is an example of colliquative necrosis caused by the enzymatic action of polymorphonuclear leucocytes.

GANGRENE

This is a complication of necrosis. In certain circumstances necrotic tissue is liable to be invaded by putrefactive organisms which are both saccharolytic and proteolytic. Foul-smelling gases are produced and the tissue becomes green or black due to breakdown of haemoglobin.

Obstruction of the blood supply to the bowel is almost inevitably followed by gangrene, e.g.:

Thrombosis or embolism

Intussusception

Strangulated hernia

Volvulus

Gangrene also occurs on the skin surface following arterial obstruction. It is particularly liable to affect the limbs, especially the toes in diseases such as diabetes.

A special type of gangrene follows infection with clostridial organisms (gas gangrene; see p.56).

NECROSIS

CASEOUS NECROSIS (CASEATION)

The necrotic tissue assumes a cream-cheesy appearance, slightly greasy to the touch. It is commonly seen in tuberculosis (see p.58).

FAT NECROSIS

Adipose tissue is damaged in pancreatitis and occasionally due to trauma. The special appearances are due to the action of lipases on triglycerides as follows:

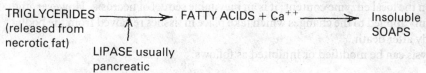

TRIGLYCERIDES ⟶ FATTY ACIDS + Ca^{++} ⟶ Insoluble
(released from   ↑   SOAPS
necrotic fat)   LIPASE usually
              pancreatic

E.g. Appearances in omentum and mesenteries.

Naked eye

Opaque white patches

Microscopic

Normal fatty tissue

Necrotic

Note loss of nuclei and cell structure, and deposition of insoluble **soaps**.

FIBRINOID NECROSIS

This is a descriptive term in which connective tissues and especially arterial walls are infiltrated by a strongly eosinophilic hyaline material which shows some of the characteristics of fibrin. Any actual necrosis is usually inconspicuous (see p.221).

NECROSIS — AUTOLYSIS

SEQUELS OF NECROSIS

1. When small numbers of cells are involved, the cellular debris is removed by PHAGOCYTOSIS (see p.34).
2. With larger numbers of dead cells, there is an inflammatory response with **organisation** and fibrous repair (see p.40).
3. When the necrotic tissue cannot be completely removed or organised, deposition of **calcium** may be an additional feature, for example in TUBERCULOUS CASEOUS NECROSIS and the ARTHEROMATOUS AORTA. This feature is important in radiological diagnosis.

AUTOLYSIS

The process of 'self digestion' begins after the death of the cell (as described above) and proceeds at a rate dependent on the local enzyme content; it is an inevitable sequel of necrosis. However, the term is more commonly applied to the changes which take place in tissues removed from the body and in the whole body after death.

In practice, autolysis can be modified or inhibited as follows:

(1) by REFRIGERATION
↓
ENZYME activity
slowed down
↓
Whole body
'preserved'
↓
AUTOPSY performed
without undue
haste

(2) by FIXATION
↓
CHEMICALS added
(e.g. formalin)
or HEAT
↓
ENZYMES and PROTEINS
DENATURED
↓
AVAILABLE for PATHOLOGICAL
PROCESSING

APOStosIS

APOPTOSIS (formerly called 'Necrobiosis')

This term has been used for a mechanism of cell death affecting single cells scattered in a population of healthy cells. It differs from necrosis and represents a physiological process by which effete and abnormal cells die and are eliminated.

Apoptosis is rapid (completed in a few hours) and is considered in two stages:

Stage 1
The dying process

(a) Active metabolic changes in the cell cause — cytoplasmic and nuclear condensation

Plasma membrane intact

(b) Cell disintegrates into apoptotic bodies — each surrounded by a plasma membrane

Some contain nuclear material

Stage 2
The elimination process

Phagocytosis by surrounding cells (e.g. liver cells, tumour cells) followed by rapid digestion

Note
1. The surrounding cells move together to fill the vacant space leaving virtually no evidence of the process.
2. The presence of intact plasma membranes around the apoptotic bodies explains the absence of inflammation.

Significance

The process is important physiologically in balancing cell proliferation and elimination. It is associated with:

      (a) maintenance of the organ size in the adult
      (b) organ development and modelling in the embryo
      (c) physiological atrophy and involution.

It is important in pathological processes particularly associated with organ atrophy and cell elimination (e.g. in tumour growth and leukaemia).

CELL DAMAGE — HYDROPIC SWELLING

The various agents which can cause cell necrosis may also cause lesser cell damage which is reversible when the injurious agent is removed.

The appearances and effects are considered under these headings: (1) **hydropic swelling,** (2) **fatty change,** (3) **radiation** and (4) **atrophy.**

HYDROPIC SWELLING

Hydropic swelling — formerly called Cloudy swelling — proceeds to hydropic vacuolation.

Normal tubules **Hydropic swelling** **Hydropic vacuolation**

Toxin

Cells swell
Cytoplasm contains
coarse granules

Cytoplasm contains
watery vacuoles

The damaged organs become swollen and on section may have a 'par-boiled' appearance.

Electron microscopic (E.M.) appearances indicate the mechanisms:

Toxic
action

Normal plasma
membrane and
mitochondria

Damaged plasma
membrane:
diminished ATP
diminished Na⁺ pump

Mitochondria
rounded, beaded:
cause granularity
and eosinophilia.

Na^+ into
cell

WATER into
cell

Vacuolation
of endoplasmic
reticulum

CELL DAMAGE — FATTY CHANGE

This is the accumulation of fat in non-fatty tissues, especially the parenchymatous organs, skeletal muscles and the heart, which have a high metabolic rate.

The essential problem is the inability of the non-fatty tissues to metabolise the amount of fat presented to them, resulting in its accumulation within the cells. There are numerous individual causes but essentially they can be considered in two main groups:

Group A

The agents in this group interfere with enzyme action in the cells. They can be further divided into two sub-groups and their action can be visualised as follows:

(1) Bacterial toxins or chemical poisons (chloroform, alcohol)
↓
Reduced ability to form enzymes

(2) Clinical conditions resulting in anoxia (anaemia, cardiac failure, extensive respiratory disease)
↓
Cellular energy impaired
↓
Diminished enzyme activity

Inability to metabolise fat
↓
Often marked ← Accumulation of fat in cells → Usually moderate

Frequently both sub-groups may be in action; for example, in respiratory disease there may be infection-releasing bacterial toxins and, at the same time, oxygenation may be much diminished.

Group B

Under this heading are conditions where there is a metabolic upset resulting in lack of substances necessary for the utilisation of fat. Two examples and the mode of action are shown in the flow diagram.

Diabetes
↓
Impaired carbohydrate metabolism

Starvation
↓
Lack of other essential food substance including carbohydrate

Cellular energy impaired → Mobilisation of depot fat ← Cellular energy impaired
↓
Incomplete utilisation of fat
↓
Accumulation of fat in cells

Note: Impaired cellular energy is basic in both groups.

CELL DAMAGE — FATTY CHANGE

In non-fatty tissues the intracellular fat is not visible by light microscopy using conventional fat stains.

In fatty change, the accumulated fat is visualised using frozen sections and fat-soluble dyes: in routine paraffin sections the fat has been dissolved and is indicated by clear vacuoles.

LIVER

Since this organ plays a central role in fat metabolism, the accumulation of fat in toxic conditions can be very considerable. Equally, because of the large normal turnover of fat, the amount which accumulates is not directly related to the degree of cell damage.

The increase of deposited fat causes enlargement of the organ. Its distribution varies with the cause, e.g. —

(1) **Lack of Oxygen** — in anaemia and cardiac failure

Fats tend to be deposited furthest from the arterial blood supply (hepatic arteriole) around the efferent vein (hepatic venule)

(2) **Poison, Toxins etc** — alcohol, infections, organic solvents

Fat is found nearest the afferent blood supply (portal venule and hepatic arteriole)

HEART

The heart is enlarged due to dilatation. In most cases there is a general pallor, but occasionally in severe anaemia there may be a rather speckled appearance especially over the papillary muscles. Microscopically, fine fat globules form in rows within the muscle fibres.

Transvers striation is obscured

KIDNEY

In most cases fatty change is confined to the epithelium of the convoluted tubules, but in severe poisoning it may affect all structures including the glomeruli.

CELL DAMAGE — FATTY CHANGE

EFFECTS OF FATTY CHANGE

Impairment of cellular function is usually due to the pathological process causing the fatty change (e.g. anoxia in severe anaemia) and not to the physical presence of fat within the cell. In the liver, for example, very large accumulations of fat do not impair basic liver functions.

A possible exception is the myocardium in certain circumstances.

(a) **Rapid or large transfusion** → Increased ventricular pressure → Dilatation of right heart → Cardiac failure

+

Fatty myocardium → Weak muscle fibres

(b) **Sudden excessive exertion** → Rise in blood pressure → Temporary left sided cardiac embarrassment

+

Fatty myocardium → Weak muscle fibres

OBESITY must be distinguished from intra-cellular fatty change described above.

Gross degrees of obesity lead to increased **adipose tissue** in abnormal sites, e.g. between myocardial fibres. In addition, parenchymal cells are unable to deal with the excessive intake of fat and a degree of fatty change occurs in them. The myocardium is under strain due to the circulatory resistance in the excessive adipose tissues.

The main controllable cause of obesity is increased intake of food, but other factors, both genetic and environmental, exert an influence. The diagram illustrates how the Food/Energy balance may be upset.

DECREASED

EXERCISE   ENDOCRINE STATUS

HEAT PRODUCTION   ↓ hypothalamus and thyroid function

DECREASED ENERGY UTILISATION

EXCESSIVE FOOD

INTAKE   ABSORPTION

particularly refined carbohydrate and fat

INCREASED DEPOSITION

Balance tipped towards **OBESITY**

Effects: Obesity reduces life expectancy mainly due to its association with cardiovascular disease.

CELL DAMAGE — RADIATION

High energy (ionising) radiation, particularly in the form of gamma (α) or X-rays can cause serious cellular and tissue damage.

At cellular level there are 2 mechanisms involving:

1. The cell CYTOPLASM

A large dose of radiation hydrolyses water producing damaging hydroxyl radicals: acute cell death follows

2. The cell NUCLEUS

Lower doses damage DNA with 2 results:
(a) failure to replicate
(b) mutation with variable genetic abnormalities

These effects will be considered under 3 headings:

1. The **localised effects** complicating radiotherapy in the tissues adjacent to the therapeutic field.

   Following any reparable acute damage a latent period precedes persistent injury. This is caused by:

   (a) damage to blood vessels ⎫ leading to (a) *ischaemia*
   (b) damage to fibroblasts ⎭ (b) *dense fibrosis*

   Injury to organs which are difficult to shield is seen, for example, in skin, eyes, alimentary tract, bladder, lungs, gonads and spinal cord.

   In surgical practice, wound healing is seriously impaired.

2. Some of the **mutations** may lead to **cancer** (at most 2% of all malignancies are associated with radiation).

   The mechanisms are described on page 196.

3. **Whole body radiation** is usually the result of atomic explosion. The acute effects which are related to large doses are summarised below.

Dose (rads)	Result	Mechanism
over 2,000	Death in a few hours	All cells damaged but particularly **CNS**: CEREBRAL OEDEMA ↓ COMA
1,000	Death 3 – 7 days	Mucous lining of **intestine** destroyed: DIARRHOEA: SEPTICAEMIC SHOCK
300	Death 2 – 3 weeks	**Bone marrow** destroyed: LEUCOPENIA THROMBOCYTOPENIA ↓ INFECTION: HAEMORRHAGE
40	Damage to fetus in early pregnancy	**Fetal** abnormalities

ATROPHY

This is a simple decrease in cell size or number, resulting in a shrinkage of affected tissues and organs. The most common example is atrophy of old age (see p.14)

Causes

(1) Gradual diminution in blood supply → Reduction in oxygen supply and nutrients → General fall in cell activity and shrinkage, e.g. narrowing of coronary arteries → myocardial atrophy

Normal

Accumulation of lipofuscin around nucleus

Lipofuscin ("wear and tear" pigment) is a golden yellow pigment representing undigested lipid material derived from cellular metabolism.

(2) Reduced functional activity (disuse atrophy) → Diminished demand for nutrition → Atrophy of cells

E.g. Obstruction of gland duct → Atrophy of gland

(3) Interrupted nerve supply → Reduced reflex and metabolic activitites, e.g. atrophy of skeletal muscles after destruction of motor nerves as in poliomyelitis.

← Normal

← Loss of structure and shrinkage

(4) Endocrine deficiency → Loss of regulating mechanism → Reduced metabolic activity in dependent tissues

E.g. Pituitary deficiency → Atrophy of → Thyroid
Adrenals
Gonads and genital organs

(5) Pressure → Interruption of blood supply and interference with function, e.g. neoplasm pressing on surrounding tissues.

Atrophy is reversible provided the cause is eliminated or deficiencies restored.

13

AGEING

The distinction between 'true' ageing and ageing complicated by disease processes may be difficult; since therapy can be directed at the latter the distinction is important in clinical practice.

The changes associated with *true* ageing would be seen in a theoretical 'ideal' environment (minimal stress).

The following diagram is illustrative. The main controlling factors are *intrinsic,* i.e. genetic.

In the real environment this theoretical concept of ageing is accelerated and aggravated by two groups of *extrinsic* factors:

N.B. Death is only very rarely, if ever, due to 'pure' ageing. It is the result of disease — either a single process or, with increasing age, more often several causes.

DEPOSITIONS

AMYLOID DEPOSITION

In this condition, a 'waxy' substance composed essentially of an abnormal protein is deposited in the extracellular tissues, particularly around the supporting fibres of blood vessels and basement membranes. Amyloid is resistant to degradation and removal by the usual processes so that the deposition progresses relentlessly.

Detection

Amyloid may be suspected when the organs are pale and enlarged and have a firm waxy texture at post-mortem, but in clinical practice, chemical tests on microscopic preparations and even electron microscopy are required using biopsy material.

Post-mortem organs

LUGOL'S IODINE
→ Amyloid — deep brown
→ Normal tissue — yellow

Biopsy materials 1. Light microscopic sections

CONGO RED
→ Amyloid — red and specific apple green fluorescence in polarised light
→ Normal tissue — pale pink or yellow: no fluorescence

2. E.M. — specific appearance: closely packed interlacing fibrils 70 to 100 Å in diameter

Nature of amyloid

Chemical — the fibrils are composed of one major and two minor components:
1. Protein — variable (see p.17)
2. (a) Protein — constant normally found in serum:
   called SERUM AMYLOID PROTEIN (SAP).
   (b) Carbohydrate — a glycosaminoglycan (e.g. heparin sulphate) – this gives the iodine stain.

Physical — the fibrils are organised uniquely — ß-pleated.

This accounts for the specific staining properties and the inability of the body to degrade the substance.

Pathological effects

AMYLOID DEPOSITION

Pressure on adjacent cells

Blood vessels

Narrowing

Increased permeability

ATROPHY

TRANSUDATION OF PROTEIN
out of vessels

AMYLOID DEPOSITION

Almost any tissue in the body may be affected by amyloid deposition, but the most important changes occur in the kidney, gastrointestinal tract and the heart. Other organs, such as the liver and spleen, may also be grossly affected without serious functional impairment.

KIDNEY

In severe cases the kidneys are pale, firm and waxy, and with the iodine test the glomeruli stand out as brown dots to the naked eye.

Renal biopsy is useful in the diagnosis of amyloidosis.

Deposits around glomerular capillaries

Thickened basement membranes of tubules

Atrophic tubules

Effects: Glomerular capillary permeability altered:

GROSS PROTEINURIA ⟶ NEPHROTIC SYNDROME

GASTROINTESTINAL TRACT

Due to altered permeability of the capillaries, the patient suffers from diarrhoea and protein loss. There may also be malabsorption, nutritional deficiencies and electrolyte imbalance.

Rectal biopsy is useful in the diagnosis of amyloidosis.

Amyloid in capillary walls

HEART

Amyloid deposition occurs around the cardiac muscle fibres and the capillary basement membranes. The heart is enlarged with apparently thick muscular walls but much of the thickness is due to amyloid deposition.

Amyloid

Shrunken atrophic muscle fibres

Effects: Cardiac failure develops mainly due to the mechanical effect of amyloid, preventing proper muscular contraction, and partly to malnutrition of the muscle fibres caused by poor blood supply.

AMYLOID DEPOSITION

MECHANISMS OF AMYLOID DEPOSITION

The essential element in amyloid deposition is the production of a protein which is either amyloidogenic itself or can be modified to become amyloidogenic.

Amyloidogenic proteins

1. *Amyloid A protein (AA)*
This protein is closely related to acute phase reactive protein which appears in the serum in many inflammatory conditions.

2. *Amyloid Light China derived protein (AL)*
This protein is derived from fragments of immunoglobulin molecules (particularly lambda light chains) and is essentially a product of plasma cells.

The important facts about these proteins is that they form specific amyloid fibrils in which the molecules of constituent polypeptides are arranged in a most unusual fashion, called ß-pleating. This imparts to amyloid its specific chemical staining characteristics and accounts for its resistance to degradation.

The mechanism of amyloid deposition is shown thus:

Amyloidogenic proteins and polypeptides may also occur in other circumstances, e.g. in tumours of endocrine glands producing polypeptide hormones (e.g. calcitonin, insulin) and in cases of rare familial amyloidosis.

In old age, minor deposits of amyloid may occur in the heart and brain; the amyloidogenic protein in these cases is related to prealbumin.

AMYLOID DEPOSITION

CLASSIFICATION

Amyloidosis was previously classified into two main types, and the distribution of amyloid among various organs was observed to be different in these types, although considerable overlapping occurred.

1. **Primary,** i.e. without known cause.
2. **Secondary,** i.e. associated with chronic inflammatory diseases such as tuberculosis, osteomyelitis, rheumatoid arthritis.

Modern knowledge of the mechanisms underlying amyloid deposition have made this classification obsolete. The classification which emerges from knowledge of the mechanisms of amyloid deposition and the more usual associated precursor diseases is shown as follows:

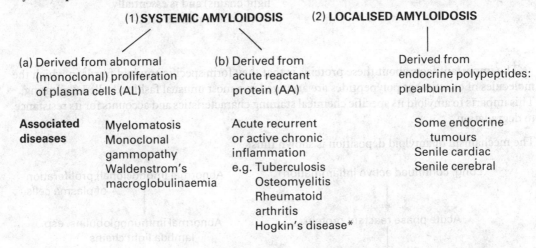

	(1) **SYSTEMIC AMYLOIDOSIS**		(2) **LOCALISED AMYLOIDOSIS**
	(a) Derived from abnormal (monoclonal) proliferation of plasma cells (AL)	(b) Derived from acute reactant protein (AA)	Derived from endocrine polypeptides: prealbumin
Associated diseases	Myelomatosis Monoclonal gammopathy Waldenstrom's macroglobulinaemia	Acute recurrent or active chronic inflammation e.g. Tuberculosis Osteomyelitis Rheumatoid arthritis Hogkin's disease*	Some endocrine tumours Senile cardiac Senile cerebral

Note: Not all cases of these diseases are associated with amyloid; e.g. certain chronic inflammatory diseases are not associated with amyloid, such as ulcerative colitis and systemic lupus erythematosus, since the serum acute reactant protein is minimally raised.

*Hodgkin's disease is considered to be a tumour with a marked inflammatory reaction (see p.598)

CALCIFICATION

Abnormal deposits of calcium salts occur in two circumstances: dystrophic calcification and metastatic calcification.

1. DYSTROPHIC CALCIFICATION
Local deposits of calcium may occur in:

(a) Necrotic tissue which is not obsorbed,
e.g. old caseous lesions of tuberculosis; old infarcts; old collections of pus; dead parasites; old thrombi.

An important variation of this is the accumulation of calcium around dead cells in ducts, leading to stone formation.

(b) Tissues undergoing slow degeneration,
e.g. hyaline areas in simple tumours; tissues in old age, especially fibrous tissue, cartilage and in arteries due to atheromatous degeneration.

The mechanism may be as follows:

Necrosis or degeneration of tissue → Release of enzymes → Breakdown of organic phosphates / Alteration of pH → Favour deposition of calcium

Note: The presence of radio-opaque Ca^{++} is of diagnostic use particularly in old healed disease (e.g. tuberculosis) and also in some tumours, e.g. breast cancer where very small deposits of calcium may be present.

2. METASTATIC CALCIFICATION
In this case the essential feature is an increase in the blood calcium. The 2 usual mechanisms are as follows:

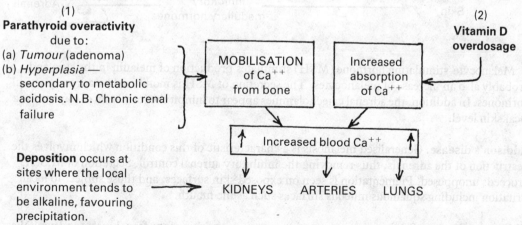

(1)
Parathyroid overactivity
    due to:
(a) *Tumour* (adenoma)
(b) *Hyperplasia* — secondary to metabolic acidosis. N.B. Chronic renal failure

(2)
Vitamin D overdosage

MOBILISATION of Ca^{++} from bone

Increased absorption of Ca^{++}

Increased blood Ca^{++}

KIDNEYS   ARTERIES   LUNGS

Deposition occurs at sites where the local environment tends to be alkaline, favouring precipitation.

About 5% of MALIGNANCY cases — particularly with carcinoma of the breast and lung — have HYPERCALCAEMIA, although most do not live long enough to have significant systemic deposition.

The mechanisms are (1) secretion by the tumour of a protein which mimics the action of parathormone and (2), of less importance, the local release of bone resorbing cytokines by tumour metastases in bones.

19

ENDOGENOUS PIGMENTATION

MELANIN PIGMENTATION

Melanin is a normal pigment found in the form of fine brown granules in the skin, choroid of the eye, adrenal medulla and sometimes in the meninges. It is produced by melanocytes embryologically derived from the neural crest and which have a dendritic branching form. After secretion of the pigment, it is taken up by adjacent epidermal cells and phagocytic melanophores in the underlying dermis.

Melanocytes   Melanophores

Local melanin pigmentation
This is seen in tumours derived from the melanocytes of the skin and choroid coat of the eye.

Generalised melanin pigmentation
Suntan is a temporary general melanin pigmentation of the skin due to ultraviolet rays. The mechanism and its control are as follows:

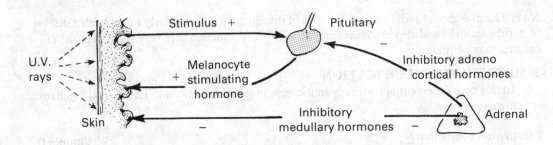

Melanocyte-stimulating hormone (MSH) stimulates production of melanin in the skin and probably also an increase of melanocytes. The secretion of MSH is monitored by adreno-cortical hormones. In addition, the adrenal catecholamines appear to inhibit the formation of pigment at a local skin level.

Addison's disease. Generalised melanosis is a characteristic of this condition which involves the destruction of the adrenals, thus removing the inhibitory adrenal control. Secretion of M.S.H. proceeds unopposed. Pigmentation is seen on exposed skin surfaces, and those subject to local irritation including squamous mucous surfaces such as the mouth.

Chloasma. Patches of melanotic pigmentation appear on the skin of the face, breasts and genitalia due to increased secretion of MSH. It is most common in pregnancy.

ENDOGENOUS PIGMENTATION

Haemoglobin is broken down and the main products, haem and its derivatives and the protein fraction GLOBIN, are re-used or excreted as follows:

(A) Destruction of effete red cells by the MACROPHAGES in the SPLENIC RETICULUM (also in other tissues, e.g. bone marrow and liver)

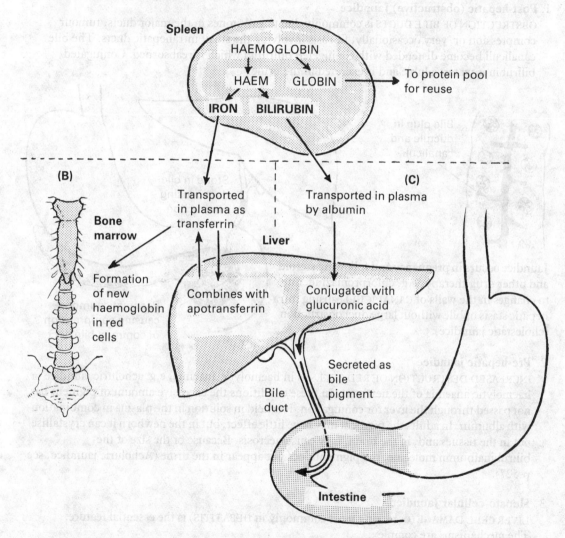

Abnormalities arising at various stages may be associated with the accumulation of pigments as illustrated in the following examples.

ENDOGENOUS PIGMENTATION

JAUNDICE due to BILIRUBIN (IRON-FREE PIGMENT)
When the bilirubin content of the serum rises above 34µmol/l, jaundice appears. This can be brought about by an abnormality in one of 3 main ways:

1. **Post-hepatic (obstructive) Jaundice**
   OBSTRUCTION OF BILE DUCTS is commonly due to gall stones in the major ducts, tumour compression or, very occasionally, fibrosis involving the small intrahepatic ducts. The bile canaliculi become distended with conjugated bilirubin which is reabsorbed. Conjugated bilirubin is water-soluble and is excreted in the urine.

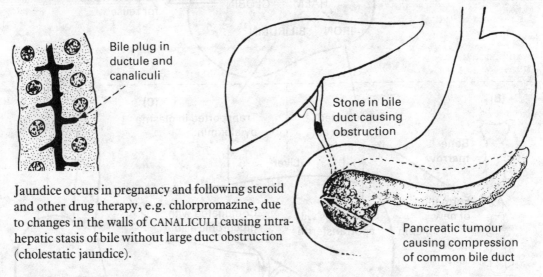

Bile plug in ductule and canaliculi

Stone in bile duct causing obstruction

Pancreatic tumour causing compression of common bile duct

Jaundice occurs in pregnancy and following steroid and other drug therapy, e.g. chlorpromazine, due to changes in the walls of CANALICULI causing intra-hepatic stasis of bile without large duct obstruction (cholestatic jaundice).

2. **Pre-hepatic jaundice**
   INCREASED DESTRUCTION OF RED CELLS as in haemolytic anaemia, e.g. acholuric jaundice or haemolytic anaemia of the newborn. In these conditions the excessive amount of pigment has not passed through the liver for conjugation. It is held in solution in the plasma in combination with albumin. In adults the pigment may have little effect, but in the newborn it can crystallise out in the tissues and, in the brain, may cause necrosis. Because of the size of the bilirubinalbumin molecule, the pigment does not appear in the urine (Acholuric jaundice, see p.527).

3. **Hepato-cellular Jaundice**
   LIVER CELL DAMAGE (occurring most commonly in HEPATITIS) is the essential feature. The mechanisms are complex:

Liver cell damage ⟶ Failure to conjugate bilirubin
Swelling ⟶ Necrosis ⟶ Architectural disturbance
Local cholestasis   Reabsorption of conjugated bilirubin

ENDOGENOUS PIGMENTATION

IRON-CONTAINING PIGMENTS

Haemosiderin

The iron derived from red cell breakdown is held in the spleen, liver and marrow, combined with apoferritin. In the plasma it is transported by transferrin. The two mechanisms maintain an equilibrium between the iron contents in these three sites. When the amount of iron within the cells becomes excessive and overloads the ferritin system, it is deposited in a brown granular form — haemosiderin.

This occurs in two situations:-

1. **Local breakdown of red cells in tissues e.g. in**

The colour changes in a 'black' eye exemplifiy this mechanism

Internal haemorrhage

Extravasated red cells

↓

Phagocytosis of red cells by macrophages

↓   ↓

Haemosiderin   Iron free pigments

RED

↓

GREENISH BLUE

↓

Yellow

2. **Visceral siderosis**

This is seen in the liver, spleen and sometimes the kidneys in cases of haemolytic anaemia, and in patients requiring repeated blood transfusion. The change is most strikingly seen in the liver, which becomes deep brown. Iron is found in the liver parenchyma, in Kupffer cells and in liver cells. Easily demonstrated by the Prussion Blue reaction.

Granules of haemosiderin in liver cells and Kupffer cells

ENDOGENOUS PIGMENTATION

Haemosiderin (continued)

Haemochromatosis (Bronzed diabetes)
The absorption of iron from the intestine is controlled by the ferritin-transferrin mechanism already mentioned.

The ferritin content of the intestinal epithelium, iron saturation of the plasma, stores of iron in the liver and spleen and the demand for iron by the bone marrow form a balancing mechanism preventing overloading of any part of the system.

In haemochromatosis, a genetic disorder, the absorption of iron is virtually uncontrolled. The system becomes overloaded and iron is deposited as haemosiderin in many sites, the main ones being:

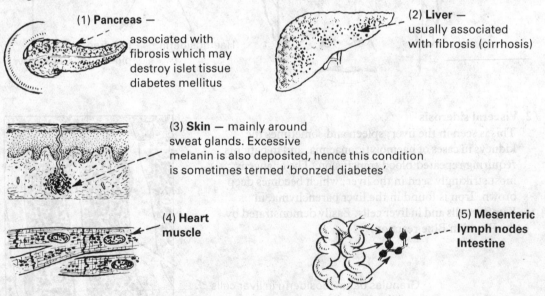

(1) **Pancreas** — associated with fibrosis which may destroy islet tissue diabetes mellitus

(2) **Liver** — usually associated with fibrosis (cirrhosis)

(3) **Skin** — mainly around sweat glands. Excessive melanin is also deposited, hence this condition is sometimes termed 'bronzed diabetes'

(4) **Heart muscle**

(5) **Mesenteric lymph nodes Intestine**

Haemosiderin may be found in almost any site in the body.

ENDOGENOUS PIGMENTATION

IRON-CONTAINING PIGMENTS (continued)

Haemoglobin

Occasionally, intravascular haemolysis occurs.
Haemoglobin appears in the urine, giving it a dull red
colour. If the condition is chronic, as in paroxysmal
haemoglobinuria, some of the haemoglobin is
reabsorbed and subsequently broken down so that iron,
as haemosiderin, appears in the renal tubular epithelium.

(Demonstrated by the
Prussian blue reaction)

Haematin (or haemazoin)

This is a brown pigment produced by malarial parasites
from haemoglobin. It is taken up by the monocytes in
the blood and subsequently deposited in the liver and
spleen.

Red-cell – containing malarial parasite

Monocyte – containing haematin

Lipofuscin

This is a yellowish brown pigment having a high lipid content, often found in the atrophied cells
of old age — 'wear and tear' pigment. It is particularly common in the heart muscle, and the term
'brown atrophy' is often applied.

Thin myocardial fibre
Pigment granules around nucleus

It is also found in liver cells, testes and nerve cells.

EXOGENOUS PIGMENTATION — DEGENERATIONS

EXOGENOUS PIGMENTATION

Pigments may be introduced by inhalation, ingestion or injection. The most important are those introduced by inhalation of dusts in industrial processes.

Inhalation

The commonest substances inhaled are COAL DUST (carbon) — black, and STONE DUST (silica) — grey.

    The particles reach the alveoli especially if the bronchial ciliary action is disturbed by chronic bronchitis.

Particles taken up by macrophages in alveoli

Transported into lymph channels and deposited in small focal aggregates throughout lungs and hilar lymph nodes

    The effects are described in detail under PNEUMOCONIOSIS (p.341).

Ingestion

Pigmentation can be caused by chronic ingestion of metals such as silver or lead. In both, the skin has a metallic hue, and in the case of lead a blue line appears on the gums due to interaction between lead and sulphuretted hydrogen. Excessive intake of carrots can lead to yellowish red skin pigmentation caused by carotene.

Injection

Tattooing is the most striking example of pigmentation following injection.

DEGENERATIONS

1. Hyaline

This is a descriptive term meaning a glossy, refractile appearance, seen in sections stained with haematoxylin and eosin. It does not denote any specific substance. It is most commonly encountered in the form of dense collagen, particularly in simple tumours such as fibromyomata where the collagen may replace muscle fibres. Cytoplasmic hyaline substance is sometimes seen when cells are severely damaged, e.g. in alcoholic hepatitis.

    The term 'hyaline' is used in many situations where degeneration is not a feature, e.g. old fibrin thrombi often assume a glossy appearance.

2. Mucoid

This is a common change in epithelial tumours which secrete mucin. In these cases the epithelial cells undergo degeneration and appear to dissolve in the mucin.

    Occasionally connective tissue appears to secrete mucin. Spaces filled with mucopolysaccharides appear between the fibres. The change is not uncommon in some tumours. In these cases the term 'myxomatous' may be used.

STORAGE DISEASES

These diseases are due to inherited errors of metabolism. There is a deficiency of an intra-cellular enzyme, leading to an abnormal accumulation of unmetabolised material. There are many such disorders; the anatomical sites of the deficient cells determine the distribution of affected organs.

The following are historically interesting and illustrative.

CARBOHYDRATE DISORDERS

Two main forms of these diseases exist:

1. Those due to a defect in the breakdown of glycogen to glucose for release into the blood stream. This reaction takes place mainly in the liver, but also the kidney. The missing enzyme is glucose-6-phosphatase. The result is hypoglycaemia and increasing storage of glycogen, which causes great enlargement of the liver and kidneys (Von Gierke's disease). The lack of glucose induces changes in lipid metabolism, leading to ketosis and growth retardation.

2. Diseases due to an inability to deal with carbohydrate in peripheral tissues. In these, there is no hypoglycaemia but a generalised accumulation of locally formed glycogen, e.g. in myocardium, muscle, nervous system, lymphoid tissues etc., (Pompe's disease) resulting in cardiac failure, mental deficiency and muscle weakness.

LIPID DISORDERS

These can be considered in 2 groups:

1. **Disorders of lipid transport** resulting in hyperlipidaemia and hypercholesterolaemia. They are either due to abnormalities of α and ß lipoproteins, or to an inability to clear chylomicrons from the plasma. The excess cholesterol is taken up by macrophages which accumulate in the organs, marrow and lymph nodes and sometimes cause yellowish deposits in the skin (xanthoma). These disorders are closely associated with the pathogenesis of ATHEROMA (see p. 212).

2. **Inborn errors of lipid metabolism,** e.g.

Gaucher's disease in which there is an inability to deal with glucocerebrosides, normal breakdown products of red cells. The cerebrosides are phagocytosed by macrophages which accumulate in organs, causing enlargement — enormous in the spleen but less so in the liver and lymph nodes. Bone marrow deposits can cause pancytopenia and pathological fractures. Usually a chronic adult disease, an acute fatal form occurs in infancy due to accumulation of lipid in neurones.

Niemann-Pick's disease is a fatal disease of childhood, causing mental deficiency. There is a deficiency of enzymes involved in the metabolic turnover of myelin, causing accumulation of a phospholipid, sphingomyelin, in almost all organs including the brain.

CELLULAR PATHOLOGY

The complexity and detail of intra-cellular structure and function and their disorders, as revealed by recent research, is such that only the basic principles can be illustrated.

In many respects, cellular pathology mimics organ and tissue pathology, e.g. (a) the various cellular components and activities are closely interdependent (it is of course convenient to describe them separately) (b) all activities are conducted with balancing control mechanisms and (c) very efficient compensation and repair mechanisms exist to minimise damage.

Energy

Source	Production	Utilisation
O$_2$ + Glucose →	Via MITOCHONDRIA ADP ATP (Oxidative phosphorylation)	→ Release of energy	→ For all cellular activities

Defects in source, production and utilisation can be reflected in all aspects of cellular function.

Plasma membranes

Main functions

(1) Contact with extra-cellular environment — e.g. recognition receptors antigenicity

(2) Passage of complex chemicals in and out of cell by
(a) pinocytosis or phagocytosis
(b) selective permeability

Any disorder may initiate a chain reaction leading to disease.

Lysosomes — These membrane-bound organelles contain hydrolytic enzymes and are responsible for digestion and disposal of complex substances. → Disorder may lead to enzyme escape or to cellular overloading, e.g. storage disorders.

Nucleus

The nucleus contains at least 50,000 genes and through them exercises control of all cellular activities. Each gene is responsible for a single specific chemical product, e.g. a protein, an enzyme or a complex lipid.

Nuclear damage occurs usually during cell replication and is greatly potentiated by ionising radiation. Repair mechanisms are very effective.

Germ cell nuclear damage

(1) Severe damage to chromosomal structure → Prevention of conception.
Early abortion.

(2) Less severe damage affecting groups of genes, single genes or DNA sequences within genes → Developmental and HEREDITARY DISEASES and SUSCEPTIBILITY to disease.

Stem cell nuclear damage

This is acquired during life.

The development of cancer is the best example — nuclear changes induced by carcinogens — activation of oncogenes — chain of events leading to malignancy.

CHAPTER 2

INFLAMMATION

INFLAMMATION

Inflammation is the dynamic processes by which living tissues react to injury. They concern vascular and connective tissues particularly.

Causes:
Various agents may kill or damage cells:

PHYSICAL

Trauma   Heat or cold   Radiation

CHEMICAL

Simple chemical poisons, e.g. acids   Organic poisons, e.g. paraquat

INFECTIVE

Bacteria   Viruses   Parasites

IMMUNOLOGICAL

Antigen-antibody   Cell-mediated

... and any other circumstance leading to tissue damage, e.g. VASCULAR or HORMONAL DISTURBANCE.

The inflammatory reaction takes place in the surviving adjacent vascular and connective tissues; the specialised parenchymal cells do not directly participate.

The initial stages are known as the **acute** inflammatory reaction. Where the process is prolonged the inflammation may be **subacute** or **chronic.**

ACUTE INFLAMMATION
The classical signs are:

e.g. Boil

REDNESS (rubor)
HEAT (calor)
SWELLING (tumor)
PAIN (dolor)
LOSS OF FUNCTION (functio laesa).

These gross signs are explained by changes occurring at microscopic level.
Three essential features are:

    1. **HYPERAEMIA**
    2. **EXUDATION**
    3. **EMIGRATION OF LEUCOCYTES**

ACUTE INFLAMMATION

HYPERAEMIA

The hyperaemia in inflammation is associated with the well known microvascular changes which occur in Lewis' triple response — a FLUSH, a FLARE and a WEAL. It occurs when a blunt instrument is drawn firmly across the skin and illustrates the vascular changes occurring in acute inflammation.

The stroke is marked momentarily by a white line due to VASOCONSTRICTION.

The flush, a dull red line, immediately follows and is due to CAPILLARY DILATATION.

The flare, a bright red irregular surrounding zone, is due to ARTERIOLAR DILATATION.

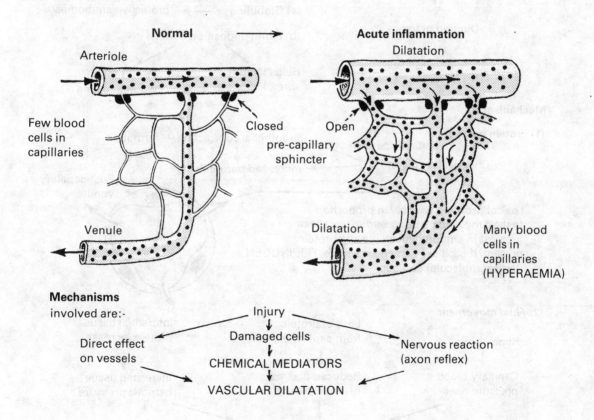

Normal

Arteriole

Few blood cells in capillaries

Closed pre-capillary sphincter

Venule

Acute inflammation
Dilatation

Open

Dilatation

Many blood cells in capillaries (HYPERAEMIA)

Mechanisms
involved are:-

Injury
↓
Damaged cells
↓
CHEMICAL MEDIATORS
↓
VASCULAR DILATATION

Direct effect on vessels →

Nervous reaction (axon reflex) ←

HYPERAEMIA explains the classical signs of REDNESS and HEAT.

ACUTE INFLAMMATION

EXUDATION

Exudation is the increased passage of protein – rich fluid through the vessel wall into the interstitial tissue. It explains the **weal** in Lewis' triple response.

Advantageous results

Fluid increase
↓
Dilution of toxins

Protein increase

(a) Globulins ⟶ protective antibodies

(b) Fibrin deposition

Helps to limit
spread of bacteria

Important in
wound healing

Mechanism

(1) **Protein passage**

Chemical mediators ⟶ Endothelial contraction — formation of gaps
⟶ Increased permeability
↓

Leak of **proteins,** roughly in proportion to their molecular size: *albumin* (smallest) greatest in amount, but all plasma proteins present. If capillary damage is severe, FIBRINOGEN (largest molecule) escapes.

Post-capillary venule

(2) *Fluid movement*

Hyperaemia
↓
Capillary blood pressure rises

Loss of protein from capillaries
↓
Reduced plasma osmotic pressure

Interstitial tissue protein increase
↓
Increased tissue osmotic pressure

INCREASED FILTRATION PRESSURE
↓
Local swelling (OEDEMA) — 3rd classical sign
↓
Increased lymph flow from area

ACUTE INFLAMMATION

EMIGRATION OF LEUCOCYTES

Polymorphs and mononuclears pass between the endothelial cell junctions by amoeboid movement through the venule wall into the tissue spaces.

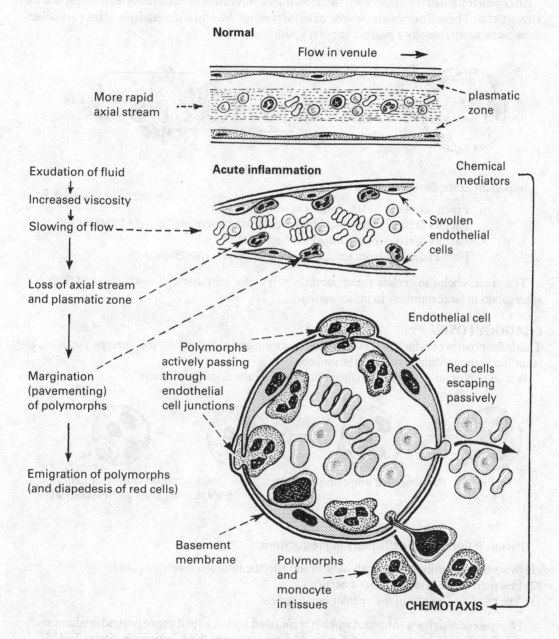

Normal

Flow in venule →

More rapid axial stream

plasmatic zone

Exudation of fluid
↓
Increased viscosity
↓
Slowing of flow

Acute inflammation

Chemical mediators

Swollen endothelial cells

Loss of axial stream and plasmatic zone

Margination (pavementing) of polymorphs

Polymorphs actively passing through endothelial cell junctions

Endothelial cell

Red cells escaping passively

Emigration of polymorphs (and diapedesis of red cells)

Basement membrane

Polymorphs and monocyte in tissues

CHEMOTAXIS

33

ACUTE INFLAMMATION

CHEMOTAXIS

The initial margination of polymorphs and mononuclears is potentiated by slowing of blood flow and by increased 'stickiness' of the endothelial surface.

After penetration of the vessel wall, the subsequent movement of the leucocytes is controlled by CHEMOTAXIS. The cell moves in response to an increasing concentration gradient of the particular chemotactic agent, usually a protein or polypeptide.

Important examples of chemotactic agents are:

Fractions of the COMPLEMENT system (esp. C5a)
Factors derived from arachidonic acid by the polymorphs — LEUKOTRIENES
Factors derived from pathogenic BACTERIA
Factors derived from sensitised lymphocytes — LYMPHOKINES.

The process helps to explain the apparently purposeful movement of leucocytes and their aggregation in large numbers in inflammation.

PHAGOCYTOSIS

This is the process by which polymorphs and macrophages ingest debris and 'foreign' particles. It is similar to the feeding process of the amoeba.

It is an important defence mechanism in bacterial infections particularly.

Factors influencing the efficiency of phagocytosis:

(1) OPSONINS — antibodies of both natural and specific immune type (see p.103)
(2) Fractions of the COMPLEMENT system
(3) The PHYSICAL STATE of the cellular environment

The opsonic activity is enhanced when it is confined within a solid organ or rigid medium such as a fibrin network; where the conditions are looser and more fluid, activity is diminished.

ACUTE INFLAMMATION

Sequels of phagocytosis
POLYMORPH *(natural life span 1 – 3 days)*

Discharge of
lysozomal enzymes +
into vacuole

Activation of
powerful
oxidising
agents (H_2O_2,
HOCl etc.)

Successful kill (a)   or (b) Failure to kill

Bacteria killed
and digested.
Polymorph
degranulated.

Bacteria resist attack. Polymorph
dies and cell membrane
disintegrates. Living bacteria
liberated to cause further damage.
Bacterial virulence is
the most important factor. Occasionally
the polymorphs are
defective.

MACROPHAGE *(natural life span — months to several years)*

(a) Successful kill may be accomplished.
(b) Failure to kill may allow bacteria to continue to live within
    the cell which may move via lymphatics to adjacent parts.
    This partly explains the spread of tuberculosis in the
    body.

(c) All debris (including dead polymorphs) which has been ingested by macrophages is gradually
    removed from the site of the inflammation.
(d) Antigenic material from bacteria available for presentation to the immune system.

Side effects: The liberation of enzymes and oxidising agents into adjacent tissues contributes in
varying degree to the tissue damage seen in several diseases, e.g. rheumatoid arthritis, progressive
pulmonary emphysema.

ACUTE INFLAMMATION

THE ROLE OF CHEMICAL FACTORS

Various substances are credited with roles in the inflammatory process; they have complex overlapping actions, many of which are only imprecisely defined.

Agents associated with vascular dilatation and increased permeability include:

1. Vaso-active AMINES — these appear early and their action is short.

2. Vaso-active POLYPEPTIDES formed by specific enzyme action (breakdown products of proteins and tissues.)

3. MISCELLANEOUS AGENTS influencing in inflammatory processes include:

- Toxins from bacteria
- Complement factors C3a and C5a
- Prostaglandins
- Leukotrienes ⎫
- Lysosomal enzymes ⎬ (from polymorphs)
- Interleukins (macrophages)
- Globulin permeability factor
- Lymph node permeability factor
- Products of DNA and RNA breakdown
- Antigen-antibody complexes
- Tumour necrosis factor

SEQUELS OF ACUTE INFLAMMATION

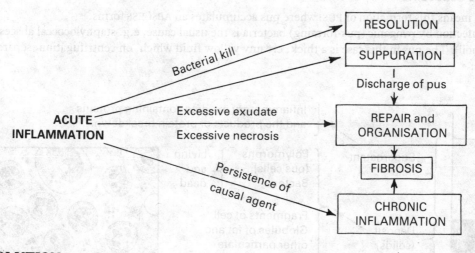

```
                                              ┌─────────────────┐
                              Bacterial kill   │   RESOLUTION    │
                                               └─────────────────┘
                                               ┌─────────────────┐
                                               │   SUPPURATION   │
                                               └─────────────────┘
                                                        │ Discharge of pus
                                                        ▼
                              Excessive exudate  ┌─────────────────┐
  ACUTE  ──────────────────────────────────────►│  REPAIR and     │
  INFLAMMATION                                   │  ORGANISATION   │
                              Excessive necrosis └─────────────────┘
                                                        │
                                                        ▼
                                                 ┌─────────────┐
                                                 │   FIBROSIS  │
                                                 └─────────────┘
                           Persistence of        ┌─────────────────┐
                           causal agent           │    CHRONIC      │
                                                   │  INFLAMMATION  │
                                                   └─────────────────┘
```

RESOLUTION

This means the complete restoration of normal conditions after the acute inflammation.

The three main features which potentiate this sequel are:

1. minimal cell death and tissue damage
2. rapid elimination of the causal agent, e.g. bacteria
3. local conditions favouring removal of fluid and debris.

Resolution of lobar pneumonia (bacterial inflammation of lung alveoli) is a good example:

Lymphatics

Blood vessel

Alveolar capillary

Inflammatory exudate:
fibrin network
many polymorphs
and bacteria

Note proximity of exudate to alveolar
capillaries and septal lymphatics.

Following bacterial kill the mechanism is as follows:

1. Solution of fibrin by enzyme action (polymorphs and fibrinolysin)
2. Removal of fluid by blood vessels and lymphatics
3. Removal of all debris by phagocytes to hilar lymph nodes
4. The capillary hyperaemia diminishes and restoration to normal is complete

37

SEQUELS OF ACUTE INFLAMMATION

SUPPURATION

This means this formation of PUS; where pus accumulates an ABSCESS forms.

Infection by pyogenic (pus-forming) bacteria is the usual cause, e.g. staphylococcal abscess (or boil). The pus in this case is a thick, creamy yellow fluid which, on centrifugation, separates thus:

Evolution of an abscess

The usual evolution of an abscess is as follows:

SEQUELS OF ACUTE INFLAMMATION

Evolution of an abscess (continued)
When the abscess is deep-seated, the process may be modified as follows:

```
                    Deep-seated abscess
        ↙                                        ↘
Chronic discharging sinus              Localised collection of pus
        ↓                                  ↙            ↘
Discharge via long                     Small          Large
   tortuous track                        ↓              ↓
                                    Absorption of   Inspissation of pus
                                        pus         and walling off by
                                                     fibrous tissue
                                         ↓              ↓
                                       Scar        Calcium salts
```

Pyogenic membrane

Failure to discharge all the abscess contents, especially if foreign matter is retained

CHRONIC INFLAMMATION

This follows the acute inflammatory reaction if the causal agent is not removed.
The essential changes superimposed upon and replacing the acute reaction are:

Diminution in numbers of polymorphs; appearance of *lymphocytes* and *plasma cells*.
Macrophages play an increasingly important role
(see Granulomas, p.43).
In some cases, *giant cells* form.
Proliferation of vascular endothelium by 'budding' — formation of *new capillaries*.
Proliferation of *fibroblasts* with *collagen* production —

Plasma cells

Capillary bud

Macrophage

Lymphocytes cuffing vessel

Fibroblast

Giant cell

Fibrosis.
Frequently the local vessels show thickening of their walls with diminution in the lumina, due to intimal proliferation — endarteritis and endophlebitis (see page 43).

Commonly chronic inflammation is *primary*, i.e. there is no preceding acute inflammatory reaction.

The pathological processes following abscess formation and chronic inflammation are very closely allied to and merge with those occurring when repair of damaged tissue commences.

SEQUELS OF ACUTE INFLAMMATION

ORGANISATION

Organisation occurs when, during the acute inflammatory process, (a) there is excessive exudation or necrosis or (b) when local conditions are unfavourable for the removal of exudate and debris. The term also applies to the local reaction to the presence of thrombus and also the necrosis associated with infarction.

The changes are similar to those described in wound healing viz — the growth of new capillaries into the inert material (exudate or thrombus), the migration of macrophages and the proliferation of fibroblasts resulting in FIBROSIS.

A good example of organisation following acute inflammation is seen in the pleura overlying pneumonia. The inflammation of the lung tissue proper usually resolves completely (p.324); in contrast the pleural exudate is not easily removed and organisation takes place.

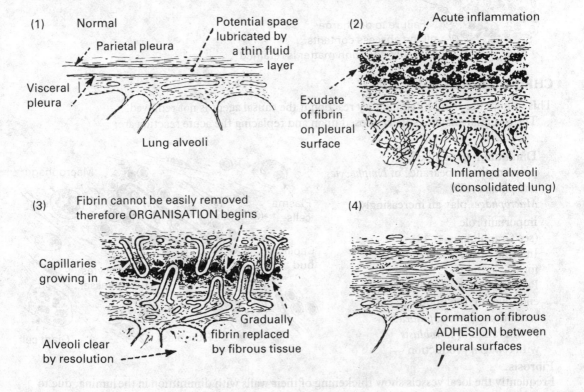

(1) Normal
Parietal pleura
Potential space lubricated by a thin fluid layer
Visceral pleura
Lung alveoli

(2) Acute inflammation
Exudate of fibrin on pleural surface
Inflamed alveoli (consolidated lung)

(3) Fibrin cannot be easily removed therefore ORGANISATION begins
Capillaries growing in
Gradually fibrin replaced by fibrous tissue
Alveoli clear by resolution

(4) Formation of fibrous ADHESION between pleural surfaces

Other good examples of organisation are seen after infarction (see p.130).

INFLAMMATION — SPECIAL TYPES

NOMENCLATURE

Inflammation is indicated by adding the suffix 'itis' to the Latin name of the organ or tissue involved, e.g. gastritis, colitis, cholecystitis and hepatitis indicate inflammation of the stomach, colon, gall-bladder and liver respectively. Pneumonia and pleurisy — inflammation of the lung and pleura — are examples of exceptions.

The inflammatory process is influenced by the SITE, the CAUSATIVE AGENT, the SEVERITY and DURATION.

CATARRHAL INFLAMMATION

A surface inflammation associated with greatly increased secretion of clear mucus. Later, polymorphs appear.

Good examples are the common cold and some forms of colitis.

EXUDATIVE INFLAMMATIONS

Excess of a particular component of the inflammatory exudate imparts distinctive features.

Serous inflammations

In this type, excessive clear watery fluid, with a variable protein content but no fibrin, is formed. Good examples are blister formation following burning (acute) and the pleural effusion associated with tuberculosis (chronic).

Note that the exudate remains fluid and resolution is not impeded.

41

INFLAMMATION — SPECIAL TYPES

EXUDATIVE INFLAMMATION (cont)
Fibrinous exudation
In this type, the formation of fibrin
is striking. An example is acute pleurisy,
complicating pneumonia, where the fibrin can
be seen as an amorphous dull deposit on the
pleural surface. Note that the presence of
solid fibrin tends to inhibit resolution,
and *organisation* with *adhesion formation*
often follows.

Parietal layer

Inflamed alveoli

A membranous film consisting mainly of fibrin with necrotic cells admixed sometimes forms on a MUCOSAL surface (esp. respiratory and alimentary tracts.) The classical example is DIPHTHERIA affecting the pharynx and adjacent areas.

NOTE SUPERFICIAL NATURE OF INFLAMMATION

DEEP TISSUES NOT AFFECTED

Membrane — Fibrin + Cell debris + Bacteria

Epithelium

Congested capillaries and inflammatory cells

Normal connective tissue

Exotoxin

Absorbed into body

This is often referred to as pseudo-membranous inflammation (see p.399).

SUPPURATIVE (PURULENT — PYOGENIC) INFLAMMATION
In this type (usually caused by infection with pyogenic bacteria), production of pus is the main characteristic. Good examples are (a) an abscess, where an enclosed collection of pus forms (see p.38), and (b) acute appendicitis (see p.413), where a purulent exudate forms on the peritoneal surface.

HAEMORRHAGIC INFLAMMATION
Where the damage is severe, actual rupture of all blood vessels occurs, with haemorrhage the most striking feature. An example is the acute haemorrhagic pneumonia occasionally occurring in fatal cases of influenza.

These are not rigid compartments into which every inflammation can be conveniently placed; overlaps and combinations of the various types are common, e.g. sero-sanguinous, muco-purulent.

CHRONIC INFLAMMATION

GRANULOMA

When inflammation is chronic from the outset because the formation of granulation tissue is such a prominent component, the term GRANULOMA is used.

The appearances may be identical to those of chronic inflammation described on page 39, but in several disease processes the granulation tissue assumes a follicular form and macrophages (epithelioid cells) are prominent. The follicle or tubercle is the basic lesion in TUBERCULOSIS.

Caseation
Giant cell
Epithelioid (endothelioid) cells *macrophages*
Lymphocytes *+ plasma cells*
Fibrous tissue

Similar follicles are seen in:

Sarcoidosis — a rare inflammatory disease of unknown aetiology affecting especially the lymph nodes and lungs, but also many other organs
'Talc' granuloma — where particular silicates introduced into the tissues evoke an inflammatory reaction after a latent period (usually years)
Crohn's disease — a chronic inflammatory disease affecting the terminal ileum and colon (see p.403),
Lymph nodes draining ulcerated areas in which breakdown of lipid is occurring.

N.B. In all of these follicular granulomatous diseases the basic lesion may be identical, but CASEATION only occurs in tuberculosis.

The epithelioid cells of the follicular granulomas are modified macrophages, and giant cells are derived from macrophages usually by cell fusion but occasionally by nuclear division without cytoplasmic separation.

The Langhan's giant cell — seen in chronic granulomata, e.g. tuberculosis and sarcoidosis.

Nuclei in horse-shoe arrangement

The foreign body giant cell — seen in association with particulate insoluble material.

Nuclei scattered throughout cytoplasm

INFLAMMATORY ENDARTERITIS

The small arteries adjacent to a chronic inflammatory site often show **fibrous proliferation** of the **intima** with serious diminution of the lumen causing ischaemic effects, e.g. *atrophy* of specialised tissues, *necrosis* and *delayed healing*.

Occasionally the results are beneficial, e.g. in chronic peptic ulceration bleeding may be minimal.

Similar changes – ENDOPHLEBITIS – may affect veins.

Ulcer

Lumen obliterated by endarteritis

43

ULCERATION — SIMPLE

ULCERATION is a complication of many disease processes.

An **ulcer** is formed when the surface covering of an organ or tissue is lost due to necrosis and replaced by inflammatory tissue.

The most common sites are the alimentary tract and the skin.

Ulcers are divided into two main groups: (1) SIMPLE (inflammatory) and (2) MALIGNANT (cancerous).

The word 'simple' is used here in the limited sense of contrasting with 'malignant': 'simple' ulcers may have serious consequences.

Evolution of a simple ulcer

Acute ulcer

(1) Necrosis — Slough

(2) Ulcer crater — Base consisting of fibrin and debris — Acute inflammation, capillary congestion (and polymorphs)

Healing can occur at this stage with restoration to normal, but if irritation (e.g. bacterial action, slight trauma, digestive juices and acid) continues, a CHRONIC ULCER forms.

Chronic ulcer

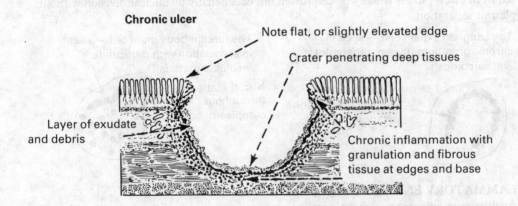

Note flat, or slightly elevated edge

Crater penetrating deep tissues

Layer of exudate and debris

Chronic inflammation with granulation and fibrous tissue at edges and base

Healing of a chronic ulcer may be impeded by the secondary obliterative changes in the blood vessels due to the chronic inflammation, and it is inevitably associated with a variable amount of scarring.

ULCERATION — MALIGNANT

Evolution of a malignant ulcer (ulcerated tumour)

Such an ulcer is the result of the growth of a malignant tumour.

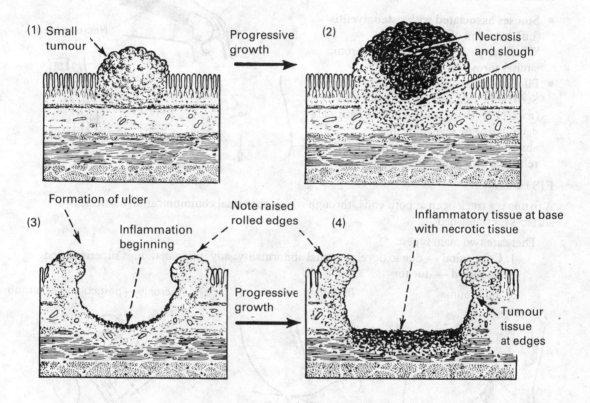

(1) Small tumour
Progressive growth
(2) Necrosis and slough

Formation of ulcer
(3) Inflammation beginning
Note raised rolled edges
(4) Inflammatory tissue at base with necrotic tissue
Progressive growth
Tumour tissue at edges

The differences between simple and malignant ulcers are most prominent at the edges — from which a diagnostic biopsy should be taken.

Simple ulcer
Edge
Base
Biopsies from edge and base both show inflammation

Malignant ulcer
Biopsy from edge likely to show malignant tumour
Biopsy from base may miss malignant tumour

45

INFLAMMATION — ANATOMICAL VARIETIES

SINUS

A sinus is a tract leading from a cavity to the surface.
Examples include:

Sinuses

Necrotic bone

- **Sinuses associated with osteomyelitis** (inflammation of bone).
  Where necrosis of bone occurs, chronic sinuses form over it.
- **Pilonidal sinus** (pilonidal = nest of hairs).
  Seen in the mid-line over the sacrum (natal cleft) where hairs situated unusually deep — due to developmental abnormality — are associated with chronic relapsing inflammation.

Sinuses containing hairs

FISTULA

A fistula is a track open at both ends, through which abnormal communication between two surfaces is established.

There are two main types:
1. **Congenital** — due to developmental abnormality: any inflammation is superimposed.
2. **Acquired** — due to:

(a) Trauma

(b) Inflammation

(c) Necrosis — particularly of tumour

Biliary fistula following operation

Gastrocolic fistula in Crohn's disease (p.404)

Vesicovaginal fistula following radionecrosis in treatment of cancer of cervix

An **EMPYEMA** is a collection of pus in a body cavity or hollow organ. The term refers usually to the pleural cavity or the gall bladder.

CELLULITIS occurs when inflammation spreads in the connective tissue planes.

CHAPTER 3

INFECTION

INFECTION

Most microorganisms are harmless; a few are **pathogenic,** i.e. have the potential to produce infectious disease.

BACTERIA and VIRUSES are the most common and most important groups of pathogenic organisms in man. Fungi and other groups (e.g. Chlamydia) less commonly cause disease.

COLONISATION AND COMMENSAL GROWTH

Vast numbers of bacteria normally colonise the external body surfaces (skin, alimentary and upper respiratory tracts). Most are of low pathogenicity and some may actually be beneficial to the host, for example:

1. By producing nutrient chemicals, e.g. vit B_{12}
2. By competing with and excluding pathogens.

Common Sites of Contamination

Skin especially

Nose

Mouth

Hands

Anus

Upper Respiratory Tract

Alimentary Tract

INFECTION AND INFECTIOUS DISEASE

INFECTION occurs when microorganisms invade the sterile internal body tissues. (Multiplication usually follows invasion.)

An INFECTIOUS DISEASE occurs when infection is associated with clinically manifest tissue damage.

Routes of entry of infecting organisms

1. Through the *skin* or *mucous membranes*

    (a) By direct close contact, e.g. venereal disease.
    (b) By contamination of abrasions and wounds, e.g. wound infections, rabies.
    (c) By inoculation, e.g. insect bite — yellow fever,
        syringe — serum hepatits, AIDS.

2. By *ingestion*
   Contaminated food and water, e.g. enteric fever, infective hepatitis (A), poliomyelitis, cholera.

3. By *inhalation*
   Dust and droplets, e.g. influenza.

INFECTION

Factors influencing the establishment of infection

1. *In the HOST*

In addition to a good state of general health and nutrition, the following mechanisms operate in preventing and limiting infection.

Physical barriers

e.g. (a) **SKIN**

Cornified squamous epithelium

Secretions

Washing action by

(a) **TEARS**   (b) **URINE**

(b) **FILTRATION** by nostril hairs

(c) **MUCIN** (aided by ciliary action in respiratory tract)

Fluid layer

Cilia

Chemical action

(1) Acid secretion in stomach and urinary tract.
(2) Lysozymes — enzymes capable of dissolving bacterial capsules, e.g. in tears and saliva.
(3) Immunoglobulin A (IgA) — a specialised immunoglobulin (see p.101),
    — tears: intestinal secretions.
(4) Non-specific inhibitory substances – urine, sweat, sebum.

2. *In the MICRO-ORGANISM*

Factors potentiating invasive capacity include:
(1) **Quantity of dose** — the larger the dose the more likely that the defences are penetrated.
(2) **Virulence** — a variable factor, and often poorly defined, includes:
    (a) Capacity to resist phagocytosis and enzyme attack,
    (b) Adhesive properties,
    (c) Production of exoenzymes which act on host tissues, *e.g.* hyaluronidase (streptococci), coagulase (staphylococci) and of toxins, e.g. leucocidins, enterotoxins.

INFECTION

Factors influencing the course of infection

Once infection has occurred, important defence mechanisms operate:

1. **Inflammation** in the **acute** local reaction (see p.31) tends to limit the spread of organisms. In some important diseases, there is no acute local inflammatory response at the site of entry, e.g. Brucellosis (undulant fever) and many virus infections.
   In the **chronic** inflammatory reaction (see p.39), the formation of fibrous tissue also helps to localise infection.

2. **Phagocytosis** (see p.34) *NB* some organisms may survive or multiply within phagocytes – usually associated with chronic infection. Good examples are tuberculosis, brucellosis, leprosy.

3. **The Immune response.** (a) Humoral antibody reactions, e.g. agglutination, opsonisation, lysis via complement; (b) Cell-mediated reactions.

4. **Interferon production** (see p.70). In virus infection, interferon, a non-specific anti-viral agent produced by infected host cells, is important.

Examples of failure of protective and defence mechanisms

1. **In skin** — direct breach by wounding and burns; softening of the surface by exposure to water and sweat or due to skin disorders.

2. **In the respiratory tract** — inhibition of ciliary movement by nicotine in smokers potentiates infection.

3. **In the stomach** — in achlorhydria (no hydrochloric acid) organisms flourish in the stomach.

4. **When secretions are prevented from flowing freely** by narrowing of natural passages, bacterial growth in the 'stagnant' fluid is potentiated (e.g. enlarged prostate urethral obstruction, urinary infection).

5. **When commensal growth is impaired** by antibiotic treatment, pathogenic bacteria may colonise the 'vacant site'.

6. **Deficiency of the immunological system:**
   (a) natural deficiency due to hereditary defect,
   (b) acquired due to administration of drugs in treatment of disease, e.g. steroids, cytotoxic drugs; specific virus infection, e.g. Human Immunodeficiency Virus (HIV) causing Acquired Immune Deficiency Syndrome (AIDS).

7. **Deficiency of phagocytosis** — especially polymorphs.

8. **In debilitating diseases** such as diabetes, chronic renal failure and nutritional deficiency.

9. **Genetic susceptibility** — an important factor in some infections, e.g. the increased prevalence of several bacterial and fungal diseases in NON-SECRETORS of ABH blood group antigens (H = blood group O antigen). The mechanism remains obscure.

INFECTION

Mechanisms by which disease is produced

The local reaction to infections is usually INFLAMMATORY and is evoked by cellular damage and death. The detailed mechanisms are different in bacteria and viruses.

BACTERIA
1. Production of toxins (poisons)

Exotoxins	Endotoxins
Secreted by living bacteria	Integral part of bacterial cell wall Release on death of organism (usually Gram-negative)
Simple proteins	Lipid-polysaccharide complexes
Neutralised by specific antibody (antitoxin)	Do not stimulate antitoxin production
Often have specific enzyme activity and may act on specific organs or tissues	Act by damaging capillaries and disturbing the coagulation system as well as causing cell necrosis. Cause fever (pyrogenic) and endotoxic shock

2. Hypersensitivity reaction causing tissue injury

This is a form of the immune response in which reaction between the bacterial protein and sensitised lymphocytes initiates the inflammatory reaction (see p. 115).

3. Tissue invasion: lymphatic spread and invasion of blood stream

51

INFECTION

BACTERAEMIA

(a) Occurs commonly: usually of no serious significance

(b) An integral part of some infections, e.g. typhoid fever.

Important special cases

(1) *Dental extraction*

Infected tooth
(organisms of low
grade virulence)

↓

Bacteraemia

↓

Bacteria may settle
on previously diseased
heart valves —
bacterial endocarditis

(2) *Established bacterial endocarditis*

Mitral valve

'Vegetations'
composed of
fibrin, platelets
and bacteria

Chronic bacteraemia
(diagnosed by blood culture)

SEPTICAEMIA

Septicaemia is a very serious condition with severe toxaemia and shock. It may:

(a) be primary — usually caused by virulent organisms e.g. *meningococci, Streptococci pyogenes*

(b) complicate the shock syndrome initiated by other causes — especially when the alimentary tract is involved (coliform organisms)

(c) occur during medical treatment when immune mechanisms are disturbed (see opportunistic infections, p.71).

In septicaemia, unless antibiotic treatment is available, the infection is rapidly overwhelming and, at post-mortem, specific damage is difficult to detect. There may be massive adrenal haemorrhage and evidence of disseminated intravascular coagulation (see p.156).

PYAEMIA

Pyaemia is a serious condition with severe toxaemia — the organisms escape into the blood stream in the form of small aggregates — micro-emboli. This results in either (a) PYAEMIC ABSCESSES or (b) SEPTIC INFARCTION.

INFECTION

PYAEMIC ABSCESS

Septic focus — usually staphylococcal

$\downarrow$

Thrombosis of venules incorporating bacteria

$\downarrow$

Showers of very small (micro-) emboli,

$\downarrow$

Multiple, very small abscesses in various organs

Especially:

Cerebral cortex   Myocardium   Lungs   Renal cortex

SEPTIC INFARCTION

The lesions are larger and less numerous than pyaemic abscesses.
They are associated with:

(a) Septic thrombosis of larger veins
    (suppurative thrombophlebitis)

(b) Acute bacterial
    endocarditis

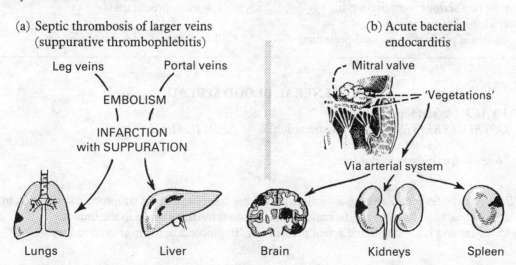

Leg veins   Portal veins

EMBOLISM

INFARCTION
with SUPPURATION

Mitral valve

'Vegetations'

Via arterial system

Lungs   Liver   Brain   Kidneys   Spleen

ACUTE BACTERIAL INFECTION

PYOGENIC BACTERIA

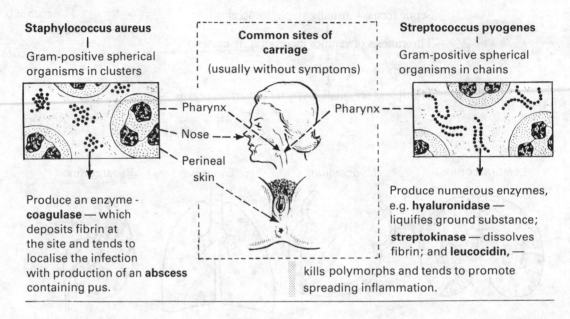

Staphylococcus aureus

Gram-positive spherical organisms in clusters

Common sites of carriage

(usually without symptoms)

Streptococcus pyogenes

Gram-positive spherical organisms in chains

Pharynx

Nose

Perineal skin

Pharynx

Produce an enzyme - **coagulase** — which deposits fibrin at the site and tends to localise the infection with production of an **abscess** containing pus.

Produce numerous enzymes, e.g. **hyaluronidase** — liquifies ground substance; **streptokinase** — dissolves fibrin; and **leucocidin,** — kills polymorphs and tends to promote spreading inflammation.

Lesions produced

Skin infections — pustules, boils, carbuncles
Wound infection
Staphylococcal broncho-pneumonia may be a serious complication in epidemic influenza
Exotoxin production → food poisoning

Skin infections — impetigo, erysipelas, cellulitis
Wound infection
TONSILLITIS and pharyngitis
Exotoxin production
↓
The skin rash of scarlet fever

GENERAL BLOOD SPREAD

PYAEMIA (and septicaemia)
OSTEOMYELITIS — acute inflammation of long bones — particularly in children

SEPTICAEMIA

NB Rheumatic fever and acute glomerulonephritis are complications of streptococcal infection in which the heart and kidneys are damaged. This is caused by disturbance in the immune mechanisms and is not due to the actual presence of streptococci in the heart and kidneys.

ACUTE BACTERIAL INFECTION

PYOGENIC BACTERIA (continued)

Meningococcus

Gonococcus

Both are Gram-negative intracellular diplococci

Carried in nasopharynx.
Causes **purulent** *meningitis* and in children, occasionally a fatal septicaemia.

Carried in genital mucous membrane.
Causes purulent inflammation of urethra in male and of uterine cervix in the female with spread to adjacent organs.

Skin rash   Massive adrenal
haemorrhage

(Waterhouse-Friderichsen syndrome)

Male

Prostatitis

Anterior urethritis

Epididymitis

Female

Acute salpingitis (inflammation of Fallopian tubes)

Massive adrenal haemorrhage   Purpuric skin rash

Cervix →

Gonococcal infection

Resultant scarring may prevent passage of ovum to uterus → sterility.

Gram-negative bacilli

These are usually commensals in the alimentary tract and include the broad group of aerobic 'coliform' organisms (*E. coli, B. proteus, Klebsiella*) as well as the anaerobic bacteroides.

They are of low grade virulence but can cause local inflammations in the alimentary tract, the urinary tract and wound infections.

The production of endotoxins is an important cause of shock.

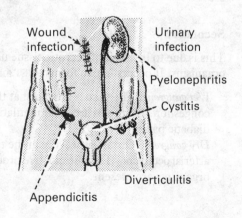

Wound infection

Urinary infection

Pyelonephritis

Cystitis

Diverticulitis

Appendicitis

ACUTE BACTERIAL INFECTION

GANGRENE

Gangrene is a form of NECROSIS in which a special type of bacterial activity is superinposed. The bacteria proliferate in and digest the dead tissues often with the production of gases.

There are two main types: PRIMARY and SECONDARY.

Primary (gas gangrene)

This occurs only occasionally in civilian practice but is a serious complication of war wounds. It is due to infection of deep contaminated wounds (in which there is considerable muscle damage) by bacteria of the *CLOSTRIDIA* group — anaerobic sporulating Gram-positive bacili which produce saccharolytic and proteolytic enzymes resulting in digestion of muscle tissue with gas formation. The infection rapidly spreads and there is associated severe toxaemia (spread of poisons in the blood).

Necrotic muscle

Gas bubbles

Secondary

This is due to invasion of necrotic tissue usually by a mixed bacterial flora including putrefactive organisms. It occurs in two forms: WET and DRY.

Wet gangrene. The tissues are moist at the start of the process either due to oedema or venous congestion. Examples are in strangulation of viscera and occlusion of leg arteries in obese diabetic patients.

Dry gangrene. Occurs especially in the toes and feet of elderly people suffering from gradual arterial occlusion. The putrefactive process is very slow and only small numbers of putrefactive organisms are present.

ACUTE BACTERIAL INFECTION

TETANUS

This is a toxigenic disease — the organism itself does not cause local tissue damage. The effects are due to a powerful EXOTOXIN secreted by the organism. This is in contrast to the usual bacterial diseases where tissue damage is important and is due to the local bacterial action.

The infecting organism, *Clostridium tetani*, a STRICT ANAEROBE, is a Gram-positive rod. Often the presence of a terminal spore gives a characteristic drum-stick appearance. The highly resistant spores are widespread in the environment due to contamination by animal faeces.

Method of Infection

Contamination of wounds in which there are anaerobic conditions, e.g. deep-penetrating wounds and wounds with severe soft tissue damage (road traffic accidents and battle casualties); only very occasionally trivial thorn punctures.

In primitive communities the umbilical stump of the newborn may be infected by faecal material.

Effects:

The exotoxin is highly potent and causes paroxysmal muscular spasm which becomes progressively more severe and is fatal in many cases.

Course

Puncture wound

Bacteria proliferate but remain localised and produce

EXOTOXIN— influences neuromuscular activity

Spread via local nerves

Spread to motor nerves generally

Local muscular spasm — triggered by minor stimuli

Spasm of jaws (trismus — lock jaw; risus sardonicus)

Convulsions with gradual muscular spasm; opisthotonos

Respiratory muscle spasm

EXHAUSTION   ASPHYXIA

DEATH

Immunity

- Active immunisation by **TOXOID** — prophylactic.
- Passive immunisation by **ANTITOXIN** — therapeutic
(only effective before toxin is fixed to nerve tissues).

57

CHRONIC BACTERIAL INFECTION (GRANULOMAS)

In these infections chronic inflammation is the basic mechanism (see p.43). The detailed evolution of the inflammatory reaction is modified by several factors of which the immune response of the host is important (see p.95).

TUBERCULOSIS

Tuberculosis is caused by the *Mycobacterium tuberculosis* (tubercle bacillus: T.B.) an organism which has a resistant waxy component in its structure and is acid and alcohol-fast (i.e. resists bleaching with strong acid and alcohol after being stained red with fuchsin).

The disease has rapidly declined in Western Europe and North America since World War II due to: (a) improved nutrition and hygiene, (b) chemotherapy and (c) BCG immunisation. It is seen now mostly as pulmonary infection in adults. It remains prevalent in developing countries, affecting both children and adults.

The tuberculous follicle (tubercle)

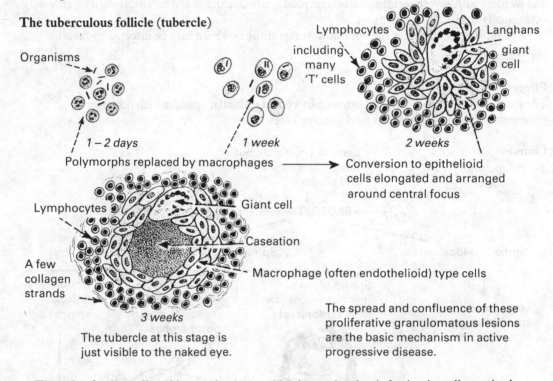

The tubercle at this stage is just visible to the naked eye.

The spread and confluence of these proliferative granulomatous lesions are the basic mechanism in active progressive disease.

The role of **cell-mediated immunity** (see p. 106) in combatting infection is well seen in the evolution of the tuberculous follicle.

The caseation is the result of the combined effects of (a) the Type IV hypersensitivity reaction, (b) bacterial activity and (c) ischaemia.

CHRONIC BACTERIAL INFECTIONS (GRANULOMAS)

TUBERCULOSIS (continued)

Primary infection

Usually seen in non-immune children in first contact with tuberculosis. A few bacilli infect the PRIMARY SITE — usually at the periphery of the lung but also occasionally in the pharynx (tonsil) or small intestine.

Inhalation of a few infecting organisms

or

(a) Healing with minimal trace or leaving a small calcified scar under the pleura.

(b) Rapid spread via lymphatics to local (hilar) lymph nodes **with caseation**

Rapid development of small aggregate of tubercles **with caseation — Ghon focus**

The **PRIMARY COMPLEX**

Healing can occur at this stage, leaving calcified lymph nodes, or occasionally the disease spreads via blood stream (a) generally or (b) to individual organs.

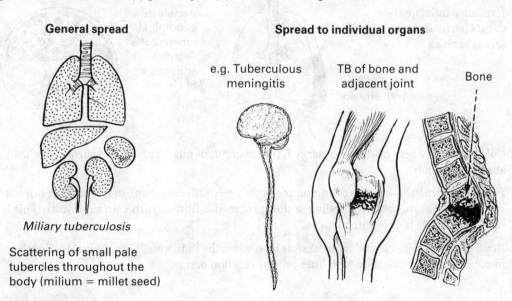

General spread

Spread to individual organs

e.g. Tuberculous meningitis

TB of bone and adjacent joint

Bone

Miliary tuberculosis

Scattering of small pale tubercles throughout the body (milium = millet seed)

CHRONIC BACTERIAL INFECTIONS (GRANULOMAS)

TUBERCULOSIS (cont)

Re-infection tuberculosis

This occurs in older children and adults who
have had a primary infection or have received
BCG vaccination by which a variable degree
of immunity to the tubercle bacillus has been
established.

    The evolution of the disease is much slower
than in the primary infection and fibrosis tends
to limit the spread, but in untreated cases gradual
extension with destruction and scarring of
tissues is usual.

The usual
site of re-
infection is
the lung apex

Gradually
progressive
disease
destroying
lung tissue

    If the individual's immunity is impaired for any reason, the disease may spread locally more
rapidly with increased caseation or in the miliary form.

NB In apparently well-healed tuberculosis, tubercle bacilli can survive for many years in scarred
and calcified tissues and are able to re-establish active disease – REACTIVATION of tuberculosis. This
is the commonest form nowadays in Western countries, occurring in late middle and old age
among people who were originally infected when tuberculosis was common.

Variations in the basic mechanism

1. *Exudative* inflammation
   occurs particulary in
   serous cavities.

e.g. Pleurisy
with effusion

Ascites in
abdominal
tuberculosis
— with
adherence
of viscera

2. *Cold abscess* — where caseation is marked, the tuberculous pus may track to a surface as a 'cold'
   abscess and sinus.

3. *Fibrotic tuberculosis* — in this condition the body's reparative mechanism is dominant but not
   sufficient to ensure complete healing; a slow progressive fibrosis with scarring results. This is
   seen particularly in lung infections.

4. *Acute caseating 'non-reactive' tuberculosis* is seen when the individual's immunity is seriously
   impaired; massive caseation with little cellular reaction occurs.

CHRONIC BACTERIAL INFECTIONS (GRANULOMAS)

SYPHILIS

Syphilis is a venereal infection; the usual sites of entry of the infection are the penis and the vulva or vagina. Extra-genital infection is uncommon.

The organism is a spirochaete *(Treponema pallidum)* with a close set, regular spiral, demonstrated by dark ground illumination, silver staining or immuno-fluorescence. Although it very rapidly dies outside the body it has a highly invasive capacity on contact with mucous membranes.

10μ

PRIMARY SYPHILIS

During the first three weeks after infection, the spirochaetes spread in the blood throughout the body without any noticeable effects. Then the primary lesion — **hard chancre** — appears at the original site of entry.

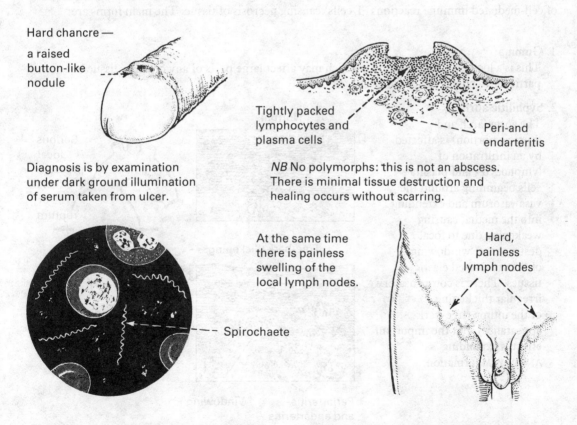

Hard chancre —

a raised
button-like
nodule

Tightly packed
lymphocytes and
plasma cells

Peri-and
endarteritis

Diagnosis is by examination
under dark ground illumination
of serum taken from ulcer.

NB No polymorphs: this is not an abscess.
There is minimal tissue destruction and
healing occurs without scarring.

At the same time
there is painless
swelling of the
local lymph nodes.

Hard,
painless
lymph nodes

Spirochaete

In the course of the next two or three months, the effects of organisms which have spread throughout the body before and during the local reaction present as the SECONDARY STAGE of the disease.

CHRONIC BACTERIAL INFECTIONS (GRANULOMAS)

SECONDARY SYPHILIS

Secondary syphilis presents as a widespread skin rash (pox) of varying appearance, ulceration of mucous membranes, generalised lymphadenopathy, damage to various individual organs and tissues. There are constitutional effects — particularly fever and anaemia.

The essential pathology is the presence of very numerous spirochaetes accompanied by focal infiltration of lymphocytes, plasma cells and macrophages with mild arteritis. Infectivity is very high. Tissue destruction is minimal and healing occurs without scarring. A latent stage of long duration is followed in 35% of cases by tertiary syphilis.

TERTIARY (Late) SYPHILIS

The lesions which may occur at any time for many years after the healing of the secondary phase offer striking contrasts. This stage is characterised mainly by local destructive lesions, the result of cell-mediated immune reactions (T cells) causing necrosis of tissue. The main forms are:

1. **Gumma**
   This is a localised area of necrosis which may affect large parts of any organ or tissue but particularly bones, testis and liver.

2. **Syphilitic aortitis**
   The aorta (arch and thoracic portion) is affected by an infiltration of lymphocytes and plasma cells beginning around the vasa vasorum and extending into the media, causing weakening due to focal destruction ('windowing') of the specialised elastic tissues. There is compensatory irregular thickening of the intima (tree-bark appearance), but the important effect is expanding ANEURYSM formation.

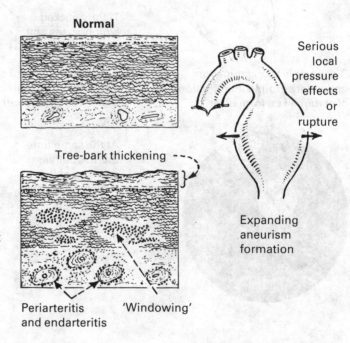

Normal

Tree-bark thickening

Periarteritis and endarteritis

'Windowing'

Serious local pressure effects or rupture

Expanding aneurism formation

CHRONIC BACTERIAL INFECTIONS (GRANULOMAS)

TERITIARY SYPHILIS (continued)

3. *Neurological syphilis*

  (a) **Meningovascular**— mainly affects the meningeal blood vessels and causes neurological impairment secondarily.

  (b) **Parenchymatous** —

    (a) General paralysis of the insane — severe destruction of cerebral tissue

Normal   Atrophy of convolutions   Enlargement of ventricles

    (b) Tabes dorsalis — the damage specifically affecting the posterior roots and columns of spinal cord — is associated with characteristic clinical symptoms due to loss of proprioceptive sensation in the legs

CONGENITAL SYPHILIS

Transplacental infection of the foetus occurs with the following possible consequences:

    (a) abortion or stillbirth — many organs damaged

    (b) birth of marasmic infant — organ and tissue damage at birth and in later childhood.

IMMUNITY IN SYPHILIS

Antibody production

1. Antibodies of uncertain origin which bind to a phospholipid (cardiolipin): these are detected in Wasserman and VDRL (Venereal Diseases Reference Laboratory) tests.
2. Specific anti-treponemal antibodies: these are detected in Treponema immobilisation, haemagglutination and fluorescent antibody tests.

Cell-mediated delayed hypersensitivity also develops

Sensitivity reactions are important in the mechanism of syphilitic damage to tissues.

CHRONIC BACTERIAL INFECTIONS (GRANULOMAS)

ACTINOMYCOSIS

Actinomycosis is a localised but gradually spreading chronic suppuration affecting the lower jaw particularly; the ileocaecal region of the bowel and occasionally the lung.

The organism – *Actinomyces* – widespread in nature, is a Gram-positive branching, filamentous anaerobe found around the teeth and in the pharyngeal crypts (the human variety is *Actinomyces israeli*). In the tissues, it forms densely felted together spherical colonies just visible to the naked eye: the pus is said to contain 'sulphur granules'.

Sites of infection

Jaw

Ileocaecal region

Lung

Sinuses to the exterior or to internal adjacent surfaces develop

Sulphur granules

The essential lesion, progressively destructive, is a loculated abscess containing.

Polymorphs

Macrophages

Fibrous tissue

Occasional spread by the blood stream starts abscesses in remote sites

LEPROSY

This slowly progressive disease which causes serious effects by damage to peripheral nerves is still widespread in the tropics and subtropics. The infection is acquired by close, prolonged contact and is due to a slender acid and alcohol-fast bacillus. The disease presents in two contrasting extreme forms and with cases of intermediate type.

1. Lepromatous leprosy

- Disfiguring nodularity of the skin — 'leonine facies'.
- Peripheral nerves affected late.
- The lesions contain lymphocytes, plasma cells and macrophages — filled with organisms.
- Organisms +++ in tissues.

2. Tuberculoid leprosy

- Focal areas of skin pallor and anaesthesia due to early involvement of nerves.
- Basic lesion is a follicular granuloma (tubercle) not unlike the true tubercle follicle.
- Organisms are scanty.

These differences are due in the main to differences in the immune reaction of the host.

- Cell-mediated immunity is markedly diminished.

- Cell-mediated immunity is well developed.

VIRUS INFECTIONS

Viruses, the smallest microorganisms in nature (measured in nm), are not visible by light microscopy but can be studied using the electron microscope (EM). The virus particle (*viron:* elementary body) consists of a central core of genetic material, either ribonucleic acid (RNA) or deoxyribonucleic acid (DNA) surrounded by a protein coat (capsid). The virus particle in itself does not contain the biochemical mechanism for replication; it is wholly dependent on the resources of the infected cell.

The diagram shows how, by taking control of and utilising the nucleic acid of the invaded cell, replication is accomplished.

Classical mechanism of disease production and viral replication

The diagram indicates the direct cytopathic effects of the virus. An alternative and important cause of damage to the host cell is the side effects associated with antibody and cell-mediated immune reactions.

RETROVIRUSES

An important variation occurs in a small group of RNA viruses. These contain an enzyme – **reverse transcriptase** – which, within the cell cytoplasm, is able (using the virus RNA as the REVERSE TRANSCRIPTASE – which, within the cell cytoplasm, is able (using the virus RNA as the (note that messenger RNA is not required).

The virus DNA may remain there inactive for long periods. When activity is resumed, replication and cytopathic changes are effected as indicated in diagram.

Retroviruses are important agents in carcinogenesis and AIDS (see p.113).

VIRUS INFECTIONS

ACUTE VIRUS INFECTION

The evolution of a typical acute virus infection can be understood in terms of virus replication, release and spread within the body, and of the host's reaction.

Typical evolution

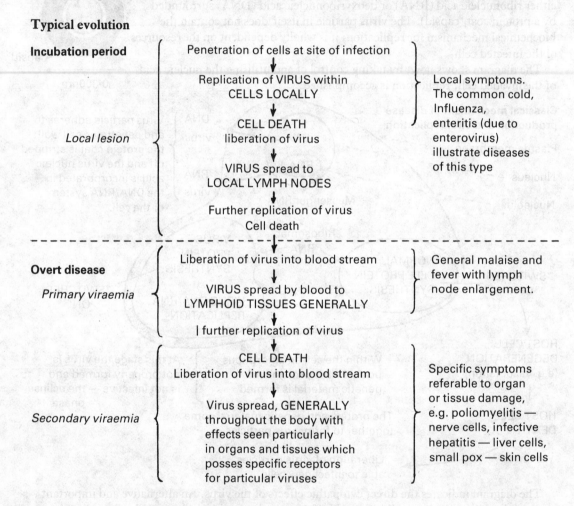

Incubation period

Local lesion

Penetration of cells at site of infection

↓

Replication of VIRUS within
CELLS LOCALLY

↓

CELL DEATH
liberation of virus

↓

VIRUS spread to
LOCAL LYMPH NODES

↓

Further replication of virus
Cell death

Local symptoms.
The common cold,
Influenza,
enteritis (due to
enterovirus)
illustrate diseases
of this type

- -

Overt disease

Primary viraemia

Liberation of virus into blood stream

↓

VIRUS spread by blood to
LYMPHOID TISSUES GENERALLY

↓

| further replication of virus

General malaise and
fever with lymph
node enlargement.

Secondary viraemia

CELL DEATH
Liberation of virus into blood stream

↓

Virus spread, GENERALLY
throughout the body with
effects seen particularly
in organs and tissues which
posses specific receptors
for particular viruses

Specific symptoms
referable to organ
or tissue damage,
e.g. poliomyelitis —
nerve cells, infective
hepatitis — liver cells,
small pox — skin cells

This typical evolution is produced by successive waves of virus. However, the great majority of virus infections are clinically latent or mild because virus replication and spread are prevented by the body's defence mechanisms. Severe overt disease occurs when there is a specially virulent virus or when the body's resistance is inadequate, especially in a primary infection.

Not all virus infections cause disease in this way. 3 important variations are:

(1) LATENT   (2) ONCOGENIC   (3) SLOW

VIRUS INFECTIONS

LATENT VIRUS INFECTION

A good example is the common 'cold sores' of the lips and face caused by the virus **Herpes simplex** (an enveloped DNA virus).

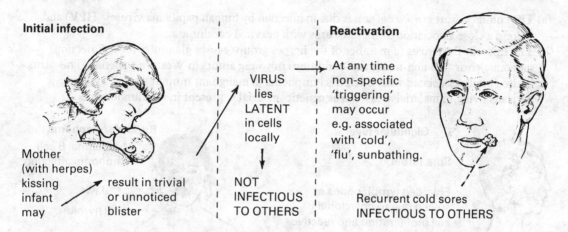

Initial infection

Mother (with herpes) kissing infant may → result in trivial or unnoticed blister

VIRUS lies LATENT in cells locally ↓ NOT INFECTIOUS TO OTHERS

Reactivation

At any time non-specific 'triggering' may occur e.g. associated with 'cold', 'flu', sunbathing.

Recurrent cold sores INFECTIOUS TO OTHERS

Another example is **herpes zoster (shingles)**.

This is a painful affection of segmental sensory nerves and root ganglia due to infection by CHICKEN POX VIRUS **Varicella**.

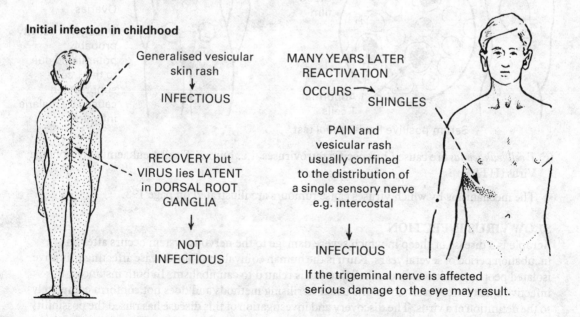

Initial infection in childhood

Generalised vesicular skin rash → INFECTIOUS

RECOVERY but VIRUS lies LATENT in DORSAL ROOT GANGLIA ↓ NOT INFECTIOUS

MANY YEARS LATER REACTIVATION OCCURS → SHINGLES

PAIN and vesicular rash usually confined to the distribution of a single sensory nerve e.g. intercostal ↓ INFECTIOUS

If the trigeminal nerve is affected serious damage to the eye may result.

VIRUS INFECTIONS

ONCOGENIC VIRUS INFECTION

In animals, viruses have been clearly proved to cause malignant tumours, and there is good evidence that some tumours in man are caused by viruses (see also p.198).
Examples include the following:

(a) **The common wart** *verruca vulgaris* is due to infection by human papilloma viruses (HPV) and there is a close association of these viruses with **cervical carcinoma.**

(b) **The Epstein-Barr virus** (a member of the herpes group) causes glandular fever (infectious mononucleosis — a non-malignant condition) in young adults in Western societies. This virus is also closely associated with Burkitt's lymphoma (a malignant tumour) found in young Africans living in malarial areas. Virus genetic material is present in the tumour cells.

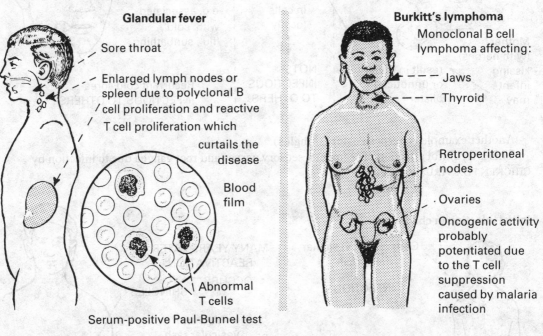

Glandular fever

Sore throat

Enlarged lymph nodes or spleen due to polyclonal B cell proliferation and reactive T cell proliferation which curtails the disease

Blood film

Abnormal T cells

Serum-positive Paul-Bunnel test

Burkitt's lymphoma

Monoclonal B cell lymphoma affecting:

Jaws

Thyroid

Retroperitoneal nodes

Ovaries

Oncogenic activity probably potentiated due to the T cell suppression caused by malaria infection

(c) *T cell leukaemias* are caused by specific retroviruses, i.e. human T cell Leukaemia-Lymphoma Virus (HTLV)

The mechanisms by which viruses cause tumours are illustrated on page 198.

SLOW VIRUS INFECTION

Scrapie is a disease of sheep in which severe damage to the nervous system occurs after an incubation period of several years. **Kuru** is the human equivalent of the disease affecting primitive isolated peoples in New Guinea: the infection is related to cannibalism. In both instances, the infective agent is very resistant to the usual sterilising methods and does not conform completely to the definition of a virus. The discovery and investigation of this disease has raised the possibility that other chronic diseases of the nervous system may be of similar origin. The progress of the disease caused by certain retroviruses (lenti-viruses) may be extremely slow. AIDS due to HIV infection is the prime example (see p.113).

HOST/VIRUS INTERACTION

The reactions occurring in the host are important.

1. Changes in the infected cells

(a) Cell degeneration
(with loss of function)
leading to cell death.

Vacuolation

Rapid degeneration and lysis

Nuclear and cytoplasmic condensation

Slow lysis

(b) Fusion of adjacent infected cells — giant cell formation, e.g. the Warthin-Winkeldy cell of measles,

Lymphocytes

(c) Cell proliferation.

Proliferation of skin epithelial cells causing a warty growth

(d) Formation of 'inclusion' bodies within cytoplasm or nucleus: they consist of aggregates of virus and/or products of cell degeneration.

Diagnostic eosinophilic intracytoplasmic Negri bodies in nerve cells of the hippocampus in **RABIES**

Nuclear and cytoplasmic inclusion in cytomegalic virus infection of salivary ducts

(e) No apparent change in cell but virus remains latent — reactivation later with continuous and slow release associated with gradually progressive disease.

(f) No apparent change but later malignant proliferation occurs, i.e. oncogenic infection.

HOST/VIRUS INTERACTION

REACTIONS IN HOST (continued)

2. Interferon production by the infected cell

Virus

Virus penetration
and replication

The presence of
foreign nucleic acid
almost immediately
switches on the
production of **INTERFERON (↑)**

Inhibition
of virus
replication

Interferon release
from cell
to inhibit
virus
replication
in other
cells

Interferon is a protein but not an antibody. It acts against any virus by interfering with the synthesis of viral protein. This is the first and very important line of defence.

3. The immune response (see p.94).

    (a) Antibodies to virus
    (b) Cell-mediated immunity
    (c) Occasionally virus/antibody complexes cause special types of reaction in the host, *e.g.* inflammatory necrosis of arteries (arteritis) and some forms of kidney damage.

4. The inflammatory response

The vascular and exudative elements follow the usual pattern; polymorphs are not a feature unless there is considerable tissue necrosis or secondary bacterial infection. However, macrophage phagocytic activity is important in the defence against virus infection.

OPPORTUNISTIC INFECTIONS

This term is used for infections caused by organisms which are often nonpathogenic or of low grade virulence, occurring in individuals whose resistance to infection is impaired. They are occurring more frequently in modern medical practice because of the increasing use of powerful immunosuppressive drugs.

CAUSES OF LOWERED RESISTANCE

1. Congenital immunological deficiences (rare).
2. Acquired
    (a) *the result of disease:* HIV infection (AIDS);
                uraemia; liver disease; malignant tumours,
                particularly Hodgkin's disease and leukaemias;
    (b) *the result of therapy:* e.g.
                immunosuppression in transplant surgery;
                immunosuppression — a side effect of tumour therapy;
                antibiotics — changing commensal populations;
                introduction of foreign material, e.g. heart valve prostheses;
                I.V. long lines in intensive care; tracheostomy.

Examples of infecting organisms

Bacteria → Acinetobacter wound infections: septicaemia

Staph. albus on heart valves: low grade septicaemia

Vegetations

Protozoa

Pneumocystis carinii: a severe pneumonia

Foamy exudate

Viruses - - - - - - - → Wart viruses: crop of warts around genitalia, e.g. Vulvar condylomata

Herpes virus group: generalised infections or severe organ damage

e.g. Herpes encephalitis

Necrosis

Fungi   Aspergillosis — lungs: septicaemia

Monilia (candidiasis) — mouth, oesophagus, bowel, anus: septicaemia: endocarditis.

'Thrush'

Mycelial cells

Monilia

INFECTION — GENERAL EFFECTS

The more general body reactions in infection are: FEVER and CHANGES IN METABOLISM.

FEVER (PYREXIA)

The body temperature rises above normal initially due partly to an imbalance between heat production and loss, but mainly due to a resetting at a higher level of the 'thermostat' mechanism in the hypothalamus. This results in:

1. Increased HEAT PRODUCTION
due to
INCREASED METABOLISM

Heat-sensitive nerve endings in skin

Muscle

2. Increased HEAT LOSS

Skin blood vessels dilate

} WARM MOIST SKIN

Sweat glands secrete

In early stages, when the temperature is rising internally, there may be a paradoxical feeling of cold with shivering (rigor).

Thermostat setting at higher level due to **pyrogens** derived from infecting organisms, polymorphs and macrophages mediated by prostaglandin E.

These changes are associated with an **INCREASED PULSE RATE** and a tendency to **DEHYDRATION.**

Pyrexia also occurs when there is:

    (a) Considerable tissue necrosis, e.g. infarction and tumours

    (b) Cerebral disease — especially in the region of the pons

    (c) Heat-stroke — where the environmental temperature and humidity are high and there is excessive water and salt loss.

Hyperpyrexia [when the temperature exceeds 41°C (106°F)] is extremely dangerous because of damage to the nerve cells in the brain.

INFECTION — GENERAL EFFECTS

CHANGES IN METABOLISM

Tissue breakdown is greatly increased, and in some infectious fevers there is a marked loss of body weight.

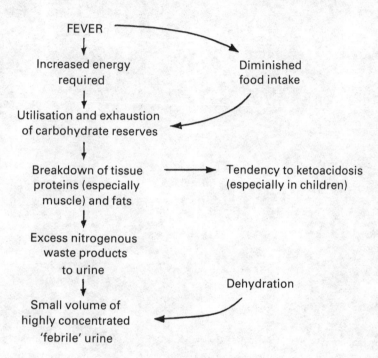

FEVER

Increased energy required

Diminished food intake

Utilisation and exhaustion of carbohydrate reserves

Breakdown of tissue proteins (especially muscle) and fats

Tendency to ketoacidosis (especially in children)

Excess nitrogenous waste products to urine

Dehydration

Small volume of highly concentrated 'febrile' urine

Plasma proteins

In chronic infections there is often a rise in the amount of immune globulins — **hypergammaglobulinaemia.**

These changes in the blood protein content are also reflected in a rise in the **ESR** (Erythrocyte Sedimentation Rate).

CHAPTER 4

HEALING

HEALING

In almost all situations repair is brought about by the formation of 'granulation tissue'.
WOUND HEALING is a good example of this process.

Healing by first intention (primary union)
This occurs in clean, incised wounds with good apposition of the edges — particularly planned surgical incisions.

Immediately: Blood clot and debris fill the small cleft.

2 – 3 hours: Early inflammation close to edges. Mild hyperaemia and a few polymorphs.

Movement of epithelial cells across wound

Mitotic activity

Epithelium growing across

2 – 3 days: Macrophage activity removing clot. Fibroblastic activity.

10 – 14 days: Scab loose and epithelial covering complete. Fibrous union of edges, but wound is still weak.

Weeks: Scar tissue still slightly hyperaemic. Good fibrous union, but not full strength.

Months – years: Devascularisation. Remodelling of collagen by enzyme action. Scar is now minimal and merges with surrounding tissues.

WOUND HEALING

WOUND HEALING (continued)

Healing by second intention (secondary union)

This occurs in open wounds, particularly when there has been significant loss of tissue, necrosis or infection.

Early

Cavity fills with blood and fibrin clot

Acute inflammation commences at junction of living tissue

A few days

Scab dries out

Mitotic activity in epithelium

A single sheet of epithelial cells is being pushed between the surface debris and the underlying living tissue

Note contraction of wound size due to action of fibro blasts at edges

New capillary loops bring macrophages, polymorphs and fibroblasts

1 week approximately

Epithelium continues to grow across

Capillary loops form small 'granulations' in the base of

Note contraction continuing

Surface debris has to been shed

Loose connective tissue formed by fibroblasts

the wound. These can be seen by the naked eye and, historically, are the origin of the term 'granulation tissue'. This term is now used in a wider context to describe tissue consisting of newly formed capillaries with fibroblasts and macrophages and occurring in many circumstances in addition to wounds.

WOUND HEALING

Healing by second intention (continued)

2 weeks onwards

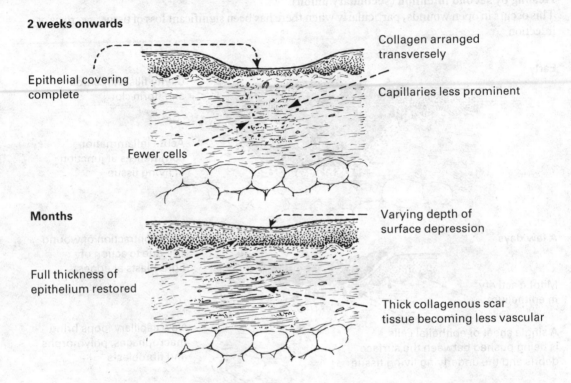

Epithelial covering complete

Collagen arranged transversely

Capillaries less prominent

Fewer cells

Months

Varying depth of surface depression

Full thickness of epithelium restored

Thick collagenous scar tissue becoming less vascular

Note that the differences in the two types of wound healing are quantitative: the essential pathological processes are the same.

Wound contraction

Wound contraction which is beneficial and begins early, is due mainly to the young, specialised 'myofibroblasts' in the granulation tissue exerting a traction effect at the wound edges. The exposed surface is reduced by gradual regeneration of the surface epithelium. The remodelling of the collagen continues for many months.

WOUND HEALING — COMPLICATIONS

Contracture

Later CONTRACTURE with distortion due to thickening and shortening of collagen bundles may cause serious cosmetic and functional disability, particularly in deep and extensive skin burns and around joints if muscles are seriously damaged.

Contracture following burn of neck and jaw

Occasional complications

1. At the edges and base of a wound granulation tissue may form in excess and prevent proper healing ('exuberant granulations': 'proud flesh').

2. The formation of excess collagen in the form of thick interlacing bundles which causes marked swelling at the site of the wound is known as a KELOID. The essential cause is unkown but it may be due to deficient polymerisation of fibrin (factor XIII deficiency): the condition is more common among negroes.

HEALING — FIBROSIS

FIBROSIS is the end result of WOUND HEALING, CHRONIC INFLAMMATION and ORGANISATION.

Formation of fibrous tissue

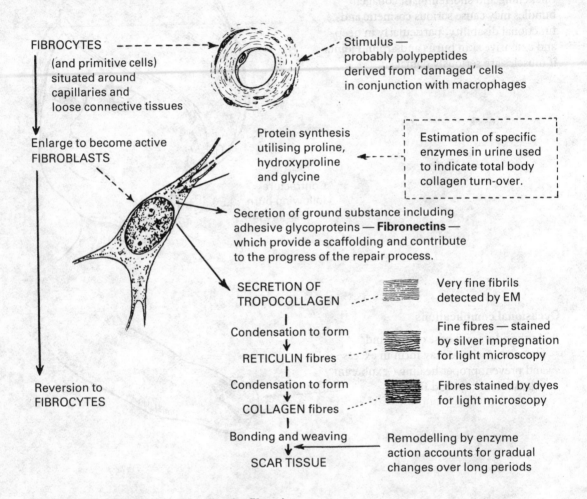

FIBROCYTES
(and primitive cells)
situated around
capillaries and
loose connective tissues

Stimulus —
probably polypeptides
derived from 'damaged' cells
in conjunction with macrophages

Enlarge to become active
FIBROBLASTS

Protein synthesis
utilising proline,
hydroxyproline
and glycine

Estimation of specific
enzymes in urine used
to indicate total body
collagen turn-over.

Secretion of ground substance including
adhesive glycoproteins — **Fibronectins** —
which provide a scaffolding and contribute
to the progress of the repair process.

Reversion to
FIBROCYTES

SECRETION OF
TROPOCOLLAGEN

Very fine fibrils
detected by EM

Condensation to form

RETICULIN fibres

Fine fibres — stained
by silver impregnation
for light microscopy

Condensation to form

COLLAGEN fibres

Fibres stained by dyes
for light microscopy

Bonding and weaving

SCAR TISSUE

Remodelling by enzyme
action accounts for gradual
changes over long periods

Factors influencing wound healing by fibrosis

1. *Local*
   INFECTION and a POOR BLOOD SUPPLY to the wound DELAY HEALING.
2. *General*
   DEFICIENCY of VITAMIN C
   DEFICIENCY OF AMINO ACIDS (in malnutrition)   } Failure of proper collagen
   EXCESS OF ADRENAL GLUCOCORTICOIDS   } synthesis with delayed
   Traces of ZINC are beneficial   } healing and weak scars.

HEALING

REGENERATION

In the examples of wound healing, the restoration of the epithelial surface of the skin was effected by movement and proliferation of the surviving epithelial cells. Such regeneration of the specialised cells occurs in most organs and tissues to a varying degree, and the healing process consists of combinations of regeneration and repair by granulation tissue in varying proportions.

The capacity to regenerate is related to the amount of proliferation and replacement which takes place in physiological conditions. It is convenient to consider three broad groups of cells:

1. *Labile cells* — normally a continuous process of active replacement is occurring; the chances of restoration by regeneration are excellent, e.g. the covering epithelium (both external and internal), the bone marrow cells and the lymphoid cells.

2. *Stable cells* — although normally the replacement requirements are minimal, they have not lost the capacity to proliferate in response to damage. Chances of regeneration are good, e.g. liver, endocrine glands, renal tubular epithelium.

3. *Permanent cells* — normally are unable to multiply after the growth phase early in life. Such cells cannot regenerate and healing is by granulation tissue with permanent loss of function, e.g. nerve cells.

The process of regeneration can be divided into two main components:

1. *Movement* of surviving cells into the vacant space made available by loss due to wounding or necrosis.

2. *Proliferation* of surviving cells to replace the loss.

The factors which control these processes are extremely complex and their roles somewhat speculative.
Probable mechanisms are:

    (a) Removal of contact inhibition allows movement of cells
    (b) Presence of chemical factors promoting proliferation
    (c) Removal of chemical factors inhibiting mitosis

HEALING

REGENERATION (continued)

1. **Removal of contact inhibition**

    Messages passing between cells in close contact inhibit cell migration.

Normal skin

NO CONTACT INHIBITION ON SURFACE

Cells move vertically to replace surface loss

CONTACT INHIBITION prevents lateral movement

After wounding

LOSS OF CONTACT INHIBITION IN WOUND

Cells move laterally to cover wound surface

2. **Presence of chemical factors promoting proliferation**

    Many growth factors, usually polypeptides, have been defined. For example, platelet-derived growth factor (PDGE) and growth factors derived from epidermal cells (EGF) and macrophages (MDGF) are likely to be involved in healing and regeneration.

3. **Removal of chemical factors inhibiting mitosis**

    These factors called **CHALONES**, manufactured by healthy cells, inhibit mitosis in neighbouring cells of the same type. When cells are destroyed by wounding or necrosis, the absence of chalones allows proliferation of the surviving cells.

Normal skin

All cells producing chalones inhibiting undue proliferation

Cells missing — no chalones produced, therefore mitotic activity

Other important factors which influence regeneration and restoration to normal are (a) the availability of a good blood supply and (b) the survival of the supporting framework allowing the cells to grow in an organised way.

When regeneration of specialised cells is occurring, they may lose some of their specialised qualities (dedifferentiation), but usually these are restored after regeneration is complete.

HEALING — SPECIAL SITUATIONS

INTERNAL SURFACES

The regeneration of the covering epithelium is very similar to that of the skin, as seen for example in the alimentary tract.

Superficial damage   **Deep damage**

Debris

Cells moving across from edges

Mitotic activity in mucous cells

Granulation tissue

Organisation

Surface cells budding downward to form new glands

Restoration to normal including reappearance of specialised cells

Contracting scar tissue which may cause serious effects due to stricure, e.g. pyloric stenosis

HEALING — SPECIAL SITUATIONS

SOLID EPITHELIAL ORGANS

1. **Following gross tissue damage — including supporting tissue.**

e.g. **Kidney**

Liver

Necrotic tissue

Progressive removal of dead tissue with organisation and COARSE SCAR formation

2. **Following cell damage with survival of the supporting (reticular) tissues**

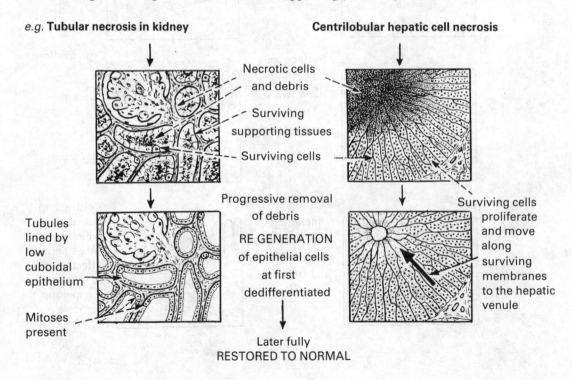

e.g. **Tubular necrosis in kidney**

Centrilobular hepatic cell necrosis

Necrotic cells and debris

Surviving supporting tissues

Surviving cells

Progressive removal of debris

RE GENERATION of epithelial cells at first dedifferentiated

Tubules lined by low cuboidal epithelium

Mitoses present

Surviving cells proliferate and move along surviving membranes to the hepatic venule

Later fully RESTORED TO NORMAL

HEALING — SPECIAL SITUATIONS

MUSCLE

Muscle fibres of all 3 types — skeletal, cardiac and visceral — have only limited capacity to regenerate.

When a MASS of muscle tissue is damaged, repair by SCARRING occurs. This is particularly important in the HEART after infarction.

If the damage affects individual muscle fibres diffusely and with varying severity, then regeneration of the specialised fibres is possible (e.g. the myocardium may recover completely from the effects of diphtheria toxin and virus infection).

NERVOUS TISSUE

Central nervous system

Regeneration does not occur.

In cases of acute damage, the initial functional loss often exceeds the loss of actual nerve tissue because of the reactive changes in the surrounding tissue. As these changes diminish, functional restoration commences.

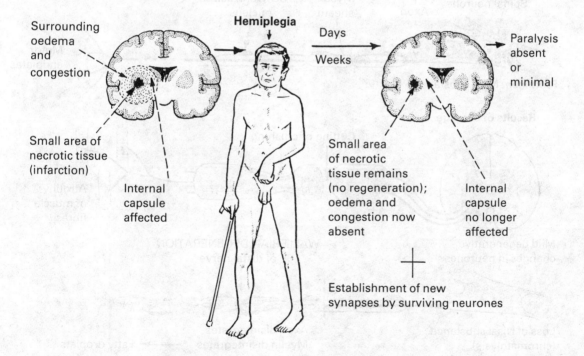

Surrounding oedema and congestion

Small area of necrotic tissue (infarction)

Internal capsule affected

Hemiplegia

Days

Weeks

Paralysis absent or minimal

Small area of necrotic tissue remains (no regeneration); oedema and congestion now absent

Internal capsule no longer affected

Establishment of new synapses by surviving neurones

HEALING — SPECIAL SITUATIONS

NERVOUS TISSUE (continued)

Peripheral Nerves

When a peripheral nerve is damaged, the axon and its myelin sheath rapidly degenerate distally. The supporting tissues of the nerve (neurilemma) degenerate slowly.

Regeneration can occur because the central neurone of which the axon is a peripheral extension is remote from the site of damage.

A spinal motor nerve is taken as an example.

Normal Spinal cord

Motor impulse

Anterior root

Nerve trunk

Muscle fibres

Spinal neurone

Axon

Myelin sheath

Schwann cell nucleus

Motor endplates

Prominent Nissl substance

Results of damage

Cutting or crushing

Atrophy of muscle fibres

Mild degenerative changes in neurones

WALLERIAN DEGENERATION of distal nerve

Loss of Nissl substance (chromatolysis)

Axon disintegrates
Myelin disintegrates ⟶ Fatty droplets
Schwann cells survive

HEALING — SPECIAL SITUATIONS

PERIPHERAL NERVES (continued)

Regeneration takes the form of a sprouting of the cut ends of the axons.

Sprouting of
axons

Growth along the
track of the degenerate nerve
(about 20 mm per week)

The results depend on the apposition of the distal remnant with the sprouting axons.

Good apposition   **Good restoration**

The best results are seen in crushing injuries where the sheaths remain in continuity.

Poor apposition

6 — 12
months

Distal nerve remnant
disappears

Irregular sprouting of
axons and proliferation
of Schwann cells

Formation of
**TRAUMATIC
'NEUROMA'**

Severe atrophy
of muscle

HEALING — SPECIAL SITUATIONS

BONE

A fracture is usually accompanied by damage to or haemorrhage into adjacent soft tissues which are repaired by the process of organisation already described, while the bone fragments are reunited by regeneration.

Events following a fracture

(1) *Immediate effects*

Periosteum

Medulla

Cortex

Necrosis of ends of bone

Damage to soft tissues with haemorrhage (haematoma) and fibrin deposition

(2) *Early reaction — inflammatory*
   First 4-5 days

Phagocytosis of debris and necrotic tissues

Early organisation: capillaries and fibroblasts

(3) *Early bone regeneration*
   After 1st week,

Osteoblastic activity

Periosteal

Medullary

Provisional callus bridges the gap — first, osteoid tissue (may include cartilage) then woven bone

Resorption in healthy bone (seen on X-ray as rarifaction)

HEALING — SPECIAL SITUATIONS

Events following a fracture (continued)

(4) *Well-formed callus*
From 3 weeks onwards

Firm union by callus mineralisation

Osteoblastic and osteoclastic activity proceeding

(5) *Remodelling of callus*
Definitive — weeks into months

Osteoblasts and osteoclasts active

Lamellar bone

Medullary early reopening

(6) *Final reconstruction*
Months later

Fracture site may be almost invisible

Island cartilage

Osteoid tissue — woven bone

Background of granulation tissue

Calcified

Osteoblasts

Osteoclasts 'eating away' bone

Dense lamellar bone: trabeculae orientated along lines of stress.
Osteoblasts and osteoclasts now scanty.

HEALING — SPECIAL SITUATIONS

EVENTS FOLLOWING A FRACTURE (continued)

Complications

1. *Fat embolism* may occur in fracture of long bones due to entry of fat from the marrow cavity into the torn ends of veins.

2. *Infection*

If the overlying skin is breached in any way, i.e. the fracture is 'compound', the risk of infection is greatly increased; this is an important adverse factor in the healing process.

E.g.

By sharp bone ends

Penetrating injury from outside

PATHOLOGICAL FRACTURE

When the break occurs at the site of pre-existing disease of the bone, the term 'pathological fracture' is applied.

A common condition is a secondary tumour growing in and destroying the bone

Mixture of tumour and haematoma — healing inhibited

Very easily fractured

HEALING — SPECIAL SITUATIONS

FACTORS INFLUENCING HEALING OF FRACTURES

ADVERSE	FAVOURABLE

1. Local factors

(a) *Infection* ⎱ See previous
(b) *Pathological fracture* ⎰ page

(c) *Poor apposition and alignment* . . . .   *Good apposition*

There may be interposition
of soft tissue, *e.g.* muscle

Large irregular callus:
slow repair, permanent deformity of bone

*Small callus,
quick repair*

(d) *Continuing movement of bone ends* . . . .   *Good immobilisation*

Callus formation
inhibited

Fibrous union

In extreme cases, a rudimentary joint
(pseudoarthrosis)
may form

*Small callus, good
bone formation*

(e) *Poor blood supply.* . . . .   *Good blood supply*

This is largely influenced by the anatomical site
of the fracture, for example:
(a) Nutrient artery entering remote from the
fracture or damaged by fracture (*e.g.* scaphoid,
femoral head)
(b) Fracture through area devoid of periosteum
(*e.g.* neck of femur)
(c) Minimal adjacent soft tissue (*e.g.* tibia).

In favourable conditions
blood supply is derived from:
(a) periosteal arteries
(b) nutrient artery
(c) adjacent soft tissues.

2. General factors

(a) *Old age* . . . .   *Youth*

(b) *Poor nutrition* — e.g. famine conditions, ...   *Good nutrition* — especially
malabsorption lead to lack of   protein, calcium, vit D and vit C.
protein, calcium, vit D and vit C.

CHAPTER 5

IMMUNITY

IMMUNITY

It has been known from historical times that a person who has recovered from an infectious disease, e.g. smallpox, is most unlikely to suffer from it again — even when exposed maximally — although he would remain susceptible to other infections.

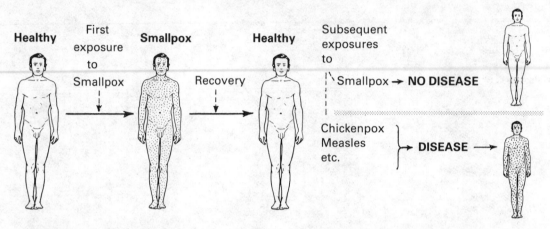

That is, during the recovery period he has ACQUIRED SPECIFIC IMMUNITY to smallpox but not to other infections.

Of course, in its literal meaning, immunity — the inability to be infected — includes NON-SPECIFIC mechanisms, some of which have been mentioned previously.

Many of these mechanisms are innate or may be associated with species or race — **NATURAL IMMUNITY** — but some are acquired.

Note: CO-OPERATION. The specific and non-specific mechanisms are conveniently separated but they have important influences on each other.

The modern science of IMMUNOLOGY is engaged mainly in the study of the mechanisms involved in the establishment of specific immunity, i.e. the IMMUNE RESPONSE and its CONSEQUENCES.

THE SPECIFIC IMMUNE RESPONSE

The sequence of events in an infection is as follows:

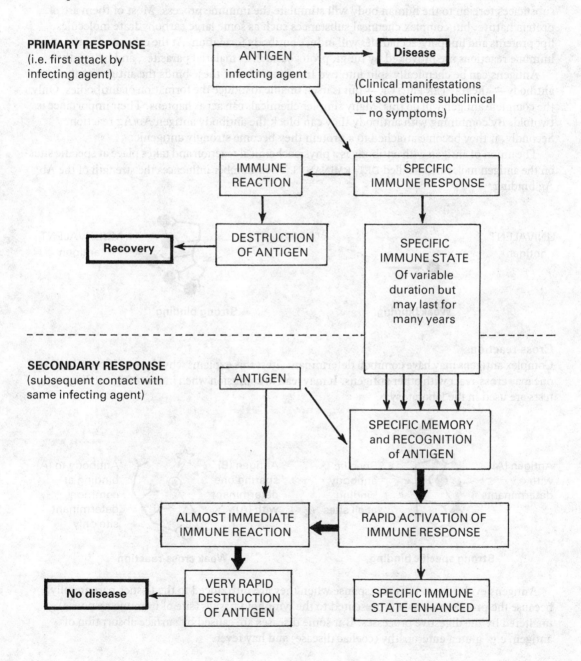

PRIMARY RESPONSE
(i.e. first attack by
infecting agent)

ANTIGEN
infecting agent

Disease

(Clinical manifestations
but sometimes subclinical
— no symptoms)

IMMUNE
REACTION

SPECIFIC
IMMUNE RESPONSE

DESTRUCTION
OF ANTIGEN

Recovery

SPECIFIC
IMMUNE STATE
Of variable
duration but
may last for
many years

SECONDARY RESPONSE
(subsequent contact with
same infecting agent)

ANTIGEN

SPECIFIC MEMORY
and RECOGNITION
of ANTIGEN

ALMOST IMMEDIATE
IMMUNE REACTION

RAPID ACTIVATION OF
IMMUNE RESPONSE

VERY RAPID
DESTRUCTION
OF ANTIGEN

No disease

SPECIFIC IMMUNE
STATE ENHANCED

ANTIGEN

The most familiar antigens are infectious agents such as bacteria and some viruses, but other substances foreign to the human body will stimulate the immune process. Most of them are of protein nature, but complex chemical substances such as some large carbohydrate molecules, lipoproteins and lipopolysaccharides will induce antibody formation. At the other end of the scale, immune reactions are provoked by fungi, protozoa such as malarial parasites, and helminths.

Antigens can be chemically split into two fractions. One of these binds the antigen to the antibody — the HAPTEN FACTOR — but is itself unable to induce the formation of antibodies. Only the complete antigen will do this. Many simpler chemicals can act as haptens. Their importance is twofold. By combining with antibody they can block the antibody antigen Ab/Ag reaction. Secondly, if they become attached to a protein they become strongly antigenic.

The union of antigen with antibody is a physicochemical reaction and takes place at specific sites on the antigen molecule — called DETERMINANTS. Their number influences the strength of the Ab/Ag binding.

Cross-reactions

Complex antigens may have common determinant sites; this explains why the specific antibody to one may cross-react with other antigens. It may lead to confusion when immunological diagnostic tests are used in the laboratory.

Antigens evoke the strongest response when they are introduced to the tissues parenterally, because the protein molecule is presented to the lymphoid tissues (site of immune response) unaltered by the digestive processes. But some diseases are caused by surface absorption of antigen, e.g. gluten enteropathy (coeliac disease) and hay fever.

THE SPECIFIC IMMUNE RESPONSE

The process is essentially an activity of the small lymphocytes of which there are two main types. They are indistinguishable by light microscopy using conventional stains but show clear differences, under the electron microscope, in their surface properties and in their function.

Stem cells in MARROW

In man, to reach functional maturity, stem cells are processed in lymphoid tissue probably in alimentary tract. (First associated with the **B**ursa of Fabricius in the bowel of chicken — ∴ called **B lymphocytes.**)

In man and most mammals, to reach functional maturity, stem cells are processed in the **T**hymus ∴ called **T lymphocytes**.

In the peripheral blood there are:
25% **B** cells

5% unidentifiable ('null') cells

70% **T** cells

Although occasional **B** cells have a nuclear cleft ......

using light microscopy and conventional stains, the majority cannot be distinguished from **T** cells.

The use of electron microscopy, surface markers and monoclonal antibodies is required.

Electron microscope (EM)

Surface

Nucleus ← Rough ← Smooth → Nucleus

Surface markers

e.g. Surface immunoglobulin (Ig)

No Ig

Possess natural receptors for sheep erythrocytes — rosette formation.

Monoclonal antibodies

Their use has greatly facilitated the identification of lymphocytes and there is now recognition of an increasing number of T lymphocyte subpopulations each with a specific function.

THE SPECIFIC IMMUNE RESPONSE

LYMPHOID TISSUES
The activities of the two cell types take place in different parts of the lymph node.

Lymph flow

B cells in cortex, especially **germinal centres**

To thoracic duct or blood stream

T cells in **paracortical area**

The introduction of an antigen results in activation and proliferation of these two lymphocyte populations.

ANTIGENIC STIMULATION

Antigen → Activation → Transformation → Enlargement → Division (Clonal proliferation) → Maturation

In germ centre (not in blood)

Blast cells

Memory cells

PLASMA CELLS

In paracortical area and blood

Blast cells

Memory cell

SPECIFICALLY SENSITISED LYMPHOCYTES

Loss of surface Ig markers but:

Synthesis of specific antibody (immunoglobulin Ig) within the cell

Secretion of (Y) Ig into tissue fluids and blood

The end result of the B cell response is the formation of *humoral* antibodies or
HUMORAL IMMUNITY

Most of the specific immune effects remain closely associated with the sensitised cells

The end result of the T cell response is the formation of
CELL-MEDIATED IMMUNITY

HUMORAL ANTIBODIES — IMMUNOGLOBULINS (Ig)

The basic immunoglobulin is a protein molecule consisting of 2 pairs of polypeptide chains arranged in a particular way.

1, 2 : 3, 4
polypeptide
chains

1 and 2 are **HEAVY** chains
Differences in structure allow separation of five main
Ig groups — Ig G; A; M; D; E

Bonding
sites

3 and 4 are **LIGHT** chains
They exist in 2 forms — Kappa (K) and Lambda (λ).
In any one molecule both chains are either K or λ.

Note that the molecule can hinge.
This allows a better fit with the
antigen surface and explains the
symbols commonly used for Ig (⋏, ⋏)

Enzymatic digestion (papain) splits the molecule into named fragments.

Papain

Fc (Fragment crystalline)

Fab (Fragments antigen binding)

Fc is the *constant* part of the molecule and does not participate in antigen binding.

However, the Fc fragment is associated with secondary effects after binding has occurred, e.g. complement activation; attraction of lymphocytes and particularly the facilitation of phagocytosis by macrophages which carry Fc receptors (see p. 103).

Antigen

Fc

Fab

Fab

Fab are the *variable* parts of the molecule and are the site of antigen binding, the variation in amino acid content allowing a wide range of specific activity.

IMMUNOGLOBULINS

MAIN GROUPS

These groups are named according to the composition of the heavy chains.

IgM

IgM (heavy chain = μ) is a polymer of five identical basic molecules, therefore called macroglobulin. Although in low concentration in the blood, 0.5 – 2 mg/ml, it is the main Ig on the surface of B lymphocytes (before conversion to plasma cells) and is active in the early phase of the immune response. It neutralises viruses. In combination with complement, it is actively bactericidal and is especially effective in bacteraemia.

Note: The numerous (10) antigen-binding sites increase its efficiency.

The natural blood group antibodies, anti-A and anti-B are M globulins.

IgG

IgG (heavy chain = γ) is a single molecule with two antigen binding sites .

It is produced mainly in **secondary response.**
IgG has the highest concentration of all immunoglobulins in the blood — within a range of 8 – 16 mg/ml dependent on antigenic stimulation at the time. Of its several activities, the important ones take place in the blood and tissue fluids and are:

IgG — Anti → Microbes

IgG — Anti → Toxins

COOPERATION with

Macrophages

Sensitised lymphocytes (T cells)

'Passive' transfer of IgG from mother to baby occurs via the placenta and colostrum. The immunity only lasts for a few months.

Transplacental passage of IgG

Colostrum, rich in IgG, absorbed from alimentary tract into the blood stream of the neonate.

IMMUNOGLOBULINS

IgA IgA (heavy chain = ∝) is a single molecule occuring in blood (concentration 1.5 – 4 mg/ml) where it is **anti-toxic.**

It is in high concentration in secretions of eyes, nose, mouth, bronchi and gut, existing as a dimer of two identical molecules with four antigen binding sites.

Local production of IgA e.g. **in alimentary tract**

Plasma cell

Synthesis and secretion of IgA dimer.

Passage through epithelial cell with secretory piece added to protect it from digestive juices.

This important immunoglobulin protects mucous surfaces from antigenic attack and prevents access to foreign substances to the circulation and general immunological system.

IgD (heavy chain △) of uncertain function: concentration in blood very low. Like IgM it is present on the surface of lymphocytes prior to transformation.

IgE (heavy chain Ɛ) — a single molecule similar to IgG and IgA.

It is sometimes called **REAGIN**: concentration in blood is low (20 – 500 ng/ml).

The serum level is raised in worm infestation and is probably protective.

Its main activity is mediated by **MAST CELLS** (or **BASOPHILS**).

Plasma cell

IgE.. attached by Fc to mast cell in tissues, leaving antigen-binding sites free on surface

Specific antigen... bound to mast cell

Degranulation with release of **vaso-active amines** (histamine, etc.)

The range of antigens is immense and B cells produce an infinite number of specific antibodies by interchanging and rearranging the shape of the terminal amino acids of the FAB fraction to suit the antigen determinants.

IMMUNE REACTIONS

The basic reaction is the combination of antigen (Ag) and antibody (Ab) to form an Ag/Ab complex.

This reaction is reversible in varying degree (Ag+Ab $\rightleftharpoons$ Ag/Ab).

IMMEDIATE AND DELAYED REACTIONS

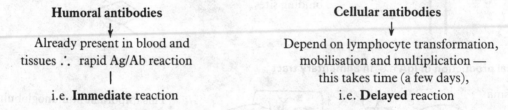

Humoral antibodies	**Cellular antibodies**
↓	↓
Already present in blood and tissues ∴ rapid Ag/Ab reaction	Depend on lymphocyte transformation, mobilisation and multiplication — this takes time (a few days),
|	
i.e. **Immediate** reaction	i.e. **Delayed** reaction

The forces binding the antigen and antibody are essentially non-specific and are the same as those operating in most situations where protein molecules are in proximity.

Attraction   or   Repulsion

Protein molecule   Protein molecule   Protein molecule   Protein molecule

Depends on the ELECTRO-CHEMICAL conditions at the molecular surfaces

In antigen/antibody binding, these forces of attraction are boosted by the shape and flexibility of the Ig molecule ensuring a good 'fit' with determinants on the antigen surface.

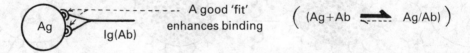

Ag   Ig(Ab)   A good 'fit' enhances binding   ((Ag+Ab) $\rightleftharpoons$ Ag/Ab)

There are several consequences of the basic Ag/Ab combination which have been extensively studied *in vitro*.

1. PRECIPITATION
2. AGGLUTINATION
3. ANTI-TOXIC effect
4. ENHANCEMENT of the natural non-specific defence mechanisms

IMMUNE REACTIONS

1. PRECIPITATION

A soluble antigen is rendered insoluble by aggregation of the Ag/Ab complexes into a lattice.

Antigen in solution + Antibody in solution → Aggregation leads to → PRECIPITATION

2. AGGLUTINATION

Particulate antigen, e.g. bacteria on red blood cells, are aggregated in the same way as in the precipitation reaction and the process is called AGGLUTINATION.

3. ANTI-TOXIC Effect

The Ag/Ab combination neutralises the toxic activity.

Toxic molecule

Anti-toxin (Ig)

4. ENHANCEMENT of the natural non-specific defence mechanisms

(a) Phagocytic activity

Macrophage

Ag/Ab

Fc receptors on surface

Rapid adherence of antigen

Efficient phagocytosis

Antibodies with this property are called **opsonins**.

(b) Complement activation

Humoral immune reactions frequently involve activation of the complement system. Complement consists of nine main protein components circulating in inactive form in the blood. Activation is affected by Ag/Ab complexes. The complex attaches itself to complement via the Fc part of the Ab (IgG or IgM). When the first protein (C1) is activated it acts as an enzyme, splitting the second protein (C2) into two parts, one an effector and the other an enzyme which splits the third protein (C3) into two parts, an effector and an enzyme and so on down the cascade.

The ultimate objective is to enhance the immune reaction particularly by killing micro-organisms, by improving phagocytosis and mediating the inflammatory response.

IMMUNE REACTIONS

COMPLEMENT SYSTEM

The sequence of the reactions and the substances produced are as follows:

Activation —
classical pathway

Ag/Ab

Fc
(IgM or IgG)

Activation —
alternate pathway,

e.g. by endotoxin and
properdin (an activator
present in blood and
tissue fluids)

The cascade augments the activation
and effects of each step to achieve
a powerful result at step 9.

Chemotactic activity (polymorphs)

Anaphylatoxin activity — release of
vasoactive agents, e.g. histamine
(*Note:* this is not related to
anaphylactic shock)

Opsonic activity (improved
adherence and phagocytic activity)

**Bactericidal
effect**

Punched out holes in
target cell membrane

Cytolytic effect

Escape of
haemoglobin

Bacterium

RBC

B lymphocytes, polymorphonuclears, monocytes, macrophages and red cells have receptors for
complement and thus concentrate the released kinins at the reaction site.

Activation of C by Ag/Ab complex is called **fixation of complement**. Antibodies with this
property are termed **amboceptors**. Using red cells as markers, this fixation can detect the presence
of antigen or antibody in serum.

E.g.   Test serum + antigen +C.
       If serum contains antibody, C is fixed, otherwise it remains free.
       Add sensitised RBC (coated with Ab).
       Lysis of RBC ≡ complement still free ∴ no Ab in original serum.
       No lysis = C was fixed by Ab serum.

MONONUCLEAR PHAGOCYTE SYSTEM

The cells of this system have important roles in many disease processes and appear throughout the book. Although their main functions are essentially *non-specific*, they have important roles in the immune response, particularly in cooperation with T lymphocytes. Found at many sites throughout the body, they are derived from **STEM CELLS** in the bone marrow.

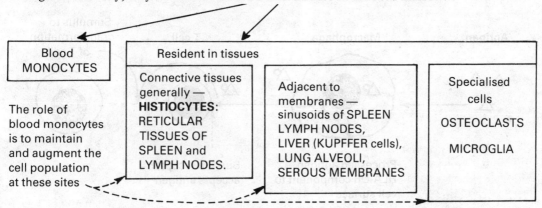

Historically, cells with varying degrees of phagocytic activity recognised at many of these sites were grouped into the **RETICULOENDOTHELIAL** system, but since reticulum cells are still ill-defined and endothelial cells have little phagocytic function the term is inappropriate and (although still used by some) is becoming obsolete.

Main functions

The System in Disease

Primary disorders of the system are extremely rare. Although participation in many disease processes is well recognised and detailed mechanisms are rapidly being elucidated, disturbances of the activities of these cells are as yet ill-defined.

CELL-MEDIATED IMMUNITY

The maximal specific T cell response is obtained when the antigen is 'processed' by macrophages and then presented to the T cell. The processing includes linkage of the foreign antigen with molecular components of the HLA-DR System.

The transformed blast cell undergoes progressive mitotic division and each cell of the resulting clone has the same specific immune potential.

The subsequent T cell activities tend to remain local at the site of the antigen concentration and this cell-mediated immunity (CMI) is delayed, i.e. at least 24 hours are required for a significant local concentration of sensitised T cells.

T cell functions and mechanisms

1. *Overall regulation of the immune response and reactions.* This is effected by **HELPER T cells** which promote, and **SUPPRESSOR T cells** which inhibit immune reactions. In the peripheral blood, 2/3 of the T lymphocytes are helper and 1/3 suppressor. Using monoclonal antibodies, helper cells carry the T_4 surface antigen and suppressor cells the T_8.

2. *Direct T cell effector immune reactions*
   (a) The secretion of locally acting mediators called **lymphokines.**
   (b) Direct cell-to-cell contact activity, e.g. **killer T cells.**

The diagrams on the following page indicate in summary the complex T cell activities.

T CELL ACTIVITIES

1. Influence on B cells

Transformed cell

T helper (T$_4$) cell → Promotes B cell activity → Plasma cell → Increased Ig production

T suppressor (T$_8$) cell → Inhibits B cell activity → Decreased Ig production

Balance controls humoral immune reaction to suit conditions in vivo

2. Lymphokines controlling cell proliferation

Transformed T cell → Secretion of

Growth inhibitory factor → Decrease in lymphocytes

T cell growth factor (Interleukin-2) → Increase in lymphocytes

Transfer factor → Unsensitised new lymphocytes transformed and capable of secreting lymphokines

Control exerted according to demands

3. Action on neutrophils and macrophages

Transformed cell

Chemotactic and phagocytic activation factors → Attracts cells to site or promotes phagocytosis

Migration inhibitory factors → Concentrates cells at site

4. Killer cells. There are at least two types of 'killer' cell: (a) a cell belonging to the T$_4$ (suppressor) group and (b) a so-called 'null' cell which does not have the usually recognised lymphocyte surface markers. Both these cell types 'kill' target cells during close cell to cell contact.

Practical tests for the detection of specific sensitised T lymphocytes in the blood are:

(a) **The lymphocyte transformation test:** During incubation with a specific antigen, the rate of transformation, as indicated by DNA synthesis or mitotic activity, is measured.

(b) **The macrophage migration inhibition test:** The migration of macrophages in the presence of specific antigen is measured and the amount of inhibition is an indicator of the specific T lymphocyte activity.

(c) **The Tuberculin test:** This is a good example of the use of T cell sensitising in diagnosis in clinical practice. In individuals who are or have been infected by mycobacterium tuberculi or BCG, sensitised T cells are present in the blood. Intradermal injection of a small quantity of tuberculoprotein results in an inflammatory reaction (papule) appearing after 24 hours and lasting for several days.

TOLERANCE

Humoral and cell-mediated immunity are specific responses with a protective function.

In certain circumstances an antigen does not evoke these specific responses. This is not a failure of immunologically competent lymphocytes but is a third type of specific activity — TOLERANCE.

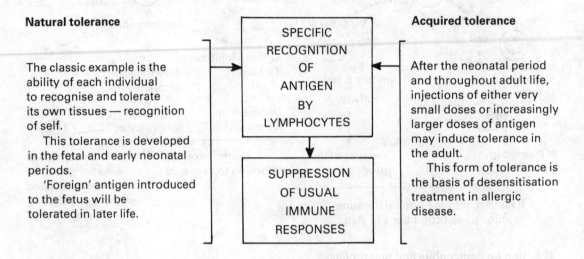

Natural tolerance

The classic example is the ability of each individual to recognise and tolerate its own tissues — recognition of self.

This tolerance is developed in the fetal and early neonatal periods.

'Foreign' antigen introduced to the fetus will be tolerated in later life.

SPECIFIC
RECOGNITION
OF
ANTIGEN
BY
LYMPHOCYTES

SUPPRESSION
OF USUAL
IMMUNE
RESPONSES

Acquired tolerance

After the neonatal period and throughout adult life, injections of either very small doses or increasingly larger doses of antigen may induce tolerance in the adult.

This form of tolerance is the basis of desensitisation treatment in allergic disease.

The mechanisms of inducing tolerance are not yet completely understood. There are three possibilities:

1. Burnet's 'forbidden clone theory' — in fetal life all lymphoid cells which could respond immunologically to 'self' antigens are eliminated.

2. In adults, acquired tolerance is associated primarily with specific SUPPRESSOR T cell activity which inhibits the response of both helper T cells and B cells.

3. Modification of antigen structure and the form of presentation to lymphoid cells — the effect may be blocking of the immune reaction.

Persisting tolerance is a function of T cells. B cell activity is of short term significance (e.g. infections) but where the antigen is persistent i.e. exists as a reservoir in the body or is repeatedly introduced, T cells are involved and long-lasting tolerance can be induced, e.g. a tissue graft with foreign cell clones.

Tolerance is an important protective mechanism. When it breaks down, the serious effects give rise to autoimmune disease.

IMMUNOPATHOLOGY

The complicated and delicately balanced immune mechanisms clearly have been developed to protect against antigens, particularly infections. When these immune reactions are upset, the protective mechanism can itself be a source of disease states.

There are three main categories: (1) hypersensitivity states, (2) immune deficiency states and (3) autoimmune diseases.

HYPERSENSITIVITY REACTIONS

Basically these consist of an exaggerated response by an individual to an antigen, following a previous exposure. The resulting Ag/Ab reaction induces the release of large quantities of chemicals, enzymes and cell stimulators. Depending on the main type of immune response concerned these are classified as follows:

(a) Those associated with
   HUMORAL ANTIBODIES
   ∴ immediate — types I, II, III

(b) Those associated with
   CELL-MEDIATED IMMUNITY
   ∴ delayed (24 – 72 hours) — type IV.

As previously stated this classification is to some extent artificial. Hypersensitivity may start as an immediate humoral reaction but end in a mixed state with both humoral and cell-mediated activities.

Type 1 Anaphylaxis, atopy, allergy

All three terms have been used for this reaction. The basic mechanism is as follows:

First exposure to Ag → Formation of IgE → Fixation of IgE to mast cells and basophils by Fc fragment

Second exposure to Ag → Ag/Ab reaction on surface of mast cell → Degranulation of mast cell → Release of mediators and vasoactive substances

Antigens and 'allergens'

While the most potent antigens are usually very large molecules with molecular weights from 15 to 40,000, they are, however, associated with other substances which may be inactive. Examples of common 'allergens' are: anti-tetanic serum, penicillin, bee venom, pollen, house mite dust, food, drugs, etc.

Antibody

This is IgE. Plasma cells forming IgE are found extensively in the internal secretory surfaces of the body — tonsils, adenoids, bronchi, gastrointestinal tract and urinary bladder.

HYPERSENSITIVITY STATES

Mast cells

These have a wide distribution but are prominent in the same areas as the IgE-producing plasma cells, plus skin, uterus and synovial membranes. This explains the frequently used term 'target organs' when discussing hypersensitivity.

Clinical examples of Type I reaction

ANAPHYLACTIC SHOCK

1st injection of e.g. horse serum (e.g. antitetanic serum, ATS) penicillin or a bee sting → General sensitisation

– – – – – – – – – –

2nd injection of above → Acute collapse: bronchial constriction; vomiting; diarrhoea; perhaps a skin rash. May be fatal. Note that the antigens are injected — enter blood stream → basophils affected → widespread reaction

HAY FEVER

1st contact with grass pollen → Local sensitisation of conjunctiva and nasal passages

– – – – – – – – –

2nd contact with above → Irritation or swelling of conjunctiva with excessive watery secretion

ASTHMA

1st contact with house mite dust or animal dander → Local sensitisation of bronchi

– – – – – – – – –

2nd contact with above → Bronchial constriction and secretion of thick mucus cause dyspnoea (difficult breathing)

Chronic asthma may involve cell-mediated immunity with tissue destruction.

Allergic conditions are often familial with a genetic basis. If both parents are allergic = 75% chance of allergic offspring; one parent = 50%.

Type II – Cytotoxic type

The antigen is on the cell surface

Specific antibody combination produces

Complement activation

Increased phagocytic activity (opsonic effect)

Increased "killer" cell activity

DESTRUCTION OF CELL

This cytotoxic reaction causes some forms of haemolytic anaemia and some blood transfusion reactions.

In some auto-immune disorders antibodies of this type are directed against specialised cell surface receptors, e.g. Graves disease or myasthenia gravis (see p. 117).

HYPERSENSITIVITY STATES

Type III – Immune complex (Arthus) type

The reaction is due to the consequences of specific direct antigen/antibody combination — particularly complement activation (p. 104) and platelet aggregation. The antibodies involved are commonly IgG or IgM.

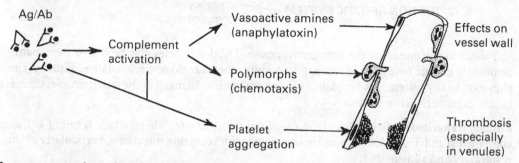

In most cases where there is Ag/Ab reaction, hypersensitivity does not develop. Where it does so, the Ag/Ab complexes tend to aggregate in small vessels and, with complement, cause tissue destruction, e.g. renal glomeruli. Serum sickness is acute short term disease of this type.

Type IV – Cell-mediated (delayed) type

This reaction is usually local and is due to the activities of specifically sensitised T cells.

The classical example of this type of reaction is the tubercle follicle; it is concerned also in other granulomatous disease processes, the rashes of virus infections and the rejection of grafts.

The skin reaction to chemicals — **contact dermatitis** — is illustrative. This condition is now common due to the increasing use of chemicals in industry and for topical application. The chemical — often of a simple nature, e.g. nickel — acts as a hapten, evoking an immune response.

Chemical + tissue protein = 'foreign' antigen → cell-mediated immunity → inflammation

Another interesting common illustration of this type of reaction is the recurrent activity at the site of an insect bite often for several days after — possibly explained by the intermittent arrival of sensitised lymphocytes.

111

IMMUNE DEFICIENCY STATES

The systems involved are:

(1) **THE SPECIFIC SYSTEM** — humoral
cell-mediated

(2) **THE NON-SPECIFIC SYSTEM** — phagocytes
complement

Failure in any one alters the immune response. The deficiencies may be of a primary nature, commonly genetic in origin, or secondary to some other disease or circumstance. Equally, the alteration in any system may be quantitative or qualitative. In many of these deficiencies there is a failure in more than one system.

Primary (inherited) deficiencies of the specific system are rare. They include B cell, T cell and combined B and T cell deficits and are associated with recurring infections, particularly of the respiratory and alimentary tracts.

Secondary deficiencies of the specific system are common. Usually T cell activity is affected, resulting in deficient cell-mediated immunity and, later, B cell deficit occurs.

Currently the acquired immune deficiency syndrome (AIDS) is causing great concern. However more common predisposing conditions and diseases are:

Malnutrition —
particularly with protein deficiency

Iatrogenic effects —
e.g. immunosuppressors: cytotoxics
corticosteroids

Infections —
acute viral
chronic bacterial
chronic protozoal, e.g. malaria

Chronic debilitating disease —
e.g. renal failure: diabetes mellitus

Malignant disease —
e.g. advanced cancer: lymphoma
Hodgkin's disease

IMPAIRED
IMMUNITY → INFECTION
often
OPPORTUNISTIC
(see p.71)

Deficiencies of the non-specific system are rare. The disorders of neutrophil function are described on page 550.

IMMUNE DEFICIENCY STATES — AIDS

The Acquired Immune Deficiency Syndrome (AIDS) is now distributed worldwide, but has assumed epidemic status in some parts of the world — particularly CENTRAL AFRICA and HOMOSEXUAL COMMUNITIES of some cities in the U.S.A.

It is due to infection by a lentiretrovirus — human immunodeficiency virus (HIV).

The disease is slowly progressive and is often fatal.

Infection
No initial symptoms

Latent and prodromal stages
(months up to several years)
Virus present in lymphocytes
– may be no signs
– may be persistent lymph node enlargement

Stages of opportunistic infection and tumours (1 – 2 years)

Infection ⟨ opportunistic / others

Malignant tumours ⟨ Kaposi's sarcoma / lymphomas

The whole range of opportunistic infection (see p.71), including disseminated virus infection (e.g. herpes simplex and cytomegalovirus), occurs.

The diagram show the more common AIDS-associated diseases and sites:

Brain
Tumours
Inflammation

Mouth, Trachea, Oesophagus
Candidiasis

Lungs
Pneumocystis carinii infection
Fungal infections, Tuberculosis

Intestines
Protozoal, Salmonella infections

Skin
Kaposi's sarcoma, Fungal infections, Herpes zoster

Blood changes

Antibodies — after infection, up to 6 months may elapse before anti-HIV antibodies appear; in the later stages the titre may drop greatly.

Immunoglobulins may be elevated in the early stages.

T4 (helper) lymphocytes are severely reduced, producing a lymphopaenia. T4/T8 ratio reversed.

IMMUNE DEFICIENCY STATES — AIDS

EPIDEMIOLOGY AND TRANSMISSION

Although the virus may be present in many body fluids and secretions, transmission is by the parenteral route, usually by (1) **sexual contact** or (2) **injection of blood** or **blood products.**

Transmission does not occur with normal social contact and there is no risk to medical or nursing personnel using normal procedures.

1. *Sexual transmission*

(a) MALE HOMOSEXUAL PRACTICE: HIV in seminal fluid → via anorectal abrasion to passive partner.

(b) HETEROSEXUAL TRANSMISSION is less common except where there is a high prevalence in prostitutes.

    Female to male — infectious genital secretions and blood → via penis to male (risk increased in uncircumcised).

    Male to female — infectious seminal fluid and blood → to female cervix uteri.

In both sexes the risks are very considerably increased where there is genital ulceration or abrasion.

2. *Transmission by blood*

- The risk from blood transfusion and blood products has now been virtually eliminated by screening and sterilization procedures.
- The communal use of contaminated syringes and needles continues to be important among drug addicts.

Cellular mechanisms

(1) HIV binds to specific receptor

(2) HIV into cell

(3) Using reverse transcriptase —
virus RNA ⟶ virus DNA

(4) Into cell nucleus

T$_4$ HELPER CELL

Results in

Cell death, *i.e.* loss of T$_4$ cells

or

Cell survives but genetic material altered

Abnormal T$_4$ cell function

T$_4$ cell deficiency

During latent phase B cells may be stimulated, allowing antibody formation and lymph node enlargement.

Gradual failure of immune effector mechanisms.

AUTOIMMUNE DISEASES

Autoimmune diseases result from, or are associated with, an immune response against the individual's own cells, or in some cases cell products. The phrase 'associated with' is used advisedly since the autoimmune response is often a phase or feature, generally of late onset, in an ongoing disease state and is not a primary cause. It involves changes in humoral, cell-mediated immunity and in tolerance.

Aetiology

The aetiology of autoimmune diseases is not established, but clues to their genesis are available.

| An increased FAMILIAL incidence of autoimmune diseases in general and of particular individual diseases | The overlapping of the incidence of antibodies and of the types of damage produced | An increased incidence of malignant tumours among affected individuals |

Suggest
an INBORN INSTABILITY OF IMMUNE TOLERANCE

The changes in the immune mechanism involve four factors, of which the two most important are (1) alteration of the cell antigenic structure and (2) deficient suppressor T cell activity.

(1) Altered cell antigens
(ACAg)

(2) T SUPRESSORS –
T helpers +

(3) B cell proliferation

Auto-antibodies produced

(4) Primed T cells
(K cells)

ACAg/Ab + complement

CELL DESTRUCTION

AUTOIMMUNE DISEASES

The absence of T cell suppressor controls remains unexplained. In some autoimmune reactions, such as systemic lupus erythematosus, antibodies to lymphocytes are formed. These may eliminate the suppressor cells or block the signals between the various components of the immune reaction so that the suppressor cells remain unstimulated.

Examples of autoimmune conditions are:

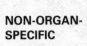

	Antibody to	Target Organ	Associated Diseases
ORGAN-SPECIFIC	(a) Thyroid cells and hormones, or (b) TSH receptor	Thyroid	Hashimoto's disease (auto-immune thyroiditis) Thyrotoxicosis (Graves' disease)
	Parietal cells	Stomach	Pernicious anaemia
	Red blood cells	Red blood cells	Haemolytic anaemia
	Pancreatic islet cells	Pancreas	Type 1 diabetes
	Adrenal cortical cells	Adrenal	Addison's disease
	Parathyroid cells	Parathyroid	Primary hypoparathyroidism
	Acetylcholine receptor	Voluntary muscle	Myasthenia gravis

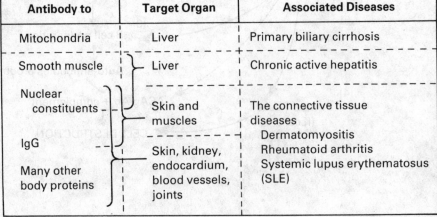

	Antibody to	Target Organ	Associated Diseases
NON-ORGAN-SPECIFIC	Mitochondria	Liver	Primary biliary cirrhosis
	Smooth muscle	Liver	Chronic active hepatitis
	Nuclear constituents	Skin and muscles	The connective tissue diseases Dermatomyositis
	IgG	Skin, kidney, endocardium, blood vessels, joints	Rheumatoid arthritis Systemic lupus erythematosus (SLE)
	Many other body proteins		

AUTOIMMUNE DISEASES

Primary thyrotoxicosis (Graves' disease) and myasthenia gravis are of particular interest. The activity of the auto-antibodies is a modification of the Type II reaction in that the specific antibody combines with antigen on the cell surface and either stimulates or blocks the action of the physiological agent which would normally turn on the activity of the cell.

Stimulatory effect

In Graves' disease, excessive amounts of thyroid hormone are produced. LATS (long acting thyroid stimulator), an IgG auto-antibody, combines with antigen on the thyroid cell surface and produces changes mimicking those produced by TSH (thyroid stimulating hormone) — (physiologically manufactured by the pituitary).

Normal production of thyroid hormone
TSH from pituitary
Receptor site on thyroid cell surface
Message to nucleus activates cell — thyroid hormone produced

GRAVES' DISEASE
LATS (IgG antibody)
Antigen
Receptor site activated by Ag/Ab combination

See also page 832

Blocking effect

In myasthenia gravis, the acetylcholine formed at the motor nerve endings is prevented from stimulating the muscle motor end plate due to the antibody blocking the specific acetylcholine receptors.

Normal
Motor end plate
Nerve ending
Acetylcholine
Receptor site
Muscle Contraction

MYASTHENIA GRAVIS
Blocking antibody
Muscle contraction diminished

See also page 784

APPLIED IMMUNOLOGY

Immunohistochemical identification

Immunohistochemical techniques are developing rapidly. They allow the clear identification of specific substances in histological sections.

Example:

Microscopic result

(1) Rabbit serum containing antibody to IgG

→ adherance to any IgG in tissue

Histological slide containing plasma cell infiltrate.

(2) Rabbit protein identified by a peroxidase/benzidine reaction (brown colour)

Only plasma cells containing IgG are coloured brown.

This or similar techniques may be used to identify a wide range of substances.

Prophylaxis and treatment of infections

1. **Passive immunisation** is the term used when antibody formed in one individual is given to another individual who is at risk of infection — the protection is temporary. Examples include:
   - Pooled human γ-globulin → general protection — particularly useful in cases of immune deficiency.
   - Horse serum containing antibodies to **tetanus** or **diphtheria** → specific protection. *NB* the foreign horse protein may itself cause immunological reactions, e.g. serum sickness or anaphylactic shock.

2. **Active immunisation** is the term used when the infective agent is modified in some way to eliminate its harmful effects without loss of antigenicity. The subject's own immune response is activated. Examples include:

   TOXOID — e.g. tetanus toxin modified chemically
   KILLED ORGANISMS — e.g. TAB (typhoid, paratyphoid A and B) vaccine
   ATTENUATED ORGANISMS — e.g. viruses; cowpox, polio, measles.

Diagnosis of disease

Diagnosis is confirmed by the detection in serum of specific antibodies using known antigens. The immune reactions, such as agglutination and specific complement fixation, are indicators.

Infections and autoimmune disease are investigated by these means. The specificity of such tests has been greatly improved by the use of **monoclonal antibodies.**

CHAPTER 6

CIRCULATORY DISTURBANCES

THROMBOSIS

A thrombus is a mass formed from the blood constituents within a vessel or the heart during life.

MECHANISM OF FORMATION

The liberation of **thromboplastin** initiates a "chemical cascade" leading to coagulation.

Platelets adhere to the endothelium and to each other, forming a projecting mass.

(1)

Release of thromboplastins

↓

Thrombin formation
+
Fibrinogen

↓

Fibrin strands

p. 560
Coagulation pathway

If the rate of flow is slow, as in a vein, red cells are entangled so that the lumen is occluded.

(2)

Platelet mass

In front of and behind the platelet mass, the blood stagnates. Further formation of fibrin takes place, resulting in a large solid coagulum. The thrombus extends in either direction to the nearest junction. At this point more platelets are deposited on the end of the mass. This gives the head of the thrombus a pale tip.

With a slow flow in the joining vessel more fibrin is formed by the platelets at the tip of the thrombus, thus occluding the joining vessel.

(4)

Blood stagnates in the joining vessel and thrombosis extends forward to the next joining vessel. There may be a succession of thrombotic episodes — a propagating thrombus.

(3)

FACTORS LEADING TO THROMBOSIS

There are THREE factors leading to thrombosis

1. ALTERATIONS OF BLOOD FLOW

The main effect is to bring platelets into contact with the vessel wall. This results from:
Slowing of blood flow, e.g. in cardiac failure or during bed rest. With slowing, the normal axial stream of blood cells is lost and white cells and platelets fall out of the main stream and accumulate in the peripheral plasma zone.

Clear plasma zone

White cells and platelets

Axial stream of cells

Red cells

Turbulence, e.g. by deformation of vessel wall or around venous valves.

Local increase in lumen, as in varicose veins or aneurysm, causes eddies and platelets and white cells fall out of main stream.

Swelling or compression of vessel wall by disease. Eddies form in front and behind obstruction.

Eddies form around valves if flow slows.

121

FACTORS LEADING TO THROMBOSIS

2. DAMAGE TO ENDOTHELIUM OF VESSEL

This leads to platelet adhesion. Common causes are:
(a) Disease in vessel wall e.g. atheroma

Atheromatous degeneration
interferes with nutrition of
vessel wall

(b) Toxins from nearby inflammatory processes
(c) Local compression of vessels (e.g. during operation).

3. CHANGES IN THE COMPOSITION OF THE BLOOD

(a) **Increase in platelets, fibrinogen and prothrombin,** e.g. after operations and childbirth.

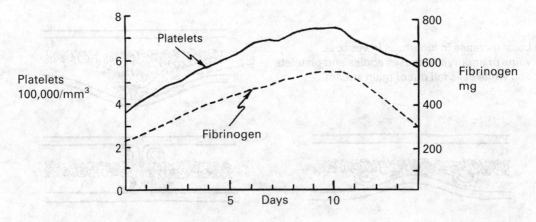

(b) **Change in platelet adhesiveness** — This increases after operations and childbirth and is most marked around the 10th day, at the same time as the other changes reach a peak.

VARIETIES OF THROMBOSIS

The following types are recognised:

WHITE
Composed mainly of platelets, they occur chiefly where the circulation is rapid, e.g. in arteries. They tend to be non-occlusive (mural).

RED
In this case the thrombus, starting as a small aggregate of platelets, produces fibrin strands entangling the blood cells.

MIXED OR LAMINATED
This type of thrombus consists of alternate layers of red and white thrombi. Commonly found in aneurysms.

Red thrombi are the commonest type and have to be distinguished from postmortem clots. The former are dry, granular, firm but friable. They are usually adherent to the vessel wall at their point of origin and a network of fine white lines of fibrin (striae of Zahn) can be seen on the surface. Postmortem clots are shiny in appearance and jelly-like in consistency.

Pulmonary trunk

AGONAL
These are formed in the last minutes of life when death occurs slowly. They are composed mainly of yellowish fibrin. Commonly found attached to the apex of the right ventricle, they form a stringy mass extending into the pulmonary arteries.

COMMON SITES OF THROMBOSIS

CARDIAC

Antemortem thrombi may be formed
in the auricles, ventricles or on the heart
valves. The auricular appendage may be
filled with red thrombus, or small pale
globular thrombi (cardiac polypi) may form
between the muscular columnae.

Similar red and pale thrombi
occur in ventricles, especially
the left. Red thrombi are frequently
secondary to infarction
of the ventricular wall.

Thrombi of pale variety occur
on the heart valves frequently due
to one type of endocarditis.

Sometimes bacterial endocarditis
occurs and the thrombi are
larger, mixed, friable and contain
bacterial masses.

COMMON SITES OF THROMBOSIS

ARTERIAL

Thrombi are common in the aorta due to disease, e.g. atheroma or arteriosclerosis. Due to high pressure and rapid flow, they are of platelet variety. An exception is the laminated thrombus in aneurysms.

In smaller arteries they may be of the more mixed type, for example:

Coronary arteries

Middle cerebral arteries

Small arteries of limbs and digits

VENOUS

Systemic vein thrombosis is common because of the slower flow, lower pressure with easy compressibility and eddy formation around valves.

They usually start in the deep veins of the calf. Frequently a propagating thrombus, it may extend along the femoral vein into the iliac vessels.

Abdominal operations, childbirth, cardiac disease, varicose veins and inflammation are potentiating conditions.

Portal thrombosis is rare and may follow disease in abdominal organs. It has special effects due to the anatomy of the region (see p.139).

CAPILLARY

Thrombi, composed mainly of fused red cells, form when capillaries are damaged, usually in acute inflammatory processes.

Capillaries are occluded by fibrin thrombi in cases of disseminated intravascular coagulation DIC — see p.565).

FIBRINOLYSIS

Clotting of blood naturally occurs in vessels, even after trivial injury. To control this process, another mechanism — the fibrinolytic system — exists which limits clot deposition by lysing fibrin.

Normally these two mechanisms are activated at the same time and are in dynamic equilibrium. The lytic activity modifies the coagulation process, preventing excessive or continued clotting.

In trivial injury the two processes are activated and together they limit the results of injury and take part in the restoration of the tissues to normal. With very large thrombi, fibrinolysis limits the extension of the thrombotic process and aids the removal of the thrombus during the period of organisation.

Fibrinolysis is also activated during repair of wounds, helping to remove the fibrin scaffold when no longer required. A similar activity is seen during the removal of inflammatory fibrin exudates.

PROSTAGLANDINS AND BLOOD COAGULATION

Prostaglandins, substances first discovered in semen, act particularly on smooth muscle but also influence blood platelets and blood clotting. Most prostaglandins cause blood platelets to clump and adhere to blood vessel walls, initiating thrombosis. One prostaglandin (prostacyclin) has an opposite effect, preventing platelet adhesion.

HORMONES AND THROMBOSIS

Artificial oestrogens, such as those used in contraceptive pills, induce deficiencies in the fibrinolytic system, especially the content of fibrinolytic activator in vessel walls. As a result, thrombosis may occur, particularly in veins.

SEQUELS OF THROMBOSIS

ORGANISATION

Capillaries grow into the point of thrombus attachment within a day or two. Fibroblasts and phagocytic cells accompany the capillaries, and gradually the thrombus material is dissolved and replaced by a fibrovascular tissue. At the same time endothelium covers the ends of the thrombus, thus limiting the thrombotic process.

— Endothelium

Capillaries

Ultimately, the branching capillaries may be converted into one or two stouter vessels which may partially restore the circulation through the vessel — 'recanalisation'.

CALCIFICATION

In diseased vessels, organisation may not take place. The thrombus shrinks, calcium salts are deposited and convert it into a phlebolith.

INCORPORATION

A mural thrombus, e.g. in a large artery, may be covered by endothelium and incorporated in the vessel wall. This process may be important in the formation of atheroma.

EMBOLISM

Part of the thrombus may be detached and carried along in the blood stream to impact in a distant vessel.

EMBOLISM

An embolus is any abnormal mass of matter carried in the blood stream and large enough to occlude some vessel. Emboli may be:

1. Generated within the vascular system, e.g. fragments of thrombus, or material from atheromatous plaques. Thromboembolism is the commonest.

2. Matter entering the vessels:
   (a) Solid e.g. tumour cells, bacterial clumps, parasites, foreign bodies
   (b) Gaseous — air
   (c) Liquid — amniotic fluid, fat.

Source and destination of emboli

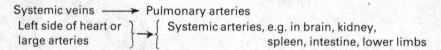

Systemic veins ⟶ Pulmonary arteries
Left side of heart or } ⟶ { Systemic arteries, e.g. in brain, kidney,
large arteries   spleen, intestine, lower limbs

Gaseous and fluid emboli, being malleable, may traverse the lung and appear in the systemic arterial circulation causing occlusion at various sites.

Gas embolism occurs mainly in two forms:

1. *Single embolism.* Atmospheric air may enter the blood when a neck or intracranial vein is incised. Inspiration induces a suction effect by causing a negative pressure in the veins. As a result of frothing in the right ventricle cardiac action is seriously impaired.

2. *Multiple 'embolism'*, in 'Caisson disease'. This occurs in persons working in barometric pressures of several atmospheres, e.g. diving to great depths. The atmospheric gases go into solution in high concentration in the blood and tissues. If decompression occurs too quickly these gases 'boil' off and appear as bubbles in the circulation. The oxygen is taken up by the tissues but insoluble gases cause widespread 'embolism', especially in the nervous system.

Fluid embolism

1. *Fat embolism.* This may occur when a long bone is fractured. Fat globules enter the veins of the bones and pass to the lungs, obstruct the pulmonary blood flow and cause anoxaemia. Cerebral symptoms are common due to this and also to the actual arrival of fat particles which have passed through the lungs.

2. *Amniotic fluid embolism.* During parturition, amniotic fluid may enter a uterine vein, especially after manipulations or with certain obstetric treatments. Vernix, hairs and squames enter the circulation. In addition to embolic phenomena, there are also coagulation disorders.

RESULTS OF ARTERIAL OBSTRUCTION

Results of vascular obstruction vary with type of vessel and anatomy of the part.

1. ARTERIES WITH GOOD COLLATERAL ANASTOMOSIS

Three phases can be recognised.

(1) Obstruction

Disappearance of distal pulse → ← Reflex contraction of other vessels in area

→ Fall in blood pressure in area

→ Tissue pale and cold

(2) Dilatation of collateral vessels

↓ Blood fills vessels distal to obstruction

↓ Pulse reappears

↓ Tissues return to normal

(3) Permanent Dilatation

↓ Increased pressure in collateral vessels

↓ Hypertrophy of muscle and elastic tissue in vessel wall

The obstruction in the artery organises and the vessel is filled by vascular fibrous tissue. Very occasionally it may effectively recanalise.

RESULTS OF ARTERIAL OBSTRUCTION

2. END ARTERIES

These may have:

(a) No collateral anastomosis e.g. splenic artery;
or (b) Capillary anastomosis, e.g. renal arteries, coronary arteries;
or (c) Arterial anastomosis, but too small to maintain circulation, e.g. superior mesenteric artery.

Result: Obstruction of end artery
                  ↓
                Dilatation of collateral vessels
                  ↓
                Stagnation of blood
                  ↓
                Anoxia of tissues
                  ↓
                Congested necrotic area = INFARCTION (Latin, *infarctire* — to stuff in)

Infarction

An infarct is an area of necrosis due to ischaemia usually found at the periphery of an organ.

After 12 hours: Area is pale. Degenerative changes already seen with electron microscope or histochemical tests.

By 24 hours: Collateral vessels have dilated. Blood fills area, stagnates and causes red swelling.

At 36 hours: Area shows coagulative necrosis. In solid organs, infarct may become increased number of small molecules → increasased number of small molecules → rise in osmotic pressure → cells swell → blood pressed out of area.

At 72 hours: Stagnant blood breaks down. Polymorphs and macrophages appear at periphery and break down dead tissue.

Healing

This takes place slowly. Capillaries and fibroblasts replace the necrotic tissue. Collagen is formed, contracts and results in a depressed scar.

IMPORTANT SITES OF INFARCTION

HEART

Infarction is almost always due to thrombosis.

Diseased coronary arteries
↓
Thrombosis
↓
Infarction of ventricle

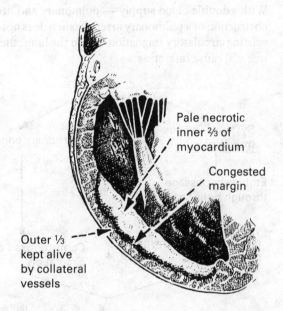

Pale necrotic inner 2/3 of myocardium

Congested margin

Outer 1/3 kept alive by collateral vessels

Cardiac action is immediately upset, eddies form, the endocardium is damaged and a thrombus may form on the inner surface of the infarcted area.

If the patients survives, the infarct heals by fibrosis.

BRAIN

Infarcts are commonly due to thrombosis of diseased vessels, e.g. MIDDLE CEREBRAL, posterior cerebral and basilar arteries.

The usual changes of infarction take place, but the necrosis is colliquative — cerebral softening.

Embolism is less common and may cause infarcts in almost any part of the brain.

Infarction may occur without arterial occlusion in severe, prolonged hypotension (shock).
Parts of the brain at the junction of arterial territories are affected (boundary zone or watershed infarcts).

Middle cerebral infarct

IMPORTANT SITES OF INFARCTION

LUNG

With a double blood supply — pulmonary and bronchial arteries — and a vast anastomosis, obstruction of a pulmonary artery branch does not necessarily cause infarction. When there is pre-existing circulatory stagnation within the lung, the arrival of an embolus in the pulmonary arterial tree will cause infarction.

Cardiac failure

Systemic venous thrombosis

Pulmonary congestion

Embolism passage through right heart

PULMONARY ARTERIAL EMBOLISM   +   Compromised collateral circulation

INFARCT of
LUNG
(red, conical and subpleural)

Occlusion

KIDNEY

Usually a complication of thrombus formation in the left side of the heart, e.g. associated with:

Auricular fibrillation or Bacterial endocarditis

Occasional bland embolus

Multiple emboli

Renal infarct

Numerous haemorrhages

Haematuria

IMPORTANT SITES OF INFARCTION

INTESTINE

Infarctions, which are relatively uncommon, are usually smaller than expected due to arterial anastomosis, and embolism is the usual cause. The sequence of changes seen in solid organs is altered in the terminal stages.

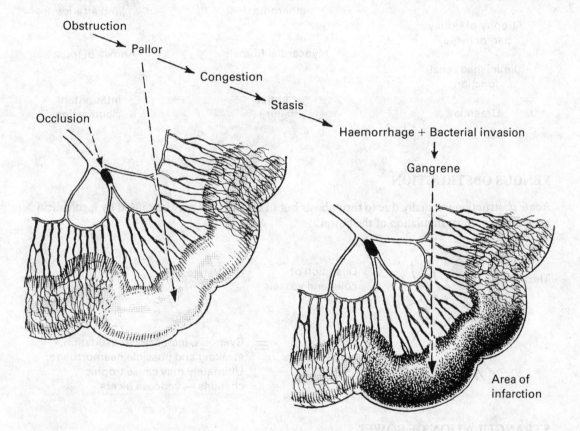

SPLEEN

Infarcts are common in arterial embolic conditions. Being true end arteries without collateral anastomosis, obstruction of splenic artery branches results in pale red infarcts becoming yellow as the stagnant blood breaks down.

PARTIAL OR SLOW ARTERIAL OCCLUSION/VENOUS OBSTRUCTION

This is common in old age and in chronic systemic arterial disease such as atheroma. Parenchymal cells atrophy and are replaced by fibrous tissue. Serious functional disturbance may result.

Renal artery narrowing
↓
Atrophy of kidney parenchyma
↓
Diminished renal function
↓
Uraemia

Coronary artery atheroma
↓
Myocardial fibrosis
↓
Cardiac failure

Narrowing of lower limb arteries
↓
Anoxia of muscles
↓
Intermittent claudication

VENOUS OBSTRUCTION

Acute obstruction is usually due to thrombosis but in certain sites may be caused by mechanical pressure, e.g. in strangulation of the bowel.

Thrombosis

Dilatation of collateral vessels ≡ Varicosities

Dilatation of small venules ≡ Cyanosis, increased transudation, swelling and possible haemorrhage. Ultimately may cause trophic changes → varicose ulcers

STRANGULATION OF BOWEL

This may follow hernia, volvulus or intussusception. The sequence of events is as follows:

Mechanical obstruction of veins
↓
Congestion and oedema
↓
Further obstruction by swelling of tissues → Arterial flow obstruction
↓
Necrosis of tissue + Bacteria
↓
Gangrene

CHRONIC VENOUS CONGESTION

General venous congestion is a condition where *all* the veins of the body are distended with blood. It is associated with disease of the heart or lungs since all the circulating blood must pass through them.

Chronic cardiac failure or lung disease which reduces the pulmonary vascular bed, e.g. fibrosis or emphysema, are the usual causes.

The basic mechanism is:

The ultimate cause is right heart failure, but progressive reduction in left ventricular output is probably the initiating factor. The sequence of events in cardiac failure is as follows:

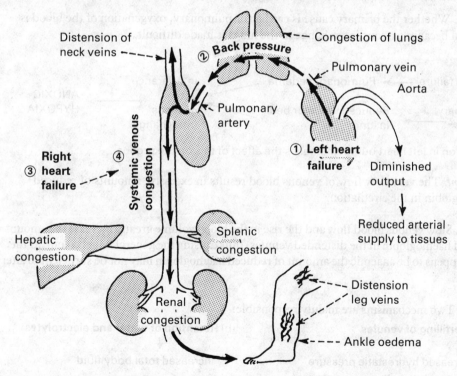

Where pulmonary disease is the primary cause, passive congestion of the lungs does not occur.

CHRONIC VENOUS CONGESTION

GENERAL EFFECTS

1. **Increased blood volume.** This is probably related to the reduced output of blood from the left ventricle. Two mechanisms may be involved:

(a) **Diminished arterial filling**
↓
Reduced renal blood supply
↓
Fall in glomerular filtrate

(b) **Diminished arterial filling**
↓
Stimulation of adrenal crotex
↓
Aldosterone secretion

Retention of sodium and water

The increasing volume is accommodated on the venous side of the circulation.

2. **Hypoxia.** There are two types: anoxic and stagnant.

   (a) *Anoxic.* Whether the primary cause is cardiac or pulmonary, oxygenation of the blood is reduced because gaseous interchange in the lungs is made difficult.

Cardiac failure ⟶ Pulmonary oedema
or
Pulmonary   Reduced vascular bed
disease ⟶   in lungs

Interference
with   ⟶   ANOXIC
gaseous   HYPOXIA
interchange

Reduction in left heart output increases the effect of this on the organs.

   (b) *Stagnant.* The very slow flow of venous blood results in excessive amounts of reduced haemoglobin in the circulation.

3. **Cyanosis.** Slow venous blood flow and the rise in the blood volume greatly increase the amount of reduced haemoglobin in the distended venules, thus causing the general 'blue' colour. If the patient happens to be anaemic the amount of reduced haemoglobin may not be sufficient to alter coloration.

4. **Oedema.** Two mechanisms are mainly responsible:

   (a) **Overfilling of venules**
↓
Increased hydrostatic pressure

   (b) **Retention of water and electrolytes**
↓
Increased total body fluid

Oedema of dependent parts
where pressure is greatest

CHRONIC VENOUS CONGESTION

PATHOLOGICAL CHANGES IN ORGANS

Because of the increase in venous blood, the organs become swollen and purplish. With long continued over-distension, the walls of the venules show reactive thickening and there is mild interstitial fibrosis of the organs, giving them a very firm consistency. These changes are seen typically in the kidney and spleen.

Important additional changes are found in the lungs and liver.

LUNGS

The lungs are bulky, congested and brownish in colour.

At post mortem, application of potassium ferrocyanide and hydrochloric acid to the lung results in a blue colour (Prussian blue reaction) indicating the presence of free iron.

CHRONIC VENOUS CONGESTION

PATHOLOGICAL CHANGES IN ORGANS (continued)

LIVER

Mechanical distension of the veins causes considerable enlargement of the liver so that it can be felt below the costal margin.

The parenchymal cells furthest from the arterial blood supply, i.e. around the hepatic venules (centrilobular), undergo degeneration with atrophy and ultimately disappear. Cells nearer the arteries show an accumulation of fat.

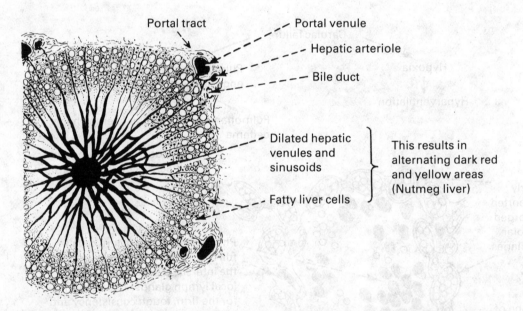

Portal tract

Portal venule

Hepatic arteriole

Bile duct

Dilated hepatic venules and sinusoids

Fatty liver cells

This results in alternating dark red and yellow areas (Nutmeg liver)

Much of the liver parenchyma may be destroyed. If the patient has periods of remission, the remaining liver cells may undergo compensatory hyperplasia. This results in small, irregular, pale nodules alternating with areas of fibrosis — so-called cardiac cirrhosis. It is not a true cirrhosis and does not cause hepatic failure.

PORTAL VENOUS CONGESTION

PORTAL VENOUS CONGESTION

This is the result of vascular
obstruction in the liver since the whole of the portal
circulation must pass through that organ. The
usual cause is hepatic cirrhosis.

Cirrhosis of liver

Obstruction of
venous blood
flow within
the liver

Congestion affects the spleen, the
gastrointestinal tract and the peritoneum. One of
the main results is ascites — accumulation of fluid
in the peritoneal cavity.

Spleen enlarged,
firm and
congested

Ascites

Fluid ---

Venous congestion
of intestines

Certain collateral anastomotic connections do exist, and these dilate and become varicose.
These include haemorrhoidal veins around the rectum and veins at the lower end of the
oesophagus. Haemorrhage may occur from these sites.

Less important are vessels around the umbilicus and over the anterior abdominal wall.

Dialated veins
at lower end
of oesophagus

Dilated vessels
around umbilicus
(caput medusae)

Dilated
haemorrhoids

BODY WATER CONTROL

NORMAL TISSUE FLUID CIRCULATION

There is a continuous interchange of fluid between blood and tissues. Some fluid enters the lymphatics before eventually returning to the blood stream.

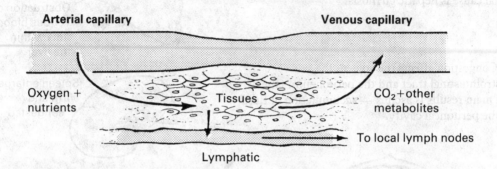

In order to maintain this normal circulation two main forces operate a pressure gradient which controls the rate and direction of fluid movement.

1. **Hydrostatic pressure**, i.e. capillary blood pressure (BP) encouraging the passage of fluid through the capillary wall, = 35 mm mercury.
2. **Protein osmotic pressure**, (OP), i.e. the plasma proteins encourage the retention of fluid in the capillaries to try and maintain osmotic equilibrium. This pressure is equivalent to 25 mm mercury.

At the arterial end the blood pressure is greater than the osmotic pressure and fluid is forced out of the capillary. The reverse is true at the venous end and fluid is attracted into the vessel.

Some fluid enters lymphatics. This may be partly the result of tissue pressure and partly due to osmotic attraction of proteins in the lymphatic system.

BODY WATER CONTROL: OEDEMA

In addition to those forces operating at capillary level, there are other mechanisms which influence the movement of fluid within the body in a general manner.

1. **Fluid intake**

   Intake via the gut or parenterally may exceed the ability of the kidneys to eliminate water.

2. **Integrity of the kidneys**

   Damage to the renal parenchyma may diminish the elimination of fluid.

3. **Hormone activity**

Aldosterone

Increases reabsorption of sodium by distal tubule ∴ retention of water

Cardiac hormone (from atria) antagonises aldosterone when there is any tendency to an increase in intracardiac pressure, e.g. in hypervolaemia. The hormone prevents reabsorption of sodium and therefore increases water excretion.

Increases reabsorption of water by distal and collecting tubules

Antidiuretic hormone

OEDEMA

This is an accumulation of excess fluid in the extravascular tissues. Conditions which interfere with the pressure gradients system result in oedema:

1. Rise in capillary hydrostatic pressure, especially at the venous end of the capillary.
2. Fall in blood osmotic pressure.
3. Rise in tissue osmotic pressure.

   Transudate formed (low protein content)

4. Alteration in capillary permeability operates especially in inflammation.

   Exudate formed (high protein content)

LOCAL OEDEMA

Oedema can occur in a very localised form for a variety of reasons. The mechanism is mainly an alteration in the pressure gradient system at capillary level and does not involve general bodily changes. Oedema fluid forming locally usually is associated only with local effects. However oedema of the lungs and brain can be life threatening and are of great importance. They are dealt with separately under 'Cerebral' oedema and 'Pulmonary' oedema.

LOCAL OEDEMA

(a) OEDEMA of VENOUS OBSTRUCTION

This is the commonest form of local oedema and is most frequently seen in venous obstruction of the lower limb.

(b) ASCITES (accumulation of fluid in the peritoneal cavity)

Ascites is a specialised form of local oedema associated most often with disease of the liver (cirrhosis) in which venous obstruction occurs. It may also be associated with tumour growth in the peritoneal cavity.

(c) INFLAMMATORY OEDEMA

In this condition there is intense local congestion and the production of complex chemical agents which alter capillary permeability (see also p.32).

Allergic oedema is a special form of inflammatory oedema. The patient is hypersensitive to particular substances, and the tissues immediately react with the formation of chemicals such as histamine. These induce congestion and alter the capillary permeability.

Both inflammatory oedema and allergic oedema have already been considered when dealing with the inflammatory reaction (p.32 and 109). A similar response is produced by stinging plants and insects.

(d) ANGIONEUROTIC OEDEMA

This is a rare form of local oedema of sudden onset but short duration and unknown cause. Very rarely it may affect the larynx and cause suffocation.

(e) LYMPHATIC OEDEMA

This occurs when there is chronic obstruction to lymphatic flow in an area.

Common causes are:

(a) Destruction of lymphatics by chronic inflammation
(b) Blockage of lymphatics e.g. by cancer cells or parasites such as filaria.

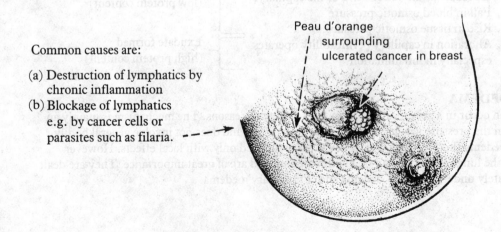

Peau d'orange surrounding ulcerated cancer in breast

LOCAL OEDEMA

PULMONARY OEDEMA

This is the most important form of local oedema since it is associated with serious disease of the heart. It differs from other forms of oedema in that fluid accumulates not only in the tissue spaces but also in the pulmonary alveoli. The results in terms of gaseous interchange are disastrous.

Normal pulmonary fluid interchange
The same factors operate as in other parts of the body. One factor, however, is more important than others — the negative tissue pressure induced by respiration.

Alveolar capillary

Venous hydrostatic pressure = 10 mmHg

Plasma osmotic pressure = 25 mmHg

Tissue osmotic pressure = 3 mmHg

Alevolar epithelium

Alevolus

Negative respiratory pressure = 5 – 10 mmHg

Filtration pressure = hydrostatic pressure + tissue osmotic pressure + negative respiratory pressure = 18 – 23 mmHg
Osmotic reabsorbing pressure = 25 mmHg

The balance between these forces is relatively fine and can be easily upset so that **OEDEMA** can occur rapidly.

Cardiac failure

Over transfusion or infusion

Increased blood hydrostatic pressure

Inhalation of irritant gases

Inflammation

Increased capillary permeability

GENERAL OEDEMA

In addition to alterations in the capillary filtration process (which have already been described), in generalised oedema there is another important factor — increase in total body water. It is particularly associated with diseases of the heart and kidneys.

CARDIAC OEDEMA

This has already been mentioned under 'Chronic venous congestion'. Three factors are involved:

In the early phases of cardiac failure, oedema is slight and is seen where the hydrostatic pressure is greatest — around the feet and ankles. Later, as the condition of the patient deteriorates, fluid gathers in the peritoneal cavity (ascites), in the pleural cavities (hydrothorax) and ultimately becomes generalised (anasarca).

RENAL OEDEMA

Two forms of renal disease are associated with oedema: (a) *acute nephritis and* (b) *nephrotic syndrome.*

The processes involved are different.

	Acute Nephritis	Nephrosis
Degree of oedema	Slight	Marked
Distribution	Loose tissues, e.g. round eyes, ankles	More generalised
Proteinuria	Moderate	Gross
Plasma osmotic pressure	Normal	Reduced
Cause	Retention of fluid	Fall in plasma osmotic pressure

FAMINE OEDEMA

In starvation there is a lack of protein building materials, particularly amino acids. The protein reserves become depleted and, ultimately, the plasma proteins are reduced below the critical level for maintaining the osmotic pressure of the blood.

A special effect of starvation may be the deficiency of vitamin B_1, (thiamine) causing Beri-Beri which is associated with cardiac failure.

SHOCK

Shock is a condition in which the vital functions of the body are depressed due to a severe and acute reduction in cardiac output and effective circulating blood volume. There is progressive cardiovascular collapse characterised by hypotension, hyperventilation and clouding of consciousness. Subsequently there is oliguria.

There are many causes, conveniently grouped under three main headings:

1. HYPOVOLAEMIC (i.e. diminished blood volume)
Associated with:

(a) **Trauma**
    (i) Severe haemorrhage — external or internal
    (ii) Severe injury — especially fractures of bones and crushing of tissues
    (iii) Surgical procedures — especially if anaesthesia is not adequate
    (iv) Burning — especially where extensive surface damage
                 allows loss of a large amount of exudate

(b) **Dehydration** — in cases of severe vomiting or diarrhoea.

2. CARDIOGENIC
Acute diseases of the heart — especially myocardial infarction — in which there is a sudden fall in cardiac output.

3. BACTERIAL (Septic, bacteraemic, endotoxic)
In serious bacterial infections (especially Gram-negative organisms, e.g. *E.coli* and *bacteroides*).

The loss of effective circulating blood causes tissue and cell damage, and, at the same time, initiates reactive changes in the circulation. These two mechanisms combine to cause the shock syndrome.

SHOCK

REACTIVE CHANGES — EARLY STAGE

These changes are concerned with the maintenance of an adequate cerebral and coronary circulation and are effected by a redistribution of the blood in the body as a whole.

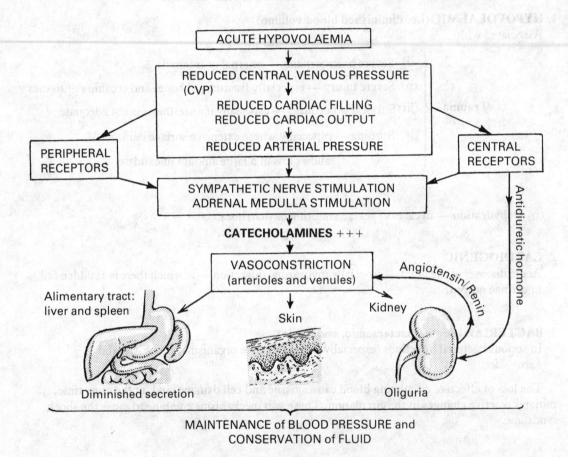

MAINTENANCE of BLOOD PRESSURE and
CONSERVATION of FLUID

At the same time, the circulations in the brain and heart are protected by autoregulatory mechanisms. They are *not* subject to the generalised vasoconstriction.

Instead:

If the loss of circulating fluid volume is great, the limits of the compensatory mechanism are exceeded and the patient goes into a state of severe shock.

SHOCK

ADVANCED STAGE

The patient is now listless, pale and cold, the face is pinched and the lips blue. The pulse is rapid and weak and the blood pressure is low.

Conditions in Vascular bed

NORMAL

Capillary bed

Arteriole   Venule

Vascular perfusion of tissues in balance

EARLY SHOCK (Compensatory phase)

CONSTRICTION

Arteriole   Venule

BP rises

Vascular perfusion of tissues diminished

ADVANCED SHOCK (Compensatory mechanism failing)

DILATATION   CAPILLARIES OPEN   CONSTRICTION CONTINUES

Arteriole   Venule

TISSUE HYPOXIA

BP falls

Fluid leaves capillaries — sludging of blood
Vascular perfusion of tissues seriously diminished

SHOCK

ADVANCED STAGE   (continued)

Thus, from the beginning of the shock process, all the body tissues, with the exception of the brain and the heart, suffer from hypoxia. This sets up vicious circles which aggravate the condition:

1.

2. When the blood pressure falls below 50 — 60 mmHg, the autoregulatory control of the cerebral and coronary circulations fails. Serious damage to the brain (p. 146) and heart may occur.

CHANGES IN THE BLOOD AND CELL METABOLISM

As well as these basic circulatory disturbances, important changes in the blood and cellular metabolism occur in shock.

Blood coagulation system

Acute hypoxia → Damaged endothelium → Coagulation cascade triggered → May proceed to formation of FIBRIN → Disseminated intravascular coagulation (DIC) syndrome

Cellular metabolism

SHOCK — INDIVIDUAL ORGANS

HEART

There are two main ways in which heart failure may be associated with shock.

1. In hypovolaemic and bacteraemic shock, heart failure is a *COMPLICATION*

Mechanisms

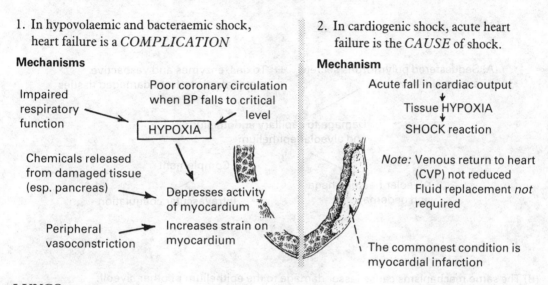

Impaired respiratory function →

Poor coronary circulation when BP falls to critical level ↘

HYPOXIA

Chemicals released from damaged tissue (esp. pancreas) →

Depresses activity of myocardium

Peripheral vasoconstriction →

Increases strain on myocardium

2. In cardiogenic shock, acute heart failure is the *CAUSE* of shock.

Mechanism

Acute fall in cardiac output
↓
Tissue HYPOXIA
↓
SHOCK reaction

Note: Venous return to heart (CVP) not reduced
Fluid replacement *not* required

The commonest condition is myocardial infarction

LUNGS

Respiratory function is seriously disturbed in 2 main ways:

1. Changes in the rate and depth of breathing

Metabolic acidosis ⟶

Respiratory centre → HYPERVENTILATION

Oxygen lack → Peripheral receptors ↗

2. Circulatory changes in the lung

These occur in late shock when compensatory mechanisms are failing. There is congestion and oedema, patchy to begin with but becoming confluent. The lungs are heavy and wet. (Called 'shock lung' or 'wet lung'.)

Alveoli full of red cells and fluid

Polymorphs are 'sequestered' in alveolar capillaries

SHOCK — INDIVIDUAL ORGANS

Circulatory changes in the lung (continued)

Several mechanisms operate to produce pulmonary changes.

(A) Sequestered polymorphs secrete superoxides + Toxins, enzymes and vasoactive materials come from damaged tissues

Damage to capillary endothelium and alveolar epithelium

Complement

Alveolar haemorrhage and oedema

Intravascular coagulation

(B) The same mechanisms cause lesser damage to the epithelium of other alveoli:

Epithelial damage

↓

Cessation of surfactant secretion

↓

Alveolar walls stick together

↓

Alveoli collapse

(C) In other parts of the lung the capillary damage can lead to hyaline membrane formation.

If the patient survives, the lesions undergo organisation with fibrosis. The end result in severe cases may be a combination of emphysema, fibrosis and bronchiolectasis.

SHOCK — INDIVIDUAL ORGANS

KIDNEYS

The secretory function of the kidneys is always disturbed in shock. This is due to the general circulatory collapse and hypotension, but it may be aggravated by the secretion of renin and angiotensin by the kidney, aldosterone by the adrenal and antidiuretic hormone by the posterior pituitary. These hormones are secreted in an attempt to retain fluid and restore the blood volume, but by inducing vasoconstriction they will tend to increase renal damage.

Mechanism

FALL in BLOOD PRESSURE

INCREASING SEVERITY

Decreased GLOMERULAR FILTRATE (GF) → retention of →

Increased breakdown of body proteins (esp. in traumatic shock)
↓
Increased formation of
↓
WASTE PRODUCTS (URAEMIA)

TUBULAR ischaemia (hypoxia)
Depression of function
OLIGURIA (less than 400ml urine/d)

INCREASING SEVERITY

TUBULAR NECROSIS
(esp. distal tubule: 'lower nephron')
GF completely reabsorbed

ANURIA
(failure of urine formation: less than 100 Ml/d) →

SEVERE PROGRESSIVE URAEMIA

In such cases, at post mortem the kidneys, are **pale** and **swollen** and the architectural markings are blurred

Normal

Shock kidney
Pale and swollen

Dilated degenerate or dead tubules separated by oedema fluid and containing debris and pigment

SHOCK — INDIVIDUAL ORGANS

ADRENALS

In addition to the release of **aldosterone** in response to changes in kidney function and fluid electrolyte balance, the adrenal CORTEX secretes increased quantities of **glucocorticoids** and the MEDULLA a great increase of **catecholamines** (adrenaline, etc.).

Occasionally in severe shock, adrenal haemorrhage occurs particularly when the blood coagulation mechanism is disturbed or if there is overwhelming bacterial infection.

ALIMENTARY TRACT

Acute ulceration of the stomach and duodenum may complicate shock — the mechanism is not known. (Curling's or stress ulcers.) Haemorrhage of varying severity may also occur, especially from the colon.

SHOCK — INDIVIDUAL ORGANS

BRAIN

During the compensated phase of shock,
relatively mild cerebral ischaemia is associated
with changes in the state of consciousness.
When the blood pressure falls
to below 50-60 mm Hg, the brain suffers serious
ischaemic damage which can amount to actual
infarction in the 'boundary zones' of
the cerebral cortex (and cerebellum).

There may also be more diffuse cerebral damage.

POST MORTEM APPEARANCES IN SHOCK

These are very variable.

Often the changes in the organs are not striking, and the continuing presence of the initating
cause of the shock is the most important finding.

SHOCK SPECIAL TYPES

FAINTING (VASOVAGAL) ATTACK — (PRIMARY SHOCK)

What used to be called 'primary shock' is in fact the common fainting attack which is brought on in susceptible individuals by emotional upset or trauma which may be minor, and is mediated by nervous mechanisms. The patient feels 'faint', becomes pale often with a cold sweat and may vomit. The pulse slows and the blood pressure falls: consciousness is lost.

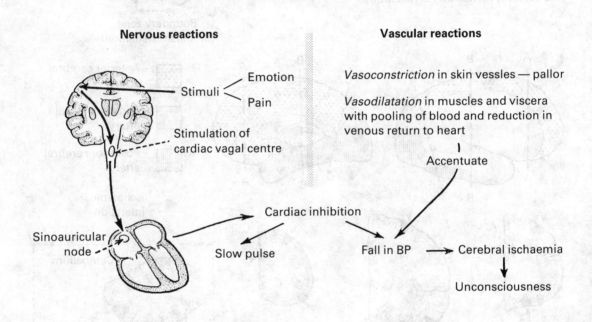

Nervous reactions

Stimuli — Emotion / Pain

Stimulation of cardiac vagal centre

Sinoauricular node

Cardiac inhibition → Slow pulse

Vascular reactions

Vasoconstriction in skin vessles — pallor

Vasodilatation in muscles and viscera with pooling of blood and reduction in venous return to heart

Accentuate

Fall in BP → Cerebral ischaemia

Unconsciousness

At this stage, nervous reaction quickly begins, and with a simple fainting attack recovery is soon complete. On very rare occasions, sudden death occurs due to complete cardiac inhibition by vagal action.

Because the nervous mechanisms of the fainting attack only play a minor part in the early stages of true shock the term 'primary shock' is now obsolete.

SHOCK — SPECIAL TYPES

SHOCK IN BURNS AND SCALDS

Mechanism

1. The immediate reaction is **NERVOUS — PAIN** and stimulation of afferent nerves, followed by

2. An **INFLAMMATORY RESPONSE** evoked by the burnt tissues.

Massive exudation and
loss of PROTEIN-RICH fluid   ⟶   HYPOVOLAEMIA   ⟶   SHOCK
(sludging of blood in capillaries)

This mechanism explains why the SEVERITY of the shock is roughly proportional to the exuding SURFACE AREA and not to the depth of the burn, and why PLASMA transfusion is indicated.
Other factors are chemical mediators derived from the burnt tissues.

3. Complications which aggravate the shock.

(a) *Infection*

Burnt tissues ⟶ Susceptible to infection ⟶ BACTERIAL SHOCK
         esp. *Staph. aureus*   may be superimposed
              Strep. pyogenes
              Gram-neg. bacilli
              (e.g. *Pseudomonas*)

(b) *Anaemia*

Haemolysis of red cells
at burnt site and later   ⟶   ANAEMIA
if sludging is severe

ANAPHYLACTIC SHOCK

This is an acute reaction caused by hypersensitivity of the host to exogenous protein and is dealt with on page 109.

SHOCK — SPECIAL TYPES

BACTERIAL SHOCK

Causes

1. *Bacteria*

   In modern practice, the GRAM-NEGATIVE BACTERIA, especially the coliform group, are the commonest causes, and the shock is caused by ENDOTOXINS.

   Other organisms which may or may not be associated with endotoxins can also produce shock, e.g. staphy lococci, streptococci and menigococci.

2. *Associated conditions*

   (a) Serious *primary* bacterial infection, e.g. septicaemia, peritonitis — potentiated by deficiency in immune status (p.50) and liver disease where detoxification is impaired.

   (b) Bacterial shock may complicate pre-existing shock due to other causes, e.g. burns.

   (c) Bacterial shock may complicate relatively trivial surgical procedures, especially in the gastrointestinal and urinary tracts in the presence of infection.

Mechanism

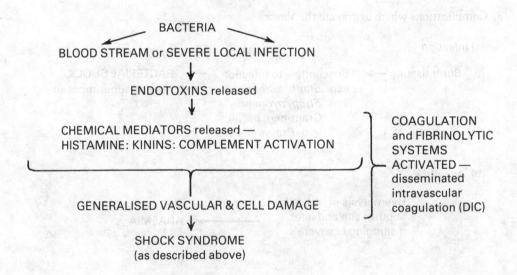

Occasionally, especially in bacterial infection where endotoxin is not produced, there is a generalised arteriolar dilatation with a fall in BP, but the cardiac output is maintained and the patient has a warm, pink skin.

SHOCK — OUTCOME

The OUTCOME of SHOCK

There are 3 possibilities, depending on several factors:

1. RECOVERY
   after convalescence,
   which may be long

2. SURVIVAL
   with permanent damage
   to various organs

3. DEATH

Factors favouring recovery	Factors favouring progression of shock
1. AVAILABILITY of EARLY TREATMENT of (a) the INITIATING CAUSE (b) the HYPOVOLAEMIA 2. Youth 3. Good general health	1. DELAY in TREATMENT 2. FAILURE to REMOVE the INITIATING CAUSE 3. Old age 4. Poor general health 5. Pre-existing Cardiovascular and Lung disease 6. Onset of Complications, esp. Infection and Organ damage

IRREVERSIBLE SHOCK

Theoretically, at some stage in its evolution, shock becomes irreversible due to the severity of vascular impairment and tissue damage. In medical practice, no certain indications are available as to when this point is reached. Measurements of blood pressure and central venous pressure indicate the severity of the vascular disturbance, but many severe cases respond to modern sophisticated treatment. However, the basic essentials remain the early transfusion of fluid and the removal of the original cause of the shock.

CHAPTER 7

NEOPLASIA

NON-NEOPLASTIC PROLIFERATION

Enlargement of an organ due to increase in the parenchymal cell mass may be due to:

(1) an increase in the size and functional capacity of the individual cells — **hypertrophy**
or (2) an increase in the number of cells — **hyperplasia**
or (3) commonly a combination of (1) and (2)

The stimuli responsible are:
    (a) increase in functional demand
    (b) increased trophic hormonal activity.

Physiological enlargement of organs is common and well illustrated by the increase in muscle bulk consequent upon training and the enlargement of uterus and breasts in pregnancy.
Pathological enlargement is the result of disease processes.

HYPERTROPHY (pathological)

Enlargement of the heart as a result of hypertension is a good example of pure hypertrophy: the result of the increased functional demands to maintain the high blood pressure is an increase in the size of the myocardial cells.

Normal   **Hypertension**

Left ventricle   Left ventricle

Heart weight: up to 350 g   Heart weight: 40 – 650 g due to hypertrophy of left ventricle.

HYPERPLASIA (pathological)

The two main causes are:

(a) In the skin *chronic irritation* (and inflammation) demands increased thickness

Normal epithelium   Hyperplastic epithelium   Chronic inflammation

(b) *Imbalance of hormonal activity*, e.g. the irregular enlargement of the prostate in old age is due to hyperplasia of the component tissues.

Normal prostate   Nodular hyperplasia of prostate   Hypertrophied muscle of bladder   Hyperplastic middle lobe   Distorted, partially occluded urethra

Note: If the abnormal stimulus is removed, the affected organ can return to normal.

NON-NEOPLASTIC PROLIFERATION

METAPLASIA

This is a change from one type of differentiated tissue to another, usually of the same broad class but often less well specialised. The change is commonly seen in lining epithelia but occurs also in connective tissues and lining of serous cavities. There is frequently an associated hyperplasia.

e.g. (a) Change from mucus-secreting epithelium to stratified squamous epithelium as in the bronchial irritation associated with smoking.

(b) Formation of bone in fibrous tissue — sometimes in healing process, e.g. prostatectomy scars.

Bone

Chronic inflammation

In some cases metaplasia is associated with chronic irritation, but the intimate causes are unknown in most instances. Lack of vitamin A however results in widespread squamous metaplasia of respiratory and salivary epithelium.

DYSPLASIA

This means disordered cellular development. It may accompany hyperplasia and metaplasia.

The changes consist of increased mitosis, the production of abnormal cells in varying numbers and a tendency to disorder in their arrangement. The true nature of dysplasia is as yet unkown, but it appears to be associated with the genesis of malignancy. It is sometimes found in epithelium of the uterine cervix.

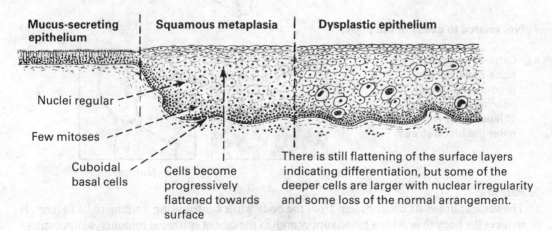

Mucus-secreting epithelium

Squamous metaplasia

Dysplastic epithelium

Nuclei regular

Few mitoses

Cuboidal basal cells

Cells become progressively flattened towards surface

There is still flattening of the surface layers indicating differentiation, but some of the deeper cells are larger with nuclear irregularity and some loss of the normal arrangement.

Note: Both metaplasia and dysplasia may be reversible, but many of the characteristics of dysplastic cells are common to malignant cells (see p. 174).

NEOPLASTIC PROLIFERATION

A tumour is a proliferation of cells which is:

1. **Progressive**

e.g. Tumour of bone

2. **Purposeless**   e.g. Tumour of fibrous tissue

The fibres of a tumour of fibrous tissue have no regular arrangement and serve no useful purpose.

In normal fibrous tissue, the strands have a definite arrangement, supporting some structure such as an epithelial surface.

NB Individual cells of a tumour may exhibit function — the fibrocytes form collagen — but it has no purpose.

3. **Regardless of surrounding tissue,**

e.g. Smooth muscle tumour of uterus compresses normal tissues and distorts uterine cavity

4. **Not related to needs of the body,**

e.g. Certain tumours of bone-marrow cells produce, needlessly, enormous numbers of leucocytes which enter the blood stream

Normal

5. **Parasitic**

The tumour draws its nourishment from the body while contributing nothing to its fuction. It induces the body to provide a blood supply and, in the case of epithelial tumours, a supporting stroma.

Since the development of a neoplasm is independent of the normal processes in the body it is *autonomous* although its growth may to some extent be influenced by these processes.

NEOPLASMS — CLASSIFICATION

Tumours may be classified in two ways: clinical and histological origin.

1. CLINICAL

The tumour is classified according to its morbid anatomy and behaviour. Two main groups are recognised — *benign* (simple) and *malignant*. The contrast between these two groups is as follows:-

	BENIGN	MALIGNANT
Spread (the most important feature)	Remains localised	Cells transferred via lymphatics, blood vessels, tissue planes and serous cavities to set up satellite tumours (metastases)
Rate of Growth	Usually slow	Usually rapid
Boundaries	Circumscribed, often encapsulated	Irregular, ill-defined and non-encapsulated
Relationship to surrounding tissues	Merely compresses normal tissue	Invades and destroys normal tissues
Effects	Produced by pressure on vessels, tubes, nerves, organs etc. Removal will alleviate.	Destroys structures and removal of tumour will not restore function

In practice, there is a spectrum of malignancy. Some tumours may grow locally and destroy normal tissues but never produce metastases. Others will produce metastases only after a very considerable time while, at the other end of the spectrum, there are tumours which metastasise very early in their development.

2. HISTOLOGICAL ORIGIN

Although tumours may arise from any tissue in the body, they can be conveniently accommodated in six groups.

      1. Mesodermic connective tissues including muscle, bone and cartilage
      2. Epithelia   3. Neuroectoderm
      4. Haemopoietic tissues   5. Blood and lymph vessels
      6. Cells originating from developmental abnormalities

In practice, tumours most often take origin from tissues which normally have a rapid turnover of cells and are active in repair — epithelia of skin and mucous membranes, breast and female reproductive organs, connective tissue, bone and haemopoietic cells.

CYTOLOGICAL DIFFERENTIATION

Tumour cells may be broadly divided into two types:

(1) Differentiated and (2) Undifferentiated.

The degree of differentiation roughly corresponds to the character of the neoplasm. Cells of simple tumours are well differentiated; those of malignant tumours tend to remain undifferentiated, and the more primitive the cells the greater the malignancy.

DIFFERENTIATED CELLS (BENIGN TUMOURS)

1. **Mimic the structure of their parent organ.**

e.g. In an adenoma (simple gland — forming tumour) of colon the cells arrange themselves in acini

In a skin papilloma (wart) the squamous epithelium still forms a covering for underlying connective tissue

2. **Resemble their cells of origin.**

e.g. The cells of a skin papilloma are squamous

The cells of a myoma are muscle cells

The cells of a chondroma are recognisable cartilage cells

3. As in normal tissue, **show a remarkable uniformity in size shape and nuclear configuration.**

4. **Show evidence of normal function even if useless.**

Mucous secretion in acinus of an adenoma

5. **Have relatively infrequent mitotic figures:** these are of normal type.

Equatorial chromosomes

Division into two identical daughter cells.

CYTOLOGICAL DIFFERENTIATION

UNDIFFERENTIATED CELLS (MALIGNANT TUMOURS):

1. **Generally show a haphazard arrangement.** $\longrightarrow$ e.g. Scirrhous carcinoma of breast

2. **Bear little resemblance to the cells of origin.**

3. **Tend to vary widely in size, shape and nuclear configuration.** $\longrightarrow$ e.g. Pleomorphic sarcoma

4. **Provide little evidence of normal function.** $\longrightarrow$ e.g. Adeno carcinoma of bowel (Secretory activity very limited)

5. **Show frequent mitoses often of abnormal type.**

Three daughter cells

Lack of differentiation is often termed anaplasia, and anaplastic tumours are highly malignant. There is a spectrum of change in neoplasms from the very slowly growing, highly differentiated simple types to the rapidly growing, undifferentiated malignant examples.

Highly differentiated	Moderate differentiation	Poorly differentiated	Undifferentiated
↓	↓	↓	↓
Simple	Simple or doubtfully malignant	Malignant	Highly malignant

SIMPLE CONNECTIVE TISSUE TUMOURS

These tumours are composed of differentiated connective tissues of the body — fibrous tissue, cartilage, bone, muscle, fatty tissue. They all tend to be rounded or lobulated, well-encapsulated and merely compress the surrounding tissues.

FIBROMA

These are relatively rare tumours, found in the subcutaneous tissues, fascia, periosteum and in the ovary and kidney. They vary in character according to the degree of the cellularity and amount of collagen. Some have abundant coarse collagen fibres and their cells are few and small. This type is firm and white. In others, cells are abundant and larger, and collagen is fine, giving a softer texture.

Spindle-shaped fibrocyte nuclei

Collagen fibres

Fascicles running in various directions ∴ no functional purpose.

The following **tumour-like growths** of fibrous tissue are also recognised:

Keloid is an overgrowth of fibrous tissue in scars. It follows radiation burns but may complicate operation scars (see p. 79).

Palmar fibromatosis, at first nodular, causes flexion deformities of fingers (Dupuytren's contracture) due to contraction of fibrous tissue within the palmar fascia. A similar condition may affect the plantar fascia.

Juvenile aponeurotic fibroma — of palms and soles in children.

Nodular fasciitis — of the subcutaneous tissues of adults.
Both of the above appear malignant in that they invade adjacent structures, but they are self-limiting and yield to local excision.

Musculoaponeurotic fibromatosis (desmoid fibromatosis) is a similar lesion but recurs frequently after excision. It grows progressively infiltrating surrounding structures.

SIMPLE CONNECTIVE TISSUE TUMOURS

MYXOMA

This is a variant of fibroma and in most instances represents a degenerative change. It is found in the same situations as fibroma. Myxomatous change may also affect chondromas and lipomas.

It is soft, translucent and frequently brownish due to old haemorrhage. The characteristic feature is the presence of a mucinous ground substance.

These tumours, although simple, may recur locally due to difficulty in achieving complete removal.

Jelly-like mucinous matrix

Stellate cells with branching processes

LIPOMA

Circumscribed masses of fat cells are commonly found in the subcutaneous tissue of the arms, shoulders and buttocks. They may also be found in the peritoneal cavity in relation to the kidney, omentum or mesentery, but very rarely in solid organs.

Lipoma on shoulder Usually lobular, well-defined and yellow

Simple fat cells

Avascular

Nuclei placed on cell membranes

Sometimes lipomas may have projections into the surrounding tissues which make complete removal difficult.

167

SIMPLE CONNECTIVE TISSUE TUMOURS

CHONDROMA

Two types are sometimes described:

1. **Solitary enchondroma.** This type is found in the metacarpals or phalanges of the fingers. It forms in the substance or at the surface of the bone and causes destruction of the bone by expansion and pressure.

Firm, bluish with fibrous capsule; sometimes central softening with brownish fluid

Hyaline, cartilagenous matrix

Regular, rounded, mononuclear cartilage cells often in pairs and quartets

Growth occurs by the proliferation and metaplastic transformation of the capsular fibrocytes.

2. **Multiple enchondromatosis.** These are cartilagenous masses which appear in children, especially in the 'cartilage' bones of the limbs. They usually cease to grow when adulthood is reached and ossify or regress; therefore they are probably in the nature of developmental abnormalities rather than true neoplasms. Occasionally they may continue to grow, and may even become malignant. Many chondromas show areas of ossification and are then termed osteochondromas.

OSTEOMA

As with chondromas, two types are described:

1. **Ivory osteoma.** This is a true tumour and is mainly found in the bones of the skull, although it may occur in the long bones. Osteomas are usually relatively small but may produce severe symptoms because of their situation.

Osteoma on floor of orbit causing protrusion of eyeball

Haversian system

Dense bone

Osteoblasts

SIMPLE CONNECTIVE TISSUE TUMOURS

OSTEOMA (continued)

2. **Cancellous bony growths.** These are found at the end of long bones and are the ossified remains of cartilagenous exostoses. They are formed from developmentally displaced epiphyseal cartilage.
Growth continues until epiphyses unite.
A cap of cartilage covers the mass and growth takes place by proliferation of the cartilage and transformation into bone.

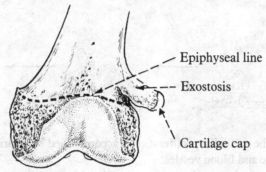

Epiphyseal line

Exostosis

Cartilage cap

MYOMA

Simple tumours of muscle are derived from smooth muscle (leiomyoma), and the majority occur in the uterus where they are extremely common. They are firm, rounded masses which usually begin in the myometrium. Subsequently, they may move inward to the uterine cavity forming polypi, or towards the serous surface.

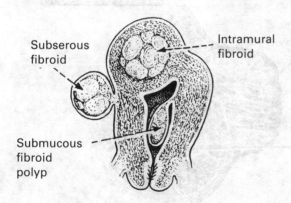

Subserous fibroid

Intramural fibroid

Submucous fibroid polyp

Fibres in parallel bundles which in turn are whorled

Occasionally, similar tumours may be found in the gastrointestinal tract, ovaries, prostate and bladder. Degenerative changes are common in myomas. Many have a large fibrous component and, in the uterus, are termed fibroids.

SIMPLE EPITHELIAL TUMOURS

Simple epithelial tumours are essentially of two types: (1) papillomas and (2) adenomas.

PAPILLOMA

Papillomas take origin from an epithelial surface. As the epithelium proliferates it is thrown into folds which become increasingly complex.

The epithelial proliferation is accompanied by a corresponding growth of supporting connective tissue and blood vessels.

Typical examples are found in the skin, e.g. the common wart.

Fibrous tissue core
Hyperplastic squamous epithelium

Nipple

Papillomas may also form within ducts, e.g. in the breast. In such a case, the papilloma is much compressed and has an apparently complex structure.

In these simple tumours:

(a) The normal arrangement of epithelial cells is maintained, e.g. in skin papillomas the surface cells are squames and proliferation is confined to the deepest layers.

(b) The relationship of epithelium to connective tissue is normal.

(c) Blood vessels are well formed.

SIMPLE EPITHELIAL TUMOURS

ADENOMA

Adenomas are derived from the ducts and acini of glands, although the name is also used to cover simple tumours arising in solid epithelial organs.

Again the proliferation of epithelium of a gland causes the formation of tubules which ramify and become increasingly compound. The original communication with the parent gland duct or acinus tends to become lost. – – – – –

In the case of a hollow viscus, such as the intestine or gall bladder, the adenomatous proliferation, instead of growing down into the subjacent connective tissue, is usually pushed upwards into the lumen of the viscus. –

The growth therefore combines the features of a papilloma and an adenoma. The term adenomatous polyp is often applied in such a case.

SIMPLE EPITHELIAL TUMOURS

ADENOMA (continued)

In the type which grows into the subjacent connective tissue, the constant budding of the epithelium results in new acini which become nipped off from the parent acini.

In cases in which retention of secretion is marked, a cyst forms and the tumour is then called a cystadenoma which may reach an enormous size, e.g. some cystadenomas of the ovary may be 30 – 40 cm in diameter, particularly those which secrete mucus.

Normal ovary

Cystadenoma

Cut surface

Tall mucus-secreting cells

As in a hollow viscus, the proliferating epithelium may be heaped to form papillomas and the tumour then becomes a papilliferous cystadenoma. These are also common in the ovary. The cyst fluid in these cases generally contains serum proteins.

Papilloma covered by cuboidal epithelium

Cysts with papillomas which may become very large and complex and fill the cyst.

SIMPLE EPITHELIA TUMOURS

ADENOMA (continued)

In some organs the supporting connective tissue of the adenoma is a
prominent component of the tumour. This is commonly seen in the breast,
and the name **FIBROADENOMA** is used. Depending on the distribution of the
fibrous tissue there are
two histological variations:

1. The fibrous tissue in some is
   condensed around the
   adenomatous acini. This
   produces a small, rounded,
   firm tumour which is termed a
   pericanalicular fibroadenoma.
   The capsule is made up of
   compressed breast tissue.

Acini and ducts surrounded by
relatively dense
fibrous
tissue

Firm, palpable,
encapsulated mass

2. A larger, softer tumour is
   sometimes produced by a
   polypoid hyperplasia of the
   fibrous tissue. It compresses
   the ducts and reduces them to
   slits — intracanalicular
   fibroadenoma.

Lobulated fibrous
tissue

Adenomatous ducts

May be large
and lobulated

Frequently both types of change may be found in the same tumour.

Simple solid epithelial tumours arise in the solid parenchymatous organs, particularly
endocrine glands. They are usually well circumscribed. The term adenoma is also applied to these
growths.

CARCINOMA IN SITU (INTRAEPITHELIAL NEOPLASIA)

This represents an intermediate stage in the production of a cancer. All the cytological features of malignancy are present, but the cells have not invaded the surrounding tissues. It is frequently found in the cervix uteri at the junction of ecto and endocervix.

Normal cervix

Stratified squamous epithelium of ectocervix

Junction

Columnar mucus-secreting epithelium of endocervix

Metaplasia

Columnar epithelium undergoes squamous metaplasia

Cells show stratification and differentiation

Dysplasia

Thickening with moderate loss of polarity and differentiation

Carcinoma in situ

No clear stratification; cells undifferentiated; mitoses

Altered cells filling crypts

Intraduct carcinoma of the breast is another example.

These premalignant conditions may revert to normal, but most commonly they become truly malignant and invade the surrounding tissues. The determining factors are unknown.

The concept of progressive premalignant proliferation applies equally in other organs (e.g. stomach, bowel, bronchus, etc.).

MALIGNANT EPITHELIAL TUMOURS

The generic term for a malignant epithelial tumour is **CARCINOMA**
(Greek: *Karkinos*, a crab). This refers to the irregular jagged shape
often assumed. It is due to the local spread of carcinoma.

The proliferating cells break
through normal barriers.

Malignant
epithelium
breaks through basement membrane
and subjacent connective tissue

Further growth is by permeation of
the tissue spaces.

Malignant
cells
permeating
spaces

Growth of malignant cells
stimulates the production of new
collagen fibres which are
sometimes converted into dense
scar tissue → contracts and fixes
the growth to surrounding
structures

e.g. Carcinoma of breast.

Retracted
nipple

Carcinoma
fixed to
underlying
muscle

Fibrous
tissue

Most breast carcinomas stimulate the formation of dense fibrous tissue and are termed *scirrhous*
(i.e. hard); less frequently, where the stroma is scanty, the carcinoma is bulky and soft —
encephaloid (brain-like). These are descriptive terms and do not indicate the histological type of
carcinoma or its malignancy.

The following diagram illustrates the basic mechanisms of cancer cell invasion.

(1) Cancer cells

Ability to secrete
lytic enzymes,
e.g. collagenases

Basement
membrane
breached

(2)

Cells are less
adhesive
than normal

(3)

Spread
and subsequent
replication

Increased amoeboid
movements — penetration
and spread

175

SPREAD OF CARCINOMA

By definition, all carcinomas spread primarily into the adjacent tissues, and after a varying period, spread to more distant structures occurs in the following ways:

VIA LYMPHATICS

This is the commonest mode of spread. The carcinoma cells easily invade lymphatic channels from the tissue spaces.

Groups of cells form *emboli* in the lymph stream and are carried to the nearest node.

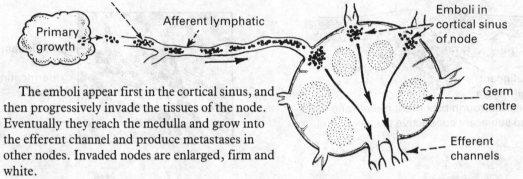

The emboli appear first in the cortical sinus, and then progressively invade the tissues of the node. Eventually they reach the medulla and grow into the efferent channel and produce metastases in other nodes. Invaded nodes are enlarged, firm and white.

These emboli are microscopic and can escape notice at operation. They account for recurrence of growth in many cases.

Growth of carcinoma cells in a node results in occlusion of afferent and efferent channels. Lymph flow is thus diverted and this has two effects:

(1) Tumour cells are diverted to neighbouring nodes and new metastatic growths are set up

(2) Lymph flow can be reversed and nodes may be invaded via the medulla

This accounts for the spread of carcinoma in a diverse and often irregular manner.

SPREAD OF CARCINOMA

VIA LYMPHATICS (continued)

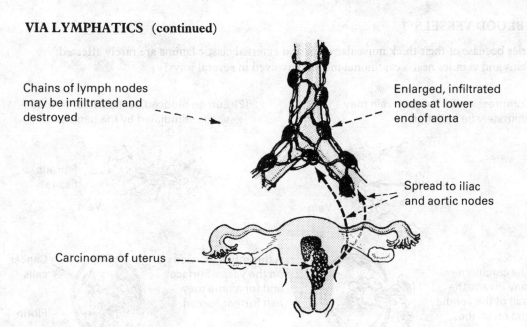

Chains of lymph nodes may be infiltrated and destroyed

Enlarged, infiltrated nodes at lower end of aorta

Spread to iliac and aortic nodes

Carcinoma of uterus

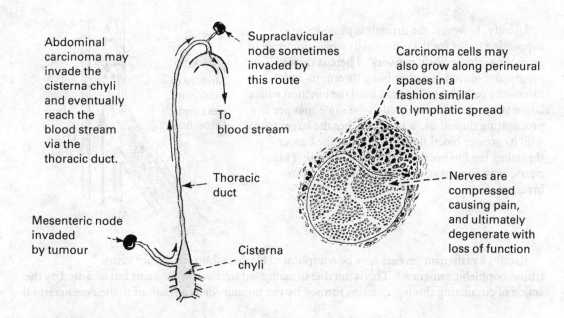

Abdominal carcinoma may invade the cisterna chyli and eventually reach the blood stream via the thoracic duct.

Supraclavicular node sometimes invaded by this route

Carcinoma cells may also grow along perineural spaces in a fashion similar to lymphatic spread

To blood stream

Thoracic duct

Mesenteric node invaded by tumour

Cisterna chyli

Nerves are compressed causing pain, and ultimately degenerate with loss of function

Although lymphatic embolism is of major practical importance, tumour cells may also grow along lymphatic channels in continuous solid columns — lymphatic permeation.

SPREAD OF CARCINOMA

VIA BLOOD VESSELS

Arteries becuase of their thick muscular walls and external elastic lamina are rarely affected.
Veins and venules near a carcinoma may be involved in several ways:

(1) Compression by tumour: vein may ultimately be obliterated.

(2) Lumen reduced by growth of fibrous tissue stimulated by the neoplasm.

Tumour

Vein

Fibrous tissue

Vein

(3) The carcinoma may invade the wall of the venule and reach the lumen.

A thrombus develops on the vessel surface and for a time may halt further spread.

Cancer cells

Fibrin

Usually, however, the thrombus provides a supporting trellis for the cancer cells which continue to grow through the fibrin network. There is thus a progressive spread of a crumbling thrombus and carcinoma cells along the vessel until the junction with a larger venous trunk is reached in the same manner as a propagating thrombus. When it reaches the larger trunk with its greater blood flow, particles of the cancer thrombus tend to break off and form emboli. This of course may happen at the original site of venous invasion.

Emboil

Mixture of malignant cells and thrombus

Main flow

Rarely, a malignant process may be complicated by thrombosis of distant veins (thrombophlebitis migrans). This is not due to malignant invasion of the veins but is caused by the action of circulating thromboplastins formed by the tumour, or as a result of tissue degeneration.

SPREAD OF CARCINOMA

DESTINATION of EMBOLI

This depends on the vessel invaded.

(1) **Portal venous system**
  — emboli pass to liver

(2) **Systemic venous system** — emboli pass to lungs. There are exceptions (see 'Retrograde Spread' below).

Liver metastases

Portal vein

Colonic cancer

SVC

Systemic veins

IVC

Emboli in lungs

Carcinoma of bronchus

(3) **Pulmonary venous system** — emboli pass to left heart and general circulation

RETROGRADE VENOUS SPREAD

As in lymphatics, growth of tumour within a vein may cause reversal of blood flow. In addition, reversal of flow is apt to happen in certain areas of the body where veins form a rich plexus and are deficient in valves, e.g. in the pelvis and around vertebrae. Changes in intra-abdominal and intrathoracic pressures easily induce changes in blood flow in these channels. It is for this reason that secondary tumours are relatively common in vertebral bodies.

Pressure

SPREAD OF CARCINOMA

FATE of CARCINOMATOUS EMBOLI

The distribution of carcinomatous emboli is determined by anatomy, but whether they give rise to a metastatic tumour depends on several factors, e.g.:

1. **Size of embolus**
   Most malignant emboli are tiny and contain few cancer cells. On impaction, the cells commonly die before they have time to multiply.

2. **Changes at site of embolic impaction**
   The malignant embolus produces the same changes as any embolus and is treated by the tissues in the same way. Thrombus is deposited on the embolus and macrophage reaction is stimulated.

3. **The organ affected**
   Metastatic tumours are **common** in:
   (a) *Lungs*. This is due to the large number of emboli reaching them in cases of malignancy. Most of the emboli are destroyed but some are bound to survive.
   (b) *Liver*. Malignant emboli seem to find this organ particularly favourable for further growth, possibly due to the high concentration of nutrient material in the portal blood.
   Metastases are **uncommon** in:
   (a) *Spleen*
   (b) *Actively moving tissues:* muscle, tendon.

4. Cancer cells may remain latent at remote sites (e.g. breast cancer cells in vertebral bone marrow) and commence aggressive growth after many months or years.

GRADING AND STAGING OF CANCER

Two important factors in assessing the prognosis in an individual case of cancer are:

   1. The histological appearance indicating the grade of malignancy
   2. The size and extent of spread of the tumour.

Grading and staging are attempts to quantify these factors.

Pathological grading

Because this assessment is subjective, a numerical assessment is not appropriate. Usually three grades are used: well, moderately and poorly differentiated.

Cinical staging

This is well exemplified in Hodgkin's disease where numerical staging has proved very useful (see p.596).

SPREAD OF CARCINOMA

VIA SEROUS SACS

This is an important and frequent route of spread in the peritoneal cavity. It also takes place in the pleural cavity and the pericardial sac.

Carcinoma cells invading wall of intestine, for example, cause irritation and interfere with nutrition of tissues.

Serous surface

Serosal cells desquamate

Carcinoma cells escape into peritoneal cavity

As malignant cells sink in peritoneal cavity, they will settle in various sites. They cause an inflammatory reaction with fibrin formation. This anchors the cells and also causes adhesions between organs, providing routes for further spread.

The inflammatory reaction can obscure the presence of carcinoma and make diagnosis difficult.

Adhesions to small intestine

Uterus

Secondary masses in ovary

INTRA-EPITHELIAL SPREAD

This form of spread may occur where carcinoma develops in a gland or its duct, e.g. in the breast.

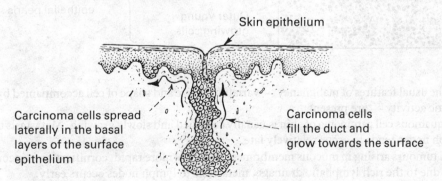

Skin epithelium

Carcinoma cells spread laterally in the basal layers of the surface epithelium

Carcinoma cells fill the duct and grow towards the surface

TYPES OF CARCINOMA

SQUAMOUS CELL CARCINOMA

This is commonly found on the skin, especially exposed surfaces, but also develops in other sites covered by stratified squamous epithelium, *e.g.* lips, tongue, pharynx, oesophagus and vagina. In addition, it may occur on surfaces covered by glandular type epithelium through metaplastic transformation as in the bronchus, gall bladder and uterine cervix.

(1) It starts as a small papular mass

Normal epithelium

Invading epithelium

(2) The surface breaks down and a characteristic irregular ulcer is produced.

Fibrinous exudate

Everted edge

Inflammatory reaction

Invading epithelial masses

Indurated base

Histologically, it is composed of irregular strands and columns of invading epithelium which infiltrate the subjacent connective tissue. If well differentiated, the central cells of the invading masses show conversion into eosinophilic keratinised squames, while the outer layer consists of young basophilic cells. In cross-section, the appearance is typical.

Inner squames — keratinised

Outer young growing cells

Often termed cell nests or epithelial pearls

The usual features of malignancy — variation in size and shape of cell accompanied by frequent mitotic activity — are present.

Squamous cell carcinoma of skin is usually cornified and slowly growing. Metastasis to the local lymph nodes tends to occur relatively late.

In tumours arising in mucous membranes, growth is more rapid, cornification is inconspicuous and, due to the rich lymphatic drainage, metastasis to lymph nodes occurs early.

TYPES OF CARCINOMA

BASAL CELL CARCINOMA (Rodent ulcer)

This tumour may arise in any part of the skin
but is most common in the face, near the
eyes and nose.

First stage
It starts as a flattened papilloma which
slowly enlarges over months or perhaps a
year or two.

Second stage
The surface breaks down and a shallow,
ragged ulcer with pearly edges is formed.

Usually the malignant tissue spreads slowly but progressively, mainly in a lateral direction. It is
composed of cells resembling those of the rete Malpighii of the skin from which it takes origin and
has a characteristic histological appearance.

Peripheral cells
cuboidal and pallisaded

Growth down to but not
beyond deeper stroma
until disease is advanced

Sometimes it seems to take origin from basal cells of skin appendages and may show
pseudoglandular structures.

It is a locally invasive growth which almost never metastasises, but nevertheless may be very
destructive.

TYPES OF CARCINOMA

CARCINOMA of GLANDULAR ORGANS

These may take origin from gland acini, ducts or the glandular epithelium of mucous surfaces. The anatomical structure varies.

(A) On mucous surfaces they may start as a polypoid growth or as a thick plaque.
e.g. Carcinoma of colon

Very quickly it ulcerates and becomes an irregular crater.

Normal mucosa

Invading carcinoma

Muscular coats

Everted edge

(B) In compound glands, e.g. the breast, the cancer forms an irregular penetrating mass — the typical crab-like appearance.

(C) Some malignant tumours are cystic. Quite commonly the malignant growth originates in a pre-existing benign cyst. This is more likely to occur when there are papillomatous structures within the cyst.

Histologically, carcinomas of glandular tissue have three basic forms.

(1) Adenocarcinoma. In this form the growth shows a varying degree of differentiation with attempts at acinus formation.

(2) The carcinoma may be undifferentiated and take the form of solid masses or columns of pleomorphic cells.

(3) Occasionally a carcinoma will produce large quantities of mucus and merit the term mucoid carcinoma. The tumour alveoli may be filled with mucus in which only a few carcinoma cells persist, the cells appearing to dissolve in the mucus. They are commonest in organs normally containing large numbers of mucus-secreting cells, e.g. large intestine, stomach, etc.

MALIGNANT CONNECTIVE TISSUE TUMOURS

These tumours are grouped under the descriptive term **SARCOMA**, from the Greek *sarkoma* meaning 'flesh'.

Sarcomas are less common than carcinomas. Next to leukaemia, they are the most common malignant tumours in children and young adults. In older age groups, 90% of malignant tumours are carcinomas.

Unlike the sinuous infiltrating carcinoma, sarcomas are large fleshy tumours. Arising from and within connective tissues means that infiltration between normal cells is not a feature. The malignant cells advance on a broad front destroying and replacing normal cells. The result is a rounded growth with fairly definite margins.

Spindle-shaped cell   Round cell   Thin-walled blood vessel

Haemorrhage

Mitosis

The neoplastic process is associated with the formation of many large, new, thin-walled blood vessels. As a result, haemorrhage and necrosis are frequent in sarcomas.

Metastatic spread

Sarcoma cells, like all connective tissue cells, are strongly motile. They easily invade the veins and commonly metastasise to the lungs. Since the vessels are thin-walled, metastases tend to occur early.

MALIGNANT CONNECTIVE TISSUE TUMOURS

FIBROSARCOMAS

These arise most commonly from fascia, intermuscular septa, subcutaneous tissue and sometimes periosteum. As usual, cellular differentiation varies with the degree of malignancy.

Spindle cell sarcoma
The cells are fairly uniform and resemble fibroblasts. Intercellular matrix varies in quantity. Considerable collagen may be formed and the term fibrosarcoma may be applied.

Myxosarcoma is a variant of fibrosarcoma

Pleomorphic or anaplastic sarcoma
Such tumours bear little resemblance to connective tissue. They are highly malignant. The commonest sites are the bones and perimysial connective tissue.

Bizarre cells
← – – and nuclei

Irregular mitotic figures

Absence of matrix

SARCOMAS arising from specialised connective tissues

These are malignant counterparts of benign mesenchymal tumours and produce a few of the features of the tissues from which they have arisen. Generally this is patchy and incomplete and is little indication of the malignancy of the growth.

CHONDROSARCOMA

This tumour is commonest at the ends of long bones but may develop from benign enchondromas in the small bones of the hands or ilium. They occur mostly in adults and tend to be lobulated.. Patches of imperfect cartilage alternate with areas of indeterminate sarcomatous tissue. Chondrosarcoma tends to be rather slowly growing. In many cases the tumour may appear to be only locally malignant. Local recurrence is the main feature and metastases only take place at a later date.

MALIGNANT CONNECTIVE TISSUE TUMOURS

OSTEOGENIC SARCOMAS

Most of these tumours occur in patients between 10 and 25 years of age. Occasionally it may complicate Paget's disease in the elderly.

They affect the metaphysial ends of long bones, especially the upper end of the tibia, lower end of the femur and upper end of the humerus.

The tumour may be endosteal in origin when it is usually solid and relatively hard. In other cases, it may arise from the periosteum and frequently presents a characteristic fir-tree appearance on X-ray due to spicules of bone radiating at right angles from the shaft.

Histologically they show irregular spicules of calcified bone and osteoid tissue among masses of pleomorphic cells.

It is a highly malignant tumour producing metastases at a relatively early stage.

Many tumours show several forms of matrix — fibrous, cartilagenous, osseous and myxomatous.

GIANT CELL TUMOUR OF BONE (Osteoclastoma)

This is a tumour found at the extremities of long bones which may involve the nearby joint. It consists of multi-nucleated osteoclasts and spindle cells.

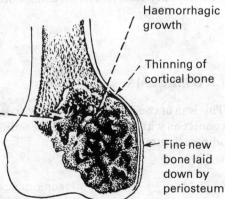

Haemorrhagic growth

Thinning of cortical bone

Begins in interior of bone

It invades local tissues and 20% produce metastases

Fine new bone laid down by periosteum

MALIGNANT CONNECTIVE TISSUE TUMOURS

MYOSARCOMA

There are two varieties:

1. **Leiomyosarcoma**
   This is a rare tumour.
   Almost all of them
   occur in the uterus and
   most arise in pre-existing
   myomas.

Thin-walled
blood vessels

Indefinite margins

Increased vascularity
at malignant change

These tumours metastasise mainly by the blood stream, but lymph node deposits are also found.

2. **Rhabdomyosarcoma**
   This is a rare tumour
   occurring mainly in
   children. They occur very
   rarely in skeletal muscles.
   More common but still rare
   are polypoid tumours in the
   bladder, uterus and vagina,
   sometimes called sarcoma
   botryoides.

Strap-like
cells
(showing
striation)

After repeated recurrences, metastases occur via the blood stream.

LIPOSARCOMA

This is an uncommon tumour. It may arise in
connection with simple lipoma. Like ordinary
adipose tissue, it is lobulated.

Pleomorphic cells with
coarse emulsion of lipid

SPECIAL TUMOURS

MIXED TUMOURS

These are tumours which appear to be composed of both epithelial and connective tissue cells. The commonest example is the mixed parotid tumour.

It is usually firm, lobulated and slowly growing

The histology is complex and variable.

Epithelium

Solid masses

Columns

Acini

Stroma

Myxomatous

Bony

Cartilagenous

It is now considered that both stroma and epithelium are derived from a single cell type, the stroma being a manifestation of metaplasia.

Malignant tumours also occur which appear to be a combination of carcinoma and sarcoma. In almost all cases, the sarcomatous element is merely a very anaplastic area of the carcinoma.

TERATOMA

This is a tumour composed of multiple tissues foreign to the site of growth. It is a true neoplasm and must be distinguished from developmental anomalies in which tissues may be displaced.

Teratomas arise in the gonads or in the midline of the body. It is now considered that they arise from totipotent germ cells. In the embryo, these appear in the mid-line beneath the coelomic epithelium, in association with the hind gut. Normally they migrate to the gonadal ridges, but it is thought that some fail to reach the gonads and remain distributed along the mid-line. The most common site of teratoma is in the ovaries.

Sites

Pineal gland

Base of skull

Mediastinum

Retroperitoneal

Gonads

Sacrococcygeal

189

SPECIAL TUMOURS

TERATOMA (continued)

Two main types are described: benign cystic and solid teratoma.

1. Benign cystic teratoma

This consists mainly of ectodermal structures such as skin and its appendages and neural tissue. Frequently respiratory epithelium, intestinal epithelium, bone and cartilage are present.

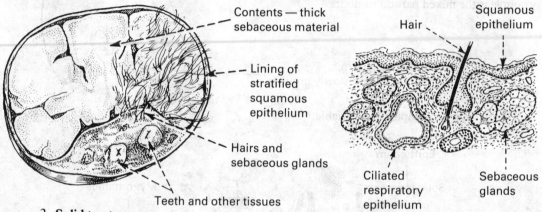

Contents — thick sebaceous material

Lining of stratified squamous epithelium

Hairs and sebaceous glands

Teeth and other tissues

Hair

Squamous epithelium

Ciliated respiratory epithelium

Sebaceous glands

2. Solid teratoma

This tumour is most commonly found in children and is frequently highly malignant. Embryonic, fetal and adult tissues of all types may be found. The malignant tumour may consist of a mixture of immature tissues, but one particular tissue may undergo malignant change and over-run the others.

HAMARTOMA

A hamartoma is a tumour-like but non-neoplastic malformation consisting of a mixture of tissues normally found at the particular site.

The commonest forms of hamartoma are those composed of blood vessels and those involving pigment cells of the skin.

HAEMANGIOMA

Two main varieties exist:

1. Capillary angioma

These are common in the skin as 'birth-marks' which vary in size. Occasionally they may be found in internal organs. They are well defined, deep red or purple. A single artery provides a supply separate from the surrounding tissue.

Prominent endothelial cells

Well formed collagen

2. Cavernous angioma

This type is confined to internal organs and quite often found in the liver. Like the capillary variety they are well defined and deep purple. Similar tumours are found involving the lymphatic system but less commonly.

SPECIAL TUMOURS

BENIGN PIGMENTED NAEVUS or LENTIGO (Melanotic naevus or mole)

This is a common congenital lesion, hence the term 'naevus',
meaning a 'birth mark'.

During fetal life melanin-pigment-forming
neuroectodermal cells migrate to the skin and are found in
small numbers in the basal layer of the skin. - - - - - - - - - - - →

The common congenital pigmented mole or lentigo is the
result of an abnormality in migration, proliferation and
maturation of these neuroectodermal cells. A continuous
layer of pigmented cells is found adjacent to the basal
epidermal cells.

The resulting naevi vary in size and appearance, varying from small flat macular brown areas or
smooth papular lesions to warty hairy excrescences. Pigmentation is variable.

Sometimes proliferation of the 'naevus' cells is a striking feature and this varies in degree and
extent:

Junctional naevus
In this case proliferation
is local and confined to
the dermoepidermal
junction.

Compound naevus
Proliferation is found
in the dermis as well
as the junctional area.

Intradermal naevus
Proliferation is wholly
in the dermis.

SPECIAL TUMOURS

BENIGN PIGMENTED NAEVUS (continued)

Another variation is the **'blue' naevus**. Melanocytes are arrested in migration in the dermis.

Active proliferative activity may extend into adult life, but the great majority of these lesions undergo a degree of involution. One feature which differentiates them from the malignant change is that the deeper the cells penetrate the dermis the smaller they become and the less active.

Continuing active junctional change is said to potentiate malignant change, but this transformation is very rare.

Hamartomas are also found involving the peripheral nerves — neurofibromatosis and its variants — the intestinal tract, congenital polypi, and in many other organs. Tuberous sclerosis is a condition in which hamartomas are found in many of the organs. Osteomas, enchondromas and lipomas are considered by many as hamartomas.

Although hamartomas are not neoplastic, true tumour growth may develop from a hamartoma.

Hamartoma	True neoplasm
Developmental abnormality.	New growth.
Present and often visible at birth.	Most occur in adults.
Enlargement continues until physiological growth ceases (i.e. on reaching adulthood).	Growth is progressive, autonomous and not related to stages of body development.
Condition is essentially benign.	May be malignant.

It will be appreciated that the borderline between hamartoma and some types of benign neoplasm is ill-defined and the distinction is often not of practical importance.

SPECIAL TUMOURS

MALIGNANT MELANOMA

Malignant proliferation of melanocytes usually arises de novo. The aetiology is unknown, but excessive exposure of white skin to sunlight is important. The exposure may be:

    1. *Chronic* — over many years — especially relevant in the elderly.
    2. *Acute* — causing burning. This may be important in the young.

Sites

    1. Skin of (a) face, soles of feet, palms of hands, nail beds,
        (b) legs (women) and (c) trunk (in men).
    2. Mucous membranes of mouth, arms and genitalia — rare.
    3. Eye and meninges — rare.

Some growths are amelanotic (non-pigmented). The rate of growth is variable.

Four types of growth may occur:

1. *Lentigo maligna* — an 'in situ' lesion occurring on the face of the elderly. It may spread at one angle and regress at another.

Aberrant melanocytes spread along basal
epidermal layer and round glands.

It may not reach the invasive stage before
the patient dies of 'natural causes'.

2. *Superficial spreading melanoma* — occurs on female leg, male trunk. It accounts for 50% of all skin melanomas in northern countries.

3. *Acral lentiginous melanoma* — found on palms of hands, soles of feet and mucous membranes.

4. *Nodular malignant melanoma* — usually on trunk. It invades early and ulceration is common.

Types 2, 3 and 4 occur in younger adults, and both 2 and 3 have an in situ stage.

The essential features of malignant melanoma are:

1. Abnormal
   melanocytes
2. Invasion of
   epidermis
3. Invasion down
   into dermis

Two-thirds are cured by excision.

The prognosis depends on depth of
invasion, measured as follows:

1.5 mm or less — good prognosis
1.5-3 mm — fair prognosis
3 mm — poor prognosis.

CARCINOGENESIS

The ultimate mechanisms which cause cancer, i.e. allow cells to proliferate continuously, break through normal bounds and invade other tissues remain unknown

There are, however, three classes of agent which will induce cell proliferation and are associated with tumour formation: 1. Chemical carcinogens, 2. Radiant energy and 3. Viruses.

Many of the changes within the cell prior to complete malignant transformation are known.

CHEMICAL CARCINOGENS

Historically, chemical agents were the first to be associated with cancer; nowadays many chemical carcinogens are known and their number is continuously increasing associated with (a) industrial process and changes in (b) diet and (c) social habits.

Industry	Tumour	Chemical responsible
Aniline Dyes	Bladder cancer	Naphthylamine
Mineral Oil and tar	Skin cancers	Benzpyrene and other hydrocarbons
Plastics	Angiosarcoma of Liver	Vinyl chloride monomer
Insulation	Mesothelioma	Asbestos (carcinogenic activity depends on the **physical** configuration of the fibres)

Diet
It is possible that chemicals in food are carcinogenic. Nitrosamines and aflotoxins are examples; some modern synthetic additives and flavourings are potential carcinogens.

Social habits
The increasing urban concentration of population increases exposure to the combustion products of organic compounds, some of which are carcinogenic, and smoking and chewing of tobacco are associated with cancers of the lung and mouth.

Note: Chemical carcinogens may act in two ways:
1. Directly at the site of application or portal of entry, e.g. skin and lung cancers
2. Through degradation products either at the sites of metabolism or excretion, e.g. liver and urinary tract tumours.

CARCINOGENESIS

CHEMICAL CARCINOGENESIS (continued)

This is a multistep process of long duration.

The stages of **initiation** and **promotion** are important and are exemplified in experimental skin carcinogenesis.

(1) **Normal skin**

Application of Benzpyrene (carcinogen)

(2) **INITIATION**
Skin appears normal but important changes have occurred in the cell nuclei

(3) **PROMOTION** — initiated by e.g. croton oil, turpentine (co-carcinogens).

Visible surface and histological changes are seen.

(a) Keratosis and papilloma formation

(b) Dysplasia

Proliferation of epithelium

Congested vessels

New fine collagen fibrils

Lymphocytes

These stages are reversible

(4) **Appearance of MALIGNANT TUMOUR** — [An irreversible change]

Breech of basement membrane: **INVASION**

In rodents these changes take months; in humans the time scale is years and is exemplified in the skin, cervix uteri, bronchus, urinary bladder, colon and breast.

CARCINOGENESIS

RADIANT ENERGY

The dangers from this source have increased greatly in recent years.

Source of radiation	Possible tumours	Type of radiant energy
X-ray workers	Skin cancer, leukaemia	X-rays (ionising)
Administration of radioisotopes (therapeutic)	Various, e.g. thyroid carcinoma due to radioactive iodine	Atomic rays (ionising)
Industrial processes involving radioactive substances	Various	Atomic rays (ionising)
Atomic explosions	Skin cancer, leukaemia, bone cancer	Atomic rays (ionising)
Mining of radioactive substances	Lung cancer	Atomic rays (ionising)
Exposure to sunlight	Skin cancer	Ultraviolet rays (non-ionising)

Effects of radiations on cells

The ionising activity of X-rays and atomic radiations produce many changes in the chromosomes of cells.

Normal chromosomes — Radiation → Dysjunction — → Random fusion of broken ends — → Mutation

New clones of mutant cells arise which may produce tumour growth.

ONCOGENIC VIRUSES

Viruses have long been known to cause cancer in animals, and for several years a few human malignancies have been associated with specific viruses.

Recently the role of retroviruses in carcinogenesis has revealed new important intracellular mechanisms leading to malignant transformation.

In addition, vaccines have been manufactured against these viruses and have proved successful in the prevention of leukaemia in ANIMALS.

CARCINOGENESIS — VIRUSES

In *animals*: Examples of viruses associated with tumours are:

Virus	Type	Host	Tumour
Shope papilloma V.	DNA	Rabbits	Skin papilloma
Polyoma V.	DNA	Rodents Hamsters	Sarcoma
Rous sarcoma V.	RNA (acute)	Chickens	Sarcoma
Onco-retroviruses	RNA (slow)	Cats Chickens, etc.	Leukaemias and lymphomas

In *humans*:

Papilloma V.	DNA	Human	Skin papilloma Cervical cancer
Herpes group Epstein-Barr v (EBV)	DNA	Human	Burkitt's lymphoma
Hepatitis B.2.	DNA	Human	Liver cancer
Onco-retrovirus group Human T cell leukaemia virus (HTLV)	RNA (slow)	Human	Leukaemia and lymphoma

The **mouse mammary tumour virus** (Bittner milk factor) — an onco-RNA virus — is of interest; it is transmitted to offspring during suckling and results in breast cancer

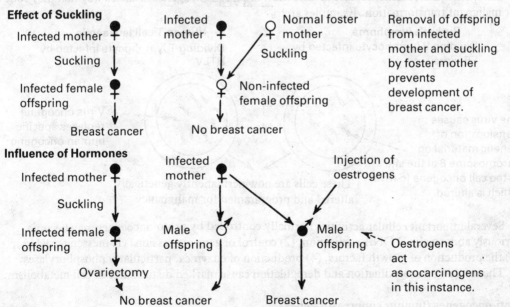

Effect of Suckling

Infected mother — Suckling → Infected female offspring → Breast cancer

Infected mother ♀ — Suckling — Normal foster mother ♀ → Non-infected female offspring → No breast cancer

Removal of offspring from infected mother and suckling by foster mother prevents development of breast cancer.

Influence of Hormones

Infected mother — Suckling → Infected female offspring — Ovariectomy → No breast cancer

Male offspring → Breast cancer

Infected mother ♀ — Injection of oestrogens → Male offspring → Breast cancer

Oestrogens act as cocarcinogens in this instance.

Comment: The development of breast cancer has been shown to be the result of the passage of the virus from the mother to the offspring. However, in addition to hormone status (illustrated above), age and the strain of mouse are other important co-factors determining the development of breast cancer. There is no clear evidence as yet linking a milk factor with human breast cancer.

197

CARCINOGENESIS — VIRUSES

Mode of action of oncogenic viruses
The essential feature is addition of new DNA to the nucleus of host cells resulting in mutants, but the way in which this is achieved differs in the two types of virus.

Oncogenes
The normal human cell nucleus contains genes — proto-oncogenes or cell oncogenes (c-onc) — which code for several important cellular activities. The oncogenic retroviruses contain genes (v-onc) which are homologous to the proto-oncogenes.

Oncogenic viruses either replace or alter the human cell oncogenes in such a way that they code for malignant transformation. Examples are:

Burkitt's lymphoma
Dividing B lymphocyte infected by EB virus

Human T cell leukaemia
Dividing T lymphocyte infected by HTLV

The virus causes translocation of genetic material on chromosome 8 at the site of the cell oncogene (c-myc) which is altered.

Virus oncogene replaces specific human oncogene

These cells are now permanently genetically altered and programmed for malignancy

Several important cellular activities normally controlled by proto-oncogenes may become seriously abnormal: (1) DNA replication, (2) control of gene expression (via messenger RNA), (3) the production of growth factors, (4) production of enzymes, particularly phosphorylases.

The resulting in-coordination and deregulation cause marked disturbance of cell metabolism.

Anti-oncogenes (tumour suppressor genes)
Another possible factor is the loss or defective functioning of these genes which are involved in normal cellular differentiation and inhibit the 'proliferative' activities of the proto-oncogenes.
Note: (a) Many abnormal cells are eliminated by the very efficient normal control mechanisms.
(b) It is not known exactly what changes are required to complete malignant transformation.

CARCINOGENESIS

CO-FACTORS (PROMOTERS) in CARCINOGENESIS

Numerous other factors appear to promote the occurence and rate of growth of cancer.

Sex. The incidence of cancer in the various organs of the body differs in the two sexes, but this is often due to environmental differences.

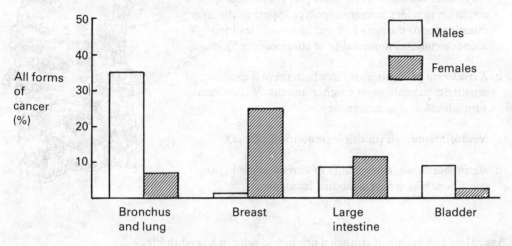

Race. The white races appear to be more susceptible to skin cancers due to lack of pigment which protects against ultra-violet radiations. Far Eastern, possibly mongol races, have an extremely high incidence of choriocarcinoma and lymphoepithelioma. Not all 'racial' incidences are genetically determined: local environmental factors are often operative.

Geography. There is undoubtedly a variation in the incidence of various cancers in different parts of the world. This is mainly a result of human activities — industrial processes, pollution, diet and social habits. In a few instances it may be related to natural background radiation in the soil, or parasites.

Hormones. In the female, the rate of growth of cancer of the breast and cancer of the uterine endometrium often appears to be dependent upon hormone secretion, usually oestrogen. Similary in the male prostate, cancer is stimulated by testosterone and depressed by oestrogen. There is however no real evidence that hormones of themselves cause cancer.

CARCINOGENESIS

CO-FACTORS in CARCINOGENESIS (continued)

Heredity. There are several well recognised genetic conditions which predispose to cancer:

(a) *Polyposis coli,* an excellent example, is a familial condition in which numerous polypi appear in the large intestine about the age of 20 and inevitably lead to adenocarcinoma (abnormality of chromosome 5).

(b) *Xeroderma pigmentosum,* in which there is excessive sensitivity to sunlight, is another hereditary condition which leads to skin malignancy.

(c) *Neurofibromatosis* (multiple tumours of nerves)

(d) *Retinoblastoma* (abnormality of chromosome 13) are conditions which have a familial incidence,

Age. Most cancers are of epithelial origin and arise in late adult life.
The possible reason for this is that normal cells of the body are recognised as 'self' and are left undisturbed by immunological mechanisms. Throughout life, abnormal mutant cells are produced during cell proliferation and these are destroyed.

- - - - - Normal cell persists

- - - - Abnormal mutant destroyed

Parent cell   Daughter cells

In later life, as control mechanisms break down, (a) the recognition and destruction of mutant cells is less active and (b) more mutant cells are produced and the chances of a malignant mutant arising are much increased.

Chronic irritation. This is rarely involved in carcinogenesis. Its role as a co-factor probably depends on the increased replication rate of damaged tissues being associated with an increased prevalence of random mutations.

Trauma. Malignant tumours are sometimes discovered after trauma but it is likely that trauma merely draws attention to a pre-existing malignant condition.

CARCINOGENESIS

CLONES and MALIGNANCY

A clone is a cell line derived from a single cell whose unique identifying characteristics are, by definition, passed to the daughter cells.

Monoclonal tumours

Certain tumours are composed of cells remarkably uniform in form and behaviour. In a few it can be shown by special methods that all of the cells are identical. A good example is plasma cell myeloma which produces multiple tumours of bone marrow. Plasma cells produce immunoglobulins, each cell producing one type of immunoglobulin. Using light chain markers it can be shown that a plasma cell myeloma is derived from a single cell — a monoclonal tumour.

Plasma Cell Myeloma

Plasma cells

Single type of immunoglobulin appears in blood

All cells identical and have arisen from a single cell — *monoclonal*

Monoclonal/multiple clone tumours

Although most tumours show a variation in cell type, and the more maligant the tumour the greater the variation is likely to be, there is strong evidence that they arise from the proliferation of a single transformed cell, i.e. they are monoclonal in origin. During subsequent tumour growth mutations account for the cellular heterogeneity. This explains why most cancers arise as a single focal lesion.

Postulated evolution of cancer

(1) Precancerous state
    e.g. dysplasia

(2)

(3) Carcinoma

Several cells show abnormality

One cell undergoes malignant transformation i.e. monoclonal proliferation.

Non-malignant neighbouring cells replaced.
Further mutation

Cells heterogeneous, malignant properties enhanced.

Field change

In a tissue or organ such as the skin and breast, precancerous cells may be present over a wide area. The chances of subsequent single cell transformation to malignancy are increased with the formation of separate tumour(s). Such a concept is important in surgical practice where the limits of excision should be wider than the field change.

201

CARCINOGENESIS — SUMMARY

A multitude of factors determine whether a proliferative lesion will progress to frank malignancy. Malignant change can be viewed as taking place by a series of steps — the *'multi-step theory of carcinogenesis'*. At each step, according to circumstances, the process can halt and may revert to normal or it may progress.

   Four stages can be recognised:

1. Stage of INITIATION

Normal cell

Chemical carcinogen

Radiation

Viruses

Two changes are involved at this stage.

(a) *Biochemical*

The 'carcinogenic' stimuli are converted into biochemically active substances.

Carcinogen

Chemical → Active biochemical molecules

Radiation → Active substances produced by ionising rays

Viruses → Viral DNA or RNA alter cell activities especially that of DNA

(b) *Interaction with cell components especially DNA*

The activated substances are positively charged molecules reacting vigorously with electrons, especially those in DNA. A variety of products are produced — altered forms of DNA. Some of these will revert to normal, but if others persist, they will be handed on to daughter cells thus forming new clones of cells with new potentialities. Viral RNA and DNA may actually be incorporated in the nuclei of cells.

An important mechanism by which these various nuclear changes may be unified is the production of abnormal oncogenic activity or the suppression of anti-oncogenes. The proliferative and control mechanisms within the cell are progressively seriously disturbed.

2. LATENT stage

These initiated cells are not yet autonomous and are still subject to normal controls. This accounts for the varying period between exposure to a carcinogen and neoplastic activity.

CARCINOGENESIS — SUMMARY

3. Stage of PROMOTION

The initiated cells may be 'promoted' be many substances. Promoters (co-carcinogens) exert a selective stimulation on initiated cells.

Initiated cell

Carcinogenic stimuli ⟶ (chemicals, viruses, etc)

Proliferation ⟵

Non-carcinogenic substances
e.g. Croton oil — skin tumours in mice.
Saccharin — bladder tumours in rats.
Prolactin — breast tumours in mice and rats.
Bile acids — colonic tumours in rats.

At the same time some of these substances may enhance the proliferative appearances by inhibiting normal cells.

In this phase there are often multiple areas of proliferation in a tissue or organ, but these lesions are focal and not yet malignant.

4. MALIGNANT CHANGES

Two possibilities exist at this point.

Promoted lesions

Reversion to normal   Persistance of lesions

The vast majority of such lesions disappear due to defence mechanisms, particularly an immune response.

In some of the lesions which persist, foci of morphologically altered cells ultimately appear. The changes are described in terms such as atypical hyperplasia, dysplasia and carcinoma-in-situ; reversal to normal is still possible.

The factors involved in the final step — the conversion of a single cell to the malignant state — remain unknown.

IMMUNOLOGY AND CANCER

It has been thought for a very long time that cancers stimulate immunological reactions. This is suggested by the following clinical observations:

(a) Some cancers do regress

(b) Secondary tumours are relatively rare in the spleen, presumably due to the ability of the spleen to destroy abnormal cells in the circulation

(c) In some tumours a lymphocyte response in the malignant tissue may be associated with a more favourable prognosis,

   e.g. some cases of carcinoma of breast.

Lymphocytic infiltration of stroma and tumour cell masses

Experimental investigations

Immunity to cancers can be induced in animals by the same methods as those used to immunise against infection. These methods include:

1. Injection of very small doses of tumour cells — too small to cause the development of neoplasm

2. Injection of tumour cells made inactive by irradiation or chemotherapy

3. Injection of parts of malignant cells especially cell membranes.

These are all forms of vaccination, but they only tend to be effective if given prior to implanting the tumour as a graft.

In the case of tumours induced by viruses, however, a vaccine of the virus can sometimes protect the animal, e.g. feline leukaemia.

IMMUNOLOGY AND CANCER

NATURAL IMMUNITY in ANIMALS

Both humoral and cell-mediated immunity can be demonstrated in animals bearing tumours.
Three features are of interest:

1. Antibodies have a protective role only when the tumour cells are in a fluid medium, e.g. leukaemic cells in the blood or tumour cells in body cavities.
2. In solid cancers, only cell-mediated (lymphocytes) immunity is effective.
3. Reaction is strongest in small tumours and disappears when they enlarge.

Blocking Factors

The observation of the third feature above and the fact that the injection of antibody may increase the rate of growth of a tumour have led to the discovery of 'blocking' or enhancement factors. The mechanism is as follows:

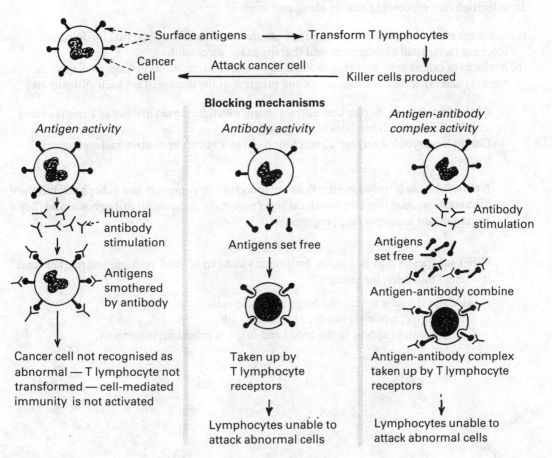

Normal cell-mediated immunity

Cancer cell — Surface antigens ⟶ Transform T lymphocytes

⟵ Attack cancer cell ⟵ Killer cells produced

Blocking mechanisms

Antigen activity

Humoral antibody stimulation

Antigens smothered by antibody

Cancer cell not recognised as abnormal — T lymphocyte not transformed — cell-mediated immunity is not activated

Antibody activity

Antigens set free

Taken up by T lymphocyte receptors

Lymphocytes unable to attack abnormal cells

Antigen-antibody complex activity

Antibody stimulation

Antigens set free

Antigen-antibody combine

Antigen-antibody complex taken up by T lymphocyte receptors

Lymphocytes unable to attack abnormal cells

IMMUNOLOGY AND CANCER

An interesting feature has been noted in experimental carcinogenesis: a virus may produce several different types of tumours, and vaccine of the cells of one tumour will induce protection against all other tumours produced by the same virus.

A chemical carcinogen can also produce several different types of tumour but immunity to one does not confer protection against another. Each tumour has its own specific antigens.

Immunological studies in man

The circumstances in man have similarities to those in animals.

1. Antibodies and specific cell-mediated immunity have been demonstrated in patients with cancer. In many cases, the antibodies react not only with the patient's tumour cells but also with the cells of similar tumours in other patients. This tends to suggest viral oncogenesis.

2. Blocking factors have been demonstrated.

   Investigations are proceeding mainly along two lines:

   (a) Attempts are being made to enhance the immune reaction in the hope that by doing so, blocking factors will be overcome and therapy made successful.
   (b) Antigens of cancer cells are being defined and these can be used sometimes as diagnostic markers and especially as a measure of the progress of the disease. Two such antigens are:

      (a) *Alpha feto-protein*. Serum concentrations are much increased in cases of hepatic cancer and certain germ cell tumours of the gonads.
      (b) *Carcinoembryonic antigen*. This is found in cases of cancer of intestinal and urinary tracts.

      Neither of these is truly specific. Both are found in other tumours and in hepatits, but the high concentration together with local signs may make them useful in diagnosis, and they are important in monitoring progress.

      Other substances may be formed by tumours and can be used as diagnostic markers and treatment monitors, for example:

      Acid phosphatase is secreted by prostatic cancers.
      5-hydroxytryptamine is produced by carcinoids.
      Catecholamines appear in the blood and urine in phaeochromocytoma.

CHAPTER 8

CARDIOVASCULAR SYSTEM

ARTERIAL DISEASES

Arterial diseases are very common and are important because of their serious effects on vital organs — particularly the brain, heart and kidneys — accounting for almost half the mortality in Western society.

The two most common are the 'degenerative' diseases.

(1) ATHEROMA (ATHEROSCLEROSIS)

(2) ARTERIOSCLEROSIS

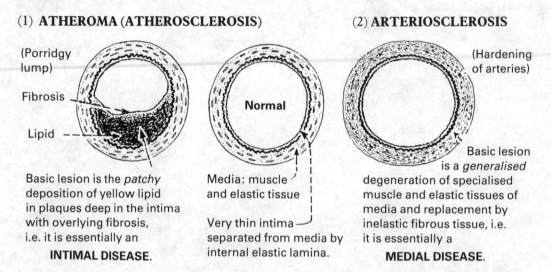

(Porridgy lump)

Fibrosis

Lipid

(Hardening of arteries)

Basic lesion is the *patchy* deposition of yellow lipid in plaques deep in the intima with overlying fibrosis, i.e. it is essentially an
INTIMAL DISEASE.

Normal

Media: muscle and elastic tissue

Very thin intima separated from media by internal elastic lamina.

Basic lesion is a *generalised* degeneration of specialised muscle and elastic tissues of media and replacement by inelastic fibrous tissue, i.e. it is essentially a
MEDIAL DISEASE.

These diagrams illustrate the diseases in their pure state. Because both are common diseases and share aetiological factors, they often occur together. However, it is important that they are considered separately since the mechanisms of damage are essentially different. To minimise the chance of confusion we will continue to use the term 'atheroma' rather than 'atherosclerosis'.

In other arterial diseases the important basic changes occur:

in the **intima** and /or in the **media**
where fibrous proliferation is common, where inflammatory or degenerative
e.g. in *endarteritis obliterans* changes occur
— small artery in e.g. in *polyarteritis nodosa*
base of inflammatory
ulcer.

Proliferation of fibrous tissue between intima and internal elastic lamina

Focal necrosis with acute inflammation in segment of arterial media

THROMBOSIS is by far the commonest complication of arterial disease, but haemorrhage and aneurysm formation are also important.

ATHEROMA

Atheroma is a disease of Western countries, of gradual onset but progressive. It may have little effect for many years, but serious chronic disease is often the end result or at any time there may be a dramatic fatal or near fatal episode due to sudden complications such as thrombosis.

Evolution of the disease

(Vessel opened longitudinally)

Cross section

Microscopic appearances

EARLY PROLIFERATIVE PHASE

Pale yellow streaks slightly raised above surrounding intima

Internal elastic lamina

Intima

Proliferated smooth muscle cells containing lipid droplets

Normal media

PROGRESSING PHASE

Raised yellow plaques

Reduction of lumen

Atrophic media

Necrotic smooth muscle cells

Hyaline fibrous tissue

Lipid pool part extracellular with cholesterol crystals

LATE ULCERATIVE PHASE

Raised irregular rough ulcerated plaques. Partly calcified with thrombus material on surface

Lumen narrowed and distorted
Branch vessel orifice narrowed and distorted

Media atrophied and thin

Thrombus

Fibrous tissue with vessels (form of 'healing')

Partly calcified lipid. Degeneration of elastic lamina

ATHEROMA

Fibrosis in the intima and media may lead to aneurysm formation, but the most important complication of atheroma is **THROMBOSIS**.

Local factors at the site of the atheromatous plaque are important:

1. Intimal roughening or distortion with eddying of flow
2. Thin, easily damaged intimal surface
3. Rupture of new capillaries in plaque with haemorrhage into the plaque

In addition, general factors influencing blood coagulability are important, e.g. smoking affecting vessel contractility and platelet function.

Results

(1) Medium and small arteries — coronaries, cerebrals

Usually occlusion by red thrombus

Atheromatous plaque

(2) Larger arteries — aorta, carotids. lumen usually too large to be completely occluded

Paler platelet thrombus on intimal surface

Small emboli may be detached — esp. to kidney, legs and brain.

The important sites of atheroma and the effects due to complications are:

CEREBRALS (Circle of Willis or branches) CAROTIDS — Generalised chronic ischaemia of brain — senile dementia.

Acute local ischaemia — cerebral softening (infarction).

CORONARIES —— Chronic ischaemia of heart muscle with fibrosis. Acute infarction.

ABDOMINAL AORTA — ANEURYSM, embolism to legs.

RENAL ARTERIES —— CHRONIC ISCHAEMIA OF KIDNEYS.

Visceral arteries —— Chronic ischaemia of bowel.

Lower limb arteries —— (Upper limb arteries are rarely affected) *NB* Collateral circulation is usually good; atheroma must be very severe before chronic ischaemia with intermittent claudication and/or gangrene develop.

In severe cases of atheroma, most of these sites may be affected, but not uncommonly, one particular artery may be much more severely damaged than the others, e.g. coronaries, cerebrals.

ATHEROMA

MECHANISMS INVOLVED

1. Intimal smooth muscle proliferation

Actual cause is unknown, but experimental evidence suggests the following:

Mechanical stresses   Smoking   Angiotensin   Hypoxia   Antigen/antibody complexes

↓

Endothelial damage

↓

Platelet deposition

↓

Platelets release cell proliferative substance

↓

Proliferation of intimal smooth muscle

2. Patchy anatomical distribution

There is a preferential distribution of lesions, e.g. arch of aorta, coronary arteries, cerebral arteries, carotids, abdominal aorta.

This is determined by local mechanical stresses which potentiate local endothelial damage.

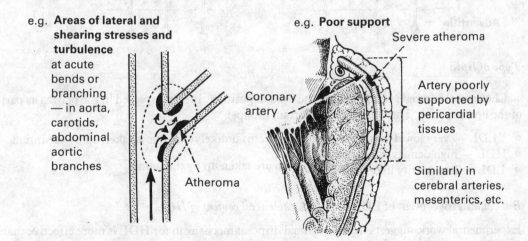

e.g. **Areas of lateral and shearing stresses and turbulence** at acute bends or branching — in aorta, carotids, abdominal aortic branches

Atheroma

e.g. **Poor support**

Severe atheroma

Coronary artery

Artery poorly supported by pericardial tissues

Similarly in cerebral arteries, mesenterics, etc.

ATHEROMA

MECHANISMS INVOLVED (continued)

3. Lipid deposition

This is related to (a) the ability of the intima to metabolise lipids, (b) the types of lipid and possibly (c) the type of smooth muscle.

1. *The ability of the intima to metabolise lipids*

Normal

Intima is metabolically active: nourished by diffusion of gases and soluble chemicals including soluble lipids from lumen under filtration pressure

Endothelium

Intima

IMPERMEABLE elastic lamina

Media

Media nourished by capillary system

Adventitia

Atheroma

Increased soluble blood lipids

Lipids are taken up by smooth muscle cells.

Failure to metabolise properly.

Aggregation against impermeable elastic lamina in insoluble forms (cholesterol or low density lipo-protein).

Watershed area — least well nourished ? Oxygen or enzyme deficiency

Type of lipid

Cholesterol is a main component of the lipid deposition. It is transported in the plasma as part of the lipo-proteins. There are three important groups:

- VLDL — very low density lipo-protein. It seems unlikely that this is taken up by the intima
- HDL — high density lipo-protein ⎫
- LDL — low density lipo-protein ⎬ Both are taken up by the intima

But cholesterol content of LDL = 22.5 × *cholesterol content of HDL.*

Experimental work suggests that the intimal disposal mechanism for HDL is more effective than for LDL.

Atheroma is common in Western countries where the *diet is rich in lipids.* These lipids are mainly of animal origin and *contain large quantities of cholesterol.*

ATHEROMA

MECHANISMS INVOLVED (continued)

Type of smooth muscle cell

An enzyme often has several different forms — isoenzymes. Normally, cells of any particular tissue are polyclonal, i.e. while each cell may possess one isoenzyme all the isoenzymes will be represented in the tissues as a whole and they will be able to deal with all the chemical variations of metabolic substances.

On this basis, an interesting suggestion has been made for which there is some evidence:

Endothelial damage
↓
Proliferative stimulus
↓
Growth of single clone of smooth muscle cells
↓
Isoenzyme deficiency
↓
Reduced ability to deal with LDL

4. Another mechanism has been suggested — **The thrombotic (encrustation) theory.**

Formation of a plaque from platelet thrombus:

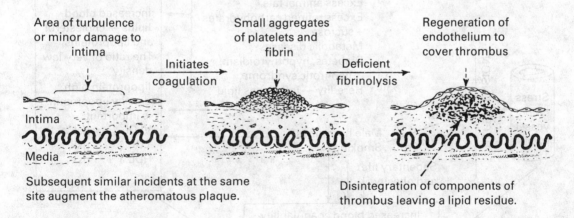

Area of turbulence or minor damage to intima → Initiates coagulation → Small aggregates of platelets and fibrin → Deficient fibrinolysis → Regeneration of endothelium to cover thrombus

Intima

Media

Subsequent similar incidents at the same site augment the atheromatous plaque.

Disintegration of components of thrombus leaving a lipid residue.

These theories are not mutually exclusive. Infiltration of lipids explains better the inital stages and the thrombotic theory is certainly relevant to the later stages.

213

ATHEROMA

BACKGROUND AETIOLOGICAL FACTORS

'Background' factors influencing the risk of or susceptibility to atheroma are multiple and interrelated.

AGE

Although there is a definite age relationship, age by itself is not a cause of atheroma; it reflects the duration over which other factors have been operative. The most important of these are illustrated in the classical victim of atheroma — the OBESE, HEAVY SMOKING, HYPERTENSIVE, SEDENTARY MALE

The major background factors may be grouped into two main categories:

1. **Endogenous** ∴ Not modifiable
   (a) SEX (i.e. male > female)
   (b) HEREDITY (evidenced
                in family history)

2. **Environmental** ∴ Modifiable
   (a) DIET — lipid and carbohydrate metabolism.
   (b) METABOLIC DISEASES.
   (c) HYPERTENSION
   (d) SMOKING

These background factors may act as follows: —

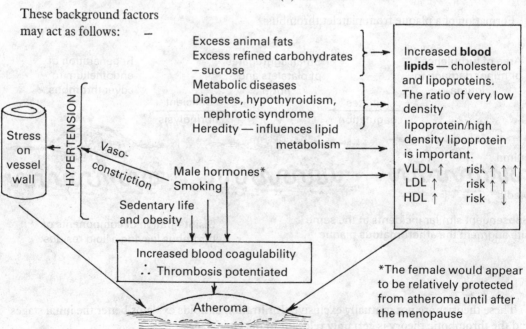

Stress on vessel wall

HYPERTENSION

Vaso-constriction

Excess animal fats
Excess refined carbohydrates – sucrose
Metabolic diseases
Diabetes, hypothyroidism, nephrotic syndrome
Heredity — influences lipid metabolism

Male hormones*
Smoking

Sedentary life and obesity

Increased **blood lipids** — cholesterol and lipoproteins. The ratio of very low density lipoprotein/high density lipoprotein is important.
VLDL ↑   risk ↑ ↑ ↑
LDL ↑   risk ↑ ↑
HDL ↑   risk ↓

Increased blood coagulability ∴ Thrombosis potentiated

Atheroma

*The female would appear to be relatively protected from atheroma until after the menopause

ATHEROMA

Population studies indicate that diet is the most important single factor related to *clinical* atheroma (e.g. patients suffering from coronary artery disease). A high intake of saturated fat involving a high cholesterol content is a constant feature in these cases. Other factors such as smoking, sedentary habits, obesity and hypertension are to some extent indicators of life style and probably act in an additive or precipitating manner in the clinical scene.

Atheroma is said to be more prevalent in soft water areas — the reason is not known.

Can modification of the environmental factors influence the progress of atheroma?

Yes, by:

(a) minimising further deposition of lipid

(b) minimising thrombotic complications

(c) perhaps allowing removal of some lipid from plaques — but, except in early cases, complete restoration to normal is not possible.

ARTERIOSCLEROSIS

ARTERIOSCLEROSIS usually affects all large and medium vessels.

Elastic and muscular tissues of media `- - -` replaced by fibrous tissue impregnated with calcium salts

Sometimes particular individual arteries are affected — e.g. arteries at wrist and temple

Normal

Soft, elastic vessel becomes harder; the collagen stretches so that lumen is **wider** and vessel becomes **tortuous;** as calcium impregnation increases the artery becomes very hard (pipe stem).

HYALINE ARTERIOLOSCLEROSIS affects the small branches of the arterial system (arterioles) — especially in the kidney.

Muscle replaced by hyaline material in media and intima

The arterioles also become tortuous

Normal

This is due to entry of blood plasma under the endothelium with protein deposition; gradual conversion to collagen occurs. The process is called **plasmatic vasculosis.**

Note that the lumen is usually narrowed so that ischaemia may be an important complication.

CONDITIONS ASSOCIATED

These changes, in mild form, represent the response of the arterial wall to wear and tear. The condition graudally progresses with **AGE,** usually in the arterial system generally, but individual arteries may be particularly affected, e.g. hard, tortuous temporal artery in old age. Certain diseases accelerate and aggravate arteriosclerosis:

1. Hypertension (high blood pressure) — a very important and common condition.
2. Diabetes (the small vessel changes are serious).

HYPERTENSION

HYPERTENSION (High Blood Pressure)

The normal BP in the large arteries of healthy young adult at the level of the heart is normally about 115/70 mmHg. These figures are means derived from a range — systolic ± 20, diastolic ± 10.

Mechanisms of normal maintenance of BP and the effect of age

The systolic pressure is governed by

(a) cardiac action
(b) the ELASTICITY and DISTENSIBILITY of the CONDUCTING ARTERIES.

AGE

normally is associated with

ARTERIOSCLEROSIS — loss of distensibility

∴ Increased SYSTOLIC pressure

The diastolic pressure is maintained by the **RESISTANCE (TONE)** of arterioles
(a subsidiary factor is blood viscosity)

ARTERIOLOSCLEROSIS — increased resistance

∴ Increased DIASTOLIC pressure

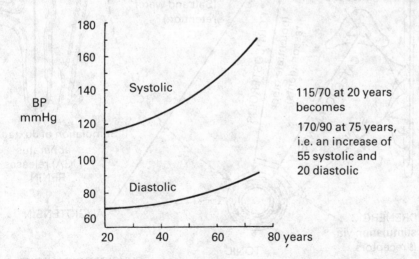

115/70 at 20 years becomes

170/90 at 75 years, i.e. an increase of 55 systolic and 20 diastolic

Because of this wide range in the normal population, the definition of hypertension is arbitrary.

Sustained DIASTOLIC pressures of 90 mmHg and above are commonly accepted as pathologically high, i.e. HYPERTENSION is present.

HYPERTENSION

AETIOLOGY

Complex interrelated effector mechanisms with feed-back controls regulate arteriolar tone. They are conveniently divided into two main groups:

(1) Nervous

Afferent stimuli from:
- External environment,
- Internal environment
  – higher cerebral centres
  – chemoreceptors
  – viscera

Vasomotor centre (VMC)

Adrenal medulla

CATECHOLAMINES

Sympathetic Nerves

'ADRENERGIC' stimulation via ß receptors

(2) Humoral (Hormonal)

(a) Pituitary

(b) SALT and water regulation

Anterior pituitary

Posterior pituitary

Kidney

Diminished afferent arteriolar perfusion

ACTH

Antidiuretic hormone (ADH)

Adrenal cortex

JGA

ALDOSTERONE

(Salt and water retention)

CORTICOSTEROIDS (potentiate other pressor agents)

Stimulation of Juxtaglomerular apparatus (JGA) releases RENIN

ANGIOTENSIN

TONIC VASOCONSTRICTION ⟶ PHYSIOLOGICAL LEVELS OF BLOOD PRESSURE

INCREASED ACTIVITY OF ANY MECHANISM ⟶ INCREASED VASOCONSTRICTION ⟶ HYPERTENSION

HYPERTENSION

In only 10 – 15% of all cases of hypertension is any disease which may be associated with disturbance of these mechanisms (see previous page) detectable — such cases are **SECONDARY HYPERTENSION.** Examples:

(a) **Kidney diseases,** especially if renal ischaemia is present, are the commonest cause of secondary hypertension.

(b) **Hyperfunction of adrenal cortex** } Cushing's syndrome — corticosteroid excess.
Conn's syndrome — aldosterone excess.

(c) **Tumour of adrenal medulla** (phaeochromocytoma) — catecholamine excess.

(d) **Drugs** may cause hypertension, e.g. the contraceptive pill, corticosteroids, sympathomimetics, monamine oxidase inhibitors if tyramine-containing foods (e.g. cheese) are eaten.

(e) Hypertension occurs in **toxaemia of pregnancy.**

(f) Miscellaneous rare diseases are:
— abnormalities of the vascular system e.g. coarctation (narrowing) of aorta
— increased blood viscosity — e.g. polycythaemia (increased RBC's).

In 85 – 90% of all cases of hypertension, no cause has been established — such cases are called **essential** or **idiopathic** or **primary.**

A plausible but speculative current theory is that in susceptible individuals the BP is unusually responsive to the afferent stressful stimuli which would normally be associated only with a mild rise.

Obesity is an important associated condition, and other background factors are relevant but the mechanism of their action is not well understood. Thus there is evidence of a FAMILIAL incidence, but the mechanism of inheritance is not clear. Although there are significant racial and geographical variations throughout the world, the explanation for them is not evident.

HYPERTENSION

CLASSIFICATION

In the classification of hypertension, in addition to the aetiology, two other main factors are considered.

(1) **Rate of Progress**		(2) **Height and rapidity of rise of the BP**	
Chronic — over many years	+	Usually only mild or moderate very slow rise. (*NB* the very old may have considerably higher BP without ill-effects)	**Benign** — during long course but eventually may have serious effects
Rapid (acute) — months or 1 – 2 years	+	Usually very high and rapidly rising BP, e.g. 120 + diastole	**Malignant** — serious damaging effects

Summary   Essential (85%)   Secondary (15%)

Benign   or   Malignant   Benign (usually endocrine type)   Malignant (often renal type)

COMPARISON of BENIGN and MALIGNANT HYPERTENSION

	Benign	Malignant
Aetiology	Usually ESSENTIAL If secondary, commonly of endocrine type	A few cases arise out of benign essential. Majority are SECONDARY TO RENAL DISEASE
Age	Begins younger than 45 years but is prolonged into 6 and 7 decades	Young adults 25 – 35 years
Sex	Female > Male	Female = Male
Incidence	VERY COMMON — at least 5% of population in Western societies	Rare
Course	VERY SLOW — many years	RAPID — months to 1 – 2 years
Blood pressure	Diastolic 90 – 120 mm Hg Very slow rise	120+ Rapid rise

HYPERTENSION

COMPARISON of BENIGN and MALIGNANT HYPERTENSION (continued)

VASCULAR CHANGES

	Benign	Malignant
Arteries	Accelerates ARTERIOSCLEROSIS; potentiates atheroma	Accelerates arteriosclerosis; causes INTIMAL FIBROUS THICKENING
Arterioles	Hyaline thickening	FIBRINOID necrosis of vessel wall and thrombosis, especially affecting kidney and abdominal viscera

Lumen narrowed but open

Necrotic media infiltrated by fibrin

Cellular reaction

Lumen occluded by thrombus

EFFECTS and COMPLICATIONS in VARIOUS ORGANS

	Benign	Malignant
Eyes	Arterial narrowing — retinal exudation.	Papilloedema; arterial narrowing; haemorrhage and exudates
Heart	Hypertrophy of left ventricle	Hypertrophy of left ventricle ± focal myocardial necrosis
Heart failure	60% of cases	Acute heart failure
Cerebral haemorrhage	Due to rupture of damaged artery — 30% of cases	Encephalopathy (fits and loss of consciousness) due to cerebral oedema
Kidney	Varying degrees of NEPHROSCLEROSIS but usually *not* serious.	Severe renal damage — death in uraemia
Other organs	No significant damage.	Focal necrosis, e.g. gut → perforation.

The effects and complications are proportional to the height of the blood pressure. Therefore drug treatment which lowers the BP lowers the incidence of complications, but the diseased vessels do *not* return to normal and organ perfusion may be inadequate at levels of BP which would usually be considered physiological.

OTHER ARTERIAL DISEASES

Compared with atheroma and arteriosclerosis, which are very common, other arterial diseases are rare. They may be considered within the following broad groups:

(a) **Degenerative,**
(b) **Inflammatory** and
(c) **Miscellaneous.**

DEGENERATIVE ARTERIAL DISEASES

Monckeberg's sclerosis (medial calcification)

This condition which affects elderly people is best regarded as a variant of the arteriosclerosis of old age. The media of the arteries of the legs particularly is the site of deposition of large amounts of insolube **calcium** salts, at first as circumferential bands but later becoming confluent so that the arteries become rigid tubes of hard chalk (pipe stem).
Note: The striking calcification, best seen on X-ray, is not associated with significant loss of lumen unless atheroma co-exists or is superimposed.

Erdheim's medial degeneration ("cystic medial necrosis")

In this rare disease the media of the proximal aorta and occasionally its major branches is abnormal: the musculoelastic tissues are patchily replaced by a weaker mucoid material. The aetiology is unknown, but similar changes in the aorta occur in Marfan's syndrome — an inherited disorder of connective tissue metabolism. Erdheim's degeneration may be an incomplete variant of Marfan's syndrome.

These changes are important becasue they are the cause of a particularly fatal form of aneurysm (see 'Dissecting Aneurysm', p. 228)

ARTERITIS

INFLAMMATORY DISEASES OF ARTERIES — ARTERITIS

(a) Associated with specific infectious diseases, e.g. tuberculosis and syphilis. The endarteritis and periarteritis, sometimes complicated by thrombosis, augment the damage caused by the infecting organisms.

(b) Arterial necrosis and inflammation of less certain or unknown aetiology.

Polyarteritis nodosa

This is a disease affecting the medium and small arteries and arterioles. In the acute phase, there are signs of generalised illness with fever, etc., but the disease often becomes chronic and relapsing so that all stages of the arterial lesion may be present at the same time.

The typical lesion is a focal necrosis of the arterial wall.

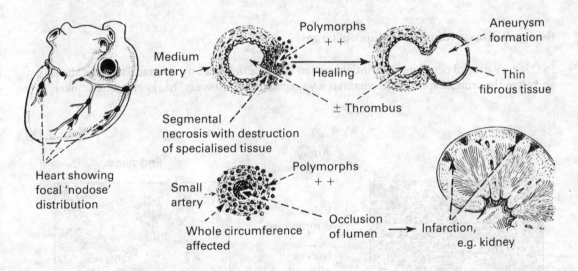

Any artery may be affected, but damage to the CORONARY or RENAL arteries is particularly important. When the arteries supplying peripheral nerves are affected symptoms of 'neuritis' may be striking.

Other forms of arteritis with some characteristics related to polyarteritis nodosa may occur as *primary disease processes*, e.g. *Wegener's granulomatosis* in which destructive lesions of the nasal mucosa, the lungs and the kidneys result from arteritis.

Arteritis may also complicate other conditions (usually the *connective tissue diseases*, see p. 820), e.g. rheumatoid arthritis, systemic lupus erythematosus (SLE).

ARTERITIS

Aetiology

In some of these conditions there is strong presumptive evidence that *hypersensitivity reactions*, due to antigen/antibody complexes (Arthus, i.e. Type III), damage the vessel wall. The antigens, a wide variety of agents, include drugs and microbial (esp. viral) components.

In some cases there is a further association with hypersensitivity reactions of the anaphylactic (atopic) type (Type I), and eosinophilia may be a feature (e.g. in some cases of allergic asthma).

Capillaries and venules may also be damaged and the more general terms VASCULITIS or ANGIITIS are then applied.

The aetiology of polyarteritis nodosa remains unproved — sensitivity to sulphonamides was the fashionable theory when these drugs were widely used. Nowadays, infection with hepatitis B virus (Australia antigen) with resultant antigen/antibody complexes has been shown to be important in some cases.

Buerger's disease (thromboangiitis obliterans)

In this very painful condition, the inflammation involves the small peripheral arteries of the legs and often the arms. Typically the victim is a young male (20-40 years) heavy cigarette smoker.

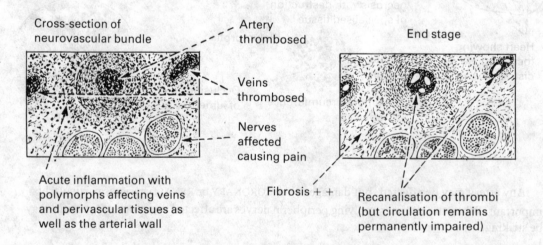

Cross-section of neurovascular bundle

Artery thrombosed

Veins thrombosed

Nerves affected causing pain

Acute inflammation with polymorphs affecting veins and perivascular tissues as well as the arterial wall

End stage

Fibrosis + +

Recanalisation of thrombi (but circulation remains permanently impaired)

GANGRENE may follow as more vessels become involved.

ARTERITIS

Temporal arteritis (Giant-cell arteritis/cranial arteritis)

This disease of unknown aetiology affects elderly people (over 60 years). It may cause severe facial pain and headache and may be associated with ocular symptoms; it very occasionally causes blindness. In a significant number of old people, there are no symptoms.

Some cases occur along with polymyalgia rheumatica — a disease in which there are generalised muscle pains and systemic malaise. Commonly, branches of the external carotid arteries are affected, but sometimes other caudal arteries and even the aortic arch may also be involved.

The arterial wall is destroyed by an acute necrosis associated with polymorph infiltration and usually thrombosis with partial organisation.

Acute — Occlusion by thrombosis — **Chronic** — **End stage**

Necrosis with polymorphs

Giant cells appearing in relation to fragments of elastic tissue

Vessel replaced by fibrous cord — no circulation.

Erythema nodosum

This condition presents clinically as red, tender subcutaneous nodules on the shins. Histologically, there is an acute vasculitis, particularly involving veins; a mixed inflammatory cellular infiltrate spreads into the subcutaneous fat.

The importance of this hypersensitivity reaction is that it is secondary to a wide range of infective processes or drug ingestion. Historically, tuberculosis or streptococcal infections were important common associations.

Takayashu's disease

In this rare disease, the typical victim is a young female (20 – 30 years). The patchy arteritis is more severe and affects the aortic arch and its primary branches, leading to ischaemia of BRAIN (cerebral arteries), EYES (ophthalmic arteries), FACE (carotid arteries), ARMS ('pulseless' disease), HEART (coronary orifices) in varying combinations.

DEATH often follows these serious effects.

ANEURYSM

A local enlargement of an artery is called an **aneurysm**. Although localised, it often reflects the presence of more widespread arterial disease.

MECHANISM of FORMATION

The two main forces concerned in the maintenance of the integrity of the shape of an artery are:

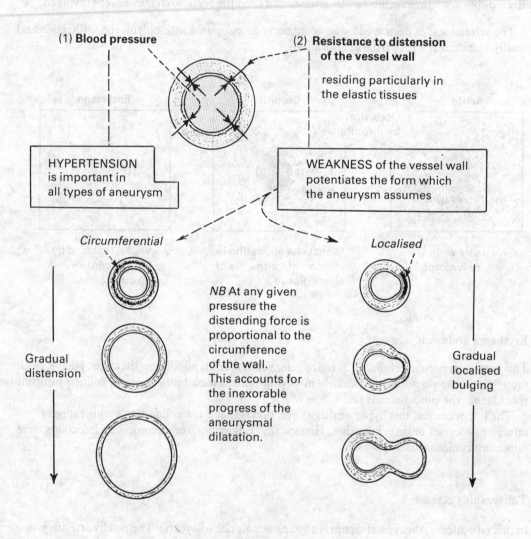

(1) Blood pressure

(2) Resistance to distension of the vessel wall

residing particularly in the elastic tissues

HYPERTENSION is important in all types of aneurysm

WEAKNESS of the vessel wall potentiates the form which the aneurysm assumes

Circumferential

Localised

Gradual distension

Gradual localised bulging

NB At any given pressure the distending force is proportional to the circumference of the wall. This accounts for the inexorable progress of the aneurysmal dilatation.

ANEURYSMS

TYPES of ANEURYSM

There are two main varieties:

(1) **Fusiform**   (2) **Saccular**

These are well illustrated in the aorta.

Fusiform aneurysm of abdominal aorta — usually due to atheroma; often below renal arteries and may also affect iliac arteries.

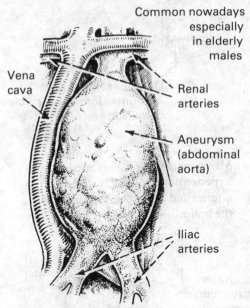

Common nowadays especially in elderly males

Vena cava

Renal arteries

Aneurysm (abdominal aorta)

Iliac arteries

Complications
1. Local pressure effects — usually not serious.
2. Thrombosis with embolism to legs.
3. Fatal retroperitoneal or intraperitoneal haemorrhage.

Saccular aneurysm of aortic arch — usually syphilitic but rare nowadays.

Vena cava

Aneurysm

Recurrent laryngeal nerve

(stretched)

Complications
1. Pressure effects
   (a) on nerves, e.g. recurrent laryngeal nerve paralysis
   (b) on bones e.g. vertebral, sternal or rib erosion
   (c) on neigbouring viscera, e.g. oesophagus, heart, lungs.
2. Fatal haemorrhage.

ANEURYSMS

OTHER VARIETIES of ANEURYSM

1. **Dissecting aneurysm**
   Classically begins in the
   arch of the aorta. Predisposing
   cause, e.g. medial
   degeneration (Erdheim).

Internal tear
through weak area

Blood tracking
proximally into
pericardium

Blood
tracking
in arterial
media — cutting off
major branches as it
proceeds

2. **'Berry' aneurysm** occurs in
   medium-sized vessels at the base of the brain,
   e.g. on Circle of Willis. Associated
   with congenital deficiency of arterial media.

Circle
of
Willis

Occasionally breaks back
into lumen forming a double-
barrel aorta

3. **Microaneurysm** — associated with
   hypertension and affects smaller
   arteries and arterioles, especially in
   the brain.

4. **Cirsoid (racemose) aneurysm**
   Tortuous complex of dilated
   arteries and veins.

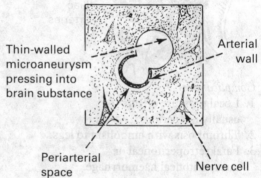

Thin-walled
microaneurysm
pressing into
brain substance

Arterial
wall

Periarterial
space

Nerve cell

ANEURYSMS

CAUSES of VESSEL WALL WEAKNESS

Congenital

(a) Potential weakness due to *deficiency of media and elastic lamina* at sites of branching — especially 'berry' aneurysms of Circle of Willis at base of brain.

Gap in elastic at site of aneurysm

(b) Developmental anomaly of arteries and veins — cirsoid type.

Traumatic —— Any type of aneurysm may result.

Acquired disease of arterial wall

(a) ATHEROMA and ARTERIOSCLEROSIS — these degeneration are the *most common and important* causes and are responsible for DIFFUSE, SACCULAR and occasionally DISSECTING aneurysms — especially in the ABDOMINAL AORTA.
(b) Syphilis — nowadays relatively rare; affects thoracic aorta.
(c) Erdheim's medial degeneration — causes dissecting aneurysm.
(d) Mycotic aneurysm — is due to bacterial infection.
(e) Arteritis — particularly polyarteritis.

COMPLICATIONS

1. Local pressure effects.
2. Rupture → haemorrhage: may be fatal,
   e.g. cerebral berry aneurysm → subarachnoid haemorrhage;
   aortic aneurysm → massive retroperitoneal haemorrhage
3. THROMBOSIS is often laminated and may be protective by preventing rupture but it often causes
4. Ischaemia in the distal territory. Ischaemia is also caused by dissection.
5. Rupture of dissecting aneurysm into pericardial cavity → cardiac failure (cardiac tamponade).

ARTERIAL DISEASES — MISCELLANEOUS

RAYNAUD'S PHENOMENON and DISEASE

Primary form

The phenomenon is essentially spasmodic attacks of pallor of the fingers (the toes, ears and nose may also be affected) due to intense constriction of the small arteries and arterioles in response to cold.

The condition is not rare and the usual sufferer is the young adult woman.

Mechanism

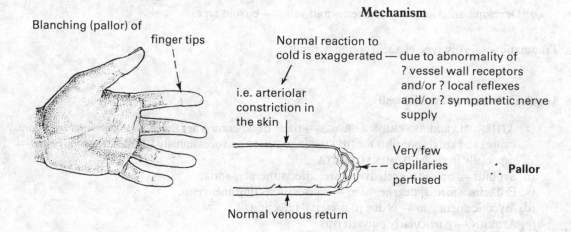

Blanching (pallor) of finger tips

Normal reaction to cold is exaggerated — due to abnormality of ? vessel wall receptors and/or ? local reflexes and/or ? sympathetic nerve supply

i.e. arteriolar constriction in the skin

Very few capillaries perfused ∴ **Pallor**

Normal venous return

In a variant, cyanosis accompanies the attack; neuromuscular control of the small veins is also disturbed.

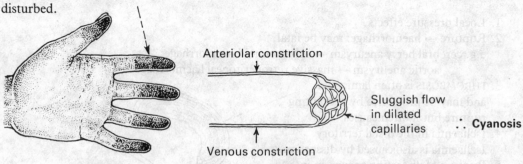

Arteriolar constriction

Sluggish flow in dilated capillaries ∴ **Cyanosis**

Venous constriction

This condition may continue for many years and NO PERMANENT DAMAGE RESULTS.

RAYNAUD'S DISEASE

The simple phenomenon is superseded by organic changes in the vessels — stenosis or occlusion — followed by degenerative changes in the skin and nerves of the fingers. Gangrene occasionally occurs. The term Raynaud's disease may be applied to this condition.

Fibromuscular thickening of wall

or

Occlusion by thrombus

or

Poor capillary circulation (permanent)

Trophic changes

Gangrene

The cause of this condition is unknown.

Secondary form

The phenomenon may occur as a symptom in other conditions, i.e. a secondary form of Raynaud's phenomenon. Examples include the 'connective tissue diseases', systemic lupus erythematosus (SLE) and systemic sclerosis (see p.821); cold agglutinins causing vascular blockage due to agglutination of red cells; the use of heavy pneumatic drills disturbing neurovascular controls in the hands.

In these circumstances the disease is serious and disabling, adding significantly to the damage caused by the primary diseases elsewhere in the body.

DISEASES OF VEINS

Diseases of the veins are important because they can be associated with:

(1) **_Acute_** severe, sometimes fatal, complications   (2) **_Chronic_** disability

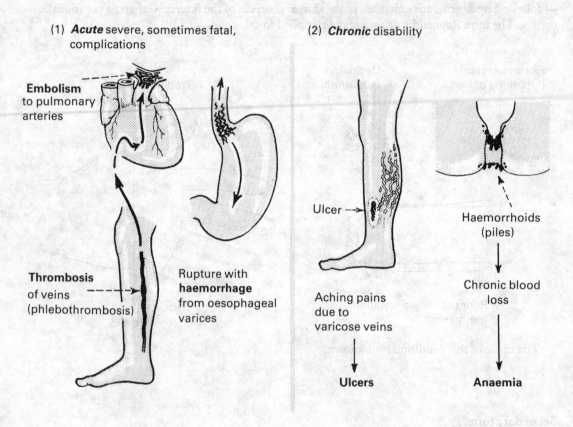

Embolism to pulmonary arteries

Thrombosis of veins (phlebothrombosis)

Rupture with **haemorrhage** from oesophageal varices

Ulcer →

Aching pains due to varicose veins

Ulcers

Haemorrhoids (piles)

Chronic blood loss

Anaemia

ACUTE PHLEBOTHROMBOSIS AND THROMBOPHLEBITIS

The veins of the lower limbs are very common sites of acute thrombosis, especially after surgical operations and during illnesses with enforced recumbancy (see p. 122).

In the majority of cases the thrombosis is the primary event and mild inflammation follows as a reaction. Phlebothrombosis is the preferred name.

Thrombophlebitis is reserved for cases in which the thrombosis is secondary to inflammation in or adjacent to the vein.

THROMBOPHLEBITIS

ACUTE PHLEBITIS

Suppurative (pyogenic)

Secondary to bacterial infection
e.g. a rare complication of
appendicitis.

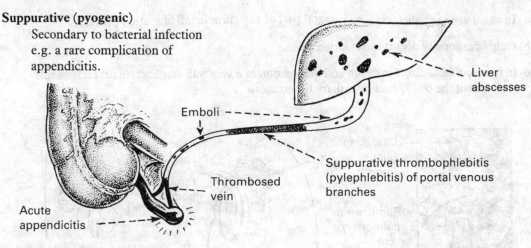

Liver
abscesses

Emboli

Suppurative thrombophlebitis
(pylephlebitis) of portal venous
branches

Thrombosed
vein

Acute
appendicitis

Migratory (thrombophlebitis migrans)

In this rare condition the thrombosis is not confined to the lower limb veins and can affect veins
anywhere in the body. A striking feature is the appearance and disappearance of thrombosis
apparently at random sites.

The mechanism is not fully understood but usually a malignant tumour is in the background —
sometimes the phlebitis is the first clinical sign of an occult tumour but more often it complicates
the terminal stages of tumour growth.

Possible mechanism

Circulating coagulation factors
derived from tumour (tumour
breakdown products or
inappropriate synthesis)

Fibrinolytic
system comes
into action

Initiation of
thrombosis in
small venous
radicles or
vasa vasorum
— local precipitating
factors not known

Formation of
loose red thrombus
in main lumen

Solution of fibrin
coagulum —
restoration to normal

233

THROMBOPHLEBITIS

CHRONIC PHLEBITIS

(a) In small venous radicles it is an integral part of any chronic inflammatory process.

(b) Only occasionally does it affect larger veins.

(c) In **tuberculosis,** direct invasion and destruction of a vein wall can liberate tubercle bacilli throughout the body, causing miliary tuberculosis.

Caseating hilar node

Rupture into pulmonary vein

Spread in blood

throughout body

Miliary tuberculosis

(d) **Hepatic venous occlusive disease** is a special type in which gradual occlusion of the hepatic veins and radicles is the result of gradual fibrous thickening of the venous intima and leads to serious disturbance in the liver. The disease is associated with the ingestion of alkaloids in 'bush' tea, particularly in the West Indies, but the mechanism is not known.

VEINS in MALIGNANT DISEASE

(a) Venules are easily invaded and infiltrated by carcinoma and are an important route in the metastatic spread of the tumour.

(b) Large veins, particularly in the mediastinum and pelvis, may be compressed from outside by the tumour — the resulting obstruction causing serious effects.

Suffusion and congestion of face

Oedema of neck

Tumour growth

Compression of superior vena cava by tumour

Compression of inferior vena cava

Oedema of legs

VARICOSE VEINS

This is a very common condition, the incidence increasing with **age,** and particularly high in **females** — often a sequel of pregnancy. The veins become prominent and tortuous and bulge outwards under the skin; the legs are particularly affected.

A **varix** is a localised bulge in a vein analogous to a saccular aneurysm in an artery. It is almost always associated with more generalised varicosity of the vein.

Aetiology

A vein wall, thin and composed of musculoelastic tissues, is designed to conduct blood at low pressures: the physiological movement of the blood is influenced mostly by pressure gradients derived from outside the vein wall.

Varicose veins arise when the vein wall is subjected to an increased expanding pressure (tension) over long periods.

Mechanism

Normal

Vein wall composed of interlacing bundles of muscle and elastic tissue

Increased pressure →

Intermediate stage of varicosity formation

Lumen dilated ∴ tension on wall increased. Moderate compensatory hypertrophy of elastic tissues

Prolonged increased pressure →

Late varicose stage

Irregular atrophy of specialised tissues (muscle and elastic) with fibrous replacement leads to stretching with tortuosity and localised bulging

VARICOSE VEINS

FACTORS WHICH INFLUENCE THE BASIC MECHANISM

(a) Acting on the vein wall

HEREDITY

OBESITY

? Weakness of
vein wall

Soft, virtually fluid
fatty tissue offers
poor support

? Defective
valves

Backflow

Normal —
no backflow

PERIODS OF
PROLONGED
STANDING

AGE

Simple
atrophy
of wall

Deprive vein of
benefits of
muscular
movement

(b) Increasing the intraluminal pressure

1. Obstruction to venous flow
   — usually in the pelvis — by:

   Pregnancy
   Tumour
   Constipation with
   loaded colon
   Thrombosis in veins
   (also may destroy valves)
   Constrictions on limbs.

2. Special anatomical considerations.

Gravitational
pressure
of a long
column
of blood

Special
communicating
veins between
deep and superficial
systems,
if not competent,
allow backflow
— greatly increasing
pressure
in superficial veins

VARICOSE VEINS

Effects

1. Symptoms of leg fatigue and aching pains.
2. Trophic changes — varicose eczema with pigmentation due to haemosiderin deposition — may proceed to ULCERATION: very slow to heal.
3. Haemorrhage is a rare complication.
4. Thrombosis is a frequent complication.
   NB Superficial venous thrombosis is not usually associated with embolism; deep venous thrombosis is the dangerous condition.

VARICOSE VEINS IN SPECIAL SITES

Oesophageal varices

Usually due to portal venous obstruction when portal-systemic venous anastomoses open up.

Haemorrhage

Complicated by serious haemorrhage which may be fatal.

Varicocele

Affects the pampiniform plexus: feels like a 'bag of worms'. It may cause dull aching and, because the increased vascularity raises the scrotal temperature, testicular atrophy is common.

The condition has been incriminated in some cases of infertility.

Haemorrhoids

Varices of the anorectal veins; usually associated with constipation.

Complications are: 1. *anaemia* due to chronic blood loss

2. acute *thrombosis* with pain (acute thrombotic pile)

237

DISEASES OF LYMPHATICS

The lymphatic vessels participate in disease processes in two main ways:

1. They afford a natural route by which diseases can spread.
2. They may become obstructed, with serious results.

1. LYMPHATICS as a mechanism by which DISEASE SPREADS

The small lympatics are delicate vessels formed by a simple endothelial layer with very little supporting tissue.

Large intercellular pores allow entry of bacteria, tumour cells and particulate matter (e.g. dust) which are subsequently transported by the flow of lymph either freely suspended or in phagocytes to the draining node.

The mechanism is important in the spread of

(a) infection and (b) tumour.

Malignant cells

Acute lymphangitis

The lymphatics draining an area infected by pyogenic bacteria (especially streptococci) may themselves become acutely inflamed.

Primary infection

Red streaks under the skin indicate inflamed lymphatics

Inflamed lymph nodes (lymphadenitis) may proceed to abscess formation

Chronic lymphangitis

This is well exemplified by tuberculosis in both the primary and reactivation types.

Primary focus (Ghon)

Spread to hilar nodes by lymphatics

Primary type

Peripheral spread from apical focus via lymphatics

Reactivation type

The lymphatics along the route of spread are thickened and show the typical histology of tuberculous granulation tissue.

DISEASES OF LYMPHATICS

LYMPHATIC SPREAD (continued)

Spread of tumours

This is an important route of spread of malignant tumours, especially carcinoma.

Disposal of particulate matter

This is well seen in the lungs where inhaled soot, especially in city dwellers, can be seen clearly indicating the lymphatic system under the pleura.

Soot (carbon) is relatively inert, but other dusts may initiate serious disease.

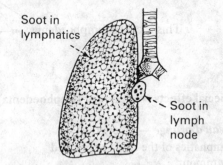

Soot in lymphatics

Soot in lymph node

2. LYMPHATIC OBSTRUCTION

This is usually secondary to acquired diseases. Only very rare cases are due to an inherited defect in the development of the lymphatics. The main causes are:

(a) Tumour growth

1. Obstruction by tumour permeation of lymphatics and/or destruction of lymph nodes, e.g. pelvic and groin nodes.

2. Direct pressure by large tumour mass.
   e.g.

3. Effects of treatment — scarring following surgery and radiotherapy.
   e.g.

Brawny oedema

Limb swollen by brawny oedema

Surgical excision and radiotherapy in axilla

(b) Relapsing chronic lymphangitis and chronic inflammation

(c) Blocking by parasites. E.g. the adult worms of FILARIA occuring in the tropics.

DISEASES OF LYMPHATICS

Effects of chronic lymphatic obstruction

1. **Accumulation of fluid** in the tissues causing brawny swelling of the affected part

2. **Low grade inflammation**

Causes fibrosis

Further damage to lymphatics and establishment of a vicious circle

This is called lymphoedema ← Aggravation

Special effects (varieties of lymphoedema)

Peau d'orange — where the lymphatics of the skin are blocked by tumour.

Elephantiasis — where a limb and/or the scrotum is massively enlarged due to filarial lymphatic blockage.

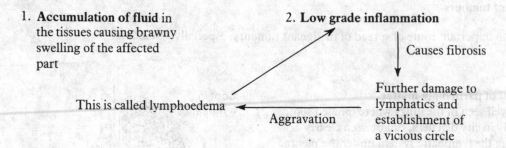

Peau d'orange surrounding ulcerated cancer of breast

Chylous ascites — where the thoracic duct is blocked either by tumour or filaria and fatty (milky) lymph accumulates in the abdominal cavity.

VASCULAR TUMOURS

The benign tumours of vessels are ANGIOMAS — the prefixes 'haem' and 'lumph' indicate the type of vessel involved. They illustrate well the difficulty of adequately defining the border line between true tumours (neoplasms) and hamartomas (developmental anomalies).

Since in many of these conditions vascular dilatation is a feature, the term ANGIECTASIS is sometimes applied and indicates clearly that neoplasia is not involved.

HAEMANGIOMAS are very common, occurring particularly in the skin as one type of birthmark but also in many solid organs. The ordinary tumours of blood vessels have been dealt with on page 190.

SPECIAL VARIETIES of ANGIOMA and TUMOUR-LIKE CONDITIONS

Occasionally specialised structures associated with blood vessels give rise to distinctive tumours:

1. (a) **GLOMANGIOMA** (glomus tumour) — arises from a specialised type of arteriolovenous junction which includes a rich neural component.
A common site is the finger tip, perhaps under the nail: a very small but often excruciatingly *painful tumour*. Microscopically it consists of a complex of blood vessels lined by endothelium but cuffed by round clear cells with contractile properties (myoid cells). It is rich in nerve fibres.

   (b) **ANGIOLEIOMYOMA** (related to glomangioma) is a tumour in which the surrounding cells are clearly of smooth muscle type.

   (c) **CHEMODECTOMA** — this benign tumour arises from specialised chemoreceptors, e.g. (1) glomus jugulare and (2) carotid body tumour.

Glomus jugulare arising from jugular bulb and growing into middle ear — may be complicated by severe haemorrhage at operation.

Carotid body tumour — a firm, smooth, ovoid, yellow-brown lump (potato-like) arising at carotid bifurcation.

Packets of small chemoreceptor cells separated by sinusoids and capillaries

VASCULAR TUMOURS

2. INFECTED ANGIOMA — PYOGENIC GRANULOMA

There is debate as to whether this is a pre-existing angioma in which infection has supervened, or whether it is granulation tissue in which exuberant capillary growth is the main feature. It is a striking lesion appearing on the skin at a site subject to trauma and infection, e.g. around the finger nails, the nostrils or the tongue.

It grows over several days to form a small red nodular excrescence up to about 1 cm in diameter and is usually ulcerated.

Pus cells

Sprouting capillaries

Narrow neck

The lesion is entirely benign despite its rapid evolution and responds to simple removal.

3. SCLEROSING ANGIOMA

This lesion, a variety of skin fibroma, is not a true vascular tumour.

4. TELANGIECTASIS

Small localised dilatations of small blood vessels. There are two main types: congenital and acquired.

(a) *Congenital.* In the rare hereditary haemorrhagic telangiectasis, the small lesions occur in the skin and mucous membranes and may be associated with bleeding (especially from the nose).

(b) *Acquired.* The small lesions, affecting the face and neck, are known as **spider naevi.**

The mechanism of their development is probably related to oestrogen excess, since they occur in pregnancy and in serious liver disease (oestrogen catabolism diminished) where they are an important diagnostic sign.

Dilated vessels

radiating from central vessel

VASCULAR TUMOURS

LYMPHANGIOMA

Lymphangiomas are much rarer than haemangiomas
and are usually without serious pathological
significance.

Sometimes the abnormal lymphatic vessels
become enormously distended and form fluctuant
swellings with local pressure effects,
e.g. 'cystic hygroma' of neck of babies and
children.

Gradually
expanding
'cyst'

SARCOMAS

The extremely rare *malignant tumours* of vessels are classified as **sarcomas** and are true neoplasms.

Haemangiosarcoma (haemangioendothelioma) of the liver is of special interest in that it has
occurred in workers in the plastics industry exposed to vinyl chloride.

Kaposi's haemorrhagic sarcoma occurs particularly in male Africans as multiple skin lumps
with eventual extensive visceral involvement. It may also occur in the 'acquired
 immunedeficiency syndrome'.

 Lymphangiosarcoma is a very rare complication of redical mastectomy for breast carcinoma.
The destruction of the axillary nodes and lymphatics at the time of operation followed by
scarring causes lymphoedema. After many years lymphangiosarcoma may supervene as
multicentre subcutaneous nodules. In some cases the differential diagnosis between recurrence
of the original breast cancer and a sarcoma of lymphatic vessels is difficult.

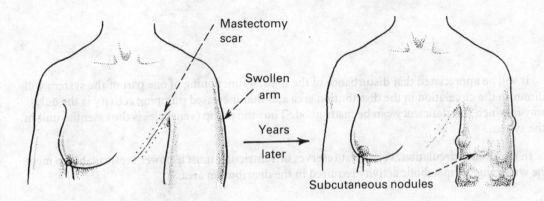

Mastectomy
scar

Swollen
arm

Years
later

Subcutaneous nodules

CARDIAC FUNCTION

The essential function of the heart is to provide the pumping action in a closed circulation.

Comparison with a simple mechanical system is useful and valid provided that it is appreciated that the animal system is infinitely more sophisticated with delicate built-in controls and balances which influence the inotropic (intrinsic contractility) activity of the heart.

It will be appreciated that disturbance of the normal functioning of one part of the system will diminish the circulation in the distribution area and that increased pumping activity is the only way in which this deficiency can be made good. Thus the pump (ventricle) is the essential unit in the system.

In the animal circulation, very great reserves of ventricular muscle power are available to meet the wide range of metabolic activity required in the distribution area.

HEART FAILURE

Heart failure occurs when the *ventricular muscle* is incapable of maintaining a circulation adequate for the needs of the body (usually assessed in terms of O_2 requirement).

Although, in the last analysis, heart failure is the result of myocardial failure, it is useful to separate the situations in which heart failure occurs into two main groups:

1. Diseases PRIMARILY affecting the MYOCARDIUM (PUMP)

(a) ISCHAEMIC HEART DISEASE
This is the most common and a very serious disease of the heart. The primary disease – atherama and thrombosis – in the coronary arteries leads to

MYOCARDIAL DAMAGE...
... FIBROSIS or INFARCTION

(b) INFLAMMATION and TOXIC DEGENERATION of the MYOCARDIUM (MYOCARDITIS)

(c) INFILTRATIONS of the MYOCARDIUM and CARDIO-MYOPATHIES

(2) Diseases of other cardiac and circulatory components leading secondarily to muscle failure.

(a) CONTROL MECHANISM DEFECTS

Nodes

Cardiac arrhythmias (inefficient pumping action)

S.A.

A.V.

Valvular disease increases work load

Bundle of His

(b) DISTRIBUTION DEFECTS

Systemic hypertension

Chronic lung disease causing pulmonary hypertension

Increased work load

LOSS OF MYOCARDIAL EFFICIENCY
INITIATION OF COMPENSATORY MECHANISMS
↓
FAILURE OF COMPENSATORY MECHANISMS
↓
Further LOSS OF MYOCARDIAL EFFICIENCY
↓
HEART FAILURE

245

HEART FAILURE

COMPENSATORY MECHANISMS

The myocardial reserve is provided by three main mechanisms:

1. Increased rate of pumping
2. **Dilatation** of the ventricular chambers (due to increased muscle stretching) ⎫ are designed to meet the normal physiological reserves
3. **Hypertrophy** is added to these when the pumping load exceeds physiological level.

    In the heart under pathological strain, all three mechanisms are operative and can compensate for considerable derangement.

DILATATION

In physiological conditions, the volume of the ventricular chamber at the end of diastole directly influences the pumping force of the ventricular muscle thus:

The larger the chamber size
(i.e. the longer the initial fibre length) ⎫------- the greater the
(i.e. the greater the fibre stretch) contracting force.

             End-diastole   Mid-systole   End-systole

Atrium

Normal

Ventricle

Physiological Dilatation

Greater cavity volume
Muscle fibres elongated   GREAT INCREASE IN EXPULSION FORCE

This physiological dilatation also compensates in cardiac disease.

HEART FAILURE

Compensatory mechanisms — Dilatation (continued)

In cardiac disease, particularly in cases of valvular incompetence, dilatation which occurs passively to accommodate the regurgitated blood is an important factor.

Aortic valve incompetence is a good example:

NORMAL HEART — DIASTOLE

Atrium

Ventricle

Aortic valve closed — back flow prevented

AORTIC INCOMPETENCE — DIASTOLE

Back flow through valve which cannot close properly

Dilated chamber to accommodate blood regurgitated from aorta as well as normal input from atrium

HYPERTROPHY involves an increase in muscle fibre bulk; the increased muscle mass is able to deal with a greater work load. In its pure form, hypertrophy is seen best in cases of increased pressure load.

RV HYPERTROPHY

(a) Most commonly seen in pulmonary hypertension due to chronic lung disease

(b) Also in mitral valve disease which causes pulmonary hypertension

Normal

LV HYPERTROPHY

(a) Most commonly seen in HYPERTENSION

(b) Also in aortic valve stenosis

At first the blood supply to the hypertrophied muscle increases to meet the increased metabolic requirements.

247

HEART FAILURE

FAILURE of COMPENSATORY MECHANISMS

The increased efficiency derived from all three mechanisms is limited, and beyond this limit serious deficiency ensues — HEART FAILURE.

Beyond the critical limit:

HEART RATE fails to compensate	DILATATION fails to compensate	HYPERTROPHY fails to compensate
At high rates there is not sufficient time for complete emptying during systole.	The increased force of contraction is lost ∴ residual blood in chamber.	(a) The muscle mass has outgrown its blood supply. Impairment of (b) utilization of nutrients, (c) response to chemical and neural stimuli, (d) inotropic activity.

Vicious circle set up

HEART FAILURE
↓
INCOMPLETE EMPTYING
↓
DILATATION AGGRAVATED

Thus in most cases of heart failure there is CARDIAC ENLARGEMENT due usually to a combination of hypertrophy and dilatation.

The **Effects** of heart failure are seen in the peripheral organs and are due to HYPOXIA and VENOUS CONGESTION.

(a) **Hypoxia** is well exemplified in the acute form of left ventricular failure where cerebral function may be seriously disturbed with transient loss of consciousness — Stokes-Adams attacks.

In the chronic forms of heart failure, the **weakness and fatigue** which are so common symptoms are probably effects mainly of **hypoxia,** but damage to organs is more difficult to define since the effects of venous congestion and water retention are added.

(b) **Venous congestion** and the more important complication, oedema, have been dealt with on page 136.

Breathlessness (dyspnoea) is almost a constant concomitant of cardiac failure and is essentially due to venous congestion and fluid retention within the lungs.

In severe failure, particularly when bed rest is obligatory, *hypostatic pneumonia* and *pulmonary embolism* (from leg vein thrombosis) may be serious and terminal complications.

HEART FAILURE

ACUTE and CHRONIC

Assignment to a particular category depends on the **suddenness of onset** and **rate of development.**

The causative diseases and the effects are different.

	Acute	Chronic
Time factors	Instantaneous Sudden (Hours — a few days)	Weeks Months
Causal diseases	(a) ACUTE CORONARY ARTERIAL OCCLUSION with infarction or arrhythmia (b) Pulmonary embolism (c) Severe malignant hypertension (d) Acute toxic myocarditis	(a) Chronic hypertension (b) Myocardial fibrosis (coronary intimal atheroma and hypertension) (c) Chronic valvular diseases (d) Chronic lung diseases (e) Chronic severe anaemia
Effects	May be no time for compensatory mechanisms to be initiated. Acute pulmonary oedema is common. May be acute ischaemic effects in brain and kidneys.	Compensatory mechanisms fully developed — hypertrophy and dilatation. Chronic oedema and chronic venous congestion.

Acute and chronic failure are at opposite ends of a spectrum but may merge into each other in two ways.

Partial but not complete recovery
(natural or response to treatment)

Acute failure   →   **Chronic failure**

Sudden deterioration
(natural or failure of treatment)

HEART FAILURE

LEFT (LV) and RIGHT (RV) and COMBINED VENTRICULAR FAILURE

The simple diagram on page 244 illustrates a single ventricle and distribution area. In the human, the system consists of two circulations in sequence (series) and the heart acts as both the pump and the connecting link. The right ventricle is the pump for the pulmonary circulation and the left for the systemic circulation. The causes and effects of right and left ventricular failure are different.

The pulmonary circulation

A low pressure system
    Mean systolic arterial pressure =
        15 mm Hg
    Pressure gradient, artery/vein =
        8 mm Hg

The systemic circulation

A high pressure system
    Mean systolic arterial pressure =
        120 mm Hg
    Pressure gradient, artery/vein =
        90 mm Hg

Right ventricular mass
and coronary blood supply

$<$

Left ventricular mass
and coronary blood supply

Approx. 1 : 4

MAIN CAUSES of:

Right ventricular failure

Usually secondary to disease elsewhere, causing obstruction to pulmonary blood flow.

(a) LUNG DISEASE
e.g. emphysema, fibrosis, malignancy

(b) Some forms of cardiac valve disease, esp. MITRAL STENOSIS

(c) Congenital heart disease

(d) As a CONSEQUENCE of LV FAILURE

Left ventricular failure

1. Muscle weakness —
ISCHAEMIC HEART DISEASE
(due to coronary artery disease)

2. Excessive work load —
SYSTEMIC HYPERTENSION
Since these causes are so prevalent, LV failure is much more common than RV failure.

Less common causes are:

Aortic valve disease

Mitral incompetence

Congenital heart disease.

RA LA
RV LV

HEART FAILURE

RV, LV and COMBINED VENTRICULAR FAILURE (continued)

The main effects are the results of:

    (a) low output
    (b) 'backward' pressure

* INCREASE IN PULMONARY ARTERIAL PRESSURE — partly due to congestion; partly due to reflex nerve action

Low output to lungs — not usually significant unless the RV failure is a sequel to LV failure when low output contributes to deficient oxygenation of blood.

Dyspnoea (cardiac asthma) is a main symptom

Congestion of pulmonary veins and capillaries

Overfilling of left atrium

RA LA

RV LV

RV FAILURE

LV FAILURE

Low output

Overfilling of:

RIGHT ATRIUM
SYSTEMIC VEINS
and CAPILLARIES

CHRONIC VENOUS
CONGESTION and
OEDEMA

Anoxia in systemic circulation → Demand for oxygen

Cyanosis is the result of excess reduced haemoglobin in capillaries and venules.

* The increase in pulmonary arterial pressure is important because in most cases of chronic LV failure it eventually leads to RV failure (combined failure).

In mitral stenosis, RV failure is caused by this mechanism without LV failure.

251

HEART FAILURE

The distinction between right and left ventricular failure is valid and certainly useful from a clinical point of view.

However, it should be remembered that in health the function of both ventricles is closely integrated in that they have the same capacity, pump virtually synchronously and are constructed in such a way that layers of muscle fibres pass from one ventricle to the other.

This simplification of a very complex arrangement of muscle fibres shows layers passing between the two ventricles.

Superficial layer RV
Deep layer LV } ——

Superficial layer LV
Deep layer RV } ----

Thus the action of each ventricle is not isolated; it both influences and is influenced by the action of the other. Therefore, in addition to the combined failure which arises as a later consequence of left ventricular failure, (see p.264), cases which begin and progress as combined failure are not uncommon.

Effects

These are a combination of the separate effects of LV and RV failure which have been described above.

In particular, PLEURAL EFFUSION (Hydrothorax) is a common effect of chronic combined heart failure.

OEDEMA fluid is contributed:

(1) Through parietal pleural lining from systemic venules and capillaries (RV failure)

(2) From lungs through visceral pleural lining

(LV failure)

Oedema fluid

HEART FAILURE

LOW and HIGH OUTPUT FAILURE

By definition, in cardiac failure, output is low in respect of body requirements, and in most cases this output is lower than the usual normal output. Such cases are called **Low Output type.**

In a few conditions, the cardiac failure complicates a pre-existing state in which the output before failure was greater than normal. In these cases, the output is not sufficient to meet the body requirements but may still be higher than the normal. Such cases are called **High Output type.**

Low Output Failure

Normal   5 l/min

Failure   3 l/min

High Output Failure

Pre-existing high output to meet body requirements   9 l/min

Failure   7 l/min

Output still greater than normal

Causes

The common types of failure:

HYPERTENSIVE
ISCHAEMIC HEART DISEASE,
VALVULAR HEART DISEASE,
MYOCARDITIS

Diseases associated with increased blood volume:

CHRONIC ANAEMIA
ARTERIOVENOUS SHUNTING
or increased vascularity of tissues,
e.g. PAGET'S DISEASE OF BONE,
HYPERTHYROIDISM,
Following TRANSFUSION OVERLOAD.

In both types of failure, venous overfilling is an important sign, but in high output failure, venous overfilling is usually present before failure ensues, reflecting the increased blood volume.

ISCHAEMIC HEART DISEASE

The effects of cardiac ischaemia are of major importance in affluent Western societies, causing severe disability and a large proportion of deaths.

The ischaemia is almost always due to *atheroma* of the coronary arteries and its complications which cause occlusion or narrowing.

The EFFECTS are mainly exhibited in the ventricles, particularly the left.

The ischaemia may be of sudden or gradual onset, depending on the nature of the coronary artery disease.

	Causes	Effects	Clinical Effects
Acute ischaemia	Usually ACUTE CORONARY ARTERY OCCLUSION due to THROMBOSIS	Myocardial necrosis, i.e. INFARCTION, depending on several factors, e.g. site, size etc.	(a) SUDDEN DEATH (b) ACUTE ILLNESS with heart failure, cardiogenic shock, chest pain. (c) ARRHYTHMIAS (d) SILENT
Chronic ischaemia	Usually CORONARY ARTERY NARROWING (STENOSIS) with or without thrombotic occlusion of small vessels	MYOCARDIAL FIBROSIS	(a) ANGINA PECTORIS (b) LV failure RV failure or combined failure from the start

Although acute and chronic ischaemia are properly separated both in respect of their causes and effects, they are often related as follows:

Acute ischaemia (acute occlusion of artery causing infarction) → Healing with scarring (fibrosis) → Local chronic ischaemia (fibrosis)

Chronic ischaemia (gradual stenosis of arteries) — fibrosis → Acute thrombosis superimposed → Acute infarction (regional)

→ Severe narrowing of all arteries beyond critical point → Acute infarction (global)

CORONARY ARTERY DISEASE

Atheroma affecting the coronary arteries is essentially the same as atheroma affecting the arteries elsewhere in the body and is subject to the same type of complication and effects. Its major importance is that serious disease of the myocardium is a direct complication.

Atheromatous artery

Complications

(1) Gradual progressive narrowing of lumen

After 70% reduction in cross-sectional area has occured the effects of CHRONIC ISCHAEMIA in the distribution area are seen

(2) Acute occlusion due to thrombosis

ACUTE ISCHAEMIA in distribution area — MYOCARDIAL INFARCTION

Plaque

(a) 'spontaneous'

or (b) at site of haemorrhage into plaque

Note: Microemboli from a ruptured plaque may compromise the circulation in the distal arterial distribution, but major coronary embolism and other types of arterial disease are very rare causes of ischaemia.

Distribution of atheromatous plaques

(1) There may be only a few plaques, but because the sites of predilection are in the proximal parts of the arteries (usually within 3 cm of the origin from the aorta), the effects of occlusion are serious.

(2) Very numerous plaques throughout the arborisation on the surface of the heart.
Note: The small terminal arteries penetrating the myocardium are usually not significantly affected.

R.cor. art.

L.circumflex artery

L.ant. desc. artery

Aortic valve

(3) any combination of (1) and (2).

The site of ischaemic damage usually represents the distribution area of the diseased arterial branch.

255

CORONARY ARTERY DISEASE

COMMON SITES WITH REGIONAL DISTRIBUTION OF EFFECTS
The following are listed in order of frequency.

(1) LEFT CORONARY ARTERY — ANTERIOR DESCENDING BRANCH

Anterior part of
IV septum

Anterior wall
of LV

Apex of heart

(2) RIGHT CORONARY ARTERY

Posterior wall
of LV

Posterior part
of IV septum

(3) LEFT CORONARY ARTERY — CIRCUMFLEX BRANCH

Lateral wall
of LV

CORONARY ARTERY DISEASE

EXTENT OF DAMAGE

This depends on:

1. The inherited individual anatomical variation in distribution area, e.g. the calibres of the right coronary artery and the circumflex branch of the left coronary artery show considerable variation and are usually inversely related.

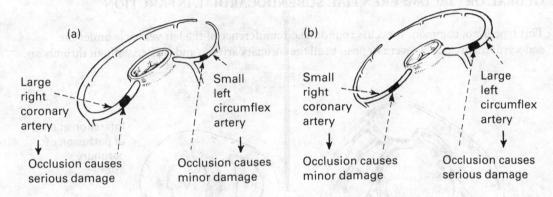

(a)

Large right coronary artery

↓

Occlusion causes serious damage

Small left circumflex artery

↓

Occlusion causes minor damage

(b)

Small right coronary artery

↓

Occlusion causes minor damage

Large left circumflex artery

↓

Occlusion causes serious damage

2. The efficiency of any anastomosis in the deprived distribution area. Gradual narrowing of an artery allows time for increased anastomosis to the deprived distribution area to develop, and so old age tends to be associated with improved anastomoses.

(a)

ACUTE OCCLUSION supervening on MINIMAL STENOSIS OF LUMEN

Left desc. branch

Minimal anastomoses

COMPLETE OCCLUSION is usually accompanied by myocardial infarction.

(b)

ACUTE OCCLUSION following GRADUAL STENOSIS of left desc. branch

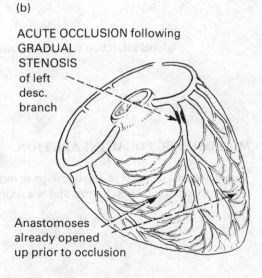

Anastomoses already opened up prior to occlusion

COMPLETE OCCLUSION may be accompanied by only minor damage.

ACUTE ISCHAEMIA — MYOCARDIAL INFARCTION

REGIONAL INFARCTION

This is the common type and is the direct result of coronary arterial occlusion usually due to **thrombosis.** (Regional infarction without thrombotic occlusion is very rare.)

GLOBAL OR CIRCUMFERENTIAL SUBENDOCARDIAL INFARCTION

This type is not common. It occurs round the circumference of the left ventricle under the endocardium in cases of severe stenosis of all the coronary arteries and is often without thrombosis.

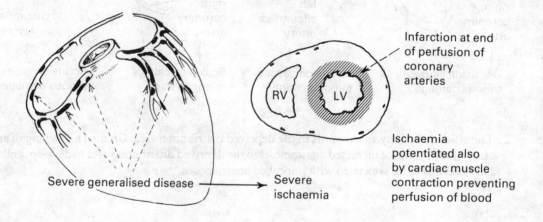

Severe generalised disease → Severe ischaemia

Infarction at end of perfusion of coronary arteries

Ischaemia potentiated also by cardiac muscle contraction preventing perfusion of blood

Global infarction is a serious, almost invariably fatal condition.

MICROSCOPIC FOCAL INFARCTION

This is necrosis of single or small groups of muscle fibres at the margins of areas of myocardium previously damaged by ischaemia and is a component of progressive chronic ischaemia.

MYOCARDIAL INFARCTION

Time			
		Normal appearance	No change
0 – 8 hrs	No change	RV / LV	
8 – 24 hrs	Minimal change	Slight blotchiness (congestion and pallor) of infarcted area RV / LV	Slight separation of fibres; slight increase of leucocytes between fibres; slight disturbance of cell cytoplasm *Normal* | *Affected fibres*
24 hrs – 3 days	Definite changes in dead muscle	Dead muscle, paler yellow Note: Usually a thin layer of healthy muscle under the endocardium RV / LV	Dead muscle fibres have lost striations and nuclei; cytoplasm glassy pink (H & E staining); capillary congestion at margin; polymorphs and macrophages increasing in number

MYOCARDIAL INFARCTION

Time			
3 – 10 days	Healing (organisation) commencing	Margin of congestion (redness) appearing round dead muscle and resorption of muscle becoming visible at the edges	Muscle fibres splitting up and being resorbed; granulation tissue at edges; polymorphs still present
10 days onwards	Healing well advanced	Broad zone of granulation tissue — translucent pink or gray; resorption of dead muscle well advanced	Well established granulation tissue with fibroblastic activity; cellularity now much less
Weeks — months	Scar tissue — healing complete	White fibrous tissue	Scar tissue — may be occasional surviving muscle fibres embedded

These changes represent the uncomplicated continuous process of healing. However, complications are frequent, producing serious, often fatal, effects.

MYOCARDIAL INFARCTION

Time	COMPLICATIONS
Minutes, hours	**1. ARRHYTHMIAS**

1. ARRHYTHMIAS

(a) *Ventricular fibrillation,* i.e. cardiac arrest (especially liable at onset of infarction and during first few days).

(b) *Block of impulse conduction in bundle of His and/or its branches* — usually causes slowing of ventricular rhythm or upsets the balance of ventricular contraction.

} **Acute heart failure —** *often FATAL*

2. CARDIOGENIC SHOCK

Associated with large infarcts.

3. THROMBOTIC COMPLICATIONS

(a) *MURAL THROMBOSIS*

Thrombus may form on endocardium over site of infarction

(b) *ATRIAL THROMBOSIS*

Thrombus may form in atrial appendages — especially if atrial rhythm is disturbed

} **Systemic embolism** (Brain, Intestine, Kidney, Lower limbs)

(c) *LEG VEIN THROMBOSIS*

Due to recumbancy and venous stasis

→ **Pulmonary embolism** may be FATAL

MYOCARDIAL INFARCTION

Time	COMPLICATIONS (continued)
3 – 14 days	**4. RUPTURE OF HEART** Potentiated by: (a) infarction of whole wall thickness (b) unusual increased polymorph activity before organisation is established → softening of dead muscle (myomalacia cordis) **Sites affected and results** (i) *MURAL MYOCARDIUM* 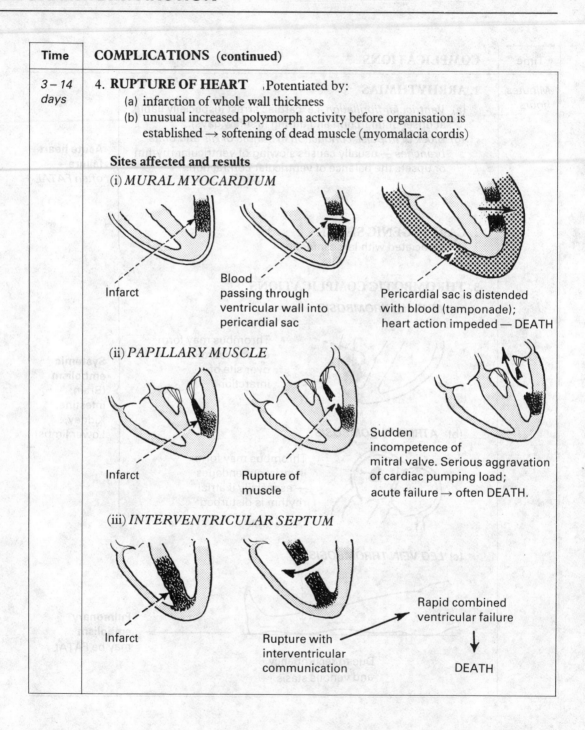

Infarct — Blood passing through ventricular wall into pericardial sac — Pericardial sac is distended with blood (tamponade); heart action impeded — DEATH

(ii) *PAPILLARY MUSCLE*

Infarct — Rupture of muscle — Sudden incompetence of mitral valve. Serious aggravation of cardiac pumping load; acute failure → often DEATH.

(iii) *INTERVENTRICULAR SEPTUM*

Infarct — Rupture with interventricular communication — Rapid combined ventricular failure ↓ DEATH

MYOCARDIAL INFARCTION

Time	COMPLICATIONS (continued)
3 – 14 days	**5. ACUTE PERICARDITIS** This may complicate the infarct.
Weeks	**6. CHRONIC HEART FAILURE** At the stage of fibrosis, chronic heart failure may supervene ($\pm$ ANGINA PECTORIS).
Months	**7. CARDIAC ANEURYSM** Laminated mural thrombus → may be embolism Gradual stretching of thin fibrous scar Bulging aneurysm formed Chronic heart failure Rupture with tamponade (rare) Sudden death
At any time	**8. RECURRENCE OF INFARCTION** Due to further thrombotic occlusion of a coronary arterial branch.

263

CHRONIC ISCHAEMIC HEART DISEASE

The basic pathological process is replacement of the myocardial fibres by fibrous tissue which is laid down in two main ways depending on whether the coronary insufficiency is due to severe generalised stenosis or is the result of local infarction following thrombosis.

(1) In severe generalised coronary artery disease

(2) The coronary thrombosis, infarction, healing sequence

A fine fibrosis separates fairly normal muscle fibres

A larger area of scar tissue with muscle fibres surviving at edges

However, in many cases both mechanisms are present and lesions merge indistinguishably into each other.

Myocardial fibrosis tends to be progressive, reflecting the progression of the atheromatous narrowing of the arteries.

Myocardial hypertrophy from any cause is an important contributory factor in many cases.

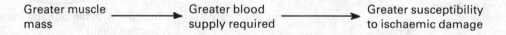

Greater muscle mass   ⟶   Greater blood supply required   ⟶   Greater susceptibility to ischaemic damage

Thus hypertension, which causes left ventricular hypertrophy, is an important background factor.

ISCHAEMIC HEART DISEASE

CLINICAL, LABORATORY and ELECTROCARDIOGRAPH (ECG) EFFECTS

Cardiac Pain is caused by muscle ischaemia as follows:

Diminished perfusion of muscle → Accumulation of pain producing chemicals (? kinins) in the area → Pain receptors stimulated

Oxygen deficiency

It is felt as a deep crushing pain in the anterior chest

May be referred in neck and jaws; the left arm and the upper abdomen

It occurs in two main circumstances:

1. **In acute infarction** — especially in the early phases before necrosis is complete. It is usually a continuous pain — *not* relieved by rest.

2. **In chronic myocardial ischaemia without infarction,** e.g. ANGINA PECTORIS — episodes of cardiac pain brought on by temporary ischaemia.

Pre-existing cardiac state
Coronary arterial disease
↓
Myocardial fibrosis and Limited perfusion reserves

Precipitating factors
Exercise
Emotional stress
Exposure to cold
A heavy meal
↓
Overloading beyond perfusion capacity but not severe enough to cause necrosis

Relieving factors
Rest, warmth, coronary arterial dilating drugs, e.g. nitrites.

ANGINA PECTORIS

Crescendo pain   Diminishing pain

Return to status quo

265

ISCHAEMIC HEART DISEASE

CLINICAL, LABORATORY and ECG EFFECTS (continued)
The blood in myocardial infarction

Leucocytosis
$12 - 15,000/mm^3$
lasting not more
than one week

Enzyme changes
Enzymes liberated from necrotic muscle.
Two commonly used in diagnosis:
1. Creatine phosphokinase (CPK) is
   fairly specific for cardiac muscle.
   Peak in 24 hours; falls in 72 hours.
2. Glutamic oxaloacetic transaminase (GOT)

Polymorphs mobilised
from marrow by
chemotaxis of necrotic muscle

Not specific for cardiac muscle.
Peak in 48 – 72 hrs; falls over 5 days.

These changes do not occur in angina pectoris since by definition necrosis has not occurred.

The Electrocardiogram (ECG)

The ventricular changes in ischaemia are reflected in the portion of ECG representing ventricular activity, i.e. the QRST complex. During excitation, contraction and restitution, the electrical potentials across the membranes of necrotic muscle fibres are strikingly different from healthy muscle. The ECG changes may be subtle but three common patterns are illustrated.

Normal

P
R
Q S
T

Ventricular excitation

Ventricular restitution

Infarction

(1) S T
Elevation of ST segment

(2) T
Inversion of T wave

(3) Q
Increased amplitude of Q wave

MISCELLANEOUS AFFECTIONS OF THE MYOCARDIUM

MYOCARDITIS

Inflammation of the myocardium may be caused by a variety of agents. The process is usually acute and may be generalised, regional or focal; the immediate effects are usually serious and cause heart failure, but full recovery is possible.

Agents	**Special features**	**Basic pathology**

Bacteria — *pyogenic.*
Direct invasion either from infected valves or by blood–stream.

Focal suppuration
Polymorphs ++

Muscle fibre damage — necrosis and lysis of individual or small groups

Toxins (incl. chemicals)
Classical example – diphtheria toxin circulating in blood.
Also in other severe infections e.g. typhoid, pneumonia

Usually generalised: muscle damage the main feature

Viruses
E.g. coxsackie B group

Usually generalised: interstitial inflammation the main feautre

Interstitial oedema and inflammatory cellular infiltrate

Immunological
E.g. rheumatic fever — myocarditis is an important component of the disease (see p.272 for details of special pathology).

Note: Nowadays the inflammation which is associated with ischaemia is *not* called myocarditis.

MISCELLANEOUS AFFECTIONS OF THE MYOCARDIUM

CARDIOMYOPATHY

This term, which strictly means 'disease of cardiac muscle' and could embrace every type of abnormality affecting the myocardium, has come to be conventionally used for conditions in which ischaemia, valve disease and inflammation have been excluded.

Primary cardiomyopathy

In this group the aetiology is not known.

Two main pathological abnormalities are present:

1. *Muscle hypertrophy* often of a particular anatomical component of the heart: histologically the enlarged muscle fibres may show a striking irregularity of orientation.

E.g.
Hypertrophy
of heart with
large septal
cushion
tending to
obstruct outflow
from left ventricle

2. *Fibrosis* may be the dominant feature. It is usually diffuse and often subendocardial, forming thick layers of fibroelastic tissue under the endocardium — disease occurs almost exclusively in Africa.

Secondary cardiomyopathy

In a second group, the cardiac muscle abnormality is associated with a miscellany of diseases and conditions. The main groups of associated conditions are:

        Nutritional — e.g. Beri-beri (thiamin deficiency)
                      Chronic alcoholism
        Drugs and Chemicals e.g. Emetrine.
        Metabolic diseases — Biochemical: (a) potassium and magnesium disturbance.
                                      (b) catecholamines, renin (acute excess).
                 — Infiltrations of heart muscle: amyloid, iron.
                 — Storage disease — glycogen.
        Endocrine disease — Thyroid abnormality.

      The changes in the heart muscle are protean, varying from subtle changes in individual muscle fibres to focal necrosis and fibrosis, and in many situations the mechanism of damage is not known.

MISCELLANEOUS AFFECTIONS OF THE MYOCARDIUM

FATTY INFILTRATION (ADIPOSITY)

The right ventricle is most commonly affected — fatty tissue penetrates between the muscle fibres but only in very severe cases contributes materially to cardiac insufficiency.

Epicardial fat

Penetrating into and separating muscle of RV

FATTY CHANGE

This reflects serious metabolic disturbance of the muscle cell and is usually caused by the action of toxins or hypoxia, particularly secondary to severe anaemia.

The muscle cells contain microscopic deposits of lipid; the change may be diffuse or in cases of severe anaemia may present as a dappled mottling under the endocardium

(thrush breast).

Lipid

ATROPHY OF HEART

This occurs in cases of starvation and generalised inanition associated with the terminal stages of cancer. The presence of lipofuscin in the muscle cells may give the heart a striking brown appearance.

Normal heart

Epicardial fat replaced by gelatinous tissue

Coronary arteries

straight

Wt 300g

Atrophy

tortuous due to muscle shrinkage

Wt 150 g

Thin muscle fibres with pigment (lipofuscin) deposition

RHEUMATIC FEVER

In Rheumatic fever (acute rheumatism), a disease of children and young adults, inflammation affects the connective tissues at many sites, of which the **heart** is the most important.

Aetiology

There is a strong association with streptococcal sore throat. The streptococcus is important because it may share antigens with human tissues, particularly heart muscle.

In the current most plausible theory, the inflammation is regarded as being due to immunological reactions since streptococci are not found at the various local sites and the disease follows some 2 – 4 weeks after the throat infection.

Mechanism

Throat infection due to:

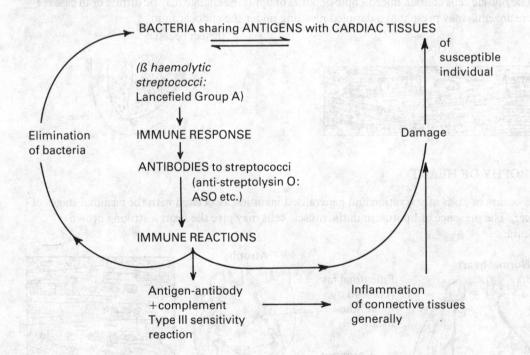

RHEUMATIC FEVER

In addition to the cardiac damage the disease is manifest in the following ways:

1. **General manifestations**
   Fever with sweating and malaise; raised ESR; polymorph leucocytosis.

2. **Indications of inflammation at local sites**

   (a) *Joints and adjacent musculofascial tissues* — causing arthritis often with effusion, muscle pains and weakness.

   (b) *Serous membranes*
   Pericardial and sometimes pleural effusion.

   (c) *Skin*
   (i) a surface rash — erythema marginatum
   (ii) small subcutaneous palpable nodules may be present over bony prominences subject to pressure. The histological appearances are striking. It is seen that the palpable nodule is an aggregation of microscopic rheumatic nodules.

The basic process is an acute non-specific inflammation in which exudation of a fibrin-rich fluid is a major component.

(a)
Serous surface
e.g. pericardium

(b)
Interstitial
connective tissues

Masses of fibrin on inflamed surface

Oedema — fibrin-rich fluid: perivascular inflammatory **cellular infiltrate** may be actual **vasculitis**

Central core of necrotic cell debris: mononuclear cells tending to a spindle shape and arranged in a pallisade. The surrounding tissues show the usual nonspecific inflammation.

   (d) *Central nervous system*
   Chorea – involuntary spasmodic muscular movements.

RHEUMATIC FEVER

CARDIAC MANIFESTATIONS

The inflammation is widespread throughout the heart, i.e. there is PANCARDITIS. It is convenient to consider the effects on the three anatomical cardiac layers separately — pericardial, myocardial and endocardial.

1. **Pericarditis** occurs during the acute phase of the illness and is an important cause of pericardial effusion.

2. **Myocarditis** is important during the acute phase and if severe can cause cardiac failure and death. The histological picture is striking and the presence of the Aschoff body is characteristic.

Oedema and lymphocyte infiltration between muscle fibres

Perivascular cellular infiltration

The Aschoff body

Central granular or hyaline debris with large mononulcear cells, some with multiple nuclei.

3. **Endocarditis.** Although there is a widespread histological inflammation, gross changes are seen usually on the endocardial sites subject to the greatest pressures and traumas, i.e. in the left side of the heart at the points of valve closure and at any sites of jet effect in the blood flow. The basic inflammation is complicated by ulceration of the valve surface followed by platelet and fibrin thrombosis in the form of small 'vegetations'.

Line of closure of valve

Valve opened up

McCallum's area on post.wall of L.atrium

Endocardium

Atrium

Swollen valve inflamed surface

Vegetation platelet and fibrin thrombus

Inflammation at base of valve

Ventricle

Rheumatic myocarditis

Vegetations

RHEUMATIC FEVER

Progression of the disease

In most cases the acute phase passes off and is followed by healing with various degrees of scarring. In a significant number of cases, no florid acute phase is noticed, and in a small number, a low grade chronic inflammation is present for long periods.

Clinical presentation	Pathology	Sequels

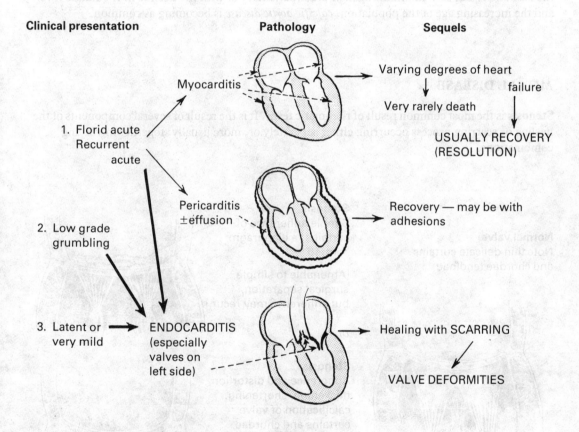

Clinical presentation

1. Florid acute
   Recurrent
   acute

2. Low grade
   grumbling

3. Latent or
   very mild

Pathology

Myocarditis

Pericarditis
±effusion

ENDOCARDITIS
(especially
valves on
left side)

Sequels

Varying degrees of heart
failure

Very rarely death

USUALLY RECOVERY
(RESOLUTION)

Recovery — may be with
adhesions

Healing with SCARRING

VALVE DEFORMITIES

Incidence

Since the advent of antibiotics (penicillin particularly), rheumatic heart disease, formerly very common in the temperate zones of the Western world, has declined. This is directly related to the decline in Type A streptococcal sore throat and to the successful prevention of recurrent attacks in susceptible individuals.

VALVULAR HEART DISEASE

The main causes are RHEUMATIC ENDOCARDITIS and DYSTROPHIC CALCIFICATION. Developmental anatomical abnormality and inherited deficiencies of the ground substance of the valve are rare causes. Nowadays, with the advent of powerful antibiotics, the late effects of healed infective endocarditis are assuming greater importance.

The MITRAL and AORTIC valves, subjected to much greater pressures, are more susceptible to damage than the tricuspid and pulmonic valves. *Rheumatic mitral disease* has been very common in the past and is still seen in middle aged or older patients, but with the decline in rheumatic fever and the increasing age of the population, *calcific aortic disease* is becoming as common.

MITRAL DISEASE

Stenosis is the most common result of rheumatic fever. It is the result of several components of the healing or scarring process occurring either separately or, more usually, together in varying combinations.

Normal valve
Note thin delicate curtains and chordae tendinae

Stenosis
Simple adherence of curtains: a diaphragm formed

[Amenable to simple surgical separation, but adherence may recur.]

or

Stenosis
Adherence and distortion, thickening, shortening, calcification of valve curtains and chordae resulting in 'funnel' stenosis

[Whole valve replacement required.]

MITRAL VALVE DISEASE

Mitral disease (continued)

Incompetence may follow from the rheumatic process by a similar slow mechanism.
In addition it may develop acutely due to other quite different causes:

1. In cases of left ventricular failure when severe dilatation occurs.

2. Necrosis with rupture of papillary muscle in acute myocardial infarction.

3. Rarely it results from abnormality of the ground substance of the valve — the 'floppy valve syndrome'. More cases of this condition are now being recognised using modern non-invasive techniques to study cardiac valve function in life.

The mechanical effects of mitral disease

Chronic stenosis — pure   *Chronic incompetence — pure (rare)*

In rheumatic heart disease, pure stenosis is not uncommon; incompetence usually occurs along with stenosis.

275

MITRAL VALVE DISEASE

Mitral disease (continued)

In mitral disease, the back pressure in the left atrium is transmitted to the pulmonary veins and by raising pulmonary arterial pressure causes effects on the right side of the heart.

(a) Compensated phase

(1) Left atrial dilatation
↓
(2) Pulmonary congestion
↓
(3) Right ventricular hypertrophy

(b) Congestive cardiac failure

(3) Right Ventricular Hypertrophy → (4) Dilated RV → (5) Dilated RA

In the acute types of mitral incompetence, the sudden change in the intracardiac haemodynamics very seriously aggravates the heart failure already present due to the primary disease.

Complications of chronic mitral disease

1. Atrial fibrillation is common.
   Fibrillation → Thrombosis in atrial appendage → Systemic embolism
2. Infective endocarditis.

AORTIC VALVE DISEASE

STENOSIS

The main causes are RHEUMATIC SCARRING and CALCIFICATION occuring in a congenitally abnormal valve or one previously damaged by rheumatism or endocarditis (bacterial), but in elderly people there may be no obvious pre-existing disease.

Changes in the valve

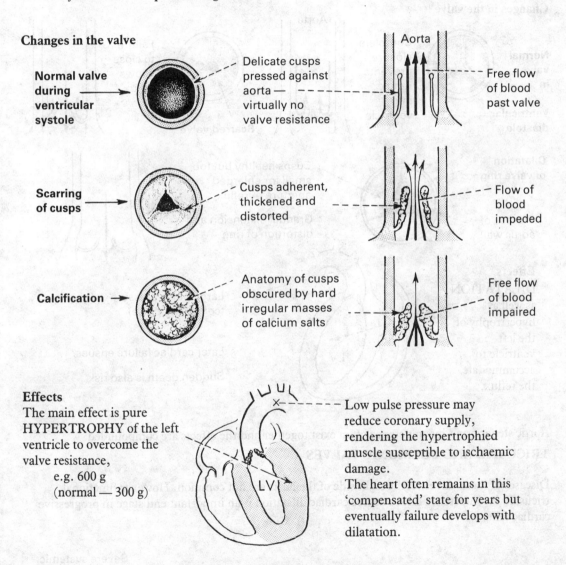

Normal valve during ventricular systole → Delicate cusps pressed against aorta — virtually no valve resistance

Aorta — Free flow of blood past valve

Scarring of cusps → Cusps adherent, thickened and distorted

Flow of blood impeded

Calcification → Anatomy of cusps obscured by hard irregular masses of calcium salts

Free flow of blood impaired

Effects
The main effect is pure HYPERTROPHY of the left ventricle to overcome the valve resistance,
    e.g. 600 g
    (normal — 300 g)

LV

Low pulse pressure may reduce coronary supply, rendering the hypertrophied muscle susceptible to ischaemic damage.
The heart often remains in this 'compensated' state for years but eventually failure develops with dilatation.

However SUDDEN DEATH (without pre-existing signs of failure) is a definite risk at any time, but particularly during exercise in cases of aortic stenosis.

AORTIC VALVE DISEASE

INCOMPETENCE

The main causes are rheumatic and infective endocarditic scarring of the cusps; rarely dilatation of the valve ring due to syphilis or hereditary disease (e.g. Marfan's syndrome).

Changes in the valve

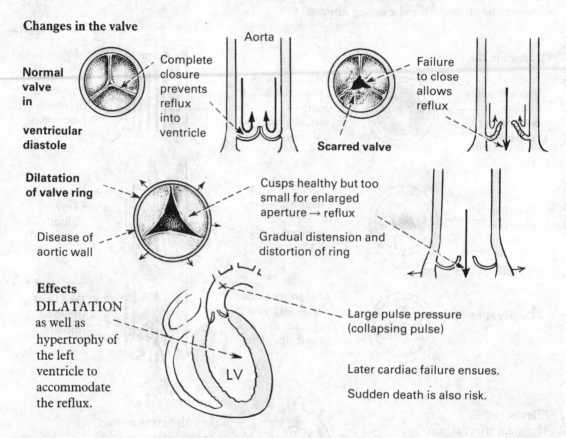

Normal valve in ventricular diastole

Aorta

Complete closure prevents reflux into ventricle

Failure to close allows reflux

Scarred valve

Dilatation of valve ring

Cusps healthy but too small for enlarged aperture → reflux

Disease of aortic wall

Gradual distension and distortion of ring

Effects
DILATATION as well as hypertrophy of the left ventricle to accommodate the reflux.

LV

Large pulse pressure (collapsing pulse)

Later cardiac failure ensues.

Sudden death is also risk.

Aortic stenosis and incompetence often exist together and the effects are compounded.

TRICUSPID AND PULMONIC VALVES

Diseases of these valves on the right side of the heart are not common. However functional tricuspid incompetence due to severe cardiac dilatation is an important end stage in progressive cardiac failure.

Progressive failure → Dilatation → TRICUSPID INCOMPETENCE → Right atrial failure → Severe systemic venous congestion (congestive cardiac failure)

INFECTIVE ENDOCARDITIS

This is a disease of the heart valves particularly: the mural endocardium is only occasionally affected by late spread from the valves.

In the classical situation, bacteria settle on previously diseased valves. The disease evolves in one of two main patterns depending on the type of bacteria.

(1)

Pyogenic bacteria, e.g. *Staph. aureus* present in local suppurating lesion

Bacteria enter blood stream

(2)

Low grade bacteria, e.g. *Strep. viridans* (mouth) coliform organisms (gut) *Staph. albus* (skin)

Many are destroyed by the body's defence mechanism — but some adhere to platelets and are deposited on the rough surface of a diseased vlave.

(a) acquired disease — usually rheumatic scarring

(b) congenital disease, e.g. bicuspid valve

The bacteria proliferate and, mixed with fibrin, platelets and leucocytes in varying proportions, form large *VEGETATIONS*.

ACUTE BACTERIAL ENDOCARDITIS
— Vegetations large and crumbling
— A loose mixture of organisms and fibrin mainly, with cellular debris

SUBACUTE BACTERIAL ENDOCARDITIS
— Large firm vegetations; fairly dense fibrin and platelet aggregations with bacterial colonies; few leucocytes

Local effects

Rapid destruction of cusps and chordae and spread of suppuration to adjacent heart muscle

Acute heart failure

Gradually increasing damage to valve cusps; minimal spread to adjacent structures.

Gradual heart failure

INFECTIVE ENDOCARDITIS

In addition to the local effects, the course of the disease is influenced by other important complications.

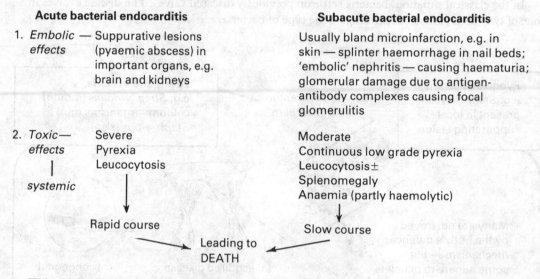

Acute bacterial endocarditis

1. *Embolic effects* — Suppurative lesions (pyaemic abscess) in important organs, e.g. brain and kidneys

Subacute bacterial endocarditis

Usually bland microinfarction, e.g. in skin — splinter haemorrhage in nail beds; 'embolic' nephritis — causing haematuria; glomerular damage due to antigen-antibody complexes causing focal glomerulitis

2. *Toxic effects* | *systemic*

Severe
Pyrexia
Leucocytosis

↓

Rapid course

Moderate
Continuous low grade pyrexia
Leucocytosis±
Splenomegaly
Anaemia (partly haemolytic)

↓

Slow course

→ Leading to DEATH ←

This classical situation is nowadays modified by immunosuppressive drugs, antibiotics and intracardiac prosthesis including catheter lines from peripheral veins.

Immunosuppression

This allows opportunistic infection by a much wider range of organisms, e.g. bacteria not usually pathogenic, and fungi.

Antibiotics

1. Their effects blur the distinction between the two types and allow healing but often with serious scarring of the valve.
2. The structure of the vegetation is important; in some cases the bacterial colonies are protected from the antibiotic.

Antibiotic in blood stream

Colonies embedded in firm fibrin, platelets and collagen

∴ Large prolonged dosage of antibiotic required

Cardiac prosthesis and catheter lines act as a focus for bacterial growth and infective endocarditis is a serious complication.

CARDIAC ARRHYTHMIAS

CARDIAC ARRHYTHMIAS and DISEASES of the CONDUCTING SYSTEM

Of the wide variety of cardiac arrhythmias which have now been studied in detail using the electrocardiograph, the majority are due to (A) functional disturbances of the intrinsic excitability of the cardiac muscle at various sites or of the cardiac neurohumoral controls; only a minority are due to (B) organic disease of the conducting system itself. Organic heart disease particularly of ischaemic type is a common concomitant.

(A) Important disorders of cardiac muscle excitability

(1) Atrial fibrillation

In this common disorder, continuous incoordinate movement of the atrial muscle completely negates its role as a priming pump and the atria become functionally inert.

There is no specific pathological change in the atrial wall, but atrial dilatation associated with cardiac disease is usually a precondition.

Predisposing conditions
Rheumatic heart disease
Ischaemic heart disease
Senile heart disease
Thyrotoxicosis
} Atrial dilatation (±atrial muscle hypertrophy) → Atrial fibrillation

Increased susceptibility to 'circus' rhythm

There are two main effects:

Dilated functionless atria

(i) *Contribution to cardiac failure*

(a) loss of atrial contraction to priming of ventricles

(b) *NB.* causes increased *irregular* ventricular rate

(ii) *Intra-atrial thrombosis and embolism*

Small thrombi forming in atrial appendages

Embolism to vital organs — brain, kidney, intestines (also legs) from left atrium.
Pulmonary embolism from right atrium.

2. Ventricular paroxysmal tachycardia and fibrillation

These very serious conditions are usually superimposed upon and aggravate pre-existing severe myocardial disease — usually ischaemic in type. In fibrillation, a form of 'arrest', cardiac function ceases; it is the terminal event in many fatal diseases.

CARDIAC ARRHYTHMIAS

Cardiac arrhythmia (continued)

B. **Diseases of the conducting system**

The usual disorder is slowing of the impulse and it is most often associated with organic disease in the adjacent cardiac tissue.

Associated conditions

Cardiac ischaemia — Acute infarction / Fibrosis — are the most common and important.

Others are — myocarditis, calcification around the valve rings and drugs, e.g. digitalis, propranolol.

Sites of disorder   **Effects**

SA node – Very rarely affected

AV node and Bundle of His

Heart block
1st degree: only mild delay in conduction
∴ no effect on ventricular rate
2nd degree: moderate delay, missed ventricular beats
3rd degree: complete block idioventricular rhythm established, 35 or less per min

Left and right bundles

Bundle branch block
Causes loss of efficiency of ventricular contraction

The 3 important components of arrhythmias are:
Tachycardia, bradycardia and irregularity.

The effect of any arrhythmia on cardiac function depends essentially on its effect on ventricular output.

Tachycardia
pulse rate over 160/min

Seriously aggravated by **Irregularity**

Bradycardia
— pulse rate less than 35/min

Diastolic time too short to allow adequate ventricular filling; also impairment of coronary flow

Low cardiac output

Failure

DISEASES OF THE PERICARDIUM

PERICARDITIS

Pericarditis is commonly a complication of diseases of the heart or adjacent structures or of generalised disorders; primary (or idiopathic) inflammation is rare.

In **acute pericarditis,** fibrin exudation is common: sometimes exudation of serous fluid is the main feature. Haemorrhage may be superadded in cases of uraemia and tumour infiltration. Purulent pericarditis complicating bacterial infections is rare.

Fibrinous pericarditis   **Pericarditis with effusion**

Cardiac surface covered by shaggy fibrinous exudate

Parietal layer

Tendency for layers to adhere and subsequently organise

Pericardial 'rub' may be heard clinically

Varying volume of yellow serous fluid (may be sufficient to embarrass cardiac action)

Very light deposit of fibrin on surfaces

Diseases which may lead to pericarditis

(a) *Intrinsic heart disease*

  (i) myocardial infarction

  (ii) acute rheumatism (pancarditis)

  (iii) trauma — esp. surgical myocarditis

(b) *Diseases in lungs, pleura and mediastinum*

  (i) tuberculosis

  (ii) carcinoma

  (iii) pneumonia complicated by empyema

(c) *Generalised disorders* (mechanism not known)

  (i) uraemia

  (ii) connective tissue diseases

283

DISEASES OF THE PERICARDIUM

CHRONIC PERICARDITIS is usually the result of recurrent attacks of rheumatism or allied diseases; occasionally it is insidiously chronic throughout. The basic changes are organisation and calcification. In extreme cases, cardiac function is impaired.

Venous ostia

Dense fibrous calcified tissues —
causing close adherence of the pericardial layers;
preventing proper cardiac filling;
causing stenosis at venous ostia leading
to severe venous congestion
— this extreme condition is called **constrictive
pericarditis**.

PERICARDIAL HAEMORRHAGE occurs most commonly as a result of cardiac rupture complicating acute infarction. The other main cause is rupture of aortic aneurysm back into the pericardium.

The pericardial sac becomes distended with blood (tamponade) and death follows rapidly due to compression of the heart.

Compression of heart

Cardiac rupture into pericardium

CARDIAC TUMOURS

Primary tumours in the heart are very rare. Secondary tumours, especially from the lungs, affecting the pericardium by direct spread and the heart by blood spread are fairly common and represent terminal stages in malignant disease.

The so-called cardiac 'myxoma' is a rare condition affecting usually the left atrium in which a smooth, pale, soft, rounded mass is attached by a pedicle to the endocardium. It can cause serious effects by occluding the mitral valve opening. It is not certain whether 'myxoma' is a true neoplasm or is the result of organisation of a ball thrombus in a particular way.

CONGENITAL HEART DISEASE

Developmental abnormalities of the heart are common; clincially significant defects occur in 6 per 1000 live births and 2 per cent of stillbirths. The severity varies from minor aberrations to complex distortions incompatible with life.

Aetiology

This is often obscure. Hereditary factors are of limited importance; possible environmental factors
    Examples include: virus infection, e.g. rubella; teratogen, e.g. thalidomide; altitude at birth (patent ductus arteriosus is commoner at high altitudes).

The initial damage which is sustained during the early formative stages in the 2nd and 3rd months of pregnancy is modified by later fetal and postnatal growth and development.

Single anatomical abnormalities occur, but often there are multiple defects which are associated in groups of which the more common are given specific names.

Abnormal development occurs:

(1) At the emergence of
   the great vessels
        ↓
   Stenoses cause impedence
   to blood flow

(2) During formation of the septa between
   right and left sides and following failure
   of closure, e.g. ductus and foramen ovale.
        ↓
   Abnormal apertures allow
   shunting of blood

Fallot's tetralogy illustrates these main points:

Pulmonary stenosis
↓
Right ventricular enlargement

Aorta over-riding
interventricular septal defect

Shunt from (R) to (L)

Mixture of venous and arterial
blood ∴ **cyanosis** —
a sign which distinguishes
one main clinical group

Often complications — pulmonary hypertension, increased blood volume polycythaemia, and occasionally infective endocarditis — increase the disability and failure is progressive.

RESPIRATORY SYSTEM

UPPER RESPIRATORY TRACT

ACUTE INFLAMMATIONS

These are the common inflammations of the nose, nasal sinuses, pharynx, larynx, trachea and bronchi. They are usually mild and self-limiting but may lead to chronic lesions. Generally they exhibit two phases according to the causal agents involved: the viral infection phase and the bacterial phase.

Viral infection phase

This phase is characterised by all the features of acute inflammation but without the cellular exudate.

Congestion of vessels

Oedema of tissues

Swelling of mucosa

Stuffiness of nose

Occlusion of ducts (partial or complete)

Excessive mucous secretion and exuded fluid

Absence of inflammatory cells

Abundant thin clear discharge

Viruses involved

A large number of viruses may cause acute inflammation of the upper respiratory tract.

1. Rhinoviruses — these are by far the commonest cause of inflammation of the nose (coryza). Coxsackie and Echo viruses may also be a cause. These three are small RNA viruses (picornaviruses).

2. Myxoviruses, e.g. parainfluenza viruses and respiratory syncytial viruses, cause laryngitis, tracheitis and bronchitis. The latter may result in severe bronchiolitis and pneumonia in infants.

   Influenza virus is also a myxovirus and may produce severe inflammation of the respiratory tract at any level.

   During the viral phase there is some loss of surface epithelium and the viral infection appears to make the mucosa susceptible to secondary infection, thus initiating the second phase.

UPPER RESPIRATORY TRACT

ACUTE INFLAMMATIONS (continued)

Bacterial phase

Bacteria, normally present in the nose and throat, invade the damaged mucosa, and the tissue reaction then shows the classical features of acute inflammation.

The infection is usually mixed; the bacteria commonly involved are *Streptococcus pneumoniae*, *Haemophilus influenzae*, *Streptococcus pyogenes* and *Neisseria catarrhalis*. In institutions where the use of antibiotics has resulted in resistant pathogenic strains colonising the environment, serious respiratory infection may result.

Since these inflammations can be caused by so many different viruses, and also since immunity is of short duration, repeated attacks are common. Chronic changes may be induced as a result.

RHINITIS

ACUTE CORYZA

This is the commonest form of upper respiratory inflammation (the 'common cold'). In almost all cases the inflammation involves not only the nose but other associated structures.

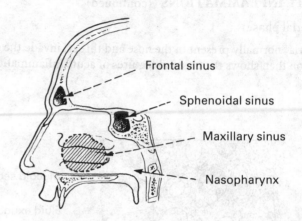

Frontal sinus

Sphenoidal sinus

Maxillary sinus

Nasopharynx

The two phases, viral and bacterial, are seen typically in this disease.

The drainage from the sinuses, especially the maxillary, is frequently obstructed by swelling of the mucosa. In such a case, a very acute suppurative condition may arise.

Rhinovirus and parainfluenza virus are the usual initiating agents, but acute rhinitis is also a feature of influenza and measles. The bacteria in the second phase are as previously stated.

Attacks are frequent in childhood and may result in a chronic condition with catarrhal discharge and nasal obstruction.

ALLERGIC RHINITIS

Acute respiratory inflammation is often of allergic type. The reaction has certain characteristics which differentiate it from ordinary, infective inflammation. The nasal form is commonly termed 'hay-fever'.

Tenacious mucus

Gross oedema of submucous tissues

Hyaline swelling of basement membrane

Very often the submucous oedema is so marked that the swelling becomes polypoid

Enlargement of mucous glands

Infiltration of eosinophils

Bacterial infection is commonly superadded and the exudate becomes mucopurulent. The repeated attacks frequently lead to chronic changes in the mucosa with polyp formation.

RHINITIS

NASAL POLYPS

These form particularly
on the middle turbinate
bones and within the
maxillary sinuses.

In the nasopharynx,
the lymphoid tissue may
be greatly enlarged
(adenoids) and contribute
to the nasal obstruction.

Gross oedema

Dilated
blood
vessels

Thickened
basement
membrane

Lymphocytes,
plasma cells
and frequently
eosinophils

Polypi

Adenoid

ALLERGIES

Seasonal allergy

This is due to pollens liberated from trees and grass.

Non-seasonal allergy

The main cause is the house dust mite,
Dermatophagoides pteronyssinus, but allergy
may develop to dust-containing animal or
human hair (dandruff), cotton or other fibres.

Feather pillow —
invisible infestation

VASOMOTOR RHINITIS

This is a clinical diagnosis. The pathological changes are, to some extent, similar to those of allergic
rhinitis, but the condition is more continuous, less spasmodic. Although the cause is unknown,
non-specific stimuli such as light or smells can precipitate an attack.

291

ACUTE LARYNGITIS AND ACUTE TRACHEITIS

These are usually mild conditions due to infection with adenoviruses or parainfluenza virus followed by secondary invaders *Streptococcus pneumoniae*, *Streptococcus pyogenes* and *Neisseria catarrhalis*. The pathological changes are as previously described. A very acute form (croup) due to the parainfluenza virus occurs in children.

Special types

Psedomembranous inflammation
This is an extremely severe form of laryngotracheitis.

Normal — Basement membrane

Membrane consisting of fibrin, necrotic epithelium and polymorphs

Congested vessels

It may be due to secondary invasion by *Staphylococcus aureus*, *Streptoccous pyogenes*, *Streptococcus pneumoniae* or more rarely *Haemophilus influenzae*. Acute fever, enlargement of the local lymph nodes and oedema are common. The larynx or epiglottis may become severely oedematous leading to respiratory obstruction. This is especially apt to happen in childhood. Spread to bronchi is frequent.

Diptheria, now uncommon in advanced countries, is a special form of pseudomembranous laryngitis. Usually it is due to spread from the pharynx. The corynebacterium diphtheriae is present in large numbers in the fibrinous membrane.

Secondary to endotracheal intubation

This can be a serious complication of treatment in intensive care units.

Prolonged intubation
↓
Excoriation of trachea
↓
Secondary infection ——————— Ulceration
(*Pseudomonas aeruginosa,*
Candida albicans)
Tracheo-oesophageal fistula ← Ulceration → Healing
↓
Tracheal stenosis

Secondary to specific infections

Serious acute oedema of the glottis (tissues above the vocal cords) may result from infection such as diphtheria, syphilis, typhoid fever, erisypelas, or spread of infection from tonsillitis. It is also a complication of agranulocytic angina. Death may occur due to suffocation.

Mild degrees of oedema of the glottis can occur in cardiac and renal disease.

CHRONIC LARYNGITIS AND CHRONIC TRACHEITIS

These lesions are characterised by two changes: (a) change in the lining epithelium and (b) increase in mucous secretion.

Vocal cords

Thickening of squamous epithelium

Hyperkeratosis

Larynx

Patchy squamous metaplasia

Lymphocytic reaction

Enlargement of mucous glands

The following sequence of events tends to take place:

Chronic laryngitis

Squamous metaplasia

Loss of ciliary action

Tendency to recurrent infection

Mucous gland hyperplasia

Increased mucous secretion

Retention of secretion

Spread of change to bronchi

Aetiology

Tabacco smoke is probably the most important factor in initiating and promoting this lesion. Once the metaplastic changes start, other factors such as atmospheric pollution and attacks of acute upper respiratory infection increase the severity of the condition.

Specific chronic inflammations

TUBERCULOSIS. This disease may cause severe ulceration of the larynx, especially in the region of the vocal cords and arytenoid cartilages. It is secondary to pulmonary tuberculosis.

SYPHILIS. Ephemeral lesions, mucous patches and superficial ulcers may be found in the larynx during the secondary phase of syphilis. Gummatous ulceration of the larynx may be caused by tertiary syphilis. Extensive ulceration can take place and the subsequent scarring may lead to stenosis.

293

TUMOURS OF UPPER RESPIRATORY TRACT

SIMPLE TUMOURS

Epithelial Epithelial tumours take the form of papillomas. They are usually single, but in children, multiple papillomas of viral origin affect various parts of the larynx.

Sites

Squamous cell

Transitional cell
(These tend to recur.)

Small non-neoplastic nodules of proliferations of both epithelium and connective tissue are common on the vocal cords (Singer's nodes).

Connective tissue

Haemangioma, occurring on the nasal septum, is the commonest and gives rise to persistent nose-bleeds. Other tumours are rare. A special form of angioma, angiofibroma, affects male children. It grows throughout childhood and may cause bone destruction; it usually regresses at adolescence.

MALIGNANT TUMOURS

These are, except in very rare instances, all carcinomata and most are of squamous cell variety.

Sites

The sites are the same as for simple papillomas. Some of them take origin from a transitional-celled papilloma. Changes resembling leukoplakia often precede and accompany malignant growths. In the larynx, those which arise on the true or false cords invade slowly and have a better prognosis. Ulceration destroys the local structures. Infected necrotic tissue may be inhaled and cause pneumonia.

Lymphoepithelioma, a carcinoma accompanied by masses of lymphocytes, is now considered as an anaplastic carcinoma invading local lymph tissue. It is common in Eastern countries and is associated with Epstein-Barr (EB) virus infection.

LUNGS — ANATOMY

ACINUS (PRIMARY LOBULE)

This is a sub-unit of pulmonary tissue consisting of respiratory bronchioles with associated alveolar ducts, atria and alveoli. Intercommunications exist between acini, and also between acini and terminal bronchioles. Thus disease can spread from acinus to acinus but, equally, functional deficiency in any part of one acinus can be compensated by by-pass mechanisms via these anastomotic channels.

SECONDARY LOBULE

This is the unit of pulmonary tissue served by a pre-terminal bronchiole. Self-contained and bounded by connective tissue septa, it has no anastomotic connections with other lobules.

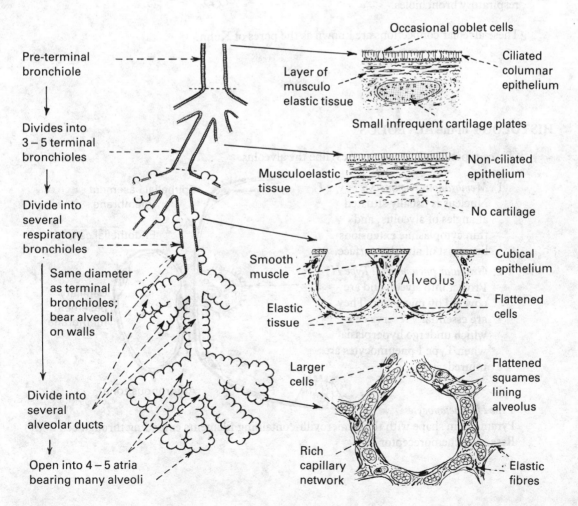

Pre-terminal bronchiole

↓

Divides into 3 – 5 terminal bronchioles

↓

Divide into several respiratory bronchioles

Same diameter as terminal bronchioles; bear alveoli on walls

↓

Divide into several alveolar ducts

↓

Open into 4 – 5 atria bearing many alveoli

Occasional goblet cells

Layer of musculo elastic tissue

Ciliated columnar epithelium

Small infrequent cartilage plates

Musculoelastic tissue

Non-ciliated epithelium

No cartilage

Smooth muscle

Elastic tissue

Cubical epithelium

Alveolus

Flattened cells

Larger cells

Flattened squames lining alveolus

Rich capillary network

Elastic fibres

295

LUNGS — ANATOMY

ANASTOMOTIC CHANNELS in ACINUS

These exist at two levels:

1. Between one or more
   atria and the related
   terminal bronchiole.

2. Between alveoli of
   atria of same
   respiratory
   bronchiole and
   between alveoli
   related to adjacent
   respiratory bronchioles.

These alveolar connections are known as the pores of Kohn.

HISTOLOGY of the ALVEOLUS

Three types of cell (pneumocytes) line the alveolus.

1. *Membranous pneumocyte (Type I)*
   Nucleus is usually situated
   at angles of alveolus, and
   thin cytoplasmic extensions
   line most of alveolar surface.

2. *Granular pneumocyte (Type II)*
   Project into alveoli and are
   covered by microvilli. They
   are essentially reserve cells
   which undergo hyperplasia
   when Type I pneumocytes are
   injured.

3. *Type III pneumocytes*
   Pyramidal in shape with thick microvilli-containing filaments extending through cell body.
   Resemble chemoreceptor cells.

RESPIRATION

The normal intake of air is around 7 litres per minute; of this, after allowing for non-functioning dead space (trachea, bronchi, etc.), approximately 5 litres per minute are available for alveolar ventilation. A definite flow of air is maintained as far as the terminal bronchiole. Beyond this point the actual flow ceases and gas exchange is effected by diffusion.

A single terminal bronchiole (TB) gives rise to

3 – 5 respiratory bronchioles (RB)
Diameter of each RB ≡ diameter of TB. Air flow stops.

Each RB gives rise to several alveolar ducts (AD) of similar diameter to respiratory bronchiole ← From this point on, air pressure falls to zero and movement of repiratory gases is by diffusion.

Three factors are involved in the maintenance of adequate respiration:
  1. Adequate intake of air
  2. Rapid diffusion along alveolar ducts and through alveolar walls
  3. Adequate perfusion of pulmonary circulation
Interference with any of these factors will result in respiratory embarrassment (dyspnoea) and even respiratory failure.

Inadequate air supply to alveoli (hypoventilation)

This may be due to lesions and diseases which interfere with the mechanics of respiration, such as central nervous lesions affecting the respiratory centre, paralysis of the muscles of respiration as in poliomyelitis, injuries and deformities of the thoracic skeleton (e.g. fracture of ribs, kyphosis) and pleural disease preventing lung expansion as in pleural effusion or pneumothorax.

Perhaps the most common cause of hypoventilation is bronchial obstruction. This may be due to retained secretions and mucous gland hyperplasia in advanced chronic bronchitis or bronchial spasm in asthma. Local bronchial obstruction can be caused by tumour growth or foreign bodies.

Effects

Fall in alveolar and blood oxygen.
Rise in blood and alveolar CO_2
The clinical changes mainly due to hypercapnia (increase in systemic arterial carbon dioxide) — rapid pulse, sweating, small pupils and rise in blood pressure.

RESPIRATION

Impaired diffusion of gases

Three mechanisms may interfere with diffusion:

1. Reduction in the total alveolar surface available for diffusion, e.g. consolidated airless lobe in pneumonia, fibrosis of lung, tumour growth, advanced tuberculosis.
2. Increase in distance over which diffusion takes place as in emphysema.

3. Increase in the thickness of the alveolar capillary membrane. Diffusion of gas across the membrane is so rapid this can be of little practical importance. CO_2 is more soluble than O_2 and diffusion through the alveolar wall is 20 times as rapid as O_2, therefore while blood O_2 progressively falls there is no retention of CO_2.

   Attacks of hypoxia and cyanosis are the usual results of defects in diffusion.

Altered pulmonary perfusion

Interference with the pulmonary circulation may occur in 4 main ways:

1. Occlusion of larger vessels by multiple emboli.
2. Slowing of the pulmonary circulation as in venous congestion due to left heart lesions or congenital left-right shunts.
3. Reduction in the pulmonary capillary bed by diffuse lung disease such as fibrosis, emphysema or extensive tuberculosis.
4. Pulmonary vascular spasm due to hypoxia. Permanent changes can occur in the vessels if the hypoxia is unrelieved.

Inadequate perfusion will tend to cause both retention of CO_2 and fall in blood oxygen, but again due to the solubility of CO_2, the effects are mainly those of lack of oxygen.

While in acute respiratory embarrassment the cause may be mainly an abnormality of one mechanism, i.e. ventilation, diffusion or perfusion; in chronic lung disease it is always due to a combination of all three. Not only so, but the relative importance of these mechanisms, one to the other, will vary from one part of lung to another according to the stage of the pathological process in the particular part of the lung. Fibrosis with destruction of capillaries may be prominent in one part of the lung, while alveolar exudation interfering with gaseous diffusion is occurring in another.

ACUTE BRONCHITIS

This is an inflammation of the large and medium bronchi. The condition may be serious if associated with pre-existing respiratory disease. Mucous and serous glands in the walls of the bronchi provide abundant mucoid secretion during the inflammation. Ciliated epithelia lining the bronchi aid passage of the exudate upward and help prevent spread down to the bronchioles.

In most cases, the process is initiated by a viral or mycoplasmal infection. It is a common complication of influenza and measles. This initial phase is followed by bacterial invasion. *Streptococcus pneumoniae* and *Haemophilus influenzae* are commonest, but *Staphylococcus aureus* and *Streptococcus pyogenes* may be found, especially in infants.

The condition is usually mild, and spread to the bronchioles is unusual in healthy adults due to the effective ciliary action of the bronchial epithelium. Spread may occur however in children and debilitated people. Bronchiolitis and bronchopneumonia result and can prove fatal. Equally important is the serious effect of repeated attacks of acute infection in patients with chronic bronchitis.

CHRONIC BRONCHITIS

CHRONIC OBSTRUCTIVE AIRWAYS DISEASE (COAD)

This is a clinical syndrome which, as the name implies, is characterised by obstruction to the flow of air in the distal airways. The pathological conditions causing this are: (1) chronic bronchitis, (2) emphysema, (3) asthmatic bronchitis and (4) some cases of bronchiectasis. These conditions usually display considerable overlap.

CHRONIC BRONCHITIS

Clinical definition is based upon the presence of a productive cough over a period of at least two years. The pathological counterpart is illustrated.

The essential feature is a change in the epithelial structure of the bronchus.

Numerous goblet cells

Reduced number of ciliated cells

Lymphocytes and plasma cells

Circular muscle

Marked increase of mucous glands: loss of serous glands

Cartilage

At first, the bronchial wall is thickened due to the increase in glandular tissue, oedema and congestion. At autopsy, the severity of the disease can be measured using the Reid Index, i.e. the ratio of the submucous layer to the whole thickness. A ratio greater than 1:2 is significant. At a later stage it can become thin as a result of atrophy of all structures.

The effect of these changes is:

Increase of goblet cells
+
Increase of mucous glands

Loss of serous glands
↓

Loss of ciliated epithelium

Large quantity of viscid secretion difficult to eliminate

The tendency to retention of secretion encourages bacterial growth and thus a vicious circle may be set up.

Chronic bronchitis

Retention of secretion

Bacterial growth

Repeated attacks of acute inflammation

Continued chronic irritation may result in squamous metaplasia of the bronchial epithelium.

CHRONIC BRONCHITIS

With repeated acute exacerbations of the inflammation and increasing retention of secretion, spread of the chronic changes along the bronchial tree is encouraged.

When the terminal bronchioles are affected, more serious changes take place:

Absence of ciliated epithelium

Terminal bronchiole

Appearance of goblet cells (normally absent)

Seepage and retention of exudate in alveoli

↓

Bacterial spread

↓

Patches of pneumonia during acute exacerbations

The lack of ciliary action makes it difficult to get rid of exudate and hinders resolution. Healing takes place by organisation. The results of this process are as follows:

Organisation

Obliteration of some alveoli and bronchioles

Stenosis of bronchioles
↓
Obstruction to expiration
↓
Emphysema

The causes of chronic bronchitis are multiple and form an interacting complex.

Atmospheric pollution

Particulate matter, e.g. chemical vapours, exhaust fumes, sulphur dioxide
↓
Irritation
↓
Stimulation of secretion
↓
Mucous gland hyperplasia

Tobacco smoke
↓
Metaplasia of epithelium

Repeated attacks of acute bronchitis

Loss of ciliated epithelium

Retention of secretion → Bacterial proliferation

Chronic Bronchitis

Chronic bronchitis is most common in industrial areas with a high rainfall. In its serious form it occurs in males over the age of 40, but the onset can be dated many years earlier.

301

BRONCHIAL ASTHMA

This condition, of allergic nature, is characterised by spasmodic attacks of severe dyspnoea with some coughing. The difficulty in breathing is mainly related to exhalation due to the plugging of bronchioles with viscid mucus. The lung is rather voluminous but without any real emphysema.

Histological changes are a combination of allergic reaction and muscular hypertrophy, the result of prolonged spasm.

The asthmatic attack begins with difficulty in breathing, particularly exhalation, producing loud wheezing noises. Coughing which is non-productive may occur. At the end of the attack, thick viscid sputum is produced.

Sputum

In some cases the following may be seen:

1. *Curschmann's spirals* — appear as small white granules in sputum.

2. *Charcot-Leyden crystals* — in association with eosinophils.

BRONCHIAL ASTHMA

COMPLICATIONS

The repeated attacks of coughing and excessive mucus production may induce a chronic bronchitic condition. This in turn may result in emphysema. An attack may be prolonged and unremitting — **status asthmaticus** and death may occur.

Aetiology: Although two mechanisms are recognised they are not completely seperable.

Extrinsic Immune reaction — Type I hypersensitivity	Intrinsic Abnormal autonomic regulation of airways
Family history of hypersensitivity common	No family history
Starts in childhood	Starts in adult life
Preceded by infantile eczema and hypersensitivity to foods	No evidence of atopy
Predisposition to form IgE antibodies	IgE antibodies may be formed but no particular predisposition
Allergens recognised — pollen, dandruff, house dust mite	No recognisable allergens
Attacks often diminish in later years	Attacks increase in severity
Chronic bronchitis seldom develops	Associated with nasal polypi and chronic bronchitis
Emphysema unusual	Emphysema commonly develops
No drug sensitivity	Drug sensitivity may develop (aspirin, penicillin)

BRONCHIECTASIS

Bronchiectasis means a permanent dilatation of one or more bronchi.

The main bronchi up to the 4th division posses large supporting cartilage rings and the condition only affects bronchi beyond this point. Two main anatomical varieties are described but these may have similar causes and frequently both are found in the same lung.

1. Cylindrical

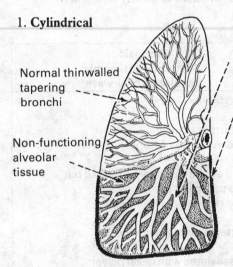

Normal thinwalled tapering bronchi

Non-functioning alveolar tissue

This type is almost always found in the lower lobes. The bronchi are grossly dilated throughout their length. Intervening lung tissue is much reduced and much of it is fibrosed.

The pleura is usually fibrotic and thick with dense adhesions to the chest wall.

There is a foul smell due to the large quantities of secretion containing putrefactive bacteria.

A variation of this type is called 'fusiform' where the bronchi are spindle-shaped, the dilatation affecting part of the length while either end is of normal calibre.

2. Saccular

Saccular dilatations usually containing pus

As the name suggests the dilatations tend to be more localised and exaggerated. They are roughly rounded and may be single or multiple. Sometimes they are associated with bronchial obstruction due to tumour, enlarged glands or foreign body. They may also occur in chronic tuberculosis. In these cases, the bronchiectasis may be found in the upper lobe.

BRONCHIECTASIS

Microscopical changes

BRONCHI. The condition usually follows a viral pneumonia in childhood and the initial change is the production of lymphoid aggregations in the bronchial wall.

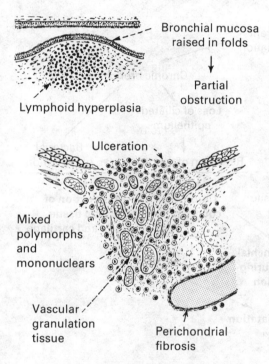

Bronchial mucosa raised in folds

↓

Partial obstruction

Lymphoid hyperplasia

Ulceration

Mixed polymorphs and mononuclears

Vascular granulation tissue

Perichondrial fibrosis

The partial obstruction causes retention of secretion and a progressive chronic bronchitic condition arises.

Recurrent inflammation

Bacterial proliferation

Metaplasia of epithelium

Increasing retention of secretion

With infection, the secretion becomes purulent and destruction of tissues occurs. The specialised tissues such as muscle, epithelium, elastic tissue, glands and cartilage are progressively destroyed until the whole wall is converted virtually into fibrous tissue with areas of ulceration.

BRONCHIOLES. Frequently these are obliterated by pre-existing disease or may become so due to spread of the inflammatory process along the bronchus. Bands of fibrous tissue are created during healing of these lesions.

ALVEOLAR TISSUE. The alveoli associated with the terminal bronchioles are also obliterated by the inflammatory process or secondary to collapse. In addition, much of the alveolar tissue adjacent to the dilated bronchi is compressed, rendered non-functional and may also be involved by spread of infection.

PLEURA. The inflammatory changes in terminal bronchioles and alveoli extend to the pleura, both layers of which become adherent and fibrotic. More or less continuous bands of fibrous tissue may be formed between the wall of the bronchus and the pleura.

BRONCHIECTASIS

Mechanism of formation

This involves a combination of mechanical factors and concomitant inflammatory changes. The process may be visualised as follows:

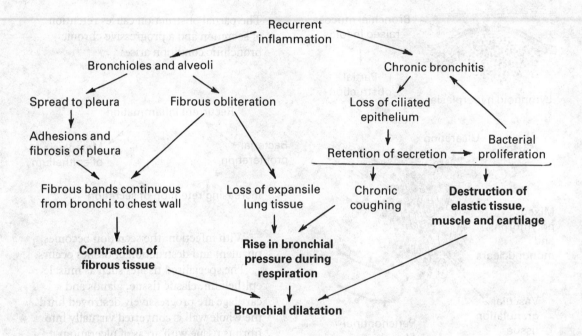

Aetiology

INFECTION. Most cases are initiated by bronchopneumonia which fails to resolve. In children this may be of primary bacterial origin or a complication of specific infections, e.g. measles, whooping cough. Other virus infections, e.g. adenovirus, may be important.

BRONCHIAL OBSTRUCTION. Partial bronchial obstruction by neoplastic growth, enlarged lymph nodes or foreign body, causes retention of secretion and infection leading to localised bronchiectasis.

PNEUMOCONIOSIS. Very occasionally lung fibrosis leads to bronchiectasis.

CONGENITAL DISEASE. Bronchiectasis may complicate maldevelopment of part of the lung or follow acute purulent infections complicating fibrocystic disease (mucoviscoidosis). See page 496.

BRONCHIECTASIS

Effects

(1) Large quantities
of secretion are
retained in the
bronchi and
putrefactive
bacteria produce
a foul smell

(2) Suppuration is
common in the
cavities and local
complications arise,

    e.g. lung abscess
    bronchopleural
    fistula

    empyema

(3) Pyaemia giving
rise to brain abscess
or meningitis may
result from involvement
of a pulmonary
vein branch by the
suppurative process

(4) Much of the lung
tissue may be destroyed
and haemodynamic
changes follow.

    Pulmonary
    hypertension
    ensues and right
    ventricular failure
    is apt to occur

(5) Clubbing of fingers
(hypertrophic pulmonary
osteoarthropathy)

(6) Development of amyloid
disease, e.g. in kidney

Amyloid
around
glomerular
capillaries
and tubule
basement
membranes

EMPHYSEMA

In this condition there is a permanent increase in the size of air spaces distal to the terminal bronchiole with destructive changes in their walls. It causes dyspnoea and is associated with chronic coughing.

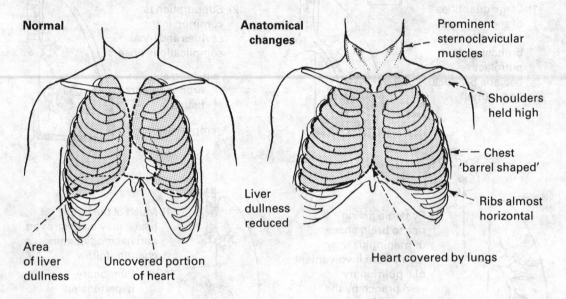

Normal

Area of liver dullness

Uncovered portion of heart

Anatomical changes

Prominent sternoclavicular muscles

Shoulders held high

Chest 'barrel shaped'

Ribs almost horizontal

Liver dullness reduced

Heart covered by lungs

Pulmonary pathology

At post mortem, the lungs are voluminous and pale. They contain little blood.

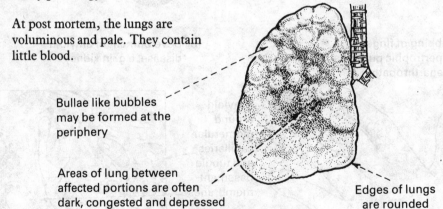

Bullae like bubbles may be formed at the periphery

Areas of lung between affected portions are often dark, congested and depressed

Edges of lungs are rounded

Section of the lung can reveal two separate patterns:

(1) **alveolar emphysema** and (2) **centrilobular emphysema**.

EMPHYSEMA

ALVEOLAR EMPHYSEMA

This is the condition which produces the
striking anatomical changes characteristically
associated with emphysema.

Limits of ⊱
enlarged secondary lobules

General distension of lung parenchyma

Histology shows distension of the alveolar tissue.

Normal

Ruptured
alveolar walls
are retracted
with bulbous
ends

Alveoli and
alveolar ducts
distended

Alveolar walls
stretched and
thin

Special stains show loss of elastic tissue. The capillaries are stretched and thinned. The
reduction in blood supply is probably a factor in leading to rupture of alveoli.

There is little evidence of bronchiolitis. The voluminous lungs produce characteristic
radiological changes. The distension eventually spreads to involve the respiratory bronchiole, i.e.
the whole acinus is affected — panacinar emphysema.

Respiratory
bronchiole

Alveolar
duct

Alveoli

Normal

Normal respiratory
bronchiole

Alveolar
emphysema = Distended alveolar
ducts and alveoli

Panacinar
emphysema = Distended respiratory
bronchiole, alveolar
ducts and alveoli

EMPHYSEMA

CENTRILOBULAR EMPHYSEMA

In centrilobular emphysema, there is no enlargement of the lung and the condition tends to be most marked in the upper lobes. A characteristic pattern is only obvious in cross section of the lungs.

Microscopically, the condition is seen to affect the respiratory bronchioles.

The chronic inflammation of the terminal bronchioles is an important feature. In this type of lesion, there is little radiological evidence of emphysema since the alveolar tissue is normal for a considerable time.

Eventually, in many lobules the distension extends to involve the alveolar tissue producing panacinar emphysema.

EMPHYSEMA

Aetiology

ALVEOLAR EMPHYSEMA

Two factors may operate:

1. Acute pulmonary inflammation but no suggestion of chronic bronchitis.

2. Possible deficiency of α_1 antitrypsin. In individuals with a hereditary deficiency, alveolar emphysema is common.

The compound α_1 antitrypsin protects tissues during inflammatory processes by limiting proteolysis which might destroy essential structures. Its relationship to emphysema may be visualised as follows:

CENTRILOBULAR EMPHYSEMA

The basis of this lesion is repeated bronchitis and chronic irritation, causing chronic coughing. The mechanism is probably as follows:

311

EMPHYSEMA

FUNCTIONAL CHANGES

1. In **alveolar emphysema** the effects on oxygen/carbon dioxide interchange which would tend to take place are offset by the structural changes and compensatory adaptations.

The patient has a normal colour but appears to be dyspnoeic. Clinically, the term 'pink puffer' is used to describe this type of patient. Ultimately with the progressive destruction of alveolar tissue the compensatory mechanism fails.

2. The functional changes in **centrilobular emphysema** are more serious and cause increasing disability.

The alveolar tissue is normal. There is no increase in lung capacity and therefore no compensatory mechanism.

The clinical effects of these changes are cumulative. Poor oxygenation results in cyanosis and severe dyspnoea. Clinically this patient is often described as a 'blue bloater' (contrast with 'pink puffer').

Chronic hypoxia always leads to pulmonary hypertension. The peripheral pulmonary vessels become thickened and muscular, increasing peripheral resistance. Ultimately, the increasing respiratory distress is complicated by right ventricular failure.

EMPHYSEMA — OTHER FORMS

FOCAL DUST EMPHYSEMA

This is found in coal miners and is associated with deposition of dust in the walls of bronchioles which become fibrotic and inelastic. Chronic coughing induces stretching of the inelastic bronchiolar walls and a mild form of centrilobular emphysema ensues.

Normal alveoli

Dilated respiratory bronchioles

ATROPHIC or SENILE EMPHYSEMA

This condition occurs in old age and wasting diseases. The lungs are not enlarged and no bullae are formed. The alveolar septa atrophy due to deficient nutrition. It is doubtful if the term emphysema is justified in this condition.

INTERSTITIAL EMPHYSEMA

Air may penetrate into the connective tissue framework surrounding the secondary lobules of the lung. It may travel along the septa to the pleura of the lung producing a fine white beaded appearance on the surface. If a large amount of air penetrates the tissues, it can spread via lymphatics and tissue spaces to the mediastinum and to the subcutaneous regions of the neck.

Blood vessel

Air separating peribronchial connective tissue fibres

There are two main causes:

1. Over distension of alveoli due to coughing as in whooping cough, bronchiolitis or Caisson disease or to forced inspiration, e.g. during positive pressure ventilation in the newborn.

2. Trauma. Penetrating and crush injuries of the chest wall.

313

ATELECTASIS

This means failure of the lung to expand at the time of birth.

— Large pleural space

— Lungs small and collapsed against vertebral column: cyanotic colour

— Heart and great vessels fully exposed

Histological pattern

Atelectasis

Slitlike air spaces

Fluid

Lining of cuboidal cells in air spaces

Air spaces with flattened inconspicuous cells

Normal

The condition is due to lack of proper inspiration at birth. It occurs in premature infants. Two factors probably operate in varying degree.

(1) Inefficiency of respiratory centre
↓
Lack of respiratory movement
↓   ↘
Blood flow continued through ductus arteriosus, by-passing lungs
↓
Loss of erectile effect on alveolar walls

Poor negative pressure effect

(2) Lack of surfactant
↓
High surface tension
↓
Difficulty in separating alveolar walls

HYALINE MEMBRANE DISEASE

This is a condition of absorption collapse affecting the newborn, with a mortality rate of at least 30 percent. It differs from atelectasis in its time of onset, the mechanism involved and the bronchiolar changes.

Associated factors

These include prematurity, caesarean section and maternal diabetes.

Respiration is apparently normal at birth, but there is increasing difficulty within a short time, minutes to hours. X-ray examination shows loss of expansion until almost complete collapse occurs.

Clinical effects

These are the result of:

1. Increasing difficulty in obtaining alveolar expansion leading to laboured respiration with use of accessory muscles such as sternomastoid.

2. Lack of oxygenation, hypoxia and cyanosis.

Due to the lack of expansion and the consequent lack of negative alveolar pressure, little blood is drawn into the lungs and there is a continuation of the fetal circulation, i.e. largely a right to left shunt via the foramen ovale and ductus arteriosus.

Pathology

The lungs are very often similar in appearance to those seen in atelectasis. If the changes are less diffuse, the lung shows 'geographical' markings — collapsed congested areas surrounded by more normal lung tissue.

Histologically, the alveoli are collapsed, while the respiratory bronchioles tend to be distended and lined by a prominent pink-staining hyaline membrane of proteinaceous character.

HYALINE MEMBRANE DISEASE

Mechanism of production

The main factor is probably immaturity of the lung tissue which, prior to the 34th week of pregnancy, has little ability to secrete lecithin. This is the main component of surfactant, which lowers surface tension. This has two effects:

1. Prevents alveolar walls sticking together and thus allowing easy opening by inspiratory pressure.

2. Allows alveolar fluid to spread as an even film over the walls. This protects surfaces from direct exposure to the air and the cells only have to deal with dissolved gases.

Secondary changes arise as a result of hypoxia — tendency to haemorrhage and disseminated thrombotic episodes.

ADULT RESPIRATORY DISTRESS SYNDROME (ARDS)

The adult lung may show similar changes secondary to a wide variety of disorders: severe shock, inhalation of irritant gases and pure oxygen, paraquat ingestion and uraemia are a few examples.

The condition is illustrated as **shock lung** (see p.149).

COLLAPSE OF LUNG

ABSORPTION COLLAPSE

This is a common condition and
is due to bronchial obstruction

↓

Absorption of air from
non functioning air spaces

↓

Collapse

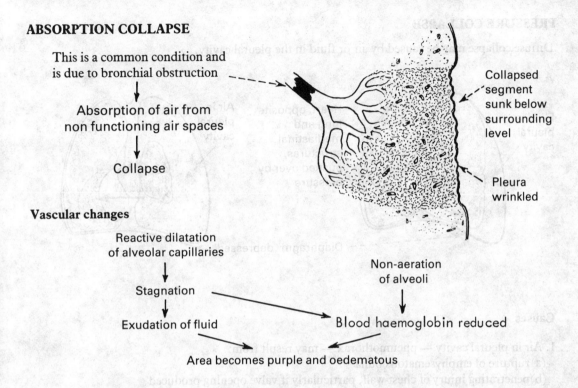

Collapsed
segment
sunk below
surrounding
level

Pleura
wrinkled

Vascular changes

Reactive dilatation
of alveolar capillaries

↓

Stagnation

↓

Exudation of fluid

Non-aeration
of alveoli

↓

Blood haemoglobin reduced

Area becomes purple and oedematous

Subsequent development

1. Secretions accumulate behind the obstruction. These frequently become infected and
   suppuration with abscess formation occurs.

2. In the absence of infection, and if the collapse persists, the granular pneumocytes of the alveoli
   proliferate and this is followed by progressive fibrosis. Local pulmonary artery branches show
   narrowing of the lumen due to intimal fibroelastosis.

Causes of obstruction

Acute obstruction

Large bronchi may be blocked by foreign bodies. Small bronchi are frequently blocked by mucus
during pulmonary infections.

Chronic obstruction

1. Tumours in the wall of bronchus.
2. Tumours or enlarged lymph nodes pressing on bronchus.

COLLAPSE OF LUNG

PRESSURE COLLAPSE

Diffuse collapse may be caused by air or fluid in the pleural cavity.

Fluid in pleural cavity

Heart, opposite lung and mediastinal structures, pushed over by pressure

Air in pleural cavity

Diaphragm depressed

Causes

1. Air in pleural cavity — pneumothorax — may result from:
   (a) rupture of emphysematous bulla
   (b) penetrating injury of chest wall, particularly if valve opening produced
   (c) fistulous communication with stomach or oesophagus due to injury or cancer.

2. Pleural effusion due to infection, often tuberculous, or malignant growth on the pleural surface.

3. Empyema. This condition, now rare in developed countries is usually due to spread of infection from the lung.

4. Haemothorax. Trauma, rupture of a mediastinal aneurysm or haemorrhage from a local cancerous growth may cause effusion of blood into a pleural cavity.

Subsequent development

1. Unlike absorption collapse there is no obstruction to the drainage of pulmonary secretions and therefore no development of new pulmonary inflammation.

2. Inflammation is, however, the main problem. Even in pneumothorax, effusion of fluid quickly takes place and secondary infection follows.

3. If the tension within the pleural cavity is unrelieved, healing can occur by organisation of the exudate. Collapse of the lung becomes permanent and pulmonary fibrosis results.

PNEUMONIA

Pneumonia is an inflammatory
process involving the alveolar tissue
of the lungs. Three main types
exist:

1. Bronchopneumonia
2. Lobar pneumonia
3. Interstitial pneumonia

Bronchopneumonia   Lobar pneumonia

BRONCHOPNEUMONIA

Bronchopneumonia caused by a variety of bacteria, is the commonest form. It may affect all ages,
but it is particularly frequent in four circumstances:

1. as a terminal event in a chronic debilitating disease
2. in infancy
3. in old age
4. as a manifestation of secondary infection in viral conditions, e.g. influenza, measles.

Bronchopneumonia is primarily a spreading inflammation of terminal bronchioles and
their related alveoli.

The lesions are initially focal,
involving one or more lobules.
First red, then grey, they show a
central bronchiole containing pus.

Being a spreading inflammation,
the foci are not all at the same
stage of the inflammatory process.

The disease starts as a
bronchiolitis.

Lesions are
usually in the
lower lobes

At the lung base
the changes are
more advanced,
coalesce and
become
confluent

Bronchiole becomes
inflamed; ciliated
epithelium is destroyed

Congestion of vessels and
emigration of polymorphs

319

BRONCHOPNEUMONIA

After the initial bronchiolitis, spread to the alveoli quickly follows.

1. In the early stages, the alveolar walls are congested giving a red colour to the tissues.

Polymorphs

Dilated capillaries

2. At a later stage the exudate becomes fibrinous and polymorphs are extremely numerous. Congestion is less marked and the lesions become pale grey.

Inflammation spreads through pores of Kohn to adjacent lobules.

Lobule directly affected by spread of inflammation from bronchiole

The onset is insidious, but marked toxaemia develops. Pneumococci are the common infecting organisms. When the inflammation subsides, resolution may take place. The fibrin is dissolved and the exudate is partly absorbed and partly removed by coughing.

BRONCHOPNEUMONIA — COMPLICATIONS

1. **Death** is common since the pneumonia commonly complicates debilitating disease (hypostatic pneumonia).

2. **Resolution** is often incomplete, even if the patient survives. Many consolidated patches end in fibrosis. Granulation tissue is formed as in a healing wound.

Macrophages gradually clear the exudate while fibroblasts and blood vessels grow in from the alveolar septa.

Pore of Kohn

Granulation tissue formed in bronchioles and alveoli

If the resulting fibrosis is gross, the lung structure may be distorted and changes in the larger bronchi cause bronchiectasis. A vicious circle may be set up:-

Bronchiectasis

Fibrosis

Re-infection

Repeated bronchopneumonia

3. **Suppurative Changes**

These are less common with specific antibiotic treatment, but lung abscess and empyema occur in debilitated patients, and especially in cases of aspiration pneumonia.

LOBAR PNEUMONIA

As the name suggests, in this condition a complete lobe or even two lobes of a lung are affected. The most striking changes occur in the alveolar tissue. Although spread of the inflammatory process is via the ducts and not through alveolar walls, changes in the bronchioles are of minor importance. The disease is seen in adult males previously healthy, mainly between 30 and 50 years. It is rare in Western countries but still occurs frequently in underdeveloped countries. One attack gives little immunity. Repeated attacks are common. The sudden onset and pathology suggest an element of hypersensitivity.

Four distinct phases are recognised:

1. Congestion (1 — 2 days)
2. Red hepatisation (2nd — 4th day)
3. Grey hepatisation (4th — 8th day)
4. Resolution (8th — 9th day).

1. Congestion (1 — 2 days)

The lobe of lung shows the usual early changes of acute inflammation. It is dark red, and frothy, blood-stained fluid can be squeezed from it. Large numbers of the causative bacteria are present in the fluid. Microscopically, the alveolar capillaries are engorged and contain an increased number of polymorphs.

The onset is sudden with fever and rigors.

Increase in polymorphs

Bacteria

Fluid exudate

Extravasated red cells

Congested capillaries

LOBAR PNEUMONIA

2. Red hepatisation (2nd — 4th day)

The lobe is dry, solid, red and granular. It contains no air. Some fibrin is present on the pleural surface. In addition to the congestion of the previous stage, there is now a well-marked fibrinous exudate, and there are polymorphs in the alveoli.

Clinically, there is pain on breathing, due to the pleural exudate, and a productive cough with brown sputum. Leucocytosis occurs early and a positive blood culture is obtained in most cases.

3. Grey hepatisation (4th — 8th day)

The affected lobe is even more solid, and the pleural surface is covered by a confluent fibrinous exudate. The cut surface is dry and granular but of a greyish white colour. The alveolar exudate is increased in amount, with dense fibrin strands and very numerous polymorphs. It is this exudate which gives the grey colour to the affected lobe. The congestion of capillaries is now much reduced.

Antibodies to the bacteria appear in the blood at this stage, and the organisms disappear quite rapidly. Coughing is not so marked and less productive. Pain and high fever persist.

LOBAR PNEUMONIA

4. Resolution (8th – 9th day)

With elimination of the bacteria, the inflammatory process subsides, and since there is no tissue destruction, the lung returns to normal apart from the pleura where the fibrinous adhesions between the visceral and parietal layers tend to undergo organisation with the formation of fibrous adhesions. The fibrin is liquefied by proteolytic enzymes possibly produced in part by the polymorphs. The liquid products together with polymorphs are coughed up — macrophages from the lung tissues invade the alveoli.

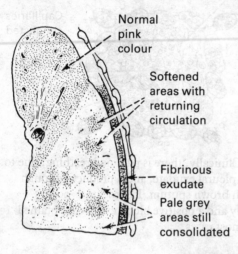

Normal pink colour

Softened areas with returning circulation

Fibrinous exudate

Pale grey areas still consolidated

Macrophage

Increased circulation of blood in alveolar capillaries

Strands of fibrin breaking up and disappearing

Polymorphs diminishing in number

The disease ends in a "crisis" with sudden drop in temperature.

Bacteriology of lobar pneumonia

The cause of the disease is *Streptococcus pneumoniae*, which has a distinctive morphology.

Gram positive diplococcus

Capsule containing mucopolysaccharide

Eight types are recognised, but 90% of cases are caused by seven of these. The following order is an indication of their frequency: I, III, II, V, VII, VIII and IV. Almost 70% of cases are due to Types I, II and III. Type III is found mainly in patients over the age of 50 already suffering from some other disease and the mortality rate is high despite treatment. It has a large amount of capsular substance and this gives a mucoid consistency to the exudate. Complications are more common with this infection, particularly lung abscess.

Type I and II are more commonly found in younger patients.

VIRAL PNEUMONIAS

INFLUENZA

HAEMORRHAGIC PNEUMONIA

In most cases, influenzal infection is confined to the upper respiratory tract, but in debilitated persons and during epidemics, the whole respiratory tract is affected.

Trachea and bronchi

Intense inflammation with haemorrhage develops.

Proliferation of epithelium

Haemorrhage

Multinucleated epithelial cells

Mononuclear infiltration

Intense congestion

Initial necrotising changes — loss of epithelium

Reactive stage — multinucleated cells and proliferation of epithelium

Pneumonia changes

The lungs are bulky, purple red and exude blood-stained froth when cut. The microscopical changes vary from one part to another.

Hyaline formation

Swelling of basement membrane and loss of epithelium

Oedema fluid and large numbers of red cells

Intense interstitial mononuclear reaction

Fibrin

Mononuclear cells

Hyaline

Infective agents

Three main types of influenza virus exist: A, B and C. The A type is the most virulent, and mutants of this type are responsible for most epidemics and the fatalities which occur.

Secondary infection is common, the bacteria most frequently involved being *Haemophilus influenzae, Streptococcus pneumoniae, Streptococcus pyogenes* and *Staphylococcus aureus*.

325

VIRAL PNEUMONIAS

There are a number of pneumonic conditions due to viruses and virus-like agents in which a common pattern of pathological change is observed.

1. Necrotising bronchiolitis

- Inspissated secretion
- Necrosis of bronchiolar epithelium
- Mononuclear infiltrate in lumen and wall

2. Interstitial pneumonia

- Alveolar walls thickened by mononuclear infiltrate
- Alveoli may contain oedema fluid, red cells or fibrin

3. Reactive changes

The lining epithelial cells of bronchioles and alveoli are stimulated by the presence of the virus.

Cuboidal cells

Multinucleated cells

Occasionally found:

Intranuclear inclusion body

Cytoplasmic inclusion body

Variations in the basic pattern occur in different infections. Confluent consolidation is often found in psittacosis and ornithosis (viruses transmitted by birds) and in measles giant cell pneumonia. Interstitial pneumonia is produced by cytomegalovirus and in rickettsial infections such as Q fever (occurring in slaughter house workers infected by animal skins) and 'scrub typhus'. In mycoplasma pneumonia, inflammation spreads from the bronchioles into the lung parenchyma.

LEGIONNAIRE'S DISEASE

Previously confused with pneumococcal pneumonia, Legionnaire's disease occurs in small epidemics, is more common in males and is due to a tiny Gram-negative bacillus — *Legionella pneumophila*. The death rate can be high — up to 20%. Infection is associated with inhalation of aerosol from contaminated water storage systems.

Clinical features

Two phases are recognised:

Prodromal phase

> Legionnaire's disease: vague flu-like illness — lasts 5 days.
> Pneumococcal pneumonia: more acute — lasts 3 days.
> Mycoplasmal pneumonia: insidious onset — lasts 13 days.

Active phase

> A dry cough develops. Vomiting and diarrhoea may be severe.
> Patient becomes somnolent, confused and signs of consolidation appear.

Laboratory findings

> Hyponatraemia. Lymphopenia. Polymorphs normal.
> Signs of disseminated intravascular coagulation may develop.

Pathology

Both lungs are consolidated, dark red, heavy and oedematous. Fibrinous pleurisy or pleural effusion may be found.

Histology

Two stages are evident:

First stage
— Dilated, congested alveolar capillaries

— Fibrinous exudate containing red cells and a moderate number of polymorphs

Polymorphs disappear — replaced by scanty lymphocytes and macrophages

Second stage

Alveolar walls inconspicuous and avascular

Small abscesses may destroy bronchioles; and lung parenchyma may show necrosis

The exudate may organise, causing an increasing interstitial fibrosis with permanent loss of lung function.

PNEUMONIA — SPECIAL TYPES

ASPIRATION PNEUMONIA

This is due to inhalation of food or infected material from the mouth or pharynx which may occur when patients are unconscious, e.g. during anaesthesia or in coma due to epilepsy or cerebrovascular disease. It may also complicate any condition associated with frequent vomiting, e.g. hiatus hernia, pyloric stenosis or oesophageal obstruction.

There may be an initial phase of shock of cardiac type.

Acid gastric contents

↓

Irritation of pulmonary tissue

↓

Pulmonary oedema

Cyanosis   Dyspnoea   Shock (fall in BP, etc.)

In many cases, the onset is insidious following the aspiration of very small quantities of material.

If the patient survives this phase, secondary infection follows. Widespread bronchopneumonia is frequently associated with necrosis of lung tissue and abscess formation. Subsequently, the inspired material results in the formation of a granuloma with giant cell reaction. — — — — — — — — — —

A similar pneumonia can arise in a patient with an ulcerated neoplasm involving the upper respiratory tract.

PNEUMONIA — SPECIAL TYPES

LIPID PNEUMONIA

This is a non-infective pneumonic condition usually of iatrogenic origin.

Inhaled oily
nasal drops

Regurgitated
oily medicine

Vegetable oils are relatively innocuous but mineral oils are especially irritant.

The lungs present one of two appearances.

(1) Diffuse type

Focal lesions commonly in lower lobes.
These tend to coalesce until a whole lobe
becomes solid, indurated and yellowish.

(2) Localised type

Single rounded indurated mass,
pale colour. This type may be
mistaken for carcinoma.

Microscopically the process exhibits two phases:

Foamy lipid-
filled macrophages

Multinucleated
giant cells

Lymphocytes and
fibrocytes replace
macrophages

Fat cells form
in situ

A similar type of lesion may form in cases of non-resolving pneumonia, carcinoma or abscess
due to fatty residues of necrotic tissue.

329

PNEUMONIA — SPECIAL TYPES

All of the following may be primary infections but may also occur as opportunistic infections, especially when disease or therapy has diminished the immune response.

Staphylococcal bronchopneumonia

In patients receiving long-term antibiotic therapy for chronic respiratory disease, and in patients during epidemics of influenza, measles and whooping cough, staphylococci may cause bronchopneumonia.

The exudate is haemorrhagic with few polymorphs, giving the lungs a purple colour. The condition is often rapidly fatal, but survival is associated with abscess formation, empyema and pneumothorax.

Friedlander's bacillus (klebsiella)

This Gram-negative bacillus with a mucoid capsule causes bronchopneumonia particularly in men over 50 years of age, especially chronic alcoholics and diabetics. Red mucoid lesions occur in the right upper lobe. The sputum has a characteristic red, jelly-like appearance. Consolidation becomes confluent and large abscesses form in 80% of cases. Mortality rate is 40%.

Streptococcal pneumonia

This form of bronchopneumonia is usually secondary to viral infection and is rapidly fatal. The lungs are purple and, unlike most forms of bronchopneumonia, a fibrinous pleurisy is common.

Pseudomonas pneumonia

In hospital patients, this is an important cause of bronchopneumonia. *Pseudomonas aerugenosa* proliferates in water, soap solutions and some antiseptics. Instruments, anaesthetic apparatus and dressings may become contaminated. The exudate is haemorrhagic with scanty polymorphs but numerous organisms.

Other opportunistic infections

These occur in states of debilitation or immunological deficiency. Apart from the bacteria mentioned above, various other infective agents may be opportunistic:

>Viruses — *cytomegalovirus*
>Mycoplasma — *Mycoplasma pneumoniae*
>Protozoa — *Pneumocystis carinii*
>Fungi — *Aspergillus fumigatus, Candida albicans, Cryptococcus neoformans.*

LUNG ABSCESS

This is now an uncommon condition. The usual causes are:

1. Inhalation of infected material from the larynx or pharynx.

2. Obstruction of a bronchus by tumour growth or foreign body. Site depends on size of bronchus affected.

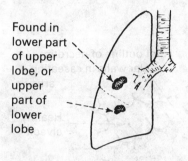

Found in lower part of upper lobe, or upper part of lower lobe

Most commonly in right lung since right bronchus is in line with trachea

Near hilum if large bronchus

At periphery if small bronchus

3. Infection of pre-existing cavities, e.g. in tuberculosis or bronchiectasis.

4. Pneumonia. Abscess is most likely to occur in debilitated persons with bronchopneumonia.

Apical abscess may occur in klebsiella infection

Usually in lower lobes, bilateral and multiple (Bacteria — Type III *Strep. pneumoniae*, staphylococcus and *Strep. pyogenes*)

Rarer causes of abscess are: pyaemia, trauma to lung, extension from suppuration in mediastinum, spinal column or subphrenic region, and infection with entamoeba histolytica.

Sequelae of lung abscess

1. Small abscesses may heal.

2. Subpleural abscesses may extend to cause empyema.

3. Bronchopleural fistula resulting in pyopneumothorax is a further complication following on 2.

4. If a large pulmonary vessel is eroded, fatal haemorrhage can occur.

5. On occasion, blood spread leads to meningitis or cerebral abscess.

TUBERCULOSIS

The lungs are more commonly affected by tuberculosis than any other organ. Where tuberculosis is common, infection usually occurs in childhood. In advanced countries where the incidence is lower, the initial lesions of tuberculosis may be delayed until adult life, and certainly the serious forms of this disease are usually found in older individuals.

PRIMARY LESION (GHON FOCUS)

1. **Infection is by inhalation**

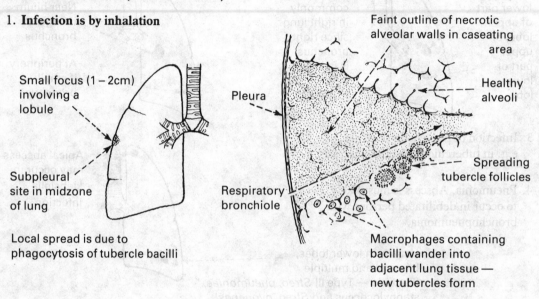

Small focus (1 – 2cm) involving a lobule

Subpleural site in midzone of lung

Local spread is due to phagocytosis of tubercle bacilli

Pleura

Respiratory bronchiole

Faint outline of necrotic alveolar walls in caseating area

Healthy alveoli

Spreading tubercle follicles

Macrophages containing bacilli wander into adjacent lung tissue — new tubercles form

2. **Lymphatic spread**

Ghon focus

Tubercles form along lymphatic tracks and spread is to tracheobronchial and mediastinal nodes. Large caseous masses may form, replacing lymphoid tissue.

The combination of the Ghon focus plus hilar nodes is termed the primary complex.

TUBERCULOSIS

SUBSEQUENT DEVELOPMENTS

1. **Healing**
   This is the commonest result.
   Small Ghon focus — complete fibrosis.
   Larger focus — caseous material is encapsulated by fibrous tissue and undergoes calcification.
   The same changes occur in the hilar nodes.

2. **Spread from the Ghon focus**

   (a) The inflammatory reaction in
   the adjacent lung tissue may
   induce an effusion in the
   pleural cavity.

   (b) Actual tuberculous infection
   of the pleura may occur resulting
   in tuberculous empyema.

   Ghon
   focus

   Lung

3. **Changes due to hilar node involvement**

   (a) **Mechanical effect.** Pressure of enlarged nodes on bronchi:
   bronchial obstruction may lead to collapse, retention of secretion and inflammatory
   consolidation.

   (b) **Spread of tubercles along bronchial lymphatics**

   (c) **Invasion of blood vessels.** This will lead to dissemination via the blood stream giving rise to
   tuberculous foci simultaneously in many organs (generalised miliary tuberculosis). A modified
   version of this is seen when tuberculous infection invades one or more branches of the
   pulmonary artery. Numerous miliary tubercles form in the lung tissue only.

TUBERCULOSIS

SECONDARY TUBERCULOSIS (POST-PRIMARY)

This is a recurrence of tuberculous infection in later life, and may be due to reactivation of the primary lesion or a re-infection by tubercle bacilli.

The lesions tend to appear in characteristic sites:

(a) posterior sub-apical and (b) upper part of lower lobes where the aeration is in relative excess over the blood flow, rendering the tissues susceptible to infection.

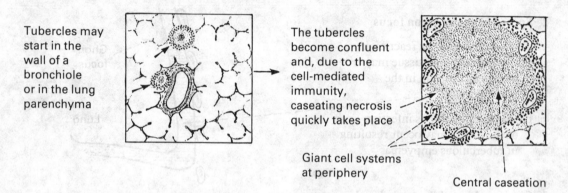

Tubercles may start in the wall of a bronchiole or in the lung parenchyma

The tubercles become confluent and, due to the cell-mediated immunity, caseating necrosis quickly takes place

Giant cell systems at periphery

Central caseation

Spread takes place by lymphatics, but the necrosis induced by the cell-mediated immunity kills many of the bacilli and the macrophages which transport them. Extension of the lesion is therefore very slow, and the hilar lymph nodes are not affected. A kind of granulation tissue heavily infiltrated by lymphocytes and macrophages forms at the periphery. Eventually the fibrous tissue becomes dense.

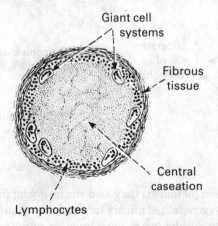

Giant cell systems

Fibrous tissue

Central caseation

Lymphocytes

At this stage the lesion:

1. May heal leaving a dense grey scar often with central calcification.
2. May become an encysted mass of caseous material and cease to spread. A few tubercle bacilli may persist.
3. May slowly extend by the formation of new tubercles and necrosis of the fibrous barrier. New successive fibrous barriers are formed in advance of the caseating process.

TUBERCULOSIS

SECONDARY TUBERCULOSIS (continued)

Further development

As the lesion extends, sooner or later the necrotising process will involve a larger bronchiole or bronchus. The lumen may become blocked by the tuberculous material, and even at this stage fibrous encapsulation with healing may take place. Commonly, however, the caseous material is discharged via the bronchus leaving a small irregular cavity behind. This is lined by fibrous tissue and contains a variable amount of caseous material. Related bronchi often show bronchiectasis.

Spread may occur by inhalation of the caseous material into other bronchi. New cavities form and coalesce to form large irregular spaces. The caseous material may be completely discharged, leaving a smooth walled fibrous cavity.

Local vessels undergo endarteritis with formation of fibrous cords. Fibrosed arteries frequently resist the caseous process and can be seen as ridges in the walls of cavities.

Fibrosis not only occurs around the cavities but also more diffusely throughout the lung. The pleura is usually thickened. This condition is often referred to as fibroid phthisis.

Thickened pleura. Often numerous adhesions to parietal pleura

Scarred apex

Fibrotic cavities

Bronchiectasis

Diffuse fibrosis

Lung shrunken

TUBERCULOSIS

SECONDARY TUBERCULOSIS (continued)

Complications

1. Haemorrhage and haemoptysis

The blood vessels in the tuberculous lesions are usually obliterated by endarteritis, but occasionally small vessels may rupture giving rise to haemoptysis. Aneurysms may form in larger vessels due to weakening of the wall. Fatal haemorrhage may ensue.

2. Acute tuberculous bronchopneumonia

This may occur in a debilitated patient when a large amount of caseous material discharges into a bronchus.

3. Acute miliary tuberculosis

Invasion of the blood stream is most likely to occur during bronchopneumonia complicating a primary infection but may also follow bronchopneumonia in post-primary tuberculosis.

4. Tuberculous ulcers of the intestine and larynx sometimes result from direct infection by sputum.

5. Secondary amyloidosis of organs is a common and serious effect of chronic tuberculosis.

Aetiological factors in secondary tuberculosis

1. Occupational hazards
   (a) Coal-miners and others exposed to silica dust.
   (b) Laboratory workers in contact with infected material.

2. Debilitating diseases — diabetes mellitus, alcoholism.

3. Diminished immunological response due to long-continued corticosteroid therapy.

4. Following gastrectomy.

ACUTE TUBERCULOUS BRONCHOPNEUMONIA

This is a complication which may occur in either (a) primary or (b) secondary tuberculous infection.

Primary tuberculous infection

Pneumonic spread may arise from:

1. Extension of the Ghon focus to involve a small bronchus. The caseous material spreads through the bronchial tree.

2. The caseous hilar nodes may ulcerate through the main bronchial wall and sudden spread to main parts of the lung occurs.

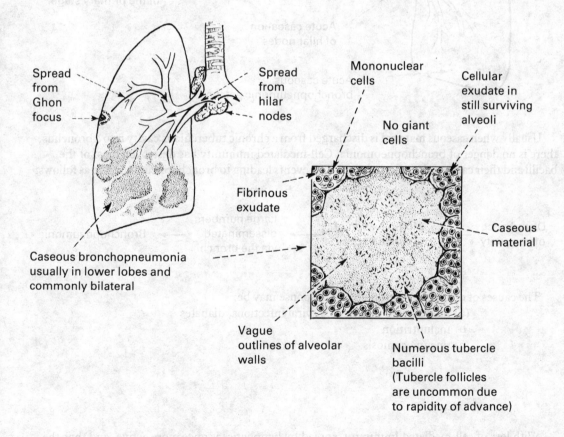

Spread from Ghon focus

Spread from hilar nodes

Mononuclear cells

Cellular exudate in still surviving alveoli

No giant cells

Fibrinous exudate

Caseous material

Caseous bronchopneumonia usually in lower lobes and commonly bilateral

Vague outlines of alveolar walls

Numerous tubercle bacilli (Tubercle follicles are uncommon due to rapidity of advance)

This condition is rapidly fatal. Pneumothorax and pleural effusion are common complications.

ACUTE TUBERCULOUS BRONCHOPNEUMONIA

Secondary tuberculous infection

Tuberculous bronchopneumonia in this instance is always due to evacuation of caseous material from a cavity into the bronchi.

Chronic cavities
in upper lobe

Evacuation of
caseous material
into bronchi

Acute caseation
of hilar nodes

Acute caseous
bronchopneumonic patches

The microscopic
features are similar
to those in
tuberculous
bronchopneumonia
of the primary stage.

Usually when caseous material is discharged from a chronic tuberculous cavity into a bronchus, there is no danger of bronchopneumonia. Cell-mediated immunity has destroyed most of the bacilli and their carriers the macrophages. The events leading to bronchopneumonia are as follows:

Disturbance
of immunity → Multiplication of
tubercle bacilli → Large numbers
disseminated
via the bronchi → Bronchopneumonia

The causes of disturbed immunological response may be:
     (a) intercurrent disease, e.g. viral infections, diabetes
     (b) malnutrition
     (c) pneumoconiosis.

With loss of cell-mediated immunity, spread by lymphatics is once more active, and thus the hilar nodes become caseous. The bronchopneumonic patches break down and discharge via bronchi, leaving ragged, soft-walled cavities and causing further spread.

ACUTE MILIARY TUBERCULOSIS

This condition is due to invasion of the blood stream by tuberculous material containing large numbers of bacilli. The distribution of the lesions depends on the vessel invaded. Usually the lesions are more numerous and most advanced in the lungs.

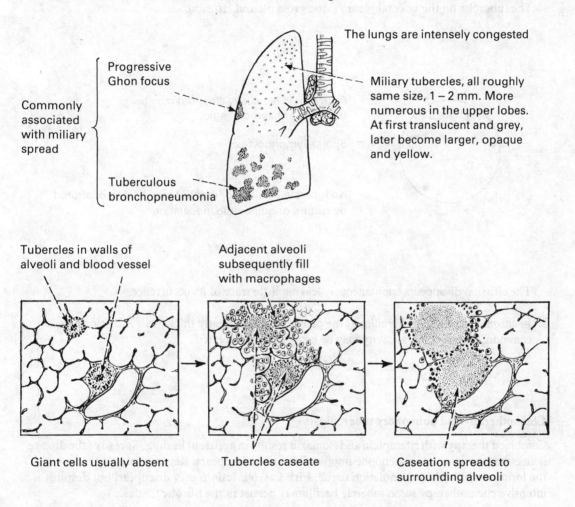

The lungs are intensely congested

Progressive Ghon focus

Commonly associated with miliary spread

Tuberculous bronchopneumonia

Miliary tubercles, all roughly same size, 1 – 2 mm. More numerous in the upper lobes. At first translucent and grey, later become larger, opaque and yellow.

Tubercles in walls of alveoli and blood vessel

Adjacent alveoli subsequently fill with macrophages

Giant cells usually absent

Tubercles caseate

Caseation spreads to surrounding alveoli

Acute miliary tuberculosis is usually a generalised condition and death is commonly due to tuberculous meningitis. If, however, the infection invades a branch of a pulmonary artery, the condition may be confined to the lungs initially.

TUBERCULOSIS AND THE PLEURA

Pleural lesions may occur in (1) primary and (2) secondary stages.

1. Infection may spread to the surface of the lung in the very early stage of tuberculous infection. The tubercles on the visceral pleura cause gross pleural effusion.

Pleural fluid is usually clear but may be fibrinous or haemorrhagic

Sparse lymphocytes

No tubercle bacilli apparent but may be demonstrated by culture or guinea-pig inoculation.

The effusion disappears spontaneously leaving little trace of its occurrence.

2. In chronic secondary tuberculosis, the pleura becomes greatly thickened. Adhesions are common, and the pleural cavity may be completely obliterated.

Chemotherapy and pulmonary tuberculosis

Combined therapy with rifampicin and isoniazid results in apparent healing. Spread of the disease is arrested even in acute bronchopneumonia. Caseation disappears. Revascularisation occurs with the formation of healthy granulation tissue. Firbocaseous lesions may disappear, but despite intensive chemotherapy some tubercle bacilli may persist in the fibrotic tissues.

PNEUMOCONIOSES (DUST DISEASES)

INORGANIC DUSTS

The reaction to inhaled dusts (e.g. carbon, silica, asbestos, haematite ore and beryllium) varies very considerably. Some are relatively innocuous; others cause severe destruction of lung tissue.

Basic pathology

Much of any dust is expectorated. Particles reaching the deeper lung tissues are ingested by macrophages. Many of these are returned to the upper respiratory tract and ejected. Those reaching the alveolar tissue accumulate in parts where movement is restricted, i.e. where alveoli are bound to more rigid structures.

Some macrophages enter lymphatics and reach local nodes. Most die in the alveoli leaving accumulations of dust. Fibrous tissue forms to enclose the particles. If marked, fibrogenesis obliterates the alveoli. Adjacent alveoli are bound down and immobilised, becoming sites for further dust accumulation and subsequent fibrosis. Thus the process becomes progressive.

The degree and site of fibrosis depends on the type of dust. Some cause intense fibrosis, others almost none. Some dusts reach the pleural surface, others are retained in the substance of the lung.

341

ANTHRACOSIS

This indicates an accumulation of carbon particles in the lung. It is found in a marked form in those who handle soft bituminous coal, particularly coal-miners. Two forms of the condition are recognised: (1) simple coal-worker's anthracosis and (2) progressive massive fibrosis.

Simple coal-worker's anthracosis

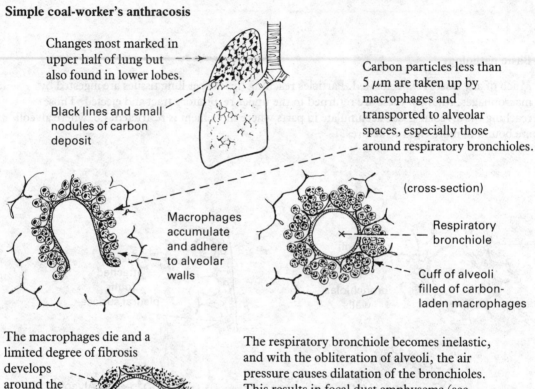

Changes most marked in upper half of lung but also found in lower lobes.

Black lines and small nodules of carbon deposit

Carbon particles less than 5 μm are taken up by macrophages and transported to alveolar spaces, especially those around respiratory bronchioles.

(cross-section)

Macrophages accumulate and adhere to alveolar walls

Respiratory bronchiole

Cuff of alveoli filled of carbon-laden macrophages

The macrophages die and a limited degree of fibrosis develops around the dust particles.

The respiratory bronchiole becomes inelastic, and with the obliteration of alveoli, the air pressure causes dilatation of the bronchioles. This results in focal dust emphysema (see p.313) which has no significant effect on respiratory function.

Alveolar epithelium grows over the fibrous masses, the alveoli are obliterated and the specialised structures such as muscle in the bronchiolar wall atrophy.

Distended respiratory bronchiole

Black, obliterated remains of alveoli

ANTHRACOSIS

Progressive massive fibrosis

In a small percentage of workers with simple anthracosis, this further serious change may develop.

Thickened pleura
often adherent to
the chest wall

Simple anthracotic
changes

Irregular masses of
black fibrous tissue
in the upper lobes

The fibrous tissue is rubbery.

Cavities are filled with black
fluid in centre of nodules.

Tuberculous infection can be demonstrated in 40% of cases. This may be the cause of cavitation in some of the fibrous nodules. In other instances, cavitation may be due to necrosis following obliteration of blood vessels. According to some observers, all of the changes — fibrosis and cavitation — are due to tuberculosis.

The functional effects are severe.

Fibrosis of lung tissue ◄——————— ? Tuberculosis

Reduction in
functional tissue

Secondary
emphysema

Vascular
obliteration

Hypoxia

**Respiratory
failure**

Pulmonary hypertension

Right ventricular failure

SILICOSIS

Workers exposed to high concentrations of silica dust over a period of years show pulmonary fibrosis of a progressive nature. This can occur in industries such as quarrying of granite, sandstone or slate; mining of anthracite, gold, tin or copper; sandblasting; boiler scaling; glass and pottery manufacture and stonemasonry.

Fine silica particles less than 5 μm are taken up by macrophages which are found in alveoli in the sites previously indicated:
- (a) Peribronchial alveoli
- (b) Perivascular alveoli
- (c) Alveoli around interlobular septa
- (d) Subpleural alveoli.

Macrophages accumulate in these sites and lie undisturbed. Silica-laden macrophages also reach the hilar lymph nodes. A characteristic fibrosis arises in all these sites.

Pleura grossly thickened

Adhesions develop to chest wall

Pleural cavity gradually obliterated

Lung tissue is nodular and gritty

Hilar nodes are enlarged, greyish black and nodular.

Nodules vary in size from 0.5 cm to several cm. They are greyish black, discrete at first and rounded.

Histology

The nodules consist of concentric laminae of hyaline, acellular collagen.

Silica granules

They are found at the sites of accumulation of the silica-laden macrophages. Most important are those which form in relation to bronchioles and vessels which are obliterated by the fibrosis.

This induces widespread secondary changes in the lungs.

SILICOSIS

Silicosis causes progressive respiratory embarrassment due to the destruction of bronchioles and alveoli and the obliteration of pulmonary vessels. Obliteration of the pleural cavity introduces mechanical difficulties in respiration. Death is commonly due to a combination of hypoxia and pulmonary hypertension causing right heart failure.

Tuberculosis and silicosis

Silicosis appears to encourage the establishment of tuberculous infection. The two conditions are commonly associated (reported incidence varies 10 – 70%). The tuberculous infection spreads rapidly; bronchopneumonia and miliary tuberculosis are common.

Mechanism of action of silica

There are three theories, none of which is entirely satisfactory:

1. *Silica solubility*
   Slow solution of the silica granules is thought to cause fibrosis. The degree of fibrosis does not appear to be related to the solubility of different forms of silica.

2. *Immunologic reaction*
   Silica has been claimed to be antigenic and fibrosis results from the antigen-antibody reaction. There is no evidence for this reaction.

3. *Phospholipid theory*
   Silica-laden macrophages die and release phospholipid which is said to stimulate fibrogenesis. Against this is the fact that macrophages die in other dust diseases, e.g. anthracosis, without causing fibrosis.

Rheumatoid pneumoconiosis

This condition arises in workers exposed to dusts (coal, silica or asbestos) who also suffer from rheumatoid arthritis. Fibrotic nodules up to 5 cm in diameter occur in the lung tissue. These are modified rheumatic lesions and frequently undergo cavitation or calcification.

ASBESTOSIS

Asbestos dust causes severe pulmonary disease. Three distinct types of lesion can be identified, but all of them may occur in the same patient: (1) asbestosis, (2) pleural fibrous plaques, and (3) malignant mesothelioma.

ASBESTOSIS

This term is generally reserved for a process which affects both lungs and leads to progressive destruction of respiratory tissue.

The particles particularly affect the lower lobes and produce a spreading fibrosis.

Fibrosis commences in subpleural zone of lower lobe

Spread occurs inwards and upwards

Destruction of lung tissue and contraction of fibrous tissue cause shrinkage of lobe

Unaffected bronchioles may undergo compensatory dilatation (one type of honeycomb lung)

Terminal bronchiole

Fibrosis first affects respiratory bronchioles

Spread occurs to ducts and alveoli

Sequelae

1. The progress is slow and symptoms may be delayed for years.
2. Progressively increasing dyspnoea appears, ending in respiratory failure.
3. Pulmonary hypertension and right heart failure complicate the process.
4. Bronchial carcinoma, usually an adenocarcinoma, arises commonly in the fibrotic lower lobe and is the cause of death in 50% of cases.

PLEURAL FIBROUS PLAQUES

Bilateral pearly white plaques of acellular collagen form on the parietal pleura and upper surface of the diaphragm. They are irregular in shape but well-defined, and circumscribed calcification may follow. They produce no symptoms and are not a precursor of mesothelioma.

ASBESTOSIS

MALIGNANT MESOTHELIOMA

This tumour can occur even when the individual is only exposed to a low concentration of asbestos dust for a relatively short space of time. There is, however, a long interval between exposure to the dust and the time of appearance of the tumour. The physical characteristics of the fibres are implicated in the initiation of the carcinogenic process.

ASBESTOS BODIES

Associated macrophages

Asbestos fibres become coated with mucopolysaccharide and iron. A typical body is brown in colour with bulbous ends. The intervening part is segmented.

These bodies are found in the sputum of individuals exposed to asbestos dust. They occur in the lung tissue whatever type of pathological lesions exists, but are rarely if ever found within the pleural fibrous plaques or in mesothelioma tumour tissue.

Types of asbestos fibres and their industrial uses

1. *Chrysotile* (white asbestos) occurs as soft curly fibres generally retained in the upper respiratory tract. It causes asbestosis but rarely mesothelioma or pleural plaques. Used in making textiles, tiles, brake and clutch linings, gaskets, roofing felt, insulation.

2. *Crocidolite* (blue asbestos)

3. *Amosite* (brown iron-rich asbestos)

Both of these are in the form of rigid fibres which reach the periphery of the lung and are associated with all three types of lesion. Crocidolite is especially associated with mesothelioma. Both are highly resistant to acids and alkalis and are used in insulation work.

Mechanism of fibrogenesis

This is unknown but two suggestions have been made:

1. Macrophages which have ingested asbestos fibres may form a fibrogenic substance.

2. An immunological mechanism may operate. Antinuclear antibody and rheumatoid factor are found in the blood in a quarter of all patients.

347

ORGANIC DUSTS PNEUMONITIS

EXOGENOUS ALLERGIC

An increasing number of occupational pulmonary diseases are being recognised in workers handling organic material. The pathological processes are of two varieties:

1. The material being handled may be itself the cause of pathological changes. Byssinosis, due to cotton, flax or hemp, is an example. Exposure to the dust induces chronic coughing. Dyspnoea develops and may end in respiratory failure. The pathological process in one of chronic bronchitis.

Chronic bronchitis ⟶ Hyperplasia of mucous glands ⟶ Bronchial obstruction ⟶ Hypoventilation ⟶ Eventual respiratory failure

Intercurrent infection

2. In a much larger group, the disease process is related to moulds and fungi contaminating the material handled. Examples are:

Disease	Causative agent
Farmer's lung	– – – Actinomycetes in mouldy hay
Bagassosis	– – – Actinomycetes in mouldy sugar cane bagasse used in paper making
Malt worker's lung	– – – Aspergillus fumigatus in barley in distilleries and breweries
Bird fancier's lung	– – – Moulds and other antigens in bird droppings

Many other industries such as mushroom growing, cork manufacture and maple bark stripping have similar dangers.

Hypersensitivity to the moulds etc. develops and the reaction termed "extrinsic allergic alveolitis" is common to all of these clinical conditions. A high level of precipitating antibody is present in the blood.

Exudation of fluid

Platelet aggregation and thrombosis

Polymorph reaction, later lymphocytes and plasma cells

Inhalation of antigens ⟶ **Antigen-antibody complexes form** ⟶ **Activation of complement** ⟶ **Inflammatory response**

Repeated attacks destroy respiratory tissue and induce a chronic spreading fibrosis. Alveoli and bronchioles are destroyed. Some unaffected bronchioles may undergo compensatory dilatation causing 'honey-comb lung'. Severe respiratory embarrassment occurs which may end in both respiratoty and right heart failure.

PULMONARY FIBROSIS

GENERALISED FIBROSIS of LUNGS (CHRONIC INTERSTITIAL PNEUMONIA)

This is the end result of a number of diseases. The pathological changes at this stage are complex, and as a result the aetiology in a large percentage of cases is obscure. Beyond a certain point, the process is not so much a chain of events as a self-perpetuating vicious circle. Three primary mechanisms can be identified:

1. **Alveolar inflammations.** Pneumonias, either bacterial or viral, particularly if attacks are repeated, are important. Toxic fumes such as cadmium and beryllium also act in this way, and prolonged administration of oxygen in high concentration. In these cases, resolution may fail and the exudate is organised.

Unresolved fibrinous exudate.

Spaces left where fibrin unattached.

Epithelium grows to line spaces thus isolating fibrin like a mural thrombus.

Remains of alveoli
Fibrin converted into fibrous tissue

2. **Immunological Reactions.** These are exemplified by the reactions to many organic dusts — bagassosis, farmer's lung etc. Pulmonary fibrosis may also occur as a manifestation of rheumatoid disease and scleroderma. An obscure condition known variously as cryptogenic fibrosing alveolitis, idiopathic diffuse interstitial pulmonary fibrosis or Hamman-Rich syndrome appears to be of this nature.

   The hypersensitivity reaction starts in the interstitial tissue but spills over into the alveolar spaces.

Fluid

Acute congestion of capillaries

Epithelial cells desquamate due to oedema

Alveolar walls swollen by protein-rich exudate

Histiocytes, plasma cells, lymphocytes and eosinophils appear in the alveolar walls. In rheumatoid disease, there may be fibrinoid necrosis with formation of a nodule.

Compressed alveoli

New reticulin fibres appear: collagen is formed and alveoli are compressed/obliterated

3. **Specific fibrogenic irritants.** The inorganic dust diseases (silicosis, asbestosis, haematite miner's lung) illustrate this type of reaction (see p. 355)

PULMONARY FIBROSIS

GENERALISED FIBROSIS of LUNGS (continued)

Once the process is initiated, secondary changes take place. In all of them, at least two factors have to be considered:

(1) Chronic coughing

↓

Chronic bronchitis

↓

Mucous gland hyperplasia
and metaplasia of epithelium

(2) Distortion of bronchioles and
bronchi by contracting fibrous tissue

↓

Weakening of
bronchiolar walls

Retention of Secretion

↓

Repeated attacks of respiratory infection

↓

Increased fibrosis

    It will be realised that in most cases, respiratory infection is a factor inducing a progressive condition whatever the initiating cause. Important changes occur in the pulmonary circulation. Many vessels are destroyed by the fibrosis, while others show endarteritis.

    The clinical effects are the same as in all chronic lung diseases which interfere with ventilation and pulmonary circulation. There is increasing respiratory failure, pulmonary hypertension and ultimately right heart failure.

Honeycomb lung

This is the name given to a complication of lung fibrosis, and therefore has the same mixed aetiology.

Cysts mainly along anteromedial
borders of lungs; 1 — 2 cm in diameter;
smooth linings but often of irregular
shape.

The cysts are 'unaffected' bronchioles
which have undergone compensatory dilatation
following obliteration of others by
the fibrosing process. They are lined by
columnar or cuboidal epithelium.

CHEMICALS AND DRUGS

Certain chemical poisons induce lung changes resulting in generalised fibrosis indistinguishable from those already described, but the time-scale is very short. The reactions to poisoning with Paraquat (1, 1-dimethy1-4, 4-bipyridilium chloride), a weed killer, are typical of this group of substances.

There is an initial period of general toxicity with mouth ulceration, temporary renal failure due to tubular necrosis, and acute alveolitis.

Hyaline membrane formation in ducts

Oedema fluid in alveoli

Pneumocytes desquamated

Swelling of alveolar walls

Several days later

Invasion of alveoli by mononuclear cells which become fibroblasts

As a result of collagen production by the invading fibroblasts, alveoli and bronchioles are obliterated causing progressive respiratory failure. A fatal outcome is common even when the amount consumed is small. It would appear that the chemical stimulates the production of fibrogenic substances.

More important than accidental poisoning is the fact that certain chemotherapeutic agents occasionally cause similar lesions, usually after prolonged treatment. Busulphan, bleomycin, methotrexate — all used in the treatment of cancer — may result in pulmonary fibrosis. Salazopyrin and hexamethonium have also been incriminated. The list of drugs which have this potential in certain patients is bound to grow but, in view of the nature of the diseases which are treated, the dangers must be accepted as a justified hazard.

Oxygen posioning

This is a hazard in intensive care units where oxygen therapy may be administered over a period of days. The lung lesions, which resemble those of paraquat poisoning, consist of oedema, necrosis of capillary endothelium and alveolar epithelium. Haemorrhagic alveolar exudates are formed which subsequently organise. The fibrous tissue becomes incorporated in the alveolar walls.

Drug sensitivity

A large range of drugs, some complex chemicals like antibiotics, others as simple as aspirin, are sometimes associated with hypersensitivity and may cause asthmatic attacks.

TUMOURS OF LUNG

SIMPLE TUMOURS

Three main varieties are described:

1. PAPILLOMA

Polypoid tumours,
usually multiple,
at mouths of
large bronchi

Papillomas are similar to the papillary tumours of the larynx. They occur in young people and, on occasion, may cause stridor due to partial obstruction or even aspiration pneumonia.

2. BRONCHIAL ADENOMA

These are relatively common and account for almost 10% of primary lung tumours. They generally appear before the age of 40 and are slightly more common in females. Usually the tumour is situated in a primary bronchus. Commonly it projects into the bronchial lumen and the surface may be ulcerated and haemorrhagic. In some instances it is submucous, growing into the wall of the bronchus and causing obstructive effects.

Histologically, there are two distinctive patterns. The majority are of the 'apudoma' series (carcinoid, see p.409). The remainder are adenomas of the bronchial glands. Very occasionally these may undergo a low-grade malignant change — adenocytic carcinoma.

Clinical features

These may simulate bronchogenic carcinoma when bronchial obstruction occurs. Cough and haemoptysis are the principal symptoms. Obstruction eventually may cause complications:

Obstruction → Local emphysema

Obstruction → Atelectasis → Bronchiectasis

Obstruction → Infection → Lung abscess

Some patients present with the signs and symptoms of the carcinoid syndrome and excrete 5-hydroxytryptamine in the urine. In these cases, multiple metastases are found in liver and elsewhere.

3. HAMARTOMA

This forms a nodule, usually close to the pleura. It consists of a jumbled mass of tissues usually found in the area — cartilage (often calcified), fibrous tissue, msucle and epithelium lining gland clefts. It usually appears in middle age, more commonly in males, and may be mistaken for carcinoma.

BRONCHOGENIC CARCINOMA

This has now become the most common form of malignancy in Western civilisation. More than 60% arise in the right bronchus or one of its main branches.

It soon
ulcerates

The lumen
of the
bronchus is
greatly
reduced

It starts as a rough area
on the mucosa near the
bifurcation of the trachea

Spread in the mucosal
lymphatics produces
other nodules

The nodules coalesce to
form a large yellowish-
white friable mass

Spread within the lung

This takes place in two ways:

1. *Direct spread.* The growth may simply destroy and replace the lung tissue. At the same time, it grows to fill alveoli and may pass from one alveolus to another through the pores of Kohn.

Hilar lymph
nodes
are involved

The growth
extends to
involve the
lung tissue

2. *Lymphatic spread.* The common mode is spread along peribronchial and perivascular lymph channels.

Bronchi and
vessels become
ensheathed by
a white collar
of growth

The finer lymphatics
of the lobules
especially in the
subpleural region
may be filled by
malignant cells
producing a network
of white lines.

BRONCHOGENIC CARCINOMA

Secondary lung changes
These are the result of bronchial obstruction and intercurrent infection.

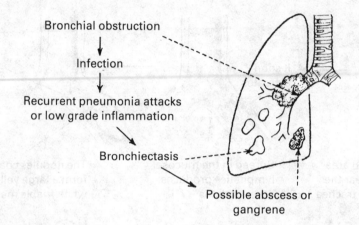

Bronchial obstruction

↓

Infection

↓

Recurrent pneumonia attacks
or low grade inflammation

↘

Bronchiectasis

Possible abscess or
gangrene

Direct spread outside lung and its effects

1. Spread may occur to the
   other bronchus and lung

2. Spread to the pleural and pericardial sacs is common.

(a) Pleural spread
resulting
in haemorrhagic
effusion.

(b) Pericardial
spread
with
subsequent
deposits in
myocardium.

BRONCHOGENIC CARCINOMA

Direct Spread outside lung and its effects (continued)

(c) The growth frequently
    encircles the great
    vessels.

Aorta

Pulmonary
venis

Pulmonary
artery

Superior
vena cava

RA

LA

LV

RV

Results

1. Constriction of vena cava:
   right atrial filling impeded.

2. Pulmonary arteries involved: upset in pulmonary circulation.

3. The pulmonary veins may also be affected, and if the growth permeates the venous wall,
   malignant thrombi may form giving rise to embolic spread. The aorta is rarely implicated due
   to the thick musculoelastic wall and the blood pressure.

(d) Nerves may be involved

1. Recurrent laryngeal ⟶ Paralysis of vocal cords

2. Phrenic ⟶ Paralysis of diaphragm

3. Vagus ⟶ Various effects on heart, lungs, etc.

4. Sympathetic ⟶ Horner's syndrome — ptosis of eyelid,
   small pupil and absence of sweating on
   same side of face.

355

BRONCHOGENIC CARCINOMA

Lymphatic spread outside of lung

This may be widespread.

Supraclavicular node

1. Hilar nodes are first to be affected.
2. Secondary masses may arise in the right adrenal by retrograde extension along lymphatics through diaphragm.

3. Invasion of thoracic duct causes chylous ascites.

4. Para-aortic nodes are sometimes affected.
5. Supraclavicular node at scalenus muscle insertion.

Haematogenous spread

This is common. It may be due to direct invasion of a pulmonary vein. Approximately 90% of cases show multiple metastases. The sites and frequency are as follows.

Site	Percentage incidence
Liver	33
Adrenal	20 – 30 — Partly lymphatic spread
Bones	15 – 20 — Mainly local (ribs, sternum and vertebrae) but may be distant
Brain	18 — Sometimes first clinical sign of a bronchial tumour
Kidneys	10

Invasion of a large vessel in the wall of a bronchus occasionally causes severe haemorrhage.

BRONCHOGENIC CARCINOMA

ASSOCIATED METABOLIC and CLINICAL SYNDROMES

Misleading symptoms and signs which suggest well-known clinical syndromes may be exhibited. Some of these are due to elaboration of hormone-like substances by the tumour:

(1) ACTH secretion ⟶ Adrenal hyperplasia ⟶ Raised blood cortisol ⟶ Cushing's syndrome

(2) 5-hydroxytryptamine secretion ⟶ Carcinoid syndrome when secondaries appear in liver and the hepatic catabolism of the amine is by-passed

(3) Antidiuretic hormone secretion ⟶ Oliguria ⟶ Hydraemia and hyponatraemia (dilution effect)

Hypercalcaemia has also been noted, possibly due to formation of parathyroid hormones. Other curious syndromes are: encephalopathies, cortical cerebellar degeneration, posterior root ganglion degeneration and other neuropathies, myopathy involving wasting of muscles of the limb, girdles and trunk.

HISTOLOGICAL TYPES

Four main varieties are recognised:

1. Squamous cell carcinoma
2. Small cell anaplastic carcinoma (oat cell)
3. Large cell anaplastic carcinoma
4. Adenocarcinoma

These are responsible for 90% of all bronchogenic cancers, and squamous cell carcinoma is the most common of these three.

BRONCHOGENIC CARCINOMA

Squamous cell carcinoma

This shows the usual characteristics of squamous cell carcinoma, but keratinisation is not common.

Lymphocyte reaction

Islands of invading squamous epithelial cells

Mitoses are not numerous

At edge of growth and in unaffected bronchi, squamous metaplasia and Ca in situ are found.

Cells of same type throughout depth of epithelium

Ca in situ cells growing into glands

Normal bronchial mucosa

Squamous metaplasia

This type of growth like all squamous cell carcinomas is relatively slow growing. It is associated with extensive destruction of local tissues, and the lung lesions due to bronchial obstruction are particularly apt to occur.

BRONCHOGENIC CARCINOMA

Oat cell carcinoma

So-called because of the resemblance of the cells to oat grains. Although the cells are relatively uniform it is really an anaplastic growth. Their appearance is characteristic.

Almost no cytoplasm

Spindle-shaped dark nuclei; may appear to be rounded or oval. May be arranged in sheets, cords or small round aggregates.

On electron-microscopy, cells show argyrophil neurosecretory granules.

This type of growth is most commonly associated with endocrine syndromes, and the neurosecretory granules are probably an indication of this activity. Metastases to lymph nodes may be difficult to recognise initially on histological material because the cells resemble lymphocytes superficially. The growth is of a highly malignant type and widespread metastases occur early. It tends to affect a younger age group more than does the squamous variety. The primary growth may be quite small although numerous blood borne metastases are present.

Large cell anaplastic carcinoma

As the name suggests this tumour shows cells of all shapes and sizes without any distinctive characteristics. Mitoses are frequent and it is highly malignant.

These three foregoing varieties almost always affect bronchi at the hilum and are most common in males. The sex incidence was until recently 8 males to 1 female.

Adenocarcinoma

This form is relatively rare, and at least 50 per cent arise in the peripheral bronchi. Another interesting feature is that there is no sex incidence, the neoplasm occuring in males and females equally. The gross appearance varies as in all glandular carcinomas.

It may be papillary ... or solid and scirrhous

Cells are cuboidal or tall columnar and mucus secreting

Despite the degree of differentiation, this is usually a highly malignant tumour.

BRONCHOGENIC CARCINOMA

AETIOLOGY

1. Bronchial carcinoma has increased by 500 per cent in the last 25 years.
2. Sex Incidence
   Previously 85% of cases occurred in males over the age of 45, with a sex incidence of 8 males to 1 female. Now the age in males is 30 and the male/female rate is 6 to 1. These facts apply to all histological types of carcinoma except adenocarcinoma which affects males and females equally.
3. Tobacco
   The increase in incidence of bronchial carcinoma is directly related to the number of cigarettes smoked per day. This is most clearly seen in females. The exact carcinogen is unknown but a component of cigarette tar is implicated.
4. Atmospheric Pollution
   Industrial vapours and combustion of oil and petrol are important factors. Bronchial carcinoma is always more frequent in towns than in rural areas.
5. Weather
   The incidence is higher in cities with a high rainfall. Noxious agents are concentrated in moisture droplets and in conditions of high humidity remain undispersed.
6. Industrial Causes
   These are related to high atmospheric pollution
   (a) Chromate industry; (b) nickel refining; (c) asbestos manufacture;
   (d) haematite mining and (e) uranium, cobalt mining. Radioactivity is important.

PROGNOSIS

1. Bronchial carcinoma causes 10% of all deaths between the ages of 45 and 64.
2. Only 20% are suitable for surgery, usually squamous cell growths. The 5 year survival rate is 25%, i.e. 5% of all cases survive 5 years. Cytological methods, e.g. brush biopsies may yield earlier diagnosis.
3. Prognosis is poorest with oat cell and anaplastic carcinoma.

SECONDARY LUNG TUMOURS

These are the commonest form of pulmonary malignancy due to the whole blood circulating through the lungs. In addition, lymphatic spread may occur from breast carcinoma and abdominal malignancies.

DISEASES OF THE PLEURA

INFLAMMATION (PLEURISY)
This takes one of three forms: (1) fibrinous, (2) sero-fibrinous and (3) empyema.
FIBRINOUS

Exudate on both
parietal and visceral
layers — pale grey

Shaggy due to
lung movement
Adhesions between
layers of pleura

Small quantity of fluid
at base of cavity

Exudate — fibrin with
entangled polymorphs.
Progress
Frequently self-limiting
disease. Much of the exudate
is subsequently absorbed,
but some fibrinous adhesions
may organise and become
permanent.

Aetiology There are two types:
1. Primary disease of the pleura. Evidence suggests that this is a tuberculous infection.
   Occasionally rheumatic fever may be the cause.
2. Secondary to an underlying pulmonary lesion, e.g. tuberculosis, lobar and bronchopneumonia,
   infarct or tumour growth. It can also be secondary to inflammation of another organ, e.g.
   pericarditis, osteitis of ribs or sub-diaphragmatic abscess.

SERO-FIBRINOUS
The appearances and effects vary according to the amount of fluid present.

Above the fluid, the
fibrin-covered layers
of pleura are adherent

Lung is collapsed
by fluid pressure

Diaphragm depressed by fluid

Pressure of fluid may displace
heart to opposite side.

Fluid contains small masses of
clot. Its specific gravity is
high, >1018, and its protein
content > 4%. These
features distinguish it from a
transudate.

Aetiology: Similar to fibrinous pleurisy.
1. Most cases are due to the tubercle bacillus. This can be demonstrated by inoculation of guinea-
   pig with fluid.
2. Occasionally other infections are responsible, e.g. pneumococci and streptococci. Rheumatic
   fever is another cause.

Progress: If the fluid is not aspirated or resorbed, lung collapse with fibrosis occurs.

DISEASES OF THE PLEURA

EMPYEMA

This is now a relatively rare condition since the introduction of antibiotics. It is usually due to spread of infection from adjacent tissues.

It is now exceptional for the whole pleural cavity to be filled with pus. Adhesions quickly localise the pus to form an abscess.

Complications
1. Local spread to lung, pericardium, myocardium.
2. Embolic brain abscess.
3. Amyloid disease if sepsis is prolonged.

Very rarely a tuberculous process in the lung ruptures into the pleural cavity causing a tuberculous empyema. Secondary infection is usual.

PNEUMOTHORAX

The introduction of air into the pleural cavity is not uncommon. Its effects depend on:-

(a) Whether the air is under pressure. This occurs when the opening into the pleural cavity is valvular, allowing the air in but not out. The lung collapses and the mediastinal viscera are displaced, and function of, e.g. the heart, may be upset.
(b) The occurrence of infection. This is almost inevitable. Empyema may be the result.

The condition occurs in three circumstances:

1. Disease of the lungs or other nearby viscera. Rupture of an emphysematous bulla is the commonest cause. Invasion of the pleural cavity by necrosing malignancies originating in the bronchus, oesophagus or stomach can also allow air to enter the cavity.

2. Penetrating wounds of the chest wall, either surgical or accidental.

3. Artificial respiration involving positive pressure.
   Occasionally, spontaneous pneumothorax occurs in healthy young adults. The cause in unknown.

DISEASES OF THE PLEURA

HYDROTHORAX

This is usually a complication of cardiac or renal disease and is more pronounced in the former. The transudate has a specific gravity <1018 and protein content <4%. Only endothelial cells are found in the fluid.

In Meig's syndrome, a rare condition, hydrothorax occurs in association with fibroma of ovary.

TUMOURS OF THE PLEURA

MESOTHELIOMA

This is the most important neoplasm of the pleura.

Growth may affect parietal pleura

Solid white tumour tissue

Usually there is pleural effusion, often haemorrhagic.

The growth spreads diffusely over the surface of the lung. It forms a thick white membrane which may envelope the whole lung, compressing it. The lung is invaded at a later stage.

Microscopically, much of the growth consists of dense connective tissue in which there are strands of large epithelial cells. They may line clefts or form acini. Papillary formations may also be seen.

Spread is initially by direct extension to neighbouring organs and tissues. Later, lymphatics and blood vessels are invaded giving rise to metastases. Apart from the effects on pulmonary function, patients may show pulmonary osteoarthropathy and arthritis.

AETIOLOGY

In almost all cases, there is a history of exposure to asbestos dust. The exposure may be of short duration — a few months — and occur many years before the appearance of tumour growth.

SECONDARY TUMOURS

Secondary carcinoma of the pleura is common and usually takes the form of small nodules scattered over the lung surface, but not usually invading the lung substance to any extent. The primary tumour is commonly in the breast.

CHAPTER 10

ALIMENTARY SYSTEM

LIPS AND MOUTH

Acute inflammation

Minor inflammations of the mouth are common due to trauma, hot food or irritants. The lips and mouth are also commonly involved as part of a more general infection such as measles.

An important lesion of modern times is infection by *Candida albicans*. Epidemics may occur in nurseries. It occurs as an opportunistic infection in adults receiving treatment with antibiotics, steroids or cytotoxic drugs.

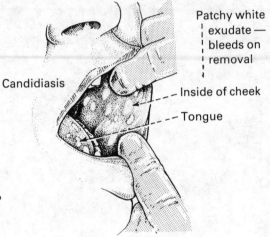

Patchy white exudate — bleeds on removal

Candidiasis

Inside of cheek

Tongue

Aphthous ulceration

Tiny ulcers, whitish in colour and extremely painful are common on the gums, tongue and inside of cheek. The aetiology is unknown.

Chronic inflammation

Specific chronic inflammation such as syphilis and tuberculosis are now rare in most developed countries but occur frequently in underdeveloped regions of the world.

Primary chancre may occur on the lips or tip of tongue. Due to moisture and secondary infection, a softer lesion is produced. In the secondary stage, white areas of cellular infiltration (mucous patches) and irregular silvery lines of ulceration (snail track ulcers) are found. Small gummata which quickly become deep punched out ulcers with a greyish base may form on the dorsum of the posterior third of the tongue.

Tuberculous ulcers are shallow and somewhat ragged with undermined edges. They are due to secondary spread from a pulmonary lesion and are found on the tip of the tongue.

Deficiency diseases associated with anaemia cause cracks and fissures at the angles of the mouth. The tongue is smooth due to loss of papillae — atrophic glossitis. The lack of B group vitamins is the usual cause.

LIPS AND MOUTH

Leukoplakia

This is an ill-understood clinical diagnosis meaning white patches on a stratified squamous epithelium in or near a mucous surface.

Hyperkeratosis gives the white appearance to the lesion

Superficial cells are swollen and oedematous

The epithelium forms downgrowths due to hyperplasia of the basal layers

The dermal papillae are elongated

The underlying tissues are heavily infiltrated by lymphocytes and plasma cells

The aetiology in many cases is obscure. Some are associated with chronic irritation, e.g. ill-fitting dentures or pipe smoking. The importance of the lesion is that in some individuals the epithelium becomes dysplastic and many cancers in this region have associated leukoplakic lesions.

Pigmentations

Dark pigmentations of the gums are seen in chronic poisoning with heavy metals lead (blue), bismuth (grey), mercury (purplish). Melanotic pigmentation of the mouth is seen in Addison's disease and the Peutz-Jegher's syndrome.

Tumours

Benign tumour masses are not uncommon in the oral cavity. Some of them are of inflammatory origin rather than true neoplasms.

Squamous papilloma is the only epithelial variety. It does not show any tendency to malignant change.

Connective tissue tumours form an interesting group. Haemangioma and lymphangioma are fairly common and give rise to cosmetic problems if on the lips. On the tongue they can interfere with swallowing and severe haemorrhage may be caused.

MOUTH

Granular cell myoblastoma

This is a rare tumour and its importance lies in the fact that it may be mistaken for carcinoma of the tongue.

Overlying epithelium shows very irregular downgrowths — but it is not neoplastic (so-called pseudoepitheliomatous hyperplasia)

Large granular cells (thought to arise from Schwann cells or nerves) between and around muscle cells of tongue

Epulis

This is a clinical term applied to swellings at the gum margin. Most of them are granulomas associated with chronic gingivitis. A few are true neoplasms.

Fibrous epulis

This is composed of fibrous tissue but frequently contains bony trabeculae. Usually in the upper jaw, it may be locally invasive and destroy bone.

Giant cell epulis

It is problematical if this is a true neoplasm. Histologically, it resembles the giant cell tumour of bone, consisting of giant cells and spindle cells. They are usually found in the mandible of children associated with primary dentition.

Congenital epulis

These tumours are very occasionally seen in the gum of the upper jaw in the newborn. Two types are seen:

1. Soft polypoid tumours containing granular cells like those of the granular myoblastoma.
2. Pigmented tumours which contain cells like neuroblasts and pigmented cubical cells.

MOUTH — MALIGNANT TUMOURS

Squamous cell carcinoma

This is the most important neoplasm, and it may arise on the lip, tongue, floor of mouth, tonsil and fauces, in that order of frequency.

Lip

Induced nodule often on lower lip, at the red margin

Breaks down to form ulcer with raised rolled edges

Histologicially it is a well-differentiated keratinizing growth

Growth is relatively slow but eventually dissemination to the submandibular nodes takes place and thence to the deeper cervical nodes

It is most common in males in the 6th decade, working in outdoor occupations. Exposure to sunlight may be a factor, and in some cases leukoplakia precedes tumour growth. In Eastern countries, cancers of the lip, tongue and inside of cheek are definitely associated with the chewing of a mixture of betel nut and tobacco.

Tongue

Carcinoma of the tongue and other sites within the mouth is a more aggressive growth than tumours of the lips. Starting as a nodule in the buccal sulcus adjacent to the tongue, it quickly

breaks down to form an irregular ulcer with ragged edges.

Local infiltration leads to fixation of the tongue. Spread may be extensive to floor of mouth, fauces and pharynx.

Lymph node involvement occurs early, usually to the deeper cervical nodes.

DISEASES OF PHARYNX

Tonsillitis

This is a common acute inflammation. It is frequently due to streptococcal infection, but viruses, particularly the adenoviruses, also cause tonsillitis and, due to the use of antibiotics, have become more important. The pharyngeal tissues including the tonsil become acutely swollen and purulent exudate appears at the mouths of the crypts. Occasionally the inflammation is very acute, resulting in suppuration in the tissues — termed quinsy. There is a marked tendency for tonsillitis to recur. Eventually a chronic condition is produced with permanent enlargement of the tonsils. The crypts are dilated and contain inspissated exudate.

During the process, various immunological phenomena arise. The importance of this disease is that it is commonly a precursor of rheumatic fever or one form of glomerulo-nephritis.

Vincent's angina

This is an acute inflammation due to the combined action of fusiform bacilli and a spirochaete — *Borrelia vincenti*. It may cause severe ulceration.

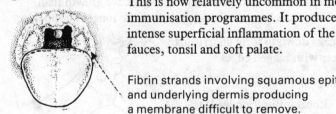

White membrane
Surrounding acute inflammation

Diphtheria

This is now relatively uncommon in most of the world, due to immunisation programmes. It produces an intense superficial inflammation of the fauces, tonsil and soft palate.

Fibrin strands involving squamous epithelium and underlying dermis producing a membrane difficult to remove.

The infection remains local and the severe clinical effects are due to the powerful exotoxin. In addition to general toxaemia there is specific damage to nerves and myocardium.

Lymphoepithelioma

This is now considered to be a squamous carcinoma heavily infiltrated by lymphocytes. It arises in the pharynx and invasion of the cervical nodes occurs early. These tumours are common in Chinese people and are associated with EB virus infection.

DISEASES OF SALIVARY GLANDS

Simple acute inflammation of these glands is uncommon. It may occur during a prolonged illness, particularly if a calculus has formed in a duct.

More commonly acute inflammation is due to the virus of *mumps,* which produces acute swelling, particularly of the parotid glands, with oedema and mononuclear infiltration of the interstitial tissue. The testes and pancreas may also be inflamed and atrophy may follow.

Parotid

Pancreas

Testes

Chronic inflammation is rare. It may occur as a manifestation of sarcoidosis. The parotid gland becomes swollen and there is an accompanying iridocyclitis. This has given rise to the term 'uveo-parotid fever'. The parotid gland shows a chronic inflammatory reaction with follicular lesions typical of sarcoidosis.

Siogren's syndrome

In this condition there is a destruction of the gland tissue of the salivary, lacrimal and conjunctival glands by an infiltrate of lymphocytes and plasma cells. The duct epithelia often undergo reactive hyperplasia. It results in dryness of the mouth, caries due to lack of saliva and ulceration of the conjunctiva caused by lack of secretion from the lacrimal and conjunctival glands. Polyarthritis is often present and the serum contains autoantibodies and rheumatoid factor.

Calculus formation

This uncommon condition mainly affects the parotid duct. Blockage of the duct leads to atrophy of the gland. Occasionally acute inflammation may be superimposed.

SALIVARY GLANDS — TUMOURS

MIXED TUMOUR

This is the commonest tumour of salivary glands, and most occur in the parotid. The mixed elements are of epithelial and 'connective tissue' types and are derived from the epithelial and myoepithelial elements of the glandular acini and ducts.

The tumours vary in size from a few millimetres to several centimetres. They are usually rounded or lobulated; consistency varies with structure.

(a) *Firm* — mainly fibrous

(b) *Fleshy* — largely epithelial

(c) *Gelatinous* — mucinous matrix

(d) *Hard* — mainly cartilagenous, sometimes with bony trabeculae

Fibrous tissue nodules

Epithelial masses

Epithelium arranged in acini or solid strands. Acini often have double layer of cells like normal salivary glands

Epithelial structures separated by large areas of mucoid stroma

Nodules of cartilage

Strands of epithelium

The epithelium may be arranged as glands, ductules, solid sheets or squamous masses. All epithelial and stromal types may be found in the same tumour.

The tumour is enclosed in a fibrous capsule, but there are frequently extensions beyond the capsule. Most are relatively benign, but they tend to recur after excision. Transition to definite malignancy is exceptional.

MONOMORPHIC ADENOMA

This is a variant consisting of epithelial elements without any specific stromal change.

SALIVARY GLANDS — TUMOURS

CARCINOMA of SALIVARY GLANDS

Approximately 30% of salivary tumours are frankly malignant, the growth taking the form of a carcinoma. The histological structure can be very varied. Some are anaplastic, others more differentiated. There are, however, four distinct forms:

1. Acinic carcinoma

Approximately ¼ of all malignant parotid tumours are of this type. It grows slowly, recurs after removal and sometimes there is late extension to the regional lymph nodes and distant organs.

Closely aggregated acinar structures. Cells often contain glycogen

2. Adenocystic carcinoma

This usually occurs in minor salivary glands and accounts for 7% of salivary gland tumours. It extends by direct spread, but metastases occur at a late stage to lymph nodes, lungs and bones. There is a special tendency to invade nerve sheaths.

Cribriform pattern. Solid masses of epithelium enclosing small cystic spaces containing mucin. The cells resemble basal cells

3. Muco-epidermoid carcinoma

The malignancy of this type varies, but all tend to recur and infiltrate locally. More malignant growths metastasise to the lymph nodes and may invade the blood stream. They are generally found in the major salivary glands and form 3 or 4% of all tumours of these glands.

Squamoid cells

Mucus-secreting cells

SALIVARY GLANDS — TUMOURS

CARCINOMA of SALIVARY GLANDS (continued)

4. *Epidermoid (squamous) carcinoma*
   This rare tumour grows rapidly and metastasises
   to regional nodes. They are thought to
   arise from duct epithelium and are found in the
   major salivary glands.

Incidence and aetiology of salivary gland tumours

1. The majority of tumours arise in the parotid gland — approximately 80%

2. Tumours of the minor salivary glands account for 12% and they are frequently malignant.

3. The smallest proportion of tumours is found in the submandibular and sublingual glands except in Malaya and Uganda. The proportion of submandibular tumours is greater in the Chinese population of Malaya, and in Uganda both submandibular and palatal tumours are common. In the West Indies, tumours occur with greater frequency in the sublingual and minor glands.

4. The over-all incidence of salivary tumours, especially malignant varieties, is greatest in Eskimos.

5. Salivary tumours are commonest in middle age.

OESOPHAGUS

The oesophagus is a muscular tube lined by stratified squamous epithelium and is highly resistant to damage.

INFLAMMATION

Infection of the oesophagus is rare and is generally due to spread from the pharynx. Herpes may affect infants and opportunistic infection with thrush can occur in states of diminished immunity.

More often, inflammation is due to chemicals and occurs in two circumstances:

1. **Caustic poisoning**

   In strong concentration, widespread necrosis and sloughing of tissues occurs. With weaker poisons, the epithelium is destroyed. Secondary infection and inflammation occur. Healing may lead to fibrous stricture.

2. **Peptic oesophagitis**

   This is the commonest form of inflammation. It is due to reflux of acid from the stomach and is especially apt to happen in any illness involving bed-rest. A more important type is associated with hiatus hernia, particularly where part of the cardia herniates into the thorax.

Acid secretion produces inflammation and superficial ulceration of the oesophageal mucosa. The two main complications are anaemia due to repeated small haemorrhages and fibrous stricture following repeated healing and relapse.

OESOPHAGUS

OBSTRUCTION is the commonest disorder. Two main types are described

1. **Organic obstruction**
   - Occlusion of lumen. This may be due to tumour growth or foreign body.
   - Compression of oesophagus by tumours and other conditions in mediastinum.
   - Stenosis may be caused by scirrhous carcinoma, or strictures following corrosive poisoning or hiatus hernia.
   - Neuromuscular incoordination due to destruction of muscle as in systemic sclerosis or of the autonomic ganglia as in South American trypanosomiasis (Chagas' disease).

2. **Functional obstruction**

 Achalasia of the oesophagus develops in young adults and may cause severe obstruction.
Above the obstruction the oesophagus is dilated, the muscle is hypertrophied and the mucosa may be ulcerated.
Narrowing occurs at the lower end.

It is due to a conduction failure in the peristaltic mechanism, preventing opening of the cardiac sphincter. Muscle spasm in anaemia of young women (Plummer-Vinsen syndrome) can cause obstruction at the upper end of the oesophagus.

DIVERTICULA

These are relatively rare and are of two varieties.

1. **Pulsion type**
Involves pharynx (pharyngeal pouch). Sac is distended during swallowing of food. By pushing down behind oesophagus, it may compress this structure. Congenital weakness of the pharyngeal muscles is said to be an aetiological factor.

2. **Traction type**
This is due to traction of fibrous tissue produced by mediastinal inflammation, e.g. tuberculosis or silicosis of lymph nodes.

Bronchus

Diseased mediastinal lymph nodes

Fibrous tissue pulling on oesophageal wall

Rarely, there may be a congenital diverticulum at the level of the bifurcation of the trachea.

OESOPHAGUS

OESOPHAGEAL VARICES

These are important lesions which occur secondarily to portal hypertension caused by cirrhosis of the liver (see p.460).

Fibrosis in the liver obstructs the flow of blood from the gastrointestinal tract in the portal system. Anastomotic channels connecting the portal and systemic venous systems open up and become distended. The most important are the oesophageal tributaries of the azygos vein which connect through the diaphragm with the portal system. They become varicose, and are easily traumatised by the passage of food, leading to haemorrhage which can be fatal.

SPONTANEOUS RUPTURE

This is a condition of unknown origin which occurs in healthy men.

A longitudinal slit appears in left posterior aspect of oesophageal wall above the diaphragm. Gastric fluid escapes causing mediastinitis and pleurisy.

It may be due to distension of the oesophagus during the act of vomiting and in some cases is associated with acute alcoholic intoxication (Mallory-Weiss syndrome). Tears without rupture but causing haemorrhage and haematemesis may also occur.

CONGENITAL ABNORMALITIES

Apart from stenosis (already mentioned), atresia is the only other congenital malformation of any note. Two anatomical forms are found:

(1) Upper part ends blindly at level of azygos vein — Fistula formed between lower part and trachea

(2) No fistulous communication. This form is very rare.

Regurgitation and inhalation of food or gastric secretions may prove fatal.

377

OSEOPHAGUS

TUMOURS

Benign tumours of the oesophagus are very rare. They are almost always of connective tissue origin and form polyps within the lumen, causing obstruction.

Carcinoma

This is the third most common malignant tumour of the digestive tract, carcinoma of large intestine and stomach taking precedence in that order.

(1) At level of bifurcation of trachea. This is the commonest site

It occurs at three levels:

(2) Upper end of oesophagus at level of cricoid cartilage

(3) Lower end of oesophagus

Seventy five per cent of those in the upper part of the oesophagus occur in females. In 80% of the remainder, males are affected. The disease is altogether more common in males. Two forms of growth are seen:

(1) Scirrhous encircling the tube and causing constriction

(2) Soft polypoidal growth filling lumen

In both instances the growth tends to extend in a longitudinal manner. Growths at the upper end and at the level of the tracheal bifurcation are usually poorly differentiated squamous cell carcinomas. At the lower end, adenocarcinoma is common.

Spread

At the common site, near the tracheal bifurcation, spread may involve the trachea or a bronchus, ulcerating the wall and resulting in aspiration pneumonia. Tumours at other levels will involve the trachea or other mediastinal structures. Death usually results from the oesophageal obstruction, but occasionally the patient may survive long enough for metastases to appear in nodes and other organs, e.g. liver.

Aetiological factors

The incidence shows a geographical variation, being common in Africa, USSR, and Caracas. The causes are unknown but may be dietetic, especially the consumption of very hot foods. Postcricoid carcinoma in women is a rare late complication of the dysphagia complicating iron deficiency anaemia.

STOMACH

The stomach is divided
into five anatomical regions:

Cardia (1)

Fundus (2)

Pylorus (5)

Body (3)

Duodenal bulb

Pyloric antrum
or canal (4)

It has three secretory areas:

Cardiac
The glands are of short
mucus secreting type.

Body
This is the main special
secreting area.

Pyloric

Chief or
pepsin
secreting
cells

Mucus
cells
of the ducts

Parietal
oxyntic cells
secreting
HCl and
intrinsic factor.

Mucus secreting cells

Vascular supply

Along the lesser curvature,
run the right and left gastric
arteries, which anastomose
directly.

The greater curvature
shows 3 arterial supplies:

Branches from the splenic
artery

Right and left gastroepiploic
arteries

The arteries anastomose freely in the muscular submucous and mucous coats, except along the lesser curvature of the pyloric antrum and including the first part of duodenum. In this area, there is little anastomosis between the terminal branches in the mucosa.

STOMACH

GASTRIC SECRETION

The secretion of gastric juice occurs in two phases under quite different controls.

1. *Reflex nervous phase*

Vagus centre

Sight, taste and smell of food

Distension of stomach by food

Juice rich in acid and enzymes

2. *Humoral phase*

Products of protein digestion

Maintenance of gastric acid secretion, poor in enzymes

Production of gastrin by pylorus and duodenum

Carried in blood stream

The stomach also produces large quantities of mucus which protects the mucosa from the action of acid and proteolytic enzymes. Both intrinsic factor (IF) which combines with vitamin B_{12} and hydrochloric acid (HCl) are secreted by the specialised parietal cells of the body. Blood group mucopolysaccharide substances are also secreted.

Apart from its secretory activity, one of the important features of the stomach and indeed the whole gastrointestinal tract is the very rapid turnover of epithelial cells.

GASTRITIS

ACUTE INFLAMMATION

Mild acute gastritis is an acute inflammation with polymorph reaction in the superficial layers of the mucosa. Pain and sickness have a multitude of causes varying from hot fluids, alcohol and aspirin which act as direct irritants, to infections such as childhood fevers, viral infections and bacterial food poisoning.

A more acute form, known as acute haemorrhagic or erosive gastritis, is occasionally seen; it is associated with ingestion of irritant drugs, particularly aspirin and is also a complication of shock states.

Haemorrhagic erosions

These are tiny ulcers, a few millimetres in diameter, which are formed by the digestion of the mucous membrane overlying small haemorrhages. They are usually multiple and affect all parts of the stomach. They occur mostly on the apex of mucosal folds and involve only the mucosa.

Note that the changes are superficial so that restoration to normal can very quickly occur.

Naked eye appearance

Stress ulcers

Occasionally, particularly in severe shock, there is deeper acute ulceration with considerable haemorrhage and even perforation.

These ulcers are described in more detail in page 384.

Erosion of mucosa with bleeding and loss of gland duct epithelium

Polymorph infiltration

Parietal cells

Muscle layer

Oedema resulting in swelling of mucosa and separation of glands

GASTRITIS

CHRONIC GASTRITIS

It is convenient to consider two pathologically distinct types:

Type I (Type A)

This is essentially an autoimmune disease. The body of the stomach is particularly affected. There is progressive destruction of the specialised chief and parietal cells ending in gastric mucosal 'atrophy'.

Normal

Phase 1 Early phase (Mild superficial chronic gastritis)

Short ducts lined by mucus-secreting epithelium

Glands lined by cells secreting pepsin (chief cells) and acid (parietal cells)

Submucosa   Muscle

Mucosa normal thickness — surface intact

Ducts long, due to replacement of damaged glandular epithelium by simple mucous cells

Gland tissue reduced

Lymphocytes, plasma cells and eosinophils

Submucosa   Muscle

Phase 2 *(Atrophic gastritis)*

This is an extension of the first phase with the inflammatory process reaching to the submucosa. The rugae become flattened giving the mucosal surface a flat, smooth appearance. Glandular may show metaplasia of an intestinal type.

Mucosa thinned
Increase of interstitial tissue

Glands reduced in number

Goblet cells may appear

Heavy infiltration by lymphocytes and plasma cells

Reduction in chief and parietal cells in deeper parts of glands

Occasional lymph follicle

Phase 3 *Gastric atrophy*

The changes are similar to those seen in atrophic gastritis, but inflammatory changes are less marked with fewer lymphocytes and plasma cells. The loss of specialised cells is complete.

GASTRITIS

Chronic gastritis (continued)
Type II (Type B)
This is much more common than Type I. It is essentially a superficial inflammatory reaction to continuing minor superficial cellular damage caused by agents within the lumen.
The pyloric antrum and adjacent distal body are particularly affected.

Mucosal surface intact

Small foci of neutrophils, some passing to surface or into superficial crypt lumen.

Increase in population of lymphocytes and plasma cells.

Note: 1. Evidence of damage (neutrophil infiltration) is superficial.
2. The population of specialised cells is minimally damaged.
3. With long-standing disease — seen in the elderly — there may be some atrophy, but it is never complete.
4. Types I and II have been described separately, but there may be some overlap, e.g. both may show intestinal metaplasia.

Complications

Type I

Complete atrophy of specialised cells

(a) Oxyntic (parietal) cells → ACHLORHYDRIA

(b) Chief cells → Absence of pepsinogen

→ Absence of INTRINSIC FACTOR → PERNICIOUS ANAEMIA

Type II — association with GASTRIC and DUODENAL ULCERS (see p.389).
Types I and II — association with gastric cancer (see p. 393).

Aetiology
Type I — evidence for auto-immune mechanisms:
1. Strongly familial (genetic component).
2. Association with other autoimmune diseases.
3. Presence of antibodies to parietal cells and intrinsic factor (IF).

Type II — see page 389.

383

PEPTIC ULCERATION — ACUTE

Peptic ulcers occur only at sites where there is acid-containing gastric juice. The common sites in order of frequency are (1) duodenum, (2) stomach, (3) lower oesophagus, and rarely with heterotopic gastric mucosa, e.g. Meckel's diverticulum.

ACUTE PEPTIC ULCER

This type may be associated with acute gastritis and particularly also with states of severe shock (Stress ulcers, see p. 381).

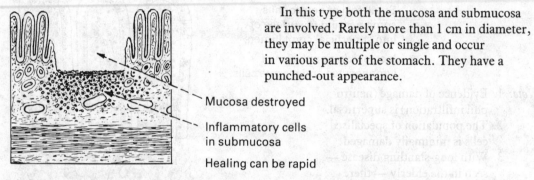

In this type both the mucosa and submucosa are involved. Rarely more than 1 cm in diameter, they may be multiple or single and occur in various parts of the stomach. They have a punched-out appearance.

Mucosa destroyed

Inflammatory cells in submucosa

Healing can be rapid

Occasionally the ulcer extends more deeply.

Erosion of a blood vessel may cause serious haemorrhage

Destruction of mucosa and submucosa

Inflammation extends to edge of muscle

Very rarely is there actual perforation (acute perforating ulcer)

Perforation with little inflammation

Peritonitis

SUBACUTE PEPTIC ULCER

384 This term is used for ulcers showing greater penetration of the muscularis with more inflammatory reaction and slight fibrosis.

PEPTIC ULCERATION — CHRONIC

CHRONIC PEPTIC ULCER

The term 'chronic' is applied when the pathological changes have penetrated and destroyed the muscle coat; they are also, of course, of much longer duration than acute ulcers. It is likely but not proven that chronic ulcers are derived from acute mucosal damage.

Gastric ulcers are typically sited on the **distal lesser curve**. Chronic ulceration of the first part of the **duodenum is the most common site** of peptic ulceration

A few occur at the cardiac end of the stomach or in the distal **oesophagus**

The ulcers are almost always single, but in 5 – 10%, a second ulcer may be found on the opposite aspect of the pyloric canal or duodenum (kissing ulcers).

The ulcer is commonly large, 2 – 3 cm, and oval. It has an overhanging lip at the proximal end.

Frequently it has a terraced structure.

The distal end slopes away from the ulcer bed.

The depth of ulceration varies. There are obviously periods of quiescence with attempts at healing and the production of scar tissue.

Muscle

Mucosa

Fibrin and necrotic debris

Granulation tissue infiltrated by lymphocytes and plasma cells

Dense scar tissue replacing muscle. Vessels show endarteritis.

Frequently the ulcerative process extends to the serous coat or even beyond.

Mucosa

Necrotic material

Muscle coat

Granulation tissue

Serous surface

Scar tissue

Extension of the inflammation to the serous coat may result in adhesion to other organs, e.g. the pancreas, and the ulceration may burrow into the affected organ.

The remainder of the stomach frequently shows chronic gastritis.

PEPTIC ULCERATION — CHRONIC

SEQUELS and COMPLICATIONS

1. **Healing** is common. This is the usual result in acute and probably subacute ulceration. Chronic ulcers frequently heal.

Healed subacute ulcer

Shallow depression

Rugae

Small amount of fibrous tissue causing depression by contraction.

Healed chronic ulcer

Deep depression

Stellate contractions

Destruction of mucosa

Large amount of contracting scar tissue

Muscle drawn up by scar tissue

Scarring in the duodenum may lead to serious stricture

Ulcers in the pyloric region. Stricture in this region may result in pyloric stenosis.

Stomach dilates leading to chronic vomiting with alkalosis and malnutrition

The constriction caused by healing of a large ulcer of the lesser curvature may draw up the greater curve producing an hour-glass stomach, with the same result as a pyloric stenosis.

Constriction at lower end of oesophagus leads to difficulty in swallowing and proximal dilatation (see p. 375).

386

PEPTIC ULCERATION — CHRONIC

SEQUELS and COMPLICATIONS (continued)

2. Perforation

Acute perforating ulcer
(This is now a rare condition.)

Ulcer has a terraced appearance.
It is probably of subacute type which
has suffered an acute ulcerative
exacerbation.

Perforation of a chronic ulcer

Acute ulceration occur diagonally
through the non-scarred soft tissues.

Perforation causes acute peritonitis. Fibrinous adhesions may result in an undiscovered loculus of pus between the liver and diaphragm — subphrenic abscess.

The advancing chronic inflammation of a chronic ulcer frequently causes adhesions to adjacent areas and this prevents perforation.

3. Haemorrhage.
As in any active ulcerative process, bleeding is frequent. Most commonly it is of minor degree — an oozing from the granulation tissue which can only be detected by testing faeces for occult blood. More marked haemorrhage may actually cause discoloration of the faeces — tarry stools due to the formation of iron sulphides. Vomiting with "coffee-grounds" vomit may also occur. Occasionally a very large haemorrhage may occur, usually from a chronic ulcer.

The pathology is as follows:

Most vessels undergo endarteritis
and serious bleeding is
thus avoided but a large patent
arterial branch in the base of
the ulcer may be attacked by
an acute ulcerative phase. The
scar tissue is an important factor
in causing continued bleeding.

- - - → Mucosa

Granulation
tissue

- - - Muscle

- - - Scar tissue

Eroded artery held in fibrous
tissue unable to contract or retract.

4. Development of carcinoma.
It is now thought that less than 1% of chronic gastric ulcers give rise to carcinoma. It always develops from the surviving mucosa at the edge of the ulcer where there is always active chronic gastritis.

Carcinoma never develops in duodenal ulcer.

PEPTIC ULCERATION

AETIOLOGY

The one essential factor in the causation of peptic ulcer is the presence of ACID, which acts as a continuing 'irritant' resulting in chronic ulceration.

For the maintenance of a healthy mucosa there are three essentials:

1. Presence of protective mucus
2. A good blood supply
3. Rapid turnover of epithelial cells to maintain surface integrity.

The diagram illustrates potentially damaging mechanisms:

In addition, there is an important genetic component.

Helicobacter pylori (formerly Campylobacter pylori)

The whole picture of the mechanism of gastroduodenal ulceration has been altered by the discovery of a specific infective agent, *Helicobacter pylori*, by Australian workers Marshall et al and since confirmed by others. There is an infestation of the gastric and duodenal mucosae in the great majority of cases of chronic gastritis (Type II) and duodenitis.

Helicobacter pylori is a Gram-negative vibrio-like (⌣, ∼) microbe which is specifically adapted to the antral mucosa. It elaborates a powerful urease and lipase.

PEPTIC ULCERATION

Helicobacter pylori (**continued**)
Infection of the antral mucosa
Chronic gastritis Type II

High magnification

Helicobacter in surface mucus

Focal epithelial cell damage

Focal neutrophil infiltration

? Infection is potentiated via glycerolipid mucus.
? Association with non-secretor status of ABO group antigens.

Infection of the duodenal mucosa
This is secondary to the gastric antral infection and depends on the presence of **superficial gastric metaplasia** in the first part of the duodenum consequent upon **hyperchlorhydria** and rapid emptying of the stomach. With the metaplasia, gastric mucus appears encouraging helicobacter colonisation.

Hyperchlorhydria

Focal metaplasia of tips of duodenal villi

Gastric type mucus and *Helicobacter* pylori

Cell damage
↓
Neutrophils
↓
Duodenitis

This continuing low grade damage establishes conditions suitable for further damage by acid and digestive enzymes.

Aetiology of duodenal ulceration

Helicobacter pylori
gastric infection

Gastric hyperacidity and hypermotility
↓
Gastric **metaplasia** in duodenum
↓
H.pylori infection of duodenum
↓

H.pylori infection of duodenum
Acid and digestive enzymes

Duodenitis

All other factors (see p. 388)

DUODENAL ULCER

Note: Cure of duodenal ulcers is obtained when *H.pylori* is eliminated and acid reduced.

GASTRIC CARCINOMA

This is a relatively common form of malignancy, although it occurs less frequently than hitherto.

Approximately 85% of these tumours occur at the pylorus or in the pyloric canal. The remainder may occur in any part of the stomach. Unlike chronic peptic ulcer, they are not confined to the lesser curvature.

Various types of growth are described:

1. Fungating carcinoma

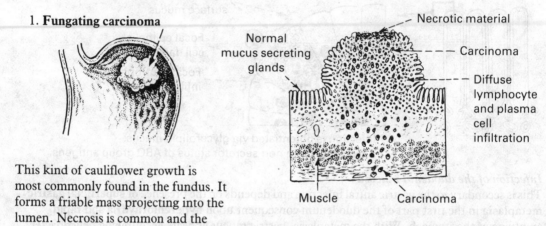

This kind of cauliflower growth is most commonly found in the fundus. It forms a friable mass projecting into the lumen. Necrosis is common and the surface is commonly ulcerated. It remains superficial for a considerable time but eventually grows through the stomach wall and spreads to adjacent structures. Histologically it is usually a typical adenocarcinoma.

2. Scirrhous carcinoma

This occurs in two forms:

1. *Localised*

Commonest at the pylorus; although it does not protrude into the lumen, constriction is caused by the fibrosis.

Necrotic material

It usually forms a large ulcer which penetrates to the muscle but not through it. The ulcer is larger and more irregular than chronic peptic ulcer.

Scirrhous carcinoma (continued)

2. *Diffuse*

Extension to the oesophagus may occur.
The stomach is reduced in size with a thickened
    firm wall (leather-bottle stomach or linitis plastica).
Ulceration is minimal.
Rugae are prominent.

The carcinoma appears to take origin from the deeper glands
and the surface is not involved. The scirrhous reaction is a
pronounced feature. Histologically, it may be an
adenocarcinoma or a signet ring carcinoma. The latter is
distinctive. The cells are rounded and contain a large globule
of mucus pushing the nucleus to one side.

3. Mucoid carcinoma

Usually found at the pylorus.
Grows diffusely in wall which
    becomes whitish and translucent.
Faint indication of muscle coat.

This growth spreads especially by direct extension and, in the
peritoneal cavity, ensheaths the other organs in a thick gelatinous
mantle. Histologically, it consists of alveoli containing small
numbers of cancer cells suspended in mucus. Sometimes they
may have a signet ring cell structure.

4. Superficial spreading carcinoma

This is an unusual type which forms serpiginous lines of growth spreading in the mucosa and
submucosa.

GASTRIC CARCINOMA

Direct spread

This is usually extensive and various structures may be involved.

Oesophagus and duodenum may be invaded by growth along the submucosa and muscle. This is seen in diffusely growing types of primary growth.

- Spleen (very rare)
- Lesser omentum
- Liver
- Greater omentum
- Pancreas

Spread also takes place to the diaphragm and abdominal wall.

Transcoelomic spread is a special type of direct spread. Cells may seed over the peritoneal cavity causing numerous small discrete tumours. The signet ring histological type sometimes causes bilateral hard ovarian tumours by this means — known as Krukenberg tumours.

In mucoid cancer, direct spread gives rise to massive growths in the peritoneal cavity.

Lymphatic spread

This occurs early and is often extensive, especially in the scirrhous variety. The gastric submucosal lymphatics are first invaded, and this may result in further nodules in the gastric wall. Penetration to the serosal lymphatics soon occurs. The omentum, mesenteries and intestinal walls may be invaded. Spread by this route to the liver is common.

Blood spread

In the first instance, this occurs via the hepatic portal system giving rise to metastases in the liver. Later the lung is involved and spread by the systemic circulation results in secondary growths in the brain and bones. Blood spread is commonest with anaplastic growths, less common in mucoid and diffuse scirrhous tumours.

GASTRIC CARCINOMA

Clinical associations

Cachexia and anaemia are usually severe. This may be related in part to the achlorhydria which is almost always present.

The anaemia is usually of microcytic or normochromic type, rarely macrocytic.
Where carcinoma develops in association with peptic ulcer there may be no achlorhydria.

The achlorhydria is possibly related more to the associated chronic gastritis (which is always present) than to the carcinoma per se.

Aetiology
The true cause of gastric carcinoma is unknown.

Incidence — Gastric carcinoma was at one time the commonest form of internal cancer in Western civilisation. It appears to be declining in most Western countries except Iceland and Finland. Japan also has a high frequency. Statistics are not available for other parts of the world.
Sex — Males outnumber females 2 to 1.
Age — It occurs most commonly between 50 and 70 years.
Social class — The condition is commoner in low income groups but is not related to any particular industry.
Blood groups A higher incidence has been noted in association with Group A.
Familial factors — Some families show a high incidence but this may be related to socio-economic factors. Pernicious anaemia which has a familial incidence is sometimes associated with gastric carcinoma. The cancer is three times commoner in these cases than in the general population.
Chronic gastritis — This is commonly present in cases of gastric carcinoma. The accompanying metaplasia in this condition produces an intestinal type of epithelium which may be the precursor to malignant transformation.
Diet — No clear relationship between type of food and gastric carcinoma has been established. More important, perhaps, may be methods of cooking which involve charring of fats etc. as in frying and grilling.
Peptic Ulcer — As previously stated carcinoma only develops in less than 1 per cent of chronic peptic ulcers.

Other forms of malignancy are rare in the stomach. Leiomyosarcoma and malignant lymphoma may occur occasionally.

GASTRIC DILATATION

Two types of **GASTRIC DILATATION** are described:

1. *Atonic*

This may be a complication of chronic gastritis. The mechanism is possibly as follows:

Chronic gastritis
↓
Reduced gastric secretion
↓
Retention of food
↓
Fermentation
↓
Atony of muscle

No obstruction

Thin smooth wall

A similar condition may also arise after acute fevers or psychological conditions. Acute dilatation may occur following abdominal operations.

2. *Obstructive*

The obstruction may be due to fibrosis caused by peptic ulceration, pyloric carcinoma or constricting adhesions to other viscera. The peptic ulcer fibrosis is commonly at the pylorus but may occur in the body of the stomach causing an hour-glass deformity (see p.386).

A special form of pyloric obstruction is congenital pyloric stenosis presenting in early infancy. It is due to hypertrophy of the muscle around the pylorus and pyloric canal. It is commoner in males. Dilatation of the stomach may occasionally occur.

Clinical effects

Repeated vomiting results in loss of fluid and upset in the body electrolytes, especially chloride. Alkalosis and dehydration are usually present. In acute cases, there may be tetany and severe prostration. In chronic cases, stomach fluid contains many organisms including yeasts. These cause fermentation with the production of lactic and butyric acids and gas.

SMALL INTESTINE

NON-SPECIFIC FORMS of ENTERITIS

Enteritis is a common condition at all ages. The pathological changes may be slight even in the most severe cases. The small intestine is most affected, but the inflammation may extend forward to the large intestine and backward to the duodenum and stomach.

Normal small intestine

Goblet cell

Lymphocytes

Swelling of villi due to inflammatory oedema

Progressive desquamation of epithelium

Polymorphs

Congestion

Submucous oedema

Inflamed bowel

After the inflammation subsides healing takes place

Villi may be temporarily atrophied

Villi covered by flattened nondifferentiated epithelium

Return to normal

Clinical effects

These are generally mild in adults, unless debilitated. In infants, the condition is often fatal.

1. Loss of fluid into intestinal lumen — diarrhoea and vomiting may be severe enough to cause shock.
2. Electrolyte loss — cardiac irregularities in severe cases, tetany.
3. In the healing stage, the temporary atrophy and loss of function may lead to temporary mild malabsorption.

Aetiology

1. Mild enteritis due to dietary indiscretion occurs in adults and children.
2. Severe enteritis may be caused by poisons such as arsenic and mercury.
3. In infants, a serious variety often assumes epidemic form in nurseries and is frequently fatal. In some instances serological types of *E.coli* have been isolated but usually only from a proportion of cases in the same epidemic. Virus particles have been found in the intestine in many of these patients.

395

TYPHOID

SPECIFIC FORMS of ACUTE ENTERITIS

Salmonella infections

These produce a number of conditions varying in severity from typhoid fever which, untreated, is often fatal, to food poisoning, usually a mild catarrhal inflammation with diarrhoea.

TYPHOID FEVER

Following ingestion of *S. typhi*, the disease process falls into three distinct phases.

Ingestion of *S. typhi*
(contaminated water or food)
↓

Phase I
Invasion of intestinal lymphoid tissue and proliferation of bacteria. This phase lasts for 2 weeks and is virtually asymptomatic.
↓

Phase II
Invasion of blood stream causing bacteraemia. General toxaemia is caused with rise of temperature. Immunological reaction occurs leading to the next phase in 10 days' time.
↓

Phase III
Localisation of bacteria in intestinal lymphoid tissue, mesenteric nodes, **GALL BLADDER,** liver, spleen and sometimes the bones. Local necrosis, probably due to antigen-antibody hypersensitivity reactions, results in characteristic lesions.

Blood vessels

Spleen

Liver

Gall bladder

Intestine

Diagnostic test

Positive blood and urine cultures obtained during febrile period.

Antibodies to *S. typhi* appear in blood.

– – Widal Test positive at end of this phase.

Widal Test rising titre.

– – – Culture of faeces.

TYPHOID

Intestinal lesions

The ileum is most affected, but lesions may be found in the jejunum and colon.

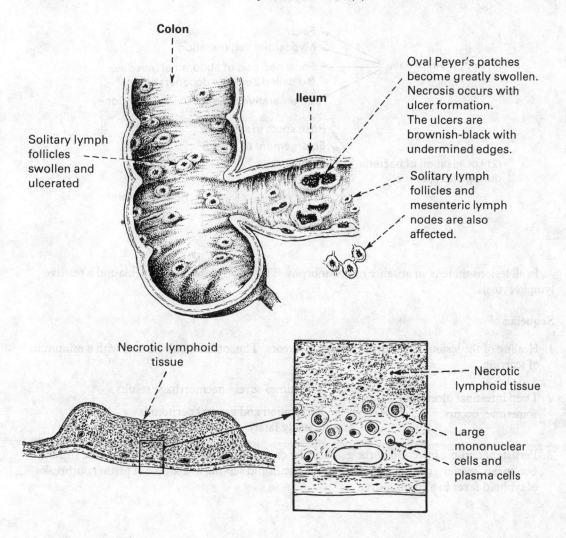

Colon

Ileum

Oval Peyer's patches become greatly swollen. Necrosis occurs with ulcer formation. The ulcers are brownish-black with undermined edges.

Solitary lymph follicles swollen and ulcerated

Solitary lymph follicles and mesenteric lymph nodes are also affected.

Necrotic lymphoid tissue

Necrotic lymphoid tissue

Large mononuclear cells and plasma cells

The features of acute inflammation are present, but, instead of polymorphs, large mononuclear cells infiltrate the tissues.

TYPHOID

Other lesions

These are very variable but can be widespread. They are due to:

In all lesions there is an absence of polymorphs. The blood shows neutropenia and a relative lymphocytosis.

Sequelae

1. Healing of the lesions is the usual pattern of events. The intestinal ulcers heal with a minimum of scarring.

2. Deep intestinal ulceration sometimes occurs
   - Sometimes severe haemorrhage results.
   - Perforation and general peritonitis (usually fatal).

3. Persistent chronic infection of the gall bladder or urinary tract. In this condition, the patient becomes a 'carrier', constantly excreting the bacilli and serving as a source of further outbreaks of typhoid fever in a community.

PARATYPHOID FEVER

This disease is clinically indistinguishable from typhoid fever but is usually much less severe.

The pathological changes resemble those of typhoid fever but are commonly limited to a small portion of the bowel. Frequently there is an absence of ulceration.

Two serological types of the paratyphoid organism are recognised, A and B. Type B is a common cause of enteric fever in Europe. As in typhoid, patients often become 'carriers'.

ENTERITIS AND ENTEROCOLITIS

SPECIAL TYPES
PSEUDOMEMBRANOUS ENTEROCOLITIS

This is a relatively uncommon acute inflammatory condition of mixed aetiology involving both small and large bowel.

The bowel wall is thickened by oedema and congestion

Irregular patches of yellow grey membrane alternate with areas of intense congestion on the mucosal surface

Membrane consisting of fibrin, necrotic cells and polymorphs

Denuded congested area

Clinical manifestations

Watery diarrhoea → Dehydration → Acute circulatory collapse → Irreversible shock and death

Aetiology Two groups appear to exist:

1. *Ischaemic enterocolitis:* This may occur in states of shock, uraemia or cardiac failure. The lesions may be related to disseminated intravascular coagulation.
2. *Superinfections of intestine:* Prophylactic antibiotic therapy may allow superinfection with *Staphy-lococcus aureus* or *Clostridium welchii.*

The use of lincomycin and clindamycin particularly may cause characteristic lesions in the colon (the small intestine is not affected).

Microscopic

Foci of mucus, fibrin, epithelial debris and a few polymorphs erupt on the mucous surface

Naked eye appearance

The lesions may coalesce forming typical adherent plaques over large areas, resulting in a fatal outcome. The lesions are caused by toxins from *Clostridium difficile* — an anaerobe normally present in small numbers which proliferate due to elimination of competing bacteria by the antibiotic.

399

ENTERITIS

SPECIAL TYPES (continued)

NECROTISING ENTEROCOLITIS OF INFANTS

This lesion occurs in newly born premature infants.

Necrosis and inflammation occur in the bowel wall

The characteristic feature is the occurrence of gas bubbles in the submucosal and muscle layers. These give rise to a characteristic X-ray picture. The gas may enter the portal venous system.

Two factors are important in the aetiology. The babies, asphyxiated at birth, have required catheterisation of the umbilical vessels. Apnoea causes bowel ischaemia and renders it liable to invasion by gas-forming bacteria. Most babies survive, but stricture may occur during healing leading to intestinal obstruction.

TOXIC ENTERITIS (Toxic food poisoning)

Food contaminated by *Staphylococcus aureus* can contain a large amount of enterotoxin. Cooking kills the bacteria, but the heat resistant enterotoxin causes acute gastroenteritis. *B.welchii* contamination can act in this way also.

CHOLERA

This is due to the exotoxin of the *Vibrio cholerae*. The equilibrium of fluid and electrolytes between gut mucosa and lumen is upset, resulting in intense diarrhoea and shock.

REGIONAL ENTERITIS (Crohn's disease)

This is a chronic disease of young adults. It is more often found in the colon but may occur in the terminal ileum (see p. 403)

TUBERCULOUS ENTERITIS

Three main pathological forms are recognised:

1. Primary infection

This is due to ingestion of infected milk, usually containing bovine tubercle bacilli, and affects the small bowel.

The reaction is similar to that seen in primary tuberculosis of the lung. A tiny lesion, often undiscovered, occurs in the bowel mucosa. This is equivalent to the Ghon focus.

The infection spreads to the local lymph nodes which are greatly enlarged and caseous (sometimes called tabes mesenterica).

Usually the condition subsides and the caseous nodes undergo calcification. Infrequently the disease spreads and causes tuberculous peritonitis.

2. Secondary infection

Swallowing of sputum containing large numbers of tubercle bacilli in cases of open pulmonary tuberculosis gives rise to tuberculous lesions in the intestine. Again the small intestine is affected. As in secondary tuberculosis of the lung, the local lesion is prominent and the lymph nodes are less affected. The lesions start in the Peyer's patches and solitary lymphoid follicles.

Caseating tubercles form in the mucosa and submucosa

Tubercle follicles in all layers

Small ragged ulcers develop which coalesce to form a large ulcer which may encircle the bowel lumen

TUBERCULOUS ENTERITIS

2. Secondary infection (continued)

As in the lung, there is a good deal of fibrous granulation tissue surrounding the caseous lesions and the vessels undergo obliteration. For this reason, perforation and haemorrhage are uncommon. Adhesions to other loops of bowel are common and the caseating process may erode through the walls and cause fistula formation with short circuiting and resulting malabsorption. If the fibrous adhesions are dense, obstruction may arise.

3. Hyperplastic caecal tuberculosis

This is a rare lesion. There is marked thickening of the wall of the caecum and ascending colon with fibrosis extending to the surrounding structures. The mucosa shows irregular ulceration and caseation extends into the wall.

Obstruction is common and may suggest carcinoma clinically.

The pathological changes may resemble Crohn's disease and it is important to demonstrate the presence of tubercle bacilli.

Pulmonary tuberculosis is usually present.

Adhesions

Ulceration

Fibrosis of peritoneum

Caseation

Thickened fibrotic wall

REGIONAL ENTERITIS (CROHN'S DISEASE)

Lymph nodes enlarged

Mesentery thick and oedematous

This is a chronic condition affecting young adults, giving rise to mild diarrhoea and abdominal pain initially.

Typically, it affects terminal 10 – 20 cm of the ileum but may be found in any part of the intestinal tract including mouth, oesophagus and anus. The wall is greatly thickened, especially in the submucosa which is oedematous and may have a gelatinous appearance. The lumen is narrowed, producing subacute or chronic obstruction. Ulceration is always present.

Ulcers are narrow and linear (fissures)

Surviving mucosa is swollen and protrudes as cobbles surrounded by ulcers

Adhesions to other structures occur, and the ulcers frequently penetrate the bowel wall and form fistulous channels.

Microscopic changes

Inflammatory reaction (polymorphs, lymphocytes and plasma cells) extends through whole wall of intestine.

non-caseating

In many cases a granulomatous reaction occurs.
Rounded accumulations of epithelioid cells with very occasionally a small giant cell. These resemble the lesions of sarcoidosis.

They occur in association with lymphatic channels causing lymphatic obstruction.

Subsequently fibrosis occurs and the mucosa undergoes metaplasia to simple mucus-secreting type resembling that of the pylorus. Secondary infection is common and is responsible for the ulceration and fissure formation.

REGIONAL ENTERITIS (CROHN'S DISEASE)

Pathogenesis

The mechanism appears to be as follows:

Focal vascular occlusion due to an immune reaction?

↓

Inflammation and granulomatous lesions

↓

Lymphatic obstruction ⟶ Gross oedema
of bowel wall

Secondary   Healing with
infection   fibrosis

↓

Ulceration,
fissures,
fistulae

Lesions may occur in the large intestine and have been reported in upper parts of the small intestine. 'Skip' lesions are also seen, i.e. discrete lesions in the bowel wall with healthy areas between them.

Complications

1. Intestinal obstruction.

2. Fistula formation either spontaneous or following operation. Perianal fistulae are common.

3. Hypochromic anaemia due to haemorrhage.

4. Macrocytic anaemia caused by interference with absorption. $B12$?

5. Signs of immunological disorders may be seen — arthritis, uveitis and dermatitis.

Aetiology

There is evidence that the disease may be due to a virus. Immunological abnormalities may determine the susceptibility of the patient, or may develop during the course of the disease. It is a disease of developed countries and it is thought that food processing and chemical additions to food may be potentiating factors.

MALABSORPTION

PRIMARY SYNDROMES

The pathological lesion is very similar in these states. It consists of an atrophy and reduction in the number of villi most marked in the jejunum.

Normal jejunum

Tall slender villi

Prominent columnar epithelium in upper part

Scattered lymphocytes in lamina propria

Cubical generative cells in crypts

The change varies from partial atrophy to almost complete disappearance of villi.

1. Partial villous atrophy

Occasional goblet cells

Numerous plasma cells in lamina propria

Villi are shorter and broader

Many of the villi fuse. To the naked eye, the mucosal surface shows a reduction in the normal folds and there are irregular ridges.

Hyperplasia of the generative cells. This suggests a more rapid turnover in the surface epithelium.

2. Complete villous atrophy

Epithelium is more cubical and shows little sign of function.

Plasma cells infiltrate

Crypt epithelium

In this stage the mucosa appears flat and thin.

405

MALABSORPTION

COELIAC DISEASE (Idiopathic steatorrhoea)

This affects both children and adults. It is associated with a sensitivity to gluten, a protein from wheat. Diffuse villous atrophy occurs in the jejunum, but the bowel returns to normal both anatomically and functionally if gluten is removed from the diet. There is a familial tendency and patients commonly possess the histocompatibility antigen HLA8. The underlying abnormality appears to be an abnormal immune response to gluten. Splenic atrophy is common and patients frequently show altered immune response to other antigens. Malignant lymphoma of the small intestine has an increased incidence in affected individuals.

TROPICAL SPRUE

This syndrome occurs in tropical countries with the exception of Africa. It can be very severe with much wasting. Anaemia of macrocytic type due to deficiency of vitamin B_{12}, and folic acid is common. Removal from the tropical country effects a cure. Oral broad spectrum antibiotics are also effective, and although the cause is unknown, it is assumed that bacterial colonisation of the small intestine is an important factor.

WHIPPLE'S DISEASE

This is a rare condition. Malabsorption is only one manifestation. There is often lymphadenopathy, arthropathy and skin pigmentation.

The lesion in the jejunum is characteristic. Large macrophages fill the lamina propria of the villi. These contain mucopolysaccharides staining strongly with periodic acid Schiff (P.A.S.). Similar cells are found in the lymph nodes and sometimes in other organs. Fat accumulates in the lymphatics, possibly due to the obstruction by the macrophages. Bacteria have been found in the macrophages and antibiotics are curative. The disease is almost confined to middle-aged males.

MALABSORPTION

SECONDARY MALABSORPTION

In this instance the malabsorption is secondary to diseases affecting digestion, absorption and transport of nutriments.

Examples are:

1. Interference with digestion

  (a) Destruction of intestinal mucosa as in regional enteritis, amyloidosis, systemic sclerosis, radiation damage.

  (b) Hepatic or pancreatic disease.

  (c) Following resection of bowel.

  (d) Congenital disaccharidase defect.

  (e) Drug influence — phenindione, neomycin, etc.

2. Diminished absorption

  (a) Intestinal stasis due to short circuits of bowel from disease or surgery.

  (b) Chronic obstruction.

Bacterial proliferation is a factor in these conditions, altering the chemical environment and the health of the bowel.

3. Altered transport

  (a) Lymphatic obstruction due to neoplasm or tuberculosis.

  (b) Disease of mesenteric blood supply.

  (c) Abetalipoproteinaemia.

The malabsorption in most of these conditions is overshadowed by the primary disease. Fatty diarrhoea, the characteristic feature of coeliac disease, is absent, and the malabsorption is manifested entirely by deficiency states.

The result of the atrophic villous changes is reduction in secretion and absorption which tends to be progressive.

MALABSORPTION

SECONDARY MALABSORPTION (continued)

Clinical features

The commonest complaint is of diarrhoea due to the bulky, fatty stools, but the presenting signs can vary and specific deficiencies may occur according to the severity and site of the lesions. For example:

Site of lesion	Function affected	Clinical manifestations
Duodenum	Iron absorption	Anaemia
Jejunum	Protein digestion Pancreatic stimulation Emulsification of fats	Wasting Fatty diarrhoea Deficient absorption of fatsoluble vitamins — rickets
	Electrolyte and fluid absorption	Dehydration Water soluble vitamin deficiencies: Vitamin B group Beri-beri, pellagra Vitamin C — scurvy Folic acid — macrocytic anaemia
Ileum	Absorption of vit B_{12}	Macrocytic anaemia
	Reabsorption of bile salts	Progressive interference with fat absorption

Vitamin deficiencies are particularly liable to occur in children.

TUMOURS OF SMALL INTESTINE

Tumours of all types are uncommon. Simple epithelial tumours are particularly rare.

POLYPI

Multiple tumours of polypoidal structure very occasionally occur as part of a genetic disorder (Peutz-Jeghers syndrome) which includes melanotic pigmentation of lips and mouth. The defect is a Mendelian dominant. The polypi are really hamartomas, consisting of glands, epithelium, muscle, etc. which are normal but arranged in a disorderly fashion.

CARCINOMA

This rare lesion is usually found in the jejunum. The pathological changes are similar to those found in carcinoma of the colon (see p.424). Very occasionally carcinoma may arise at the ampulla of Vater. Clinically, it causes obstruction of the common bile duct and jaundice.

CARCINOID TUMOURS (Agentaffinomas)

These are peculiar tumours which arise in various parts of the body, but the specific clinical features are most commonly exhibited by those found in the ileum.

Rounded tumour, often multiple, yellowish or white

Peripheral cells tend to be pallisaded

Local muscle hypertrophy

Surrounding fibrosis

Clear cells arranged in solid masses

Occasionally form trabeculae or show 'gland' forms

The cells have the capacity to reduce silver compounds and are therefore known as argentaffin cells. Cells of a similar type are normally found in the crypts of Lieberkuhn (Kulschitsky cells).

409

TUMOURS OF SMALL INTESTINE

CARCINOID TUMOURS (continued)

Sites

Appendix

The tip of the appendix is the commonest site for these tumours. They often produce symptoms of acute appendicitis, and it is not clear whether this is due to muscular spasm produced by the secretions of the tumours or to occlusion of the lumen. It is the appendicular form which gave rise to the name carcinoid, since although it infiltrates locally it almost never metastasises.

Ileum

The tumours are frequently multiple and in this case they behave like carcinoma, metastasising to the local lymph nodes and liver. Growth is slow however and the patient may live for many years although secondary spread has occurred. Spread to the liver is frequently associated with the carcinoid syndrome.

Stomach, gall bladder, colon and rectum

Carcinoid tumours are only rarely found in these sites and may be asymptomatic.

Trachea and bronchus
In this site, they may be indistinguishable clinically from carcinoma.

CARCINOID SYNDROME

These tumours tend to secrete 5-hydroxytryptamine (serotonin). This substance is destroyed in the liver and lung, and symptoms due to excessive production are unusual until secondary growths occur in the liver. The substance 5HT produces vasodilatation and stimulates smooth muscle. It may also release histamine and mucopolysaccharides from mast cells. Platelets carry 5HT and it is involved in coagulation.

The syndrome consists of diarrhoea, attacks of flushing, and right-sided cardiac failure. These changes are directly related to the action of 5HT.

TUMOURS OF SMALL INTESTINE

CARCINOID SYNDROME (continued)

The left side of the heart is rarely affected since 5HT is destroyed in the lungs.

APUDOMAS

The intestinal carcinoid is one of a group of tumours which are derived from endocrine cells scattered widely throughout the body but with common features:

1. They are of neural crest origin.
2. They synthesise and export polypeptides and in so doing utilise the enzyme *amine precursor uptake decarboxylase* (APUD).

The group includes islet cell tumours, medullary carcinoma of the thyroid and 'carcinoids' at various sites.

CONNECTIVE TISSUE TUMOURS

These are much commoner than epithelial tumours. Leiomyoma sometimes causes an intraluminal swelling which may induce intussusception or, if ulcerated, haemorrhage and anaemia.

LYMPHOMA

This may occur as a primary tumour and can be multiple. Deep ulceration, frequently with perforation, may take place. The cells are usually either of B lymphocyte or histocyte origin. The tumours sometimes cause malabsorption. They are usually extremely malignant.

Another form occurs in the East Mediterranean in young adults. The whole intestine may be infiltrated by the tumour cells which take the form of lymphocytes and plasma cells. These produce the heavy chain of IgA and the condition is sometimes called alpha-chain disease.

411

APPENDICITIS

Conventionally, three grades of severity of acute appendicitis are described:
(1) Simple acute, (2) suppurative and (3) gangrenous.

SIMPLE ACUTE APPENDICITIS

Appendix swollen, congested and curved due to tension on mesoappendix

Congestion of vessels in mesoappendix

The initial central colicky abdominal pain is due to spasmodic movements in the inflamed appendix. The subsequent localisation of pain, tenderness and rigidity are caused by the tension and irritation of the peritoneum.

Lymphoid follicles

Muscle coats

Peritoneal surface

Polymorph exudate in lumen

The acute inflammation often starts as a focus of mucosal ulceration

Fibrin on peritoneal surface

Polymorphonuclear exudate spreads in submucosa and soon affects all layers

Although the attack can be very acute and lead directly to perforation and peritonitis, the condition may be relatively mild and subside. Repeated attacks are common. The results can be:

(a) Obliteration of the whole appendicular lumen.

(b) Adhesions to surrounding structures. These may lead to complications such as intestinal obstruction.

(c) Local stenosis. By causing retention of waste material more serious inflammation may arise and lead to the second type — suppurative appendicitis.

412

APPENDICITIS

SUPPURATIVE APPENDICITIS

This may develop from simple acute appendicitis, but often there is a localising factor in the form of a faecal concretion. Less frequently it may be a swallowed foreign body, e.g. vegetable matter or very rarely thread worms which commonly inhabit the appendix.

The pathology may therefore vary.

1. *Complicating simple acute appendicitis*

2. *Associated with impacted concretion*

Most commonly the distal end is affected

Abscesses may be single or multiple

Inflammation occurs beyond site of impaction

In both instances, perforation may occur but is almost inevitable where the abscess is at the site of a concretion. The process can be visualised as follows:

Inflammation
↓
Swelling of tissues + Pressure of concretion

High tension in tissues → Vascular supply interrupted → Necrosis and perforation

GANGRENOUS APPENDICITIS

In the main, gangrene of the appendix tends to develop in two sets of circumstances:

1. *Due to vascular damage*

During inflammation the veins in the mesoappendix may become thrombosed. Haemorrhage and vascular stasis follow. Necrosis and gangrene result.

2. *Obstruction of the lumen.* This may be due to a concretion or severe stenosis of the outlet of the appendix. The main factor appears to be distension of the lumen with faecal material. Rapid multiplication of bacteria, especially anaerobes, takes place and this may account for the gangrene. General peritonitis develops early in the process.

SEQUELS OF APPENDICITIS

1. General peritonitis

This is the most important complication since it results in gross toxaemia and may be fatal. It is common with any form of acute appendicitis but almost inevitably happens in the case of gangrenous appendix.

2. Appendix abscess

This arises in the following way:

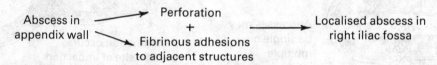

Further complications may arise due to spread of infection:

(a) Along the right paracolic gutter to produce a subprenic abscess between the diaphragm and liver

(b) Into the pelvis to form abscesses around bladder and rectum. In the female the uterus and fallopian tube may be involved.

3. Adhesions

Intestinal obstruction may result from constricting bands, or volvulus may be induced.

4. Liver abscess and portal pylephlebitis

These are now rare. They are due to spread of infection to the mesenteric veins resulting in a septic phlebitis. Liver abscesses usually arise from infective emboli, but occasionally there may be a spreading suppurating thrombosis culminating in hepatic sepsis.

APPENDICITIS

Aetiology

1. **Obstruction of the lumen:** In the majority of cases this potentiates distal infection with ulceration. In a few cases no obvious obstruction is evident.

   The usual causes of obstruction are:

   (a) Virus infection — this is part of a reaction to alimentary virus infection with reactive hyperplasia of the mesenteric lymph nodes and alimentary lymphoid tissues and is seen particularly in childhood when the lymphoid tissues are prominent. (Infection by *Yersinia enterocolitica* may cause similar changes.)

   (b) Inspissated faeces — may form small 'stones' (faecoliths) which obstruct the lumen.

(a) Hyperplastic lymphoid follicles   (b) Faecolith

Obstruction of lumen
↓
Bacterial proliferation
↓
Inflammation and ulceration

2. **Bacteria:** Those involved are of the normal intestinal flora — coliform bacilli, streptococci and anaerobic organisms.

3. **Inappropriate diet:** Appendicitis is a disease of Western society and the lack of roughage may, by causing stasis, increase the likelihood of attacks.

CHRONIC APPENDICITIS

This is a rather vague condition. In pathologocal terms, it is synonymous with fibrosis, which may be local or diffuse. The effects may be as follows:

Destruction of muscle
↓
Interference with peristalsis → Recurrent inflammation
↓
Retention of faecal matter ‒ ‒ ‒ → Danger of gangrene

If the fibrosis causes complete obstruction of the lumen, continued mucous secretion may result in cystic dilatation — mucocele. Such a cyst may rupture, giving rise to myxoma peritonei: the mucus-secreting epithelium is spilled into the peritoneal cavity and loculations of mucin and adhesions result.

415

BACILLARY DYSENTERY

This is an acute inflammation of the large intestine, varying in severity according to the infecting agent.

Shigella sonnei
Simple acute inflammation of colon.
Common in United Kingdom.

Shigella flexneri
Severe acute inflammation.
More common on the continent of Europe.

Shigella dysenteriae
Most severe type, occurs in tropics.

Irregular speading ulcers with thin shredded margins are formed by shedding of necrotic material.

Clinical Manifestations.

There is acute diarrhoea with abdominal pain, tenesmus and the passage of blood-stained mucus. *S.dysenteriae* infections are often associated with severe toxaemia and sometimes a shock-like condition. Blood mucus and polymorphs are found in the faeces, and in the early stages the bacilli can be isolated.

Healing by resolution with complete restoration of the mucosa is usual. Only in exceptional cases does relapse occur with consequent scarring.

AMOEBIC DYSENTERY

This is due to infection by *Entamoeba histolytica* in food and water.

Encysted form in food

Ingestion

Four amoebae in cyst

Cyst digested; amoebae set free

Amoebae invade wall of colon by digestive enzymes

Spread and multiply in submucosa, destroying tissue

Vessels are congested but there is almost no inflammatory reaction.

By digesting the submucosa, the blood supply to the mucosa is cut off causing necrosis. Ulcers form and ultimately large areas may be denuded of mucosa.

Necrotic mucosa is cast off

Ulcer penetrates to muscle

Amoebae spread, digesting submucosa and undermining the mucosa

Ulcers coalesce and form large eroded areas with undermined edges.

Healing of the ulcers with fibrosis occurs. The disease persists and overgrowth of fibrous tissue, adhesions to various structures and fistulae may occur. Occasionally the amoebae may invade portal venous tributaries and cause tropical abscess of the liver.

Large numbers of motile amoebae can be found in the faeces during the acute phase of the disease. Later, in the chronic state, they are frequently in an encysted form. Mucus and blood are abundant, but unlike bacillary dysentery, there are no pus cells.

Amoebic abscess

This complication affects the liver (see p.473).

ULCERATIVE COLITIS

This is an inflammatory condition of the mucosa, primarily of the sigmoid colon and rectum. Although initially the inflammation is acute, it becomes chronic.

Acute phase

Mucosa acutely congested especially over the tips of mucosal folds

Abscesses form in crypts — polymorphs and eosinophils

Muscularis mucosae

Epithelium breaks down in crypts

Inflammatory exudate spreads into lamina propria. Abscesses coalesce.

Mucosa is destroyed and ulcer forms
Often extends just into the submucosa but no further

Granulation tissue in base

Plasma cells appear in large numbers in the granulation tissue

The ulcers coalesce generally in a longitudinal direction and appear to form over the bands of longitudinal muscle.

Ulcerated areas

Swollen surviving islands of mucosa forming pseudo-polyps

Periods of remission occur when many of the ulcerated areas heal.

Granulation tissue

The crypts of Lieberkuhn do not reform completely.

Ultimately the surface may be covered by a simple layer of mucus secreting epithelium without glands

ULCERATIVE COLITIS

Clinical features

Ulcerative colitis is of chronic relapsing nature with periods of remission. It affects young adults and causes episodic diarrhoea with blood and mucus in the stool. Anorexia and weight loss are characteristic of the condition. Protein loss and haemorrhage lead to anaemia.

Complications

1. Acute fulminating cases are associated with distension of the colon and perforation is common.
2. Rectal lesions are common, but perianal fistulae are uncommon.
3. Despite granulation tissue formation, fibrosis and stricture are uncommon.
4. Hepatic cirrhosis is not uncommon.
5. In long-standing cases, carcinoma of the colon frequently develops.
6. Secondary amyloidosis may occur, causing renal and hepatic complications and at the same time exacerbating the intestinal condition.

Aetiology

The cause is unknown. Patients frequently show manifestations of hypersensitivity such as erythema nodosum, arthritis, iritis, and haemolytic anaemia and develop sensitivity to drugs easily. It is considered that the intestinal lesions may also be due to a hyperimmune state.

ISCHAEMIC COLITIS

This commonly affects one area of the colon.

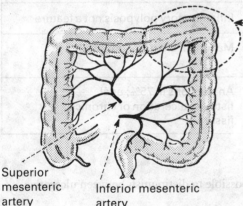

- Area of poor anastomosis — watershed zone

Damage is produced by ischaemia. The degree of damage depends upon the duration of ischaemia

Prolonged ischaemia → necrosis of intestine followed by gangrene

Less prolonged ischaemia → mucosal and submucosal necrosis → bacterial infection. Healing may result in fibrosis and stricture.

Superior mesenteric artery

Inferior mesenteric artery

The ischaemia of the bowel occurs in individuals with arterial disease who suffer a hypotensive episode, e.g. due to shock or cardiac failure.

PSEUDOMEMBRANOUS COLITIS
see page 399.

COLITIS

Macroscopic differences in the pathology of ulcerative colitis and Crohn's disease.

Ulcerative colitis	Crohn's disease
1. Lesions continuous – superficial	Lesions patchy — penetrating
2. Rectum always involved	Rectum normal in 50%
3. Terminal ileum involved in 10%	Terminal ileum involved in 30%
4. Granular, ulcerated mucosa No fissuring	Discretely ulcerated mucosa; cobblestone appearance; fissuring
5. Often intensely vascular	Vascularity seldom pronounced
6. Normal serosa	Serositis common
7. Muscular shortening of colon; fibrous strictures very rare	Fibrous shortening; strictures common
8. Fistulae rare	Enterocutaneous or intestinal fistulae in 10%
9. Inflammatory polyposis common	Inflammatory polyposis not a feature
10. Malignant change — well recognised	Malignant change – doubtful
11. Anal lesions in less than 25%; acute fissures, rectovaginal fistula	Anal lesions in 75%; anal fistulae; ulceration or chronic fissure

In about a quarter to a third of cases it may be impossible to distinguish between ulcerative colitis and Crohn's disease.

TUMOURS OF LARGE INTESTINE

Almost all of the tumours of the large intestine are of epithelial origin. Connective tissue neoplasms are rare. Lymphomas are found in the caecum and rectum but less often than in the small intestine.

POLYPI

All of the simple epithelial tumours tend to adopt a polypoidal form. Two of them are of common occurrence:

        1. Tubular adenoma (or adenomatous polyp).
        2. Villous adenoma (or villous papilloma).

The development of these can be visualised as follows.

Tubular adenoma (adenomatous polyp)

Develops from epithelium at base of crypts

Numerous glands formed

Peristalsis induces formation of pedicle composed of mucosa and muscularis mucosae

Villous adenoma (villous papilloma)

Develops from superficial epithelium

Growth becomes progressively papilliform

The tumour is superficial and sessile.

TUMOURS OF LARGE INTESTINE

TUBULAR ADENOMA
The majority of tubular adenomas occur in the rectum and sigmoid colon. In the beginning it is a sessile swelling but soon becomes pedunculated.

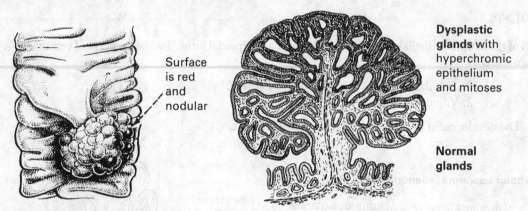

Surface is red and nodular

Dysplastic glands with hyperchromic epithelium and mitoses

Normal glands

They are common in the older age groups and are frequently multiple.

VILLOUS ADENOMA
Villous adenomas are most commonly found in the rectum. They form a sessile mass which may be quite large and have a delicate frond-like structure.

Sessile mass

Epithelium usually of clear muscus-secreting type

Broad base with no peduncle

There is an excessive production of mucus and fluid which may lead to marked loss of potassium, causing muscular weakness.

Many polypi are of mixed variety — part adenomatous, part villous. Both show a tendency to malignant change. If the tumour is of sessile variety invasion of the deeper tissues is immediate. In the pedunculated varieties, invasion of the intestinal wall is delayed.

TUMOURS OF LARGE INTESTINE

METAPLASTIC POLYPI

These are usually multiple and present as a small sessile nodule showing unusual feathery metaplastic change in the epithelium. It is found in later life but does not appear to undergo malignant transformation.

JUVENILE POLYPI

These are globular protrusions of the rectal mucous membrane in children. They are usually ulcerated and inflamed but probably represent a developmental abnormality rather than a true neoplasm.

BENIGN LYMPHOID POLYPOSIS of the RECTUM

This is not an epithelial tumour. It consists of masses of lymphoid tissue of normal structure in the submucosa of the rectum in young women. The cause is unknown.

POLYPOSIS COLI

These neoplastic adenomas are a rare hereditary condition which inevitably leads to carcinoma of the colon. Since hundreds of polyps are present, the carcinomas may be multiple and widespread. It is transmitted as a Mendelian dominant factor.

The entire colon is studded with tiny sessile adenomatous polypi. Symptoms appear in late childhood, and carcinoma arises 10 – 15 years later if colectomy is not carried out.

CARCINOMA OF LARGE INTESTINE

This has now taken the place of gastric carcinoma as the commonest form of malignancy of the gastrointestinal tract in Western civilisation.

Site and incidence

Rectum ———————————————— At least 50%
Sigmoid and descending colon ———— Up to 25%
Caecum and ileo-caecal valve ———— Approximately 10%
Ascending colon, hepatic and
　　　　　splenic flexures ———————— Around 5%
Transverse colon ————————————— Uncommon.

Types of growth

1. *Fungating polypoid carcinoma*
This form tends to be more common in the ascending
colon. It is frequently a very large, soft, friable growth.
Ulceration and haemorrhage are common, leading to
anaemia. Infiltration of the base may be slight. Occasionally
such a growth is associated with marked loss
of potassium leading to muscular weakness.

2. *Scirrhous carcinoma*

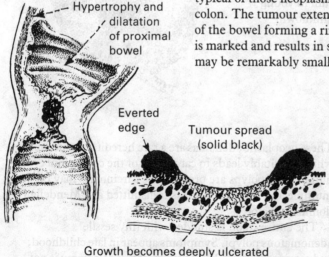

Hypertrophy and
dilatation
of proximal
bowel

Everted
edge

Tumour spread
(solid black)

Growth becomes deeply ulcerated

This is the commonest type of growth and is
typical of those neoplasms found in the descending
colon. The tumour extends round the circumference
of the bowel forming a ring. Fibrous proliferation
is marked and results in stenosis. The primary growth
may be remarkably small and circumscribed even at a late stage.

In types 1 and 2 the growth is an
abenocarcinoma.

CARCINOMA OF LARGE INTESTINE

3. *Mucoid (colloid) carcinoma*

The wall of the colon may be greatly thickened by a gelatinous growth. Almost all of the surface is ulcerated. Bulky secondary masses may form in the omentum and throughout the peritoneal cavity.

'Signet ring' cells

4. *Diffuse carcinoma*

This type produces a condition similar to that seen in the "leather-bottle" carcinoma of the stomach.

DEVELOPMENT and SPREAD

At least 50% of carcinomas start as a polyp

Growth extends to submucosa

Submucous lymphatics invaded — bowel encircled

Lymphatics are the common channel of spread

Muscularis mucosae

Mesentery

Spread to nearby lymph node

↓

Then to nodes at root of mesentery

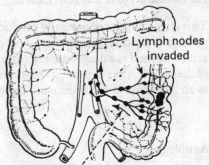

Lymph nodes invaded

Further spread follows the lymphatic drainage of the colon.

CARCINOMA OF LARGE INTESTINE

Blood spread

This may lead to secondary deposits in the liver, although these may also be due to spread from affected lymph nodes at the hilum. The lungs, bones and brain are occasionally involved.

Attempts are made to stage the disease since this has an important bearing on prognosis. The following system, which is a modification of the original proposed by Dukes, has been evolved:

Stage		5 year survival figures
A	Tumour confined to mucosa	80%
B_1	Tumour reaching muscularis propria	65%
B_2	Extension through muscularis	50%
C_1	Involvement of paracolic nodes	40%
C_2	Involvement of nodes at root of mesentery	15%

Secondary effects of colonic cancer

- Dilatation of proximal bowel
- Hypertrophy of muscle

Increasing obstruction

Increasing pressure on bowel wall with retention of faeces

Thinning of wall with ulceration

Possible perforation and peritonitis

Impairment of nutrition of mucosa

Tendency to ulceration

Carcinoembryonic antigen (CEA)

This is a glycoprotein normally produced by fetal endodermal tissues. It is also formed by a number of cancers, among them a proportion of colonic carcinomas, and appears in the blood. It cannot be used as a diagnostic test since it is found in non-neoplastic lesions such as inflammation of the bowel. After treatment, however, changes in the blood concentration of CEA may be used as an indication of recurrence of tumour growth.

Aetiology

The ultimate cause is unknown. The fact that familial polyposis inevitably leads to cancer and that simple colonic adenoma often precedes cancer indicates a genetic influence. The high incidence in Western society may be related to less fluid faeces allowing longer contact with possible carcinogens. Chronic ulcerative colitis is also associated with an increased risk of cancer.

DIVERTICULOSIS

Diverticula may form in any part of the intestinal tract but are commonest in the colon.

Small intestine

This is an uncommon site for diverticula. Their importance lies in the fact that bacterial proliferation may occur in them. Vitamin B_{12} is utilised by the bacteria, leading to deficiency and megaloblastic anaemia. Steatorrhoea may also occur. The diverticula occur near the attachment of the mesentery; their thin walls consist of mucosa, submucosa and serosa.

Large intestine

Diverticula are common, especially in the sigmoid colon. At least ten per cent of adults have this condition.

They form near the mesenteric border of the colon. Closer inspection reveals that they take origin where the blood vessels penetrate the colonic wall.

Taenia coli

Pouch pushes between muscle fibres.

The diverticula are often filled with inspissated faeces. The nearby colonic muscle is usually hypertrophied. Inflammation is common in older people. Acute attacks may give rise to symptoms resembling appendicitis but referred to the left side. Abscesses and fistulae may result. Repeated attacks can lead to marked fibrotic thickening of a segment of the colon which may be mistaken for carcinoma. Diverticula in general are only found in adult life. Their prevalence is related to a low residue diet which is thought to cause disturbance of the muscular activity of the colon.

Inspissated faeces

Inflammatory fibromuscular thickening

427

ACUTE INTESTINAL OBSTRUCTION

This most commonly affects the small intestine due to its mobility and, therefore, its liability to mechanical obstruction in conditions such as hernia, volvulus, intussusception and fibrous adhesions.

Immediately following the obstruction there is a period of very active peristalsis

This is followed by immobility and distension

Increased secretion

Decreased absorption

Bacteria tend to flourish

Retroperistalsis takes place, the fluid passes back to the stomach and vomiting occurs. The composition of the vomited fluid and the resulting biochemical changes vary with the level of obstruction.

	Pyloric obstruction	Small intestine obstruction
Content of fluid	Acid gastric juice	Saliva, gastric juice, bile, pancreatic secretion, succus entericus
Electrolytes	Chloride lost, sodium retained	Loss of sodium potassium and chloride
CO_2 combining power	Increased due to retained sodium Plasma bicarbonate increased Alkalosis produced	Normal Little change in acid-base balance.
Calcium	Alkalosis causes reduction in ionised calcium Tetany may result	Not affected
Potassium	Serum potassium may fall, causing muscle weakness and cardiac irregularity	Not a feature
Fluid balance upset	This may arise late in the process, due to loss of fluid in vomit It may cause oliguria and pre-renal uraemia	Rapid loss of fluid and electrolytes causing fall in blood volume haemocon-centration and shock

CHRONIC INTESTINAL OBSTRUCTION

In this instance the obstruction is incomplete. It is commonly due to changes in the wall of the intestine, e.g. stricture caused by inflammation such as Crohn's disease or scirrhous type of tumour growth, or obstruction of the lumen, e.g. by polypoid growth, or pressure from outside. Since tumour growth and chronic inflammation are more common in large intestine, this is the usual site of chronic obstruction.

1. As the condition develops gradually, the main local change is hypertrophy of the muscle at the proximal part of bowel.

The large bowel is the main site of water absorption therefore dehydration is not apparent in the early stages.

2. At a later date, obstruction increases and muscle hypertrophy cannot compensate. Marked distension of the proximal bowel occurs with accumulation of gas and fluid.

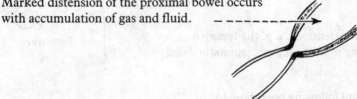

This gross distension has several effects.

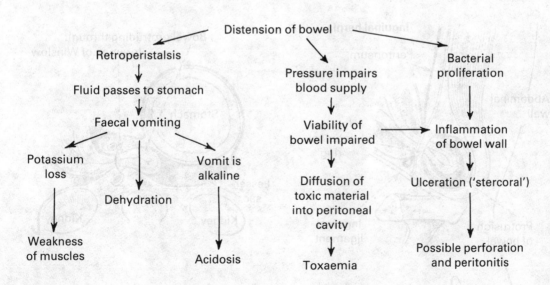

INTESTINAL OBSTRUCTION

HERNIA

This means the protrusion of bowel through an aperture.

When the hernial swelling appears on the surface of the body, it is termed 'external'; those which do not present on the body surface are 'internal'.

The protrusion of bowel may occur through:

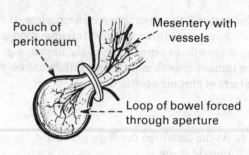

Pouch of peritoneum

Mesentery with vessels

Loop of bowel forced through aperture

1. Sites of potential weakness in the abdominal wall, e.g. inguinal canal, femoral canal, umbilicus, diaphragm. There may be congenital weakness in some individuals at these sites. In these cases a pouch of peritoneum protrudes through the aperture.

Umbilical

Inguinal

Femoral

2. Normal peritoneal extensions, e.g. the foramen of Winslow leading to the lesser sac, jejunoduodenal fossa.

3. The abdominal wall following operation due to stretching of scar tissue.

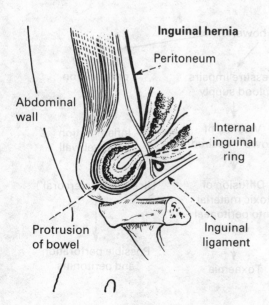

Inguinal hernia

Peritoneum

Abdominal wall

Internal inguinal ring

Protrusion of bowel

Inguinal ligament

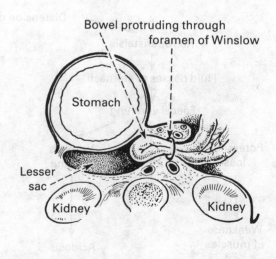

Bowel protruding through foramen of Winslow

Stomach

Lesser sac

Kidney

Kidney

INTESTINAL OBSTRUCTION

Complications of hernia

Initially, when the herniated portion of bowel is small it can be pushed back into the abdominal cavity — *reducible*.

Increased intra-abdominal pressure, e.g. during muscular exertion, coughing or straining due to constipation, helps to induce the herniation, tends to make it progressive, and secondary changes occur.

Raised abdominal pressure

↓

Increase in size of hernia

↓

Hernia impossible to return to abdomen — *irreducible*

Increasing obstruction of bowel   Partial venous obstruction

↓   ↓

Distension of bowel   Exudation into sac

↓   ↓

Hernial orifice becomes too tight for bulk passing through   Adhesions between bowel and sac

↓

Increasing venous obstruction 'strangulation'

↓

Congestion and oedema   Hernia permanently irreducible — *impacted*

↓

Increasing bulk

↓

Complete interruption of circulation   Obstructed upper bowel segment

↓

Strangulation and gangrene of bowel   Black gangrenous bowel

INTESTINAL OBSTRUCTION

INTUSSUSCEPTION

This is a condition in which the bowel is invaginated into itself.

Sites

The commonest form is the ileocaecal type, the ileum being invaginated into the large intestine with the ileocaecal valve forming the apex. Less commonly, a portion of ileum may pass through the ileocaecal valve. Other sites are occasionally affected, e.g. small intestine or parts of colon.

Clinical manifestations

The patient presents with the signs and symptoms of acute obstruction, a mass in the abdomen and blood is passed per rectum.

Aetiology

It is thought that most cases arise as a result of a swelling in the intestinal wall which is pushed distally by peristalsis, dragging the wall of the bowel with it. Most cases arise in childhood due to swelling of lymphoid tissue produced by virus infection.

Polypoidal tumours of the intestine may cause intussusception in adults.

Very occasionally, adhesions develop between the peritoneal surfaces of the invaginated portion of bowel and the external sheathing portion. The gangrenous invaginated portion may separate and the lesion heal spontaneously.

INTESTINAL OBSTRUCTION

VOLVULUS

As the name suggests, this is a rotation or revolving of the bowel. It affects bowel with a long mesentery. Another factor is the closeness of the ends of the affected loop.

The sigmoid colon has this anatomical arrangement and is the common site of volvulus. Less commonly, the small intestine is affected.

The subsequent changes are the same as in intussusception.

Twisting of the loop around its own axis
↓
Venous return interrupted
↓
Congestion and oedema
↓
Infarction and gangrene with peritonitis and shock

Acute obstruction

Aetiology

In the case of the sigmoid colon, constipation causing loading of the loop in an individual with an abnormally long mesocolon is probably the initiating factor.

Volvulus of the small intestine usually occurs in children. Commonly the mesentery is distorted by disease, e.g. tuberculous nodes.

Very occasionally two loops of bowel may become wrapped round each other.

VASCULAR OCCLUSION

Occlusion of vessels supplying the intestine will result in infarction and subsequently gangrene. The commonest vascular lesion is thrombosis or embolism of a main branch of the superior mesenteric artery causing infarction of a loop of small intestine.

Due to anastomosis the necrotic segment is usually smaller than might be expected.

Thrombosis of the mesenteric veins will produce the same result.

INTESTINAL OBSTRUCTION

PARALYTIC ILEUS

This is an ill-understood condition. The bowel is paralysed and greatly distended.
There is usually a thin peritoneal exudate.

Local and general changes take place.

Fluid and electrolytes pass into the bowel

Reduced blood volume

Blood sodium and potassium reduced

Bacterial proliferation

Diffusion of toxins

General toxaemia ← Peritoneal infection

Muscular and circulatory weakness → Shock

If the toxic contents of the bowel are not drained and the blood, fluid and electrolytes replaced quickly, death is inevitable. With this treatment the bowel may regain its normal activity.

Aetiology

1. Most commonly it follows abdominal operation, especially if bowel is abused. It may be due to overstimulation of the sympathetic nervous system.
2. Peritonitis from any cause tends to produce paralysis of the intestine.
3. Intestinal infections sometimes have the same effect.

HIRSCHSPRUNG'S DISEASE

Normal ganglion cells

Dilated bowel

Narrow segment

No ganglion cells

Hirschsprung's disease is a rare cause of chronic intestinal obstruction. It is due to a congenital absence of ganglion cells in the parasympathetic Auerbach and Meissner complexes of the rectum.

The aganglionic rectal segment and anus remain contracted due to unopposed action of the sympathetic nervous system, the bowel above becoming grossly distended and hypertrophied.

THE PERITONEAL CAVITY

There are three important features in relation to the peritoneal cavity:

1. Its enormous surface area due mainly to the coils of bowel with their mesenteries
2. A very rich blood supply associated with the abdominal organs, the vessels lying just below the serous surface
3. An equally rich lymphatic drainage.

These combine to make the area of great importance in relation to fluid exchange and absorption. They influence the pathological changes and clinical effects of any lesions involving the cavity.

Acute inflammation

There are numerous causes of acute peritonitis, almost all of them associated with lesions in the abdominal organs. Examples are:

1. Acute appendicitis
2. Perforating ulcers: peptic ulcers, ulcerative colitis, typhoid ulcers, ulcerated neoplasms
3. Devitalisation of bowel wall: intestinal obstruction, diverticulitis
4. Interference with mesenteric circulation: strangulation of herniae, volvulus, intussusception, mesenteric thrombosis
5. Cholecystitis, salpingitis, pancreatitis
6. Occasional cases arise during the terminal phases of serious debilitating disease, e.g. uraemia, with no detectable local source.

General peritonitis

This is extremely serious because of the important features mentioned above.

Widespread inflammation

Large amounts of bacterial toxins produced

Marked exudation into cavity

Great absorption from extensive peritoneal surface

Absorption and local effect on intestine

Loss of fluid, electrolytes, protein, etc.

Severe general toxaemia

Paralytic ileus with loss of fluid and electrolytes into intestine

Diminution in circulating blood volume

Hypovolaemic shock

THE PERITONEAL CAVITY

Localised peritonitis

If perforation of the appendix has been preceded by a lesser degree of inflammation on the surface of the appendix, then a localised lesion can result — appendix abscess.

Such localised lesions can be very troublesome and lead to a chronic illness with discharging sinuses or fistulas.

Fibrinous exudate on surface of appendix

Coils of bowel and omentum adhere to surface of appendix, walling it off

Similar pockets of pus may be left behind when a general peritonitis has otherwise resolved with treatment. These are apt to occur in the pelvis or between the liver and diaphragm.

Trouble may arise at a later date if fibrinous adhesions between coils of bowel or between bowel and other structures organise and fibrose. These permanent adhesions interfere with bowel function and may cause obstruction by twisting or kinking of the intestine.

The type of exudate varies with the cause. In most cases which involve the intestines, it is fibrinopurulent. Haemorrhagic exudates tend to be associated with escape of gastric contents or bile into the peritoneal cavity. The exudate is also haemorrhagic in acute pancreatitis but, in addition, opaque yellowish white flecks are seen scattered over the peritoneum. These are small areas of fat necrosis.

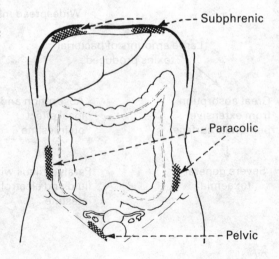

Subphrenic

Paracolic

Pelvic

THE PERITONEAL CAVITY

Chronic peritonitis

The most common type of chronic inflammation involving the peritoneum is that resulting from non-resolution of acute peritonitis.

Tuberculosis of the peritoneum is uncommon in Western civilisation, but frequent in underdeveloped countries. It commonly takes one of the following forms:-

1. **Serous effusion.** Small grey tubercles are usually scattered over the peritoneal surface. In addition, the omentum is more extensively involved with the formation of a large fibrous mass in the upper abdomen.
2. **Caseation.** This can vary in extent, from isolated small masses to diffuse caseation involving most of the cavity.
3. **Adhesive peritonitis.** The cavity may be reduced to small pockets containing serous fluid.

The source of infection may be caseous lymph nodes, tuberculous salpingitis or tuberculous ulcer of the intestine.

Chronic hyperplastic peritonitis

This is a rare condition of unknown aetiology. It results in marked hyaline thickening of the peritoneum especially over the liver and spleen.

Ascites

Accumulation of serous fluid can occur:-

1. As part of a general oedema from any cause such as cardiac or renal failure.
2. Portal venous obstruction as in hepatic cirrhosis, portal thrombosis or compression of the portal vein by tumour growth.
3. Fibroma of the ovary (Meig's syndrome).
4. Tumour of the peritoneum.

Tumours

Primary tumours are rare. Mesothelioma is the most important. It is related to the inhalation of asbestos and the pathology is similar to that of mesothelioma of the pleura, large white plaques of solid growth.

Secondary tumours are common, due to spread of carcinoma from the stomach, ovary and large intestine.

CHAPTER 11

LIVER, GALL BLADDER AND PANCREAS

LIVER-ANATOMY

Conventionally the liver is considered to be composed of regular lobules, each arranged around a central vein with portal tracts at the periphery.

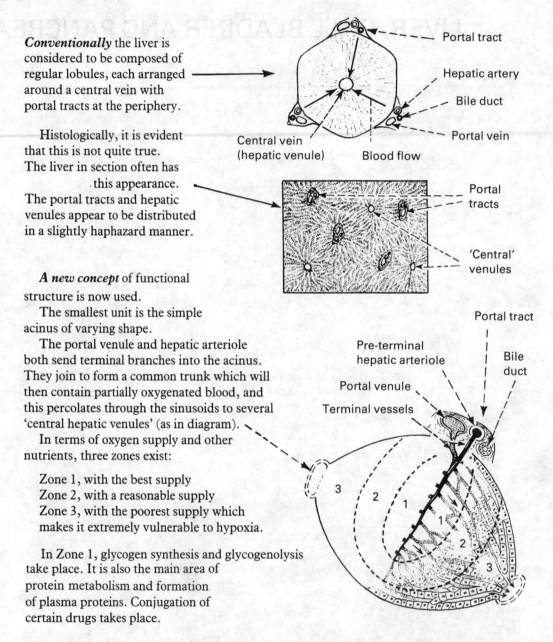

Portal tract

Hepatic artery

Bile duct

Portal vein

Central vein (hepatic venule)   Blood flow

Histologically, it is evident that this is not quite true. The liver in section often has this appearance. The portal tracts and hepatic venules appear to be distributed in a slightly haphazard manner.

Portal tracts

'Central' venules

A new concept of functional structure is now used.

The smallest unit is the simple acinus of varying shape.

The portal venule and hepatic arteriole both send terminal branches into the acinus. They join to form a common trunk which will then contain partially oxygenated blood, and this percolates through the sinusoids to several 'central hepatic venules' (as in diagram).

In terms of oxygen supply and other nutrients, three zones exist:

Zone 1, with the best supply
Zone 2, with a reasonable supply
Zone 3, with the poorest supply which makes it extremely vulnerable to hypoxia.

In Zone 1, glycogen synthesis and glycogenolysis take place. It is also the main area of protein metabolism and formation of plasma proteins. Conjugation of certain drugs takes place.

Portal tract

Pre-terminal hepatic arteriole

Bile duct

Portal venule

Terminal vessels

Zone 3 is associated with glycogen storage, lipid and pigment formation and metabolism of certain drugs and chemicals. Zone 2 shares functions with the other zones.

LIVER-ANATOMY

A complex acinus consists of at least three simple acini organised around the terminal branches of a pre-terminal portal venule, hepatic arteriole and bile duct. The blood circulates through the parenchyma and drains into two or three hepatic venules.

Zone 1, 2 and 3 form roughly concentric layers, zone 1 being the core of the complex acinus. Zone 3 is the outer layer at the periphery of the circulation and, at certain points, can come quite close to the preterminal vessels.

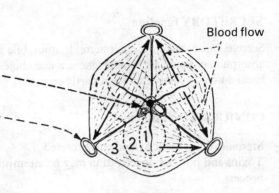

Blood flow

Complex acini (diagrammatic) — each consisting of three simple acini

Complex acinus

Portal tract

'Central' hepatic venule

Pre-terminal hepatic arteriole

Portal venule

Bile duct

'Conventional' lobule, shown by shaded area, consisting of interdigitating acini

It must be realised that the acini interdigitate in a complex way so that masses of hepatic cells are of irregular shape and the apparent regularity shown in the diagram is merely schematic. This explains the difficulty in recognising the functional units in histological sections.

441

LIVER FUNCTION

SECRETORY function

Secretes bile containing: cholesterol; lecithin; bile salts — detergent action — aid emulsification and absorption of lipids, fat soluble vitamins and cholesterol); bile pigments — products of haemoglobin breakdown — partly excreted, partly recycled.

CONJUGATING function

Steroids, drugs: inactivated and excreted.
Toxins and poisons: inactivation may be attempted but the hepatic cells can be damaged in the process.

METABOLIC function

Protein

Dietary Amino Acids

Blood → Converted to protein in tissues

Part storage in liver

Excess deaminated → Keto acid group → Conversion to glucose → Stored as glycogen / Converted to fat

Amine group excreted as urea

Protein formation → Storage / Plasma proteins (albumin, fibrinogen etc.)

Carbohydrate

Dietary glucose of fructose → Blood glucose → energy production / Glycogen stored in liver / Excess converted to fat

Fat

Dietary fat → Glycerol → Glycogen
Dietary fat → Fatty acids → Energy production / Formation of ketone bodies → Utilised in tissues

Liver damage will interfere with these functions and this will be reflected in the blood chemistry. Some substances may be increased, e.g. plasma amino acids; others may be reduced, e.g. urea. Enzymes may be released from the damaged cells and appear in the plasma.

ANATOMY HEPATIC LESIONS

The site of hepatic lesions is determined mainly by the microcirculation.
Factors involved are:
1. PO_2 of blood
2. Enzyme functions of the zones
3. Filtration function.

LIVER NECROSIS

In this text the modern description of the liver anatomy is used, providing an explanation of lesions in functional terms. The older conventional lobular nomenclature is shown in brackets.

Perivenular necrosis (Centrilobular necrosis)

This form is a feature of many apparently unrelated conditions.
It is brought about by damage in zone 3 of interdigitating
acini (A in diagram).

Thus it is a feature of
shock due to circulatory
collapse reducing
the oxygen supply
to zone 3. It also
occurs in poisoning
with chlorinated hydrocarbons (e.g. chloroform)
and drugs, e.g. paracetamol, substances
metabolised in zone 3.

It is important to realise that zone 3, particularly,
is continuous from one acinus to another,
and in severe cases, the hepatic venules
are linked together by necrotic tissues. Microscopically,
therefore, the lesions appear
irregular in distribution due to
differing planes of section.

Mid-zonal Necrosis

This is uncommon. It is seen in yellow
fever and in acute peritonitis; probably
the result of toxins affecting zones 2 and 1
(B in diagram).

Periportal necrosis (Peripheral necrosis)

This may represent damage in parts of zone 3 near the portal tracts, or changes in zone 1 due to its metabolism of drugs and chemicals; e.g. phosphorus poisoning causes marked fatty change in the peripheral parenchyma, followed by necrosis.

ANATOMY — HEPATIC LESIONS

Massive necrosis

This is an unusual lesion which can follow poisoning due to drugs, industrial chemicals or mushrooms. Rarely it is a complication of viral hepatitis.

Four factors may operate to bring about this necrosis:

1. **Personal sensitivity to the 'poison'.** This has been particularly observed in regard to drugs.

2. **Dosage.** The extent of necrosis is often related to the dose of position.

3. **Transfer of function.** If one zone becomes necrotic due to the formation of toxic substances when trying to metabolise a chemical, then the task of dealing with the chemical falls upon the adjacent zone. This occurs in paracetamol overdosage and poisoning by chloroform or carbon tetrachloride.

Zone 3 necrotic due to chloroform

↓

Zone 2 takes over function and will undergo necrosis if dose of chloroform is large enough

↓

The process may extend to zone 1

4. **Interference with circulation.** In any necrotic process, the local circulation of blood is bound to be upset, and this will tend to increase the damage which will spread in an increasingly haphazard manner if the cause is still operating.

The following substances are among the most important causing massive liver necrosis:

Drugs: monoamine oxidase inhibitors, paracetamol, halothane.
Industrial chemicals: carbon tetrachloride, tetrachlorethylene, chlorinated naphthalene and nitrobenzene compounds.

Shrunken liver

In the early stages, the liver is normal in size and is yellow. Soon the dead cells are removed, leaving collapsed dark red areas. Subsequently the surviving cells undergo hyperplasia resulting in a shrunken liver with nodules (multiple nodular hyperplasia) — a form of cirrhosis.

Early acute liver failure may prove fatal. Recovery leaves a liver with gross functional deficiency. The healing fibrotic process and complications inevitably follow.

VIRAL HEPATITIS

Viral hepatitis is the most important form of hepatitis. It is common in Eastern Europe, Africa and Asia. Hospital workers are at special risk and outbreaks are relatively common in mentally handicapped patients in institutions.

Early stage

Liver is enlarged and congested

The histology varies from case to case and from lobule to lobule in the same case.

Ballooning degeneration is the mildest change

Necrosis in some degree is always present.

Mononuclears, lymphocytes and a few plasma cells

Necrotic liver cells

Nuclei pyknotic or lysed

-- Hepatic venule

-- Normal cells

-- Councilman-like body (necrotic acidophilic cell bodies)

-- Round cell infiltrate in portal tract

This necrosis may be (a) focal (peripheral or scattered in parenchyma) or more severe (b) forming areas of bridging necrosis between vessels (portal to hepatic venule, hepatic venule to hepatic venule) or (c) panacinar: parts or the whole of many acini up to massive necrosis of a large part of the liver occasionally occurs. When it does so, it is usually most marked in the left lobe.

VIRAL HEPATITIS

Later stage

Liver is smaller, yellowish or greenish.

There is evidence of healing with mitotic activity in the hepatocytes.

Lymphocytes, plasma cells, mononuclears and pigment; collapsed stroma

Binucleate and multinucleate hepatocytes

Pigmented hyperplastic Kupffer cells (contain bile and lipofuscin derived from dead hepatocytes)

Healing stage

Resolution with complete return to normal is common, e.g. in focal and even bridging necrosis. Where necrosis has been severe and extensive with marked inflammatory reaction, the necrotic cells are cleared away, collapse of stroma occurs and fibrosis may follow. Surviving adjacent hepatocytes undergo hyperplasia. Lobular structure may become distorted so that vascular relationships, e.g. between hepatic venule and portal tracts, are disturbed and blood flow can be reversed.

Clinical effects

Pre-icteric phase

The symptoms are those of an acute infection — fever, anorexia, nausea, vomiting, epigastric discomfort, pains in muscles and joints and sometimes a rash. Hepatic enlargement and tenderness are usually present.

Icteric phase

The signs and symptoms are directly due to the changes in the liver. Jaundice increases for 1 – 2 weeks but frequently disappears in another two weeks. The urine is dark and the stool pale. Leukopenia is followed by lymphocytosis. Splenic enlargement is sometimes present.

VIRAL HEPATITIS

Biochemical changes

These changes result from liver damage

Disruption of bile canaliculi

↓

Absorption of conjugated bile into blood (levels up to 300μmol.)

Necrosis of hepatocytes

↓

Release of enzymes into blood

↓

Transferase enzymes (SGOT, SGPT) greatly increased (fall when jaundice appears)

Diminished production of special substances

↓

Coagulation mechanisms upset

↓

Prothrombin times increased

Clinical progress

1. In most cases, the disease is self-limiting and complete recovery occurs within 4 – 6 weeks.
2. Death may occur:
   (a) In the early pre-icteric stage within 10 days — fulminant hepatic failure.
   (b) In 2 – 3 weeks. The liver is reduced in size.

Capsule is wrinkled

Loss of substance

Remaining liver tissue opaque, yellowsih, without markings and is largely necrotic.

Large necrotic area

Bile duct hyperplasia

This condition is often termed 'acute yellow atrophy'.

(c) Several weeks later.
At this stage, regeneration is well advanced in places but function is inadequate and progressive failure occurs.

Pale areas of regenerating liver tissue

Gall bladder

Collapsed stroma

447

VIRAL HEPATITIS

Clinical progress (continued)

Secondary pathology due to progressive liver failure occurs in these cases:
Pleural effusion, peripheral oedema, haemorrhagic lesions often in intestinal tract due to upset in prothrombin and vitamin K metabolism, degenerative changes in brain.

3. Chronic hepatitis.

4. Cirrhosis. This may arise in the healing of acute necrosis or result from progressive chronic hepatitis.

Aetiology

Three viruses — A, B and non-A non-B – are the main causes of viral hepatitis, but the pathological changes are similar in all three. (Recently a virus in the non-A, non–B category has been isolated and named Hepatitis C virus).

	Type A	Type B	Type non-A non-B
Virus	RNA Picornavirus family	DNA. Hepadna virus family	Probably two types ?DNA
Mode of spread	Orofaecal, flies, ? parenteral	Parenteral Sexual	Parenteral. Transfusion of blood or blood products
Incubation period	15 – 40 days	40 – 180 days	Not accurately known
Age of patient	Mostly children	Mainly adults	All ages
Onset	Abrupt	Insidious	Gradual
Viraemia	Transient	Several weeks	Unknown
Severity	Mild	Commonly severe	Often mild but may be severe
Complications	Uncommon	Relatively frequent	Incidence unknown
Mortality	Less than 5%	Up to 10%	Unknown
Carriers	None	10%	Frequency unknown
Immunisation	Passive Pooled human IgG	Active Vaccine on surface viral antigen HBsAg	Not available

VIRAL HEPATITIS

ANTIGENS and IMMUNOLOGY

Hepatitis A

A small cubical RNA virus, 25 – 28 nm in diameter with a single antigen HAAg. Found in faeces before jaundice occurs. Appears in hepatocytes and Kupffer cells. IgM antibodies appear in the blood during the acute phase and IgG during convalescence. The latter confers immunity and persists for many years.

Hepatitis B

This is a complicated DNA viral structure consisting of a 'core' 37 nm in diameter, the essential infective particle containing several antigens, and a surface protein coat. The core replicates in the liver cell nuclei.

It is composed of central DNA polymerase surrounded by a layer of DNA which in turn is enclosed in a protein coat — the so-called core antigen HBcAg. Associated with this core antigen is another — the e antigen HBeAg.

The surface protein coat is formed in the liver cell cytoplasm and is applied to the core.
This protein is also antigenic — the surface antigen HBsAg. (HBsAg is produced in excess and appears in the blood forming a diagnostic marker.)

The complete virion including the surface protein coat, diameter 42 nm, is known as the Dane particle. The core antigen is never found in blood, but HBsAg, HBeAg and DNA polymerase as well as Dane particles appear during the acute phase.

Dane particle

Spheres and tubules of HBsAg in blood

VIRAL HEPATITIS

ANTIGENS and IMMUNOLOGY (continued)

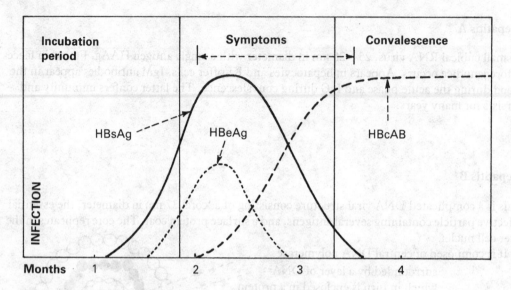

Six weeks after infection the **surface antigen (HBsAg)** appears in the blood, followed two weeks later by the **e antigen (HBcAg)**.

Core antigen (HBcAg) does not enter the blood, but the **antibody HBcAB** is found at the time symptoms appear. This antibody is of IgM variety but later, in convalescence, it changes to an IgG type.

Antibody to the e antigen (HBeAg) rapidly disappears from the blood.

Last to appear is the antibody (HBsAB) to the surface antigen two to three weeks after the symptoms subside and all trace of the antigen is lost. Antibodies to the core and surface antigens persist for many years and confer immunity.

The interpretation of these changes appears to be as follows:
Following infection an immune response is mounted in the liver which damages the hepatic cells and produces the symptoms. Antigens are released during the process and some spill into the blood. The immune response is enhanced leading to neutralisation and disappearance of the antigens with recovery from the illness. The idea that immune response is the cause of the liver damage is suggested by the delay between infection and the onset of symptoms, and by the fact that hepatic B infection in immunosuppressed patients has a very mild course or may be asymptomatic.

VIRAL HEPATITIS

OUTCOME of HEPATITIS B INFECTION

In 90% of cases, there is a vigorous antibody reaction and the patient recovers completely with liver function unimpaired. In the remaining 10%, the illness pursues a variable course, for example:

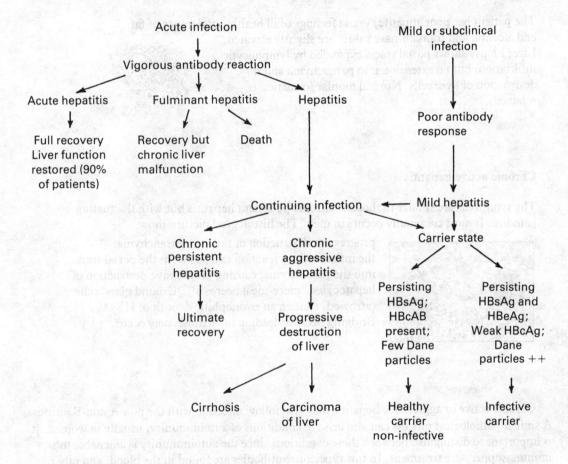

Delta agent

This is a defective RNA virus requiring the presence of HB virus for reproduction. A concomitant infection with HB and Delta agent confers a much more serious prognosis with often fulminant liver damage and subsequent chronic aggressive hepatitis.

Note: Type A rarely leads to severe complications.

Types non-A non-B are usually mild but in post-transfusion cases may be very severe especially Type C.

451

CHRONIC HEPATITIS

If the condition does not resolve within six months it can be assumed that a chronic hepatitis is present. Two types exist:

1. Chronic persistent hepatitis

The patient has poor appetite, vague feelings of ill health, intolerance of fat and alcohol, and transaminase values are slightly elevated. Liver biopsy shows portal tracts expanded by lymphocytic infiltration, but no extension into parenchyma and no destruction of liver cells. Normal lobular formation is retained.

2. Chronic active hepatitis

The symptoms are similar to those of chronic persistent hepatitis but with fluctuating jaundice. It most commonly occurs in men. The histological picture shows

progressive destruction of the liver parenchyma: the inflammatory reaction extends from the portal tract into the parenchyma, causing progressive destruction of hepatocytes ('piece-meal necrosis'). 'Ground glass' cells (arrowed) contain an eosinophilic deposit of HBsAg. Bridging necrosis leading to cirrhosis may occur.

Chronic active or aggresstive hepatitis may also follow infection with the non-A non-B viruses. A similar pathological process can also arise in conditions of autoimmunity, usually in women. It is important to distinguish between these conditions since the autoimmunity is amenable to immunosuppressive treatment. In this type, autoantibodies are found in the blood, and other systems may be affected — joints, thyroid gland, haemopoietic system, bowel and kidneys.

In both conditions there is a defective immune response, but the mechanism is unclear. Surface antigen (HBsAg) is commonly found in the blood. In the aggressive type there may be antibodies to the core antigen.

Chronic hepatitis also occurs in alcoholism, administration of certain drugs such as methyldopa, isoniazid, nitrofurantoin, the laxative oxyphenisatin, and in genetic conditions, e.g. α_1 anti-trypsin deficiency and Wilson's disease (an inborn error of copper metabolism).

ALCOHOLIC LIVER DISEASE

Excessive alcohol consumption is associated with several distinct pathological conditions in the liver: (1) **fatty liver;** (2) **alcoholic hepatitis;** (3) **hepatic fibrosis** and (4) **cirrhosis.**

It should be understood however that in many instances the pathology is mixed and all of these changes may be seen.

Fatty liver

This is due to changes in the metabolic activity of hepatocytes and occurs following even a single episode of excessive alcohol intake. The liver is enlarged and in gross cases has a yellow colour.

The accumulation of fat in the liver cells is due to diversion of hepatic enzymes to metabolise the alcohol causing a deficiency resulting in interference with fat and carbohydrate metabolism.

Swollen liver cells containing globules of fat.

Alcohol metabolism ———▶ Consumption of NAD

(nicotinamide adenine dinucleotide)

Relative deficiency of NAD

Incomplete carbohydrate metabolism → Lactic acid

Incomplete fat metabolism → Ketosis

Slowing of fat metabolism → Accumulation of fat in liver

In the early stages of alcohol abuse, the fat accumulating in the liver is mainly derived from the fat deposits of the body.

The main chemical reactions involved are as follows:

Ethanol + alcohol dehydrogenase

Acetaldehyde + acetaldehyde dehydrogenase

Hydrogen ions

Acetate (metabolised in peripheral tissues)

Hydrogen ions ———▶ NAD$^+$ / NADH

Excess H ions — introduced into various cell reactions upsetting oxidative mechanisms (esp. fat and carbohydrate).

If alcohol abuse continues, further hepatic changes quickly take place, part adaptive, part impairment. The adaptive change is indicated by an increase in the smooth endoplasmic reticulum associated with an increase in microsomal enzymes.

ALCOHOLIC LIVER DISEASE

The two processes, adaptation and impairment, act together to increase the effects of alcohol on fat metabolism in the liver.

Increased ability to metabolise alcohol utilises the phosphonucleotide cycle:

Ethanol+alcohol dehydrogenase

Acetaldehyde   H ions
+
Dehydrogenase   NADP   NADPH

Acetate   H ions

The H ions produced by this process upset further the oxidative mechanisms of the cell already unbalanced by the NAD reaction. Other enzymes associated with fat metabolism are also stimulated and the net result is as follows:

Adaptive increase
in enzymes

Increased production of lipoproteins   Production of glycerophosphate   Metabolism of alcohol

Hyperlipidaemia

Production of H ions

Interference with oxidation

Inhibitory process

Damage to mitochondria

Reduced oxidation

Conversion to triglyceride fat in cells

Diminished oxidation of fatty acids

The result is gross accumulation of fat in the liver cells. Even so this change is reversible.

Other enzymes are also increased and side-effects may be induced, for example:

(a) Increased catabolism of drugs which thus become less effective, e.g. warfarin, phenobarbitone, tolbutamide
(b) Increased catabolism of steroids, e.g. androgens which may lead to a degree of feminisation in males
(c) Conversion of potential hepatotoxins to active metabolites causing further damage to liver.

Inhibitory activities, mainly damage to mitochondria, can lead to diminished gluconeogenesis and reduced production of albumin and transferrin.

ALCOHOLIC HEPATITIS

Fatty change is reversible even when extensive. In a small proportion of cases, alcoholic hepatitis is superimposed. The essential features are hepatocellular degeneration and necrosis. A peculiar protein, Mallory's hyaline, perhaps produced by the abnormal liver cells accumulates in some of them.

Acute phase

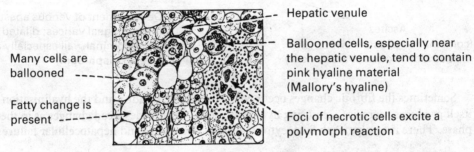

Hepatic venule

Ballooned cells, especially near the hepatic venule, tend to contain pink hyaline material (Mallory's hyaline)

Many cells are balloned

Fatty change is present

Foci of necrotic cells excite a polymorph reaction

Clinical features

The patient is acutely ill with fever, nausea, vomiting, and pain in the right upper quadrant. Jaundice may occur, partly due to cholestasis in the bile ductules. Serum transaminases are increased, but the main change is in serum alkaline phosphatase which may reach very high levels. Recently it has been suggested that the increase in glutamic dehydrogenase is directly proportional to the degree of liver damage.

Healing phase

Hyaline fibrous tissue is laid down at an early stage with disappearance of hepatocytes around hepatic venules.

The hyaline fibrosis tends to compress the hepatic venule of the lobule.

Columns of fatty liver cells

Compression of hepatic venule by hyaline fibrosis

455

ALCOHOLIC HEPATITIS

The hyaline fibrosis, if extensive, may have the following results:

Hepatic vein obstruction

↓

Portal hypertension

Ascites
(combination of ascites with
malnutrition is often characteristic)

Development of venous anastomoses
(oesophageal varices; dilated veins
on abdominal wall especially at
level of diaphragm)

Sometimes the fibrotic changes occur with remarkable rapidity and the hyalinisation process itself produces necrosis ('sclerosing hyaline necrosis') with widespread changes as in the acute phase. There is a polymorph leucocytosis, progressive ascites and hepatocellular failure.

Aetiology

The aetiology of alcoholic hepatitis is obscure. Several suggestions without adequate proof have been made.

1. Superimposed viral or bacterial infection.
2. Hypersensitivity to alcohol.
3. Delayed hypersensitive reaction to altered proteins produced in hepatocytes, e.g. Mallory's hyaline.
4. Genetic susceptibility. This has been suggested since only a small proportion of alcoholics develop the condition.

ALCOHOLIC FIBROSIS

Focal fibrosis occurs as a result of attacks of alcoholic hepatitis, but in addition there is commonly a piecemeal necrosis at the periphery of the lobules. Spurs of fibrous tissue develop around the portal tracts producing a stellate pattern.

Portal venule

Fatty liver cells

Enlargement of portal tracts by accumulation
of fibrous tissue

Fibrous tissue spurs

Fibrosis sometimes becomes progressive, leading to cirrhosis. This is most apt to happen if there are attacks of alcoholic hepatitis.

CIRRHOSIS

Three macroscopic types are described.

1. Micronodular
The liver is usually of normal size or slightly enlarged.

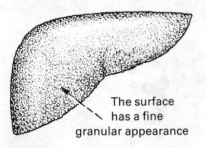

The surface has a fine granular appearance

The nodules of the liver tissue, 1 or 2 mm in diameter, are of fairly uniform size outlined by grey fibrous tissue.

2. Macronodular
Liver size tends to vary. Frequently there is irregular shrinkage in parts. The surface shows a coarse nodularity.

The nodules are larger and may be more than 1 cm in diameter. Often no hepatic venule can be seen in a lobule.

3. Mixed nodular
As the name suggests, this pattern is a mixture of the previous two.

The surface varies from part to part, according to the size of nodules

Similarly the cut surface shows variation in the diameter of the nodules.

Most cases of cirrhosis end in a mixed nodular condition.

CIRRHOSIS

Whatever the cause, four mechanisms are involved in the production of hepatic cirrhosis: (1) hepatocellular necrosis, (2) replacement fibrosis and inflammation, (3) vascular derangement and (4) hyperplasia of surviving liver tissue.

Necrosis, which is often piecemeal, may be:

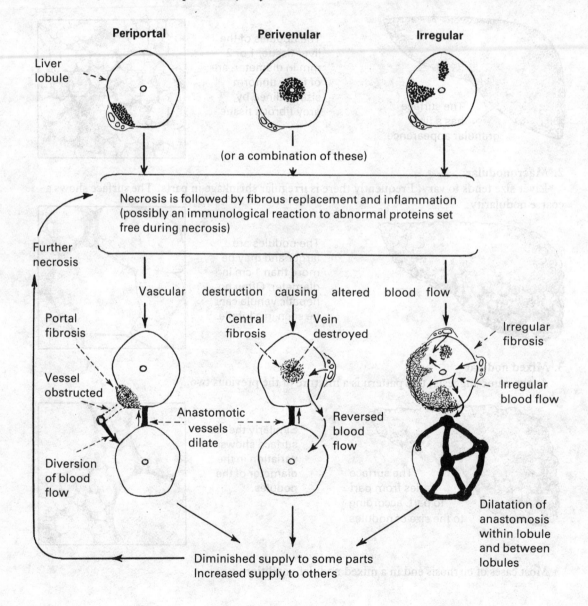

Periportal

Perivenular

Irregular

Liver lobule

(or a combination of these)

Necrosis is followed by fibrous replacement and inflammation (possibly an immunological reaction to abnormal proteins set free during necrosis)

Further necrosis

Vascular   destruction   causing   altered   blood   flow

Portal fibrosis

Vessel obstructed

Diversion of blood flow

Central fibrosis

Vein destroyed

Anastomotic vessels dilate

Reversed blood flow

Irregular fibrosis

Irregular blood flow

Dilatation of anastomosis within lobule and between lobules

Diminished supply to some parts
Increased supply to others

CIRRHOSIS

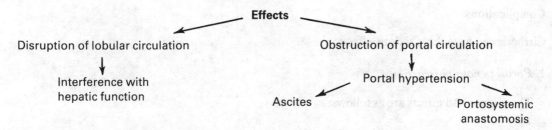

Effects

Disruption of lobular circulation → Interference with hepatic function

Obstruction of portal circulation → Portal hypertension → Ascites / Portosystemic anastomosis

The surviving liver cells undergo reactive hyperplasia forming nodules which further distort vascular distribution. Bile ducts may also undergo hyperplasia.

Cells in hyperplastic nodules are enlarged and often binucleated

Hyperplastic masses are pale and add to the nodularity of the liver

Cirrhosis is usually a slow process but inevitably progressive due to:

(a) continued action of the initial damaging factor
(b) development of cytotoxic immune reactions to proteins set free by damaged hepatic cells.

The relative importance of each of these factors varies in individual cases. A vicious circle is set up which maintains the pathological process.

Noxious agent
Liver cell necrosis
Proteins set free
Immune mechanisms stimulated
Chronic inflammation and fibrosis
Vascular damage and derangement

459

CIRRHOSIS

Complications

Cirrhosis can have three serious effects:

1. *Portal venous obstruction*

The process and effects are as follows:

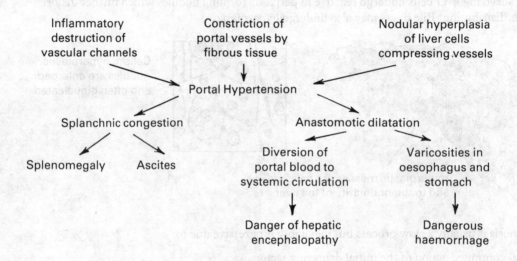

Inflammatory destruction of vascular channels

Constriction of portal vessels by fibrous tissue

Nodular hyperplasia of liver cells compressing vessels

Portal Hypertension

Splanchnic congestion

Anastomotic dilatation

Splenomegaly   Ascites

Diversion of portal blood to systemic circulation

Varicosities in oesophagus and stomach

Danger of hepatic encephalopathy

Dangerous haemorrhage

2. *Hepatocellular failure*

This is due to a combination of two factors:

(a) Continuous loss of liver cells
(b) Increasing distortion of hepatic circulation causing a reduction in effective hepatic blood flow.

The result is a progressive diminution in hepatic function.

3. *Liver cell carcinoma*

This is a late complication in just over 10% of cases of cirrhosis.

CIRRHOSIS

ACQUIRED FORMS

ALCOHOLIC cirrhosis

This is the commonest form
of cirrhosis and is most frequent
in men over 40. In its early
stages, it is a micronodular
cirrhosis affecting a large fatty
liver.

Periportal
cirrhosis with
piecemeal
destruction
of hepatocytes

Later, attacks of alcoholic hepatitis lead to centrolobular sclerosis and ultimately a small, non-fatty macronodular or mixed nodular cirrhosis results.

Periportal
fibrosis

Absence
of hepatic
venules

Hyperplastic
nodules of
surviving
liver cells

Fibrosis
spreading
between
hepatic venules

There is little inflammatory change and bile duct hyperplasia is minimal. Mallory's hyaline may be found in hepatic cells.

Clinical effects

Portal hypertension and hepatocellular failure are the main complications. Other changes are anaemia, muscle wasting, polyneuritis and mental changes. Some of these may be due to vitamin lack, especially B and C. Gastritis, peptic ulceration, pancreatitis and Dupuytren's contracture can also occur. Encephalopathy is rare.

INDIAN CHILDHOOD cirrhosis

This affects children aged 1 to 3 years of age. It is of unknown aetiology, but a mycotoxin is suspected. The pathological changes are rather similar to those of alcoholic cirrhosis, and Mallory's hyaline is usually found in the hepatocytes.

461

CIRRHOSIS

ACQUIRED FORMS (continued)

POST-VIRAL cirrhosis

This is a relatively rare condition. In viral hepatitis, although the hepatocytes undergo necrosis, there is little damage to the supporting tissues which collapse with disappearance of dead cells.

Regeneration is often remarkably complete and normal liver architecture is restored. Cirrhosis is usually the result of continuing inflammation — chronic active hepatitis. It produces a small liver showing macronodular cirrhosis.

Clinical features

It is commonest in young women. Features of chronic active hepatitis are present and various autoantibodies are found. Prognosis is poor and progress rapid with increasing portal hypertension and hepatocellular failure. Liver cell carcinoma is more common than in alcoholic cirrhosis. It appears to occur particularly in those cases showing a persistence of HB antigen in the blood.

CIRRHOSIS

ACQUIRED FORMS (continued)

BILIARY cirrhosis

Two types of this rare condition occur: primary intrahepatic biliary cirrhosis and secondary obstructive biliary cirrhosis.

PRIMARY INTRAHEPATIC BILIARY cirrhosis

The essential lesion is a chronic inflammation which destroys the small intrahepatic bile ducts.

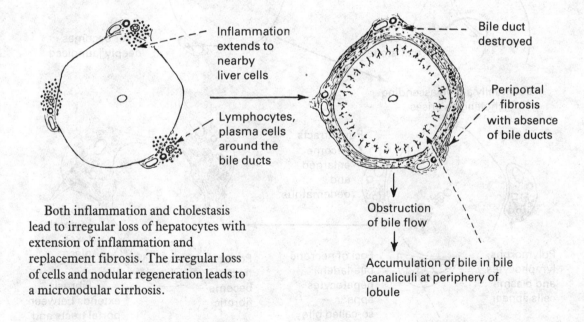

Inflammation extends to nearby liver cells

Lymphocytes, plasma cells around the bile ducts

Bile duct destroyed

Periportal fibrosis with absence of bile ducts

Obstruction of bile flow

Accumulation of bile in bile canaliculi at periphery of lobule

Both inflammation and cholestasis lead to irregular loss of hepatocytes with extension of inflammation and replacement fibrosis. The irregular loss of cells and nodular regeneration leads to a micronodular cirrhosis.

Clinical effects

The disease affects middle-aged women. Symptoms and signs are those of chronic obstructive jaundice. Malabsorption can result in osteomalacia and osteoporosis. The course of the disease is slow, but death is due to the complications of portal hypertension or encephalopathy.

The aetiology is unknown. Antibodies to mitochondria and raised IGM values suggest an immunological process. A few cases appear to be associated with use of drugs such as chlorpromazine. Cholestasis occurs in pregnancy and is known to follow the use of steroids (e.g. contraceptive pill). Some cases may be associated with similar substances.

CIRRHOSIS

SECONDARY OBSTRUCTIVE BILIARY cirrhosis

This is a rare condition which is the end result of chronic impaction of gallstones in the common bile duct or a benign stricture of the duct. The progression is as follows:

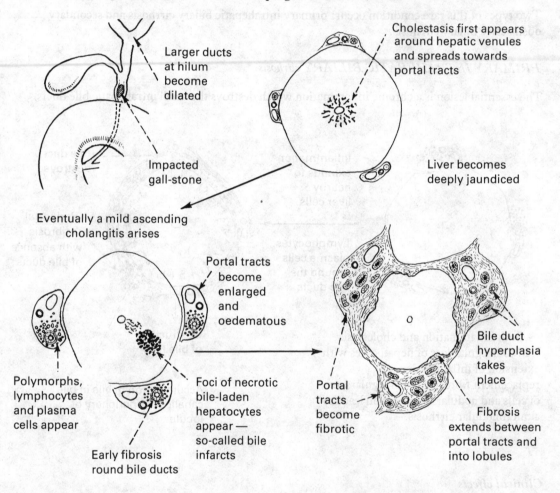

Larger ducts at hilum become dilated

Impacted gall-stone

Cholestasis first appears around hepatic venules and spreads towards portal tracts

Liver becomes deeply jaundiced

Eventually a mild ascending cholangitis arises

Portal tracts become enlarged and oedematous

Polymorphs, lymphocytes and plasma cells appear

Foci of necrotic bile-laden hepatocytes appear — so-called bile infarcts

Early fibrosis round bile ducts

Portal tracts become fibrotic

Bile duct hyperplasia takes place

Fibrosis extends between portal tracts and into lobules

Continuing erosion of the parenchyma and fibrosis lead to a true cirrhosis. The condition may be complicated by liver abscesses due to more acute ascending infection. Death is most often due to liver failure or intercurrent disease. Occasionally there is portal hypertension. Neoplasia, the other cause of bile duct obstruction, usually causes death before cirrhotic changes occur.

CIRRHOSIS

DRUG INDUCED cirrhosis

Isoniazid, methyldopa and oxyphenisat in appear to be associated with a form of cirrhosis showing features similar to those seen in the post-viral type.

Cirrhosis ASSOCIATED with GENERAL DISEASES

Cirrhosis has also been reported in ulcerative colitis, diabetes mellitus, rheumatoid arthritis, scleroderma and hyperthyroidism. A mild fibrosis is associated with chronic congestive cardiac failure. It is not a true cirrhosis and does not cause liver failure.

CRYPTOGENIC cirrhosis

This is a mixed group of conditions of unknown aetiology. The type of cirrhosis varies. As aetiological factors are progressively elucidated this group diminishes.

CONGENITAL FORMS of cirrhosis

Almost all of these are associated with inborn errors of metabolism causing infiltrations and hepatocyte degeneration. The following are examples:

Disease	Metabolic disorder	Type of cirrhosis
Hepatolenticular degeneration (Wilson's disease)	Excessive intestinal absorption of copper — deposition in liver, brain and kidney	Macronodular
Idiopathic haemochromatosis	Excessive absorption of iron — deposition in liver, pancreas and other organs	Micronodular
Galactosaemia	Inability to metabolise galactose Liver cells become distended with fat or glycogen; bile stasis	Micronodular
Glycogen storage disease	Absence of liver glucose-6-phosphate — inability to break down glycogen to glucose	Micronodular
Alpha 1 — antitrypsin deficiency	Uncontrolled action of proteases in inflammatory stasis, e.g. hepatitis	Micronodular

Biliary cirrhosis can follow congenital atresia of the bile ducts. Where the atresia affects the large extrahepatic bile ducts, death occurs in a short time before cirrhotic changes occur. Lesser degrees affecting the intrahepatic ducts have a prolonged course and cirrhosis can develop.

CIRRHOSIS

Ascites in hepatic cirrhosis

This is usually a late feature of cirrhosis and is associated with increasing hepatocellular failure. The pathogenesis is thought to be as follows:

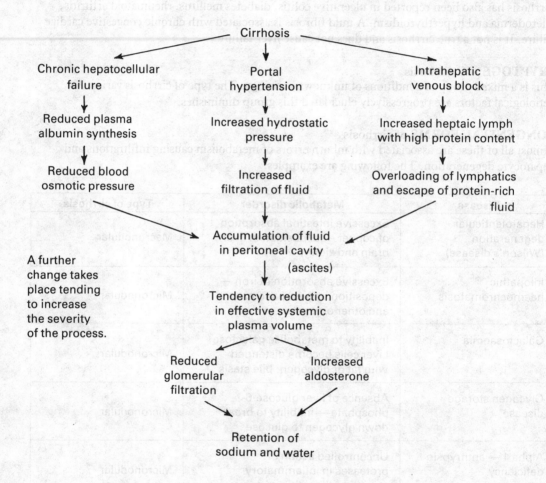

The condition is commonly one of slow accumulation of fluid, but a rapid onset is associated with those factors precipitating liver failure, e.g. haemorrhage from oesophageal varices, operations or bouts of acute alcoholic excess.

HEPATO-CELLULAR FAILURE

Failure of liver function can be:

1. **Acute** with rapid onset, e.g. in cases of massive necrosis due to poisoning (or, less commonly, acute hepatitis.)
2. **Chronic** and sometimes recurring, of slow onset, e.g. in cirrhosis or chronic hepatitis.

The mechanism is different in the two types.

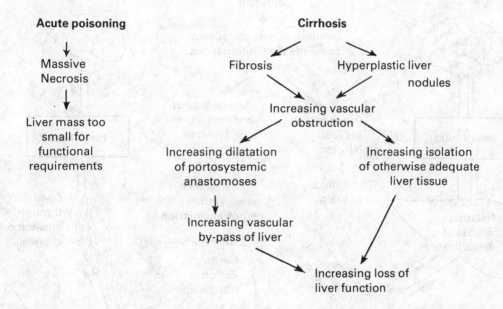

The symptoms and signs tend to be similar in both forms of liver failure but differ in degree. They consist of: jaundice, nervous system disorders, hypoglycaemia, acidosis, bleeding diathesis, renal failure, endocrine disturbances, ascites.

Jaundice

In acute liver failure, jaundice appears early and is related to the extent of liver damage. It arises as a result of lack of conjugation and excretion of bilirubin.

The time of appearance and type of jaundice in cases of chronic liver failure depend on the primary cause. In cases of biliary cirrhosis, the jaundice precedes other signs of liver failure and is of obstructive type, initially at least. Other forms of cirrhosis only give rise to jaundice at a late stage when it is of hepatic type, i.e. due to difficulties in bilirubin conjugation and excretion.

467

HEPATO-CELLULAR FAILURE

Nervous system disorders

These take the form of tremors, behavioural changes, convulsions, delirium, drowsiness and coma, and the syndrome is generally termed hepatic encephalopathy. In the acute form, severe symptoms such as convulsions, delirium and coma develop rapidly, while in chronic conditions milder changes are seen and coma is a late feature, unless a complication arises.

The basic cause is the same in both forms but the mechanism is somewhat different

↓

Diminished detoxification of toxic intestinal nitrogenous compounds

Increase in blood NH_3 etc.

↓

Toxic effect or brain

Appearance of abnormal amines in systemic circulation

↓

Interference with neurotransmission

Acute

Brain

Heart/lung

Necrosis ≡ Loss of detoxification

Toxic N₂ compounds

Chronic

Brain

Heart/lung

Diversion through anastomotic channels

Cirrhosis ≡ Portal obstruction

Toxic N₂ compounds

Despite the serious disturbances of function, pathological changes in the brain of fatal cases are surprisingly slight.

Interstitial oedema

Perivascular oedema

Protoplasmic astrocytes enlarged and increased in number. Nuclei large with prominent nucleoli.

HEPATO-CELLULAR FAILURE

Metabolic and other changes

These may be seen in both acute and chronic liver failure but are variable in their occurrence. They are again due to deficiencies in the functions of the liver and, in the chronic state, may be precipitated by some incidental factor such as bleeding, infection etc. Examples are as follows:

Defective nitrogen metabolism

Rise in blood amino acids esp. tryptophan
↓
Increased production of serotonin
↓
Drowsiness

Diminished production of plasma albumin
↓
Fall in plasma osmotic pressure
↓
Tendency to ascites and oedema

Diminished production of fibrinogen, prothrombin and factors V, VII, IX, X.
↓
Haemorrhagic diathesis

Defective carbohydrate metabolism

Increased blood insulin (non-utilisation by liver)
↓
Muscle catabolism
↓
Raised blood pyruvates, lactates, citrates
↓
Acidosis

Hypoglycaemia

In men, liver failure is associated with gynaecomastia, loss of libido and testicular atrophy. This is due to defective conjugation of oestrogens.

Renal failure

The reason for renal failure is not certain in all cases. Occasionally it may be due to shock caused by oesophageal bleeding in cases of cirrhosis, but in acute hepatic failure the mechanism is obscure.

Anaemia

Three mechanisms may be involved in the causation of anaemia in hepatic failure (usually the chronic form).

1. Repeated bleeding from oesophageal varices.
2. Hypersplenism. Portal hypertension leads to venous congestion and enlargement of the spleen which develops an increased capacity to destroy red cells.
3. Upset in folic acid and B_{12} metabolism in the liver.

HEPATO-CELLULAR FAILURE

Recurrent acute hepatic encephalopathy
This is apt to occur in cases of advanced cirrhosis and is precipitated by:

1. *Gastro-intestinal bleeding*   The mechanism is as follows:

In some patients, even a high protein diet can have the same effect.

2. *Diuretic therapy*

3. *Porta-caval shunt operations*
These are carried out for relief of portal hypertension, but untoward effects may be encountered:

4. *Narcotic and analgestic drugs*
These can be very toxic and have a cumulative action due to lack of hepatic drug metabolism.

5. *Intercurrent infections*
Dehydration, electrolyte imbalance, tissue catabolism and failure of detoxification processes all play a part.

INFECTIONS AND INFESTATIONS

PYOGENIC INFECTIONS

These are now much less common due to the efficient use of antibiotics. Abscess of the liver occurs mainly in two conditions:

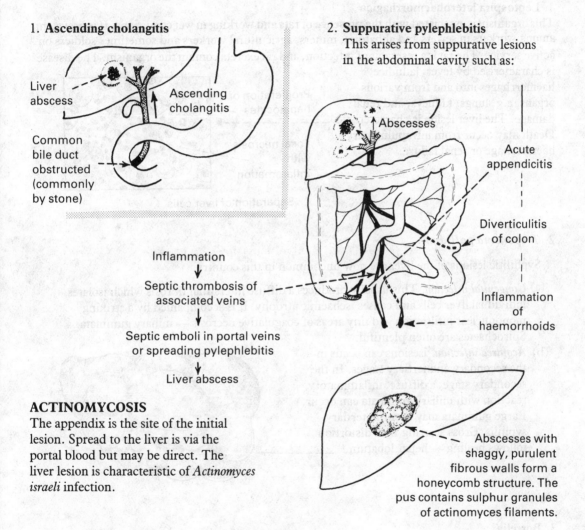

1. Ascending cholangitis

Liver abscess

Ascending cholangitis

Common bile duct obstructed (commonly by stone)

2. Suppurative pylephlebitis

This arises from suppurative lesions in the abdominal cavity such as:

Abscesses

Acute appendicitis

Diverticulitis of colon

Inflammation of haemorrhoids

Inflammation
↓
Septic thrombosis of associated veins
↓
Septic emboli in portal veins or spreading pylephlebitis
↓
Liver abscess

ACTINOMYCOSIS

The appendix is the site of the initial lesion. Spread to the liver is via the portal blood but may be direct. The liver lesion is characteristic of *Actinomyces israeli* infection.

Abscesses with shaggy, purulent fibrous walls form a honeycomb structure. The pus contains sulphur granules of actinomyces filaments.

TUBERCULOSIS

This is rare. Miliary tubercles may be seen in generalised infection.

Tuberculoid reactions

Giant cell granulomata are common in sarcoidosis and may also occur in brucellosis, histoplasmosis and early biliary cirrhosis.

INFECTIONS AND INFESTATIONS

SPIROCHAETAL INFECTIONS

Three spirochaetal infections can involve the liver.

1. **Leptospira icterohaemorrhagica**

This organism is associated with the presence of rats and working in wet conditions. It is prevalent among workers in sewers and abbatoirs, miners, agricultural workers and sometimes soldiers on active service. The rat is a reservoir of infection, and rat excreta contain the organism. The disease is characterised by fever, jaundice, haemorrhages into and from various organs, e.g. lungs, kidneys, and renal damage. The liver lesion is characteristic. Death may occur from intrapulmonary haemorrhage or renal failure.

Proliferation of hepatocytes ➝

Focal necrosis with inflammation

Separation of liver cells

2. *Treponema pallidum*

Syphilitic lesions of the liver are now uncommon in this country.

(a) *Congenital infection.* This usually produces a diffuse interstitial fibrosis which isolates individual liver cells and causes ischaemic atrophy. It is accompanied by a striking mononuclear infiltration and tiny areas of coagulative necrosis — miliary gummata. Spirochaetes are often plentiful.

(b) *Acquired infection.* Lesions can occur in the secondary and tertiary stages. In the secondary stage, a diffuse, inflammatory reaction with miliary gummata can occur. Large gummata may occur in tertiary syphilis. Gross scarring with distortion follows healing — hepar lobatum. ➝

3. **Borrelia**

Borrelia occur in many parts of the world and several species exist — *B. recurrentis* or *B. obermeieri* in Europe, and *B. duttoni* in Africa. They are transmitted by lice and ticks from animals acting as reservoirs, especially rodents. The infections produce centrilobular necrosis of the liver. Jaundice may be severe and liver failure can result in death.

INFECTIONS AND INFESTATIONS

PROTOZOAL DISEASES

Amoebic 'abcess'

This is a complication of amoebic dysentery
due to *Entamoeba histolytica*. The 'abscess' is
usually single, in the upper right lobe of liver.
An irregular fibrous wall encloses what appears
to be brownish pus. The 'pus' consists of necrotic
liver cells, debris and red cells. Amoebae may
be found in the inner wall. There are no pus
cells. It may remain localised or track through
the diaphragm into the lung, pleural or pericardial
cavities.

Venous
drainage

Chronic
amoebic
dysentery

Malaria

On initial infection, the parasites develop
within the hepatocytes but produce little damage.
In chronic malaria, red cells containing parasites
are engulfed by Kupffer cells which become
hyperplastic and contain brown malarial pigment.

In benign tertian malaria, the parasite can survive for long periods within the liver cells
(exoerythrocytic cycle).

Kala-azar

The liver is enlarged due to hyperplasia of the Kupffer cells which phagocytose many Leishman-
Donovan bodies

METAZOAL DISEASES Trematodes (flukes)

Schistosomiasis

S. mansoni is common in Egypt and other parts of
Africa. *S. japonicum* is found in China, Japan and
the Philippines. Both infections involve the liver.

The schistosomes colonise intestinal tract, the large
intestine in the case of *S. mansoni*, while *S. japonicum*
infests the small intestine. They invade the intestinal

S. mansoni

veins; ova are released into the blood stream and embolise the portal venules of the liver. There is
a focal granulomatous reaction which may lead to extensive portal fibrosis without cirrhosis. Portal
hypertension can result with its attendant dangers.

INFECTIONS AND INFESTATIONS

METAZOAL DISEASES (continued)

Two other varieties of fluke disease exist — *clonorchiasis* (Chinese fish fluke) and *fascioliasis* (sheep fluke). Both produce an ascending cholangitis. Clonorchiasis can cause biliary obstruction and marked proliferation of bile ducts. Cholangiocarcinoma may develop. Infestation in both cases is due to eating raw or insufficiently cooked food.

Flukes

Hydatid disease

This is a cystic condition caused by the embryos of *Echinococcus granulosis*, a small tapeworm. The condition is commonest in sheep and may occur in humans in close contact with them. Cattle and pigs may also be affected. Adult worms are found in dogs fed on the infected tissues of sheep, cattle or pigs. Ova are excreted by the dogs and are ingested by other animals including man. The disease is commonest in Australia, New Zealand and South America.

Digestion of the chitinous membrane by gastric juice liberates the embryos which invade the intestinal veins and reach the liver. Sometimes they pass into the systemic circulation and cysts form in the lungs, muscles, kidneys, spleen or brain.

The cyst may be very large, usually multilocular due to budding of daughter cysts.

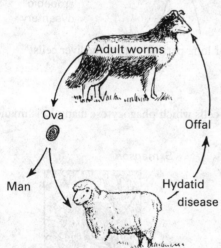

Adult worms

Ova

Offal

Man

Hydatid disease

Ingested by sheep, other domesticated animals and men

Patients show a hypersensitive reaction to an intradermal injection of hydatid antigen (Casoni test).

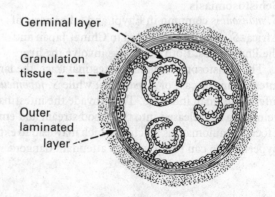

Germinal layer

Granulation tissue

Outer laminated layer

TUMOURS OF LIVER — PRIMARY CARCINOMA

PRIMARY CARCINOMA is a rare form of malignancy in Western countries but is much more common
in South Africa and South East Asia. It occurs in two main forms: hepatocellular carcinoma (75%
of cases) and cholangiocarcinoma (25%)

HEPATOCELLULAR CARCINOMA

Three main types of growth are described.

Solitary large tumour   Nodular form   Diffuse growth

In all three forms the liver is usually cirrhotic.

Histological structure

The cells grow in columns resembling normal liver.

Trabeculae
are
branched

Functional activity
is often displayed:
(a) bile secretion,
(b) fat formation,
(c) glycogen storage
(often excessive).

Basement membrane

Some tumours are anaplastic with spindle and multi-nucleated giant cells. Others may show a
part acinar structure.

CHOLANGIOCARCINOMA

Twenty five per cent of cases arise from the bile ducts. They
may develop from small intrahepatic ducts or from the main
ducts at the hilum. Two histological types occur. In most
instances, the tumour has a tubuloacinar structure. In other
cases it is a mucus-secreting adenocarcinoma with a dense
stroma. Cirrhosis is rarely present in cholangiocarcinoma.

Cells resemble bile duct epithelium.

PRIMARY CARCINOMA OF LIVER

Spread

Invasion of intrahepatic blood vessels occurs early and results in diffuse growth within the liver. Secondary growths may appear in the lungs, but the massive intrahepatic growth often results in liver failure and death before extrahepatic spread appears.

Clinical features

Many of the clinical findings are related to the underlying cirrhosis. Some unusual features are directly related to the neoplasm.

1. Hypoglycaemia, due partly to the energy requirements of the tumour and partly to its ability to store glycogen.

2. Erythrocytosis. A mild increase in red cells is common in cirrhosis, but it may be exaggerated in hepatoma due to tumour production of erythropoietin.
   Other changes are the result of destruction of liver tissue.

3. Upset in blood clotting as a result of disordered production of fibrinogen.

4. Sex hormone effects due to lack of steroid conjugation.

Diagnostic biochemical tests

The usual tests of hepatic function are of little value. Serum alkaline phosphatase may be raised, although the plasma bilirubin remains normal.

Alpha-fetoprotein
This is a protein which is normally only produced in quantity by the fetal hepatocytes. In adult life, very low levels are present in the serum (<40 ng/ml).
It is increased in:

    (a) certain gonadal tumours
    (b) liver cell damage, e.g. in hepatitis
    (c) especially some cases of hepatic carcinoma.

Values above 500 ng/ml indicate carcinoma. This is found in 80% of cases in South Africa and South East Asia, but only 40 – 50% in Western countries. It is used to monitor progress in those tumours producing the protein.

Alpha-fetoprotein is not produced by the cholangiocarcinoma form of growth.

PRIMARY CARCINOMA OF LIVER

Aetiology

Geography. There is a high incidence in South Africa and Southeast Asia.

Sex. Hepatic cell carcinoma is much commoner in men. No sex difference has been noted with cholangiocarcinoma.

Cirrhosis. Cirrhosis of macronodular type is present in 60 – 80% of cases. In Western countries 5 – 10% of cirrhosis patients develop hepatic cancer, but in South Africa the figure is 60%. Cirrhosis is only rarely associated with cholangiocarcinoma.

Aflatoxins. These are the result of contamination of food, e.g. ground nuts and rice by *Aspergillus flavus*. In Africa the consumption of contaminated food parallels the incidence of hepatic carcinoma.

Hepatitis B surface antigen. There is an association between the presence of this antigen in patients with cirrhosis and the occurrence of hepatoma. The incidence is especially high in South Africa and Far Eastern patients.

The exact relationship between cirrhosis, aflatoxins, hepatitis antigen and hepatic carcinoma is not clear. It would appear that cirrhosis is not necessarily a direct cause of carcinoma but may act as a co-carcinogen.

Liver flukes. In the Far East cholangiocarcinoma is commonly associated with liver flukes in uncooked fish (clonorchis) and mutton (fasciola).

ANGIOSARCOMA

This rare tumour is associated with the use of Thorotrast in radiology, insecticides containing arsenic used in vine cultivation and industrial processes employing vinyl chloride. There is a long latent interval up to 29 years between exposure and tumour development.

HEPATOBLASTOMA

This rare tumour is found in infancy and childhood. It contains a mixture of malignant epithelial and mesenchymal elements. Cartilage, bone and haemopoietic tissue may develop. High plasma levels of alpha-fetoprotein are produced.

TUMOURS OF LIVER

PRIMARY BENIGN TUMOURS
Very few varieties recognised.

1. **Cavernous haemangioma.** This is the commonest type. It forms a dark purple, sharply demarcated geometrical patch on the liver surface. It has the usual structure of a cavernous angioma (see p. 190).

2. **Liver cell adenoma.** These small tumours are rare, but an increased incidence has been associated with the use of contraceptive steroids. They consist of normal liver trabeculae without normal portal tracts. Intraperitoneal bleeding may occur.

3. **Bile duct adenoma.** These small tumours are extremely rare. They consist of tiny bile duct structures set in loose connective tissue. Occasionally bile duct cystadenomas form large tumours.

SECONDARY

The liver is by far the most frequent site, of all organs, of secondary tumour deposits and they form the commonest type of liver tumour. Approximately 50% of all primary tumours in the portal area spread to the liver and 33% of all disseminated tumours, whatever the source, involve the liver. Apart from the gastrointestinal tract, the lung and breast are the most frequent sites of primary growth. Leukaemic infiltration is also common.

The appearance is often characteristic. The greyish white secondary deposits are usually at the periphery of the circulation underneath the liver capsule.

Umbilication, i.e. central depression due to necrosis and fibrosis (rare in primary tumours) is common.

Variations in appearance are produced by haemorrhage, necrosis and the type of tumour, e.g. mucus-secreting carcinomas.

The secondary tumours grow rapidly and are frequently the main cause of death. An exception are the secondary deposits from a carcinoid tumour which grow slowly over a period of years.

GALL BLADDER AND BILE DUCT — ANATOMY

Anatomy

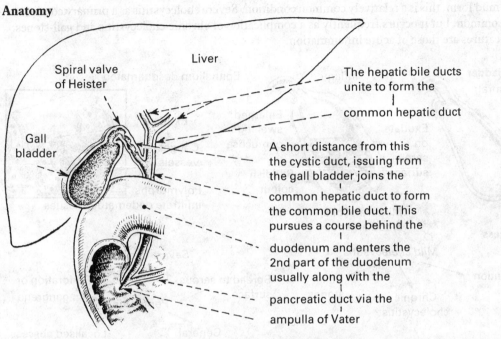

Liver

Spiral valve
of Heister

Gall
bladder

The hepatic bile ducts
unite to form the

common hepatic duct

A short distance from this
the cystic duct, issuing from
the gall bladder joins the

common hepatic duct to form
the common bile duct. This
pursues a course behind the

duodenum and enters the
2nd part of the duodenum
usually along with the

pancreatic duct via the

ampulla of Vater

The mucosa of the first part of the cystic duct is
corrugated to form the spiral valve of Heister.

Histology **Gall bladder**

The mucosa is lined by tall columnar
epithelium thrown into villous folds

Mucus-secreting glands are found
near the neck of the gall bladder

Longitudinal, circular
and oblique muscle bundles

Function

Bile is secreted continuously by the liver. The function of the gall bladder is to receive the overflow
of bile when it is not secreted into the duodenum. Overdistension is prevented by the ability of the
gall bladder to absorb water and electrolytes from the bile, up to 50% of the volume.

479

ACUTE CHOLECYSTITIS

In its mild form, this is a relatively common condition. Severe cholecystitis as a primary condition is uncommon, but it occurs frequently as a complication of chronic cholecystitis and gall-stones. The features are those of acute inflammation.

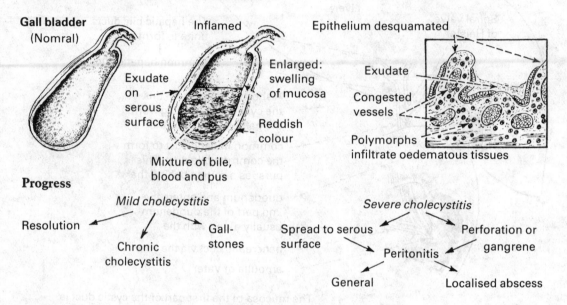

Gall bladder (Nomral)

Inflamed

Epithelium desquamated

Exudate on serous surface

Enlarged: swelling of mucosa

Reddish colour

Mixture of bile, blood and pus

Exudate

Congested vessels

Polymorphs infiltrate oedematous tissues

Progress

Mild cholecystitis

Resolution ← → Gall-stones

↓ Chronic cholecystitis

Severe cholecystitis

Spread to serous surface → Perforation or gangrene

Peritonitis

General   Localised abscess

Aetiology

1. The cause of primary acute cholecystitis is unknown.
2. Bacteria, usually streptococci and staphylococci, or enteric organisms have been isolated, but bacteria have also been isolated from normal gall bladder.
3. Most commonly acute cholecystitis follows occlusion, partial or complete, of the cystic duct by a gall-stone.

Secondary effects of cholecystitis

Inflammation upsets the function of the gall bladder and favours gall-stone formation.

Inflammation

Absorption of bile salts → Stasis of bile

Protein-rich exudate

Loss of detergent action

Lipids come out of solution

Precipitation of biliverdin

Precipitation of cholesterol

Gall-stone formation

CHRONIC CHOLECYSTITIS

Gall-stones are almost always present and this causes a variability in pathology. Two main variations occur:

1. Hypertrophic

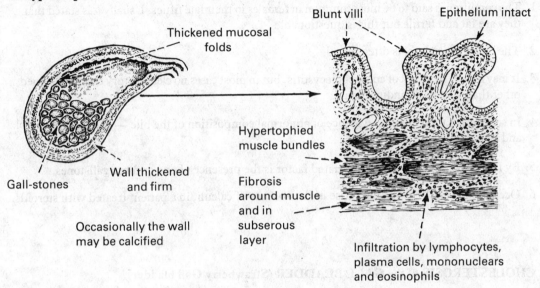

Thickened mucosal folds

Blunt villi

Epithelium intact

Hypertophied muscle bundles

Gall-stones

Wall thickened and firm

Fibrosis around muscle and in subserous layer

Occasionally the wall may be calcified

Infiltration by lymphocytes, plasma cells, mononuclears and eosinophils

2. Atrophic

This occurs when there has been long-standing obstruction of the cystic duct.

Stone blocking cystic duct

Villi tiny

Bile absent, clear, watery fluid distends sac (mucocele)

Mucosa flattened

Thin greyish wall

Inflammatory cells

Muscle almost absent: thin fibrous wall

Effects

1. Absorptive capacity of gall bladder greatly reduced. Bile is not concentrated and gall bladder is not visualised when radio-opaque substances are given.
2. Tendency to attacks of acute cholecystitis.
3. Further formation of gall-stones following exacerbations of inflammation.

CHRONIC CHOLECYSTITIS

Aetiology

The aetiology of chronic cholecystitis is inextricably associated with that of gall-stones.

1. The condition is said to be most common in females in their late fifties. Usually it is stated that they are fat and fertile but this is questionable.

2. The blood cholesterol is often raised.

3. It may follow an attack of acute cholecystitis, but in most cases no clear history can be obtained other than attacks of 'indigestion'.

4. In some cases there may be evidence of abnormal composition of the bile — excess cholesterol and lack of bile salts and lecithin.

5. By far the commonest single associated factor is the presence of one or more gallstones.

6. Occasionally cholecystitis may arise in the absence of calculi, in a patient treated with steroids.

CHOLESTEROSIS of the GALL BLADDER (Strawberry Gall bladder)

This occurs when the cholesterol content of the bile is high.

Yellow streaks and patches in mucosa

Occasional tiny polyp

Large mononuclear cells filled by cholesterol esters

The condition is most frequent in females in the 4th and 5th decades. It may be the only abnormality found in the gall bladder but is most commonly associated with the presence of a crystalline cholesterol stone. Cholecystitis frequently complicates the picture and therefore it is also found in chronic cholecystitis when the gall-bladder may contain mixed stones.

The cholesterol stone may form around protein during a mild attack of cholecystitis but it is thought that the tip of a tiny cholesterol-containing polyp may break loose and serve as the nidus around which precipitation can occur.

GALL-STONES

The mechanism of formation of gall-stones is not fully understood. Bile consists of bile acids, cholesterol and bile pigment, but it also contains mucin, phospholipids, soaps and fatty acids.

Bile acids, which are detergents and are key substances, have the following metabolic cycle.

Activities in bile

Solubility of cholesterol. A total pool of 2 – 4g of bile acids is required. Micelles soluble in water are formed:

<table>
<tr><td align="center">Cholesterol</td><td></td><td align="left">The ratio of cholesterol to</td></tr>
<tr><td align="center">+</td><td align="center">+</td><td align="left">phospholipids and bile acids is
important for keeping cholesterol</td></tr>
<tr><td align="center">Phospholipids</td><td align="center">Bile acids</td><td align="left">in solution.</td></tr>
</table>

Activities in intestine

As detergents the bile acids aid in the emulsification and absorption of lipids in the intestines.

483

GALL-STONES

In the formation of gall-stones, the concentration and solubilities of the various bile constituents are of primary importance.

Three primary types of stone exist:

1. **Cholesterol stone**

This is the commonest 'pure' stone. It is usually solitary, oval and up to 2 or 3 cm in length.

Radiating, glistening crystals of cholesterol.

Surface commonly slightly rough due to adhesion of cell debris

Often has tiny dark central deposit

Pale yellow 'soapy' feel.

Two mechanisms can operate in the formation of this stone:

(a) Excessive cholesterol, e.g. due to diet or metabolic disease such as diabetes. Treatment with 'cholesterol lowering' drugs, e.g. clofibrate, is associated with increased gall-stones.

(b) Reduction in concentration of bile salts in the bile.

2. **Bile pigment stones**

These are uncommon. They are always multiple and their presence is associated with excess concentration of pigment in the bile. This may occur in two ways:

(a) Chronic haemolysis

↓

Excessive biliverdin ⟶ excess bile pigment.
This is the mechanism when the stones are of primary type.

(b) Inflammation of gall-bladder.

Resorption of fluid ⟶ bile concentrated.
In this condition the stones are secondary to the inflammation.

 Rarely more than 1 cm in diameter, black and irregular.

3. **Calcium carbonate stones**

These are rare. They are small, greyish white and crumbling. Sometimes the gall-bladder is filled with a paste of calcium carbonate containing the stones. It has been suggested that they are associated with changes in bile pH.

GALL-STONES

Mixed stones

These account for 80% of all cases of gall-stones. Always multiple, they are irregular in shape but faceted due to contact with each other.

On section they have a laminated structure and the external colour depends on the last layer applied — cholesterol, bile pigment or calcium salts.

Frequently the gall bladder is filled with tightly packed stones. Their varying size indicates formation at different times. Often there is a much larger pure cholesterol stone present — obviously pre-dating the mixed stones.

Varying size

Single pure cholesterol stone, often impacted in the gall bladder neck

Gall bladder is usually thickened and shows chronic inflammatory changes

Whether chronic cholecystitis is a primary cause of mixed stone formation is not proved but it is an obvious factor in continuing stone formation.

Aetiological factors in stone formation

1. *Diet.* Gall-stones are common in developed countries due to diets rich in cholesterol. The highest incidence is found in North American Indians.

2. *Age.* Stones are almost confined to adult life.

3. *Sex.* It is customary to state that gall-stones occur in women who are fair, fat, forty and parous, but this is certainly wrong. Most gall-stones are discovered accidentally and appear to have little relation to sex or build. It may be that in some female patients parity is coincidentally associated with obesity and increased blood cholesterol which may add a tendency to stone formation.

4. *Cholecystitis.* There is little evidence to suggest that infection is a primary cause of gall-stones but, following formation of a stone, impaction in the gall bladder neck can encourage retrograde infection. This alters the solubility mechanisms and various substances precipitate, forming stones.

5. *Metabolic diseases.* Diabetes is associated with a high blood cholesterol and gall-stones are said to be relatively common.

6. *Haemolytic disease.* This is associated with pigment stone formation.

GALL-STONES

Clinical manifestations and complications

1. Many patients with gall-stones have no associated symptoms, and many more merely have mild dyspepsia.
2. *Impaction* This is common with single cholesterol stones. The stone impacts in the pouch of Hartmann at the neck of the gall bladder. The result depends on whether the blockage is complete or incomplete and intermittent.

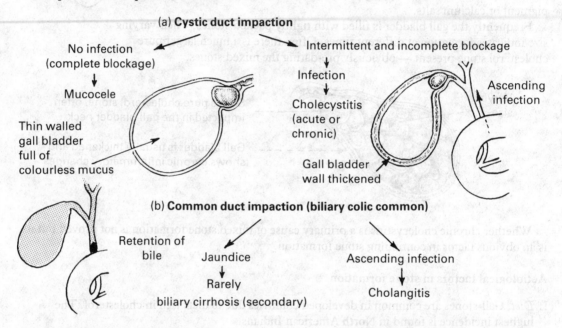

(a) **Cystic duct impaction**

No infection (complete blockage)

↓

Mucocele

Thin walled gall bladder full of colourless mucus

Intermittent and incomplete blockage

↓

Infection

↓

Cholecystitis (acute or chronic)

Ascending infection

Gall bladder wall thickened

(b) **Common duct impaction (biliary colic common)**

Retention of bile

Jaundice

↓

Rarely

biliary cirrhosis (secondary)

Ascending infection

↓

Cholangitis

3. *Fistulous Communications*. A stone may ulcerate through the gall bladder into intestine and cause obstruction.

(a) Duodenum: Contracted, inflamed gall bladder
Large barrel shaped stone
Duodenum drawn up by
inflammatory fibrosis

Wall thick and irregular

(b) Colon: In this case, inflammatory adhesions are formed between the gall bladder and the colon, and the stone ulcerates through.

Impaction of Ileum

↓

Intestinal obstruction

4. *Carcinoma of the gall bladder*. This is uncommon.
Very rarely the carcinoma arises in the common bile duct.

TUMOURS OF BILIARY TRACT

Simple tumours are exceedingly rare. Fibromas, lipomas and papillomas have been described.

CARCINOMA

This is a relatively rare tumour.

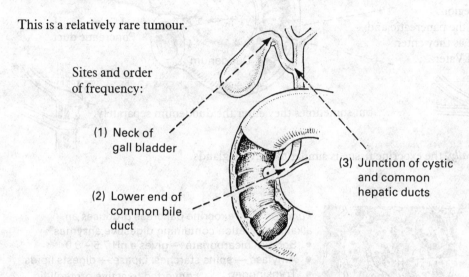

Sites and order of frequency:

(1) Neck of gall bladder

(2) Lower end of common bile duct

(3) Junction of cystic and common hepatic ducts

The tumour is usually a slowly growing adenocarcinoma. Invasion of the liver and distant metastases occur. In the case of the gall bladder, 80% of cases of carcinoma are associated with gall-stones, but only 2% or less of patients with gall-stones develop carcinoma.

THE EXOCRINE PANCREAS

This is the racemose glandular portion of the pancreas producing its digestive secretion which is delivered to the second part of the duodenum.

Anatomical variations occur in this region.

Commonly the pancreatic and bile ducts fuse as they enter the ampulla of Vater ....

Bile duct

Pancreas

Pancreatic duct

Duodenum

....but sometimes they enter the duodenum separately.

Microscopically, the exocrine tissue is similar to salivary glands.

In addition, foci of endocrine islet tissue occur throughout the pancreas

Function: The exocrine pancreas produces an alkaline secretion containing digestive enzymes.
- Sodium bicarbonate — gives a pH 7.5 – 8.0
- Amylase — splits starches. Lipase — digests lipids.
- Trypsinogen ⎫ converted to active proteolytic
- Chymotrypsin ⎭ enzymes, trypsin, chymotrypsin.

The islet tissue produces insulin and glucagon.

Exocrine secretory granules

An understanding of the microcirculation is important.
The gland has a lobular structure.
The larger arteries, veins and ducts course in the fibrous septa between the *lobules.*

This diagram shows the circulation and duct system within the lobule (*intra*lobular).

This watershed zone at the *periphery* of the lobule is susceptible when there is a circulatory perfusion deficit

Interlobular artery, vein and duct

A   V   D

This zone at the centre of the lobule is susceptible if there is damage to the intralobular duct

PANCREAS

CONTROL of EXOCRINE SECRETION

The secretory activity of the pancreas is monitored by the upper intestinal digestive activities and their products.

Bile Salts
Stimulate secretion
of enzymes plus
bicarbonate

Acid — Stimulates secretion
of bicarbonate

Products of protein digestion
Stimulate enzyme secretion only

Products of fat digestion
Stimulate both enzyme and
bicarbonate secretion.

These effects are largely mediated through three hormones produced in the intestine — secretin, pancreozymin and cholecystokinin.

Defective secretion

This may be brought about by:

(a) Permanent destruction of pancreatic tissue as in chronic pancreatitis

(b) Disease of intestine preventing formation of stimulatory hormones.

Insufficiency of exocrine secretion is uncommon. It produces maldigestion and leads to secondary changes in all other processes related to assimilation of food, e.g.

1. *Hyperphagia* which overloads digestive capacity thus exacerbating other effects

2. *Gastric hypersecretion.* Normally inhibition of gastric secretion is produced by digestive products in the intestine, especially fat. Maldigestion leads to absence of inhibition.

3. *Rapid emptying of stomach.* Lack of digestion leads to loss of the braking effect normally produced by duodenal contents. Acid and pepsin in large quantities reach the duodenum, destroying the enzymes and increasing the maldigestion.

4. *Steatorrhoea and bulky stools* due to maldigestion and lack of absorption of fats.

ACUTE PANCREATITIS

There is evidence that mild pancreatitis is not uncommon but, in a significant number of cases, progression to a severe fatal disease occurs. Clinically, there is an acute abdominal emergency with pain and shock.

The essential pathological changes are due to tissue necrosis caused by the action of liberated enzymes on the pancreatic tissues. The severity of the lesion depends on the amount of enzyme set free, the distance it diffuses and the structures affected. The pancreatic damage occurs in two forms:

1. **Periductal necrosis** — in the centre of each affected lobule.

2. **Perilobular necrosis** — affecting the periphery of lobules.

Damage to the epithelial lining of the duct allows diffusion of active enzymes into the adjacent tissues

Small areas of necrosis appear around the ducts of some of the lobules

This type is associated with gall-stones and alcohol.

Ischaemic necrosis occurs at the periphery of the lobules and is further complicated by liberation of enzymes

This type is associated with circulatory perfusion failure; severe shock; prolonged operations and hypothermia:

Both types of damage if not inhibited by antitrypsins and α_2 macroglobulins derived from the blood and pancreas itself will progress often very rapidly to the very severe form **PANLOBULAR PANCREATITIS.**

Veins thrombose

Vessels digested by enzymes. Diffuse haemorrhage results.

Diffuse necrosis

Surviving gland acini

Haemorrhage/ polymorph reaction

Thrombosed vessels

'Ghost' acini

The initial damage is severe, and large quantities of enzymes are liberated, including trypsin, chymotrypsin, lipase, elastase and phospholipase. Locally, these set up a progressive pathological process.

ACUTE PANCREATITIS

SEVERE PANCREATITIS (continued)

Damage to pancreas
↓
Release of enzymes
↓
Digestion of cell membranes

Necrosis of gland tissue   Necrosis of interstitial tissue
↓   ↓
Further release of enzymes   Thrombosis and necrosis of vessels

Extension of pancreatic damage

The released enzymes spread beyond the exocrine tissues of the pancreas:

1. *Vialymphatics to abdominal tissues* especially the omentum and mesenteries

Naked
eye
appearance

Opaque white patches of
necrotic fatty tissue — due to phospholipase
containing   and proteolytic
free   enzymes

fatty acids — lipase splits fat

2. *Locally causing destruction of islet tissue* — hyperglycaemic.

3. *Via blood stream.*

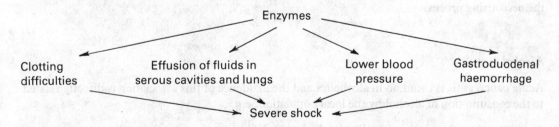

Enzymes

Clotting   Effusion of fluids in   Lower blood   Gastroduodenal
difficulties   serous cavities and lungs   pressure   haemorrhage

Severe shock

These effects are largely due to activation of thromboplastins and formation of vasoactive kinins. Hypoxia due to pulmonary oedema intensifies the shock.

Hypocalcaemia giving rise to tetany may occur due to deposition of calcium soaps in the necrotic fat cells of the omentum and peritoneum.

The appearance of amylase in the blood stream is used as a diagnostic test.

ACUTE PANCREATITIS

Aetiology

Two factors are important: (1) gall-stones and (2) alcohol.

Gall-stones

Between 50 and 60% of all cases of severe pancreatitis are associated with gall-stones. Recurrent attacks are common, and in a recent study of known gall-stone patients who developed pancreatitis, gall-stones were found in the biliary tree or stools of 80%.

Two mechanisms are postulated:

1. ***Bile reflux***
   In most patients, the bile duct and pancreatic duct have a common entrance to the ampulla of Vater. Stones passing down the bile duct could, by blocking the ampulla, cause reflux of bile along the pancreatic duct.

2. ***Bacterial infection***
   In all cases of gall-stone pancreatitis, chronic cholecystitis and cholangitis are present. Infection could spread from the bile ducts to the pancreas.

Bile and bacteria together activate the complement system which can cause cell lysis and initiate the necrotising process.

Alcohol

Acute pancreatitis is common in alcoholics and the incidence of this association is directly related to the consumption of alcohol by the local population, e.g.

> Scotland — up to 25%
> England — up to 17%
> U.S.A. — up to 70%

The causal relationship is obscure, but it is possible that in both gall-stone and alcoholic pancreatitis there is a common pathogenetic mechanism.

ACUTE PANCREATITIS

Inhibitors of pancreatic enzymes are produced by the liver — α_1 antitrypsin and α_2 macroglobulin. Large reserves are found in the normal liver. In the pancreas itself, a trypsin inhibitor is formed.

Fatty change in the liver is present in a high proportion of cases of acute pancreatitis.

Gall-stone cases — 25%

Alcohol cases — 60%

75% of all cases show hyperbilirubinaemia

It is possible that trivial damage may be followed by a necrotising chain reaction in the following way:

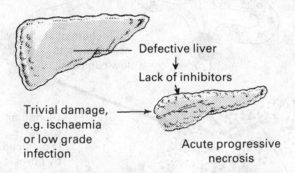

Pancreatitis has also been recorded in association with many other conditions, e.g. abdominal surgery, chronic renal failure, renal transplantation, cortisone therapy, cytotoxic therapy, mumps, hyperparathyroidism and familial hyperlipoproteinaemia.

Complications

1. With the frequent presence of cholangitis, the damaged pancreatic tissue is liable to be secondarily infected, and local suppuration is relatively common.

2. During the healing process, fibrosis may cause duct obstruction. Dilatation of the duct and cyst formation follow.

3. Recurrent attacks are common, and this may be one cause of chronic pancreatitis.

Prognosis

Death due to shock occurs in approximately 17% of cases of severe pancreatitis.

CHRONIC PANCREATITIS

The true incidence of this condition is unknown but from post mortem evidence it appears to be quite common. At least two types have been described, but the pathological changes are similar in all cases.

The process begins in the finer ductules and the associated acini

Protein rich plugs appear in the ductules

Ductule and acini become dilated behind the obstructing protein

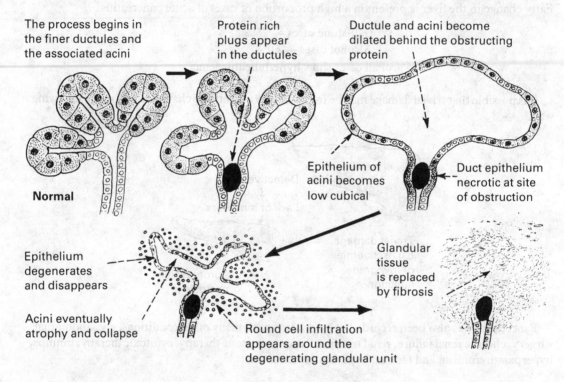

Normal

Epithelium of acini becomes low cubical

Duct epithelium necrotic at site of obstruction

Epithelium degenerates and disappears

Acini eventually atrophy and collapse

Round cell infiltration appears around the degenerating glandular unit

Glandular tissue is replaced by fibrosis

The change is focal. More and more protein plugs form, some in larger ducts. Obstruction of these may lead to production of cysts.

Ultimately, a large proportion of the exocrine tissue is destroyed.

Fibrosis with lymphocytic infiltrate

Cystic dilatation of ducts
Epithelial lining usually atrophic and incomplete

Small ducts, possibly reactive hyperplasia

This may mimic carcinoma in biopsy material

Eosinophilic protein plug in duct

Islet tissue usually survives and may appear to be increased

CHRONIC PANCREATITIS

With progress of the disease, two other developments take place:

1. *Calcification.* This occurs mainly in the protein plugs in the ducts, resulting in the formation of calculi.
2. *Rupture of the duct cysts into the surrounding tissues.* A granulation tissue reaction is set up with formation of a pseudocyst. The result depends on the site of the pseudocyst.

Rupture into the peritoneal cavity causes ascites, frequently haemorrhagic.

Progressive destruction of the parenchyma with fibrosis may ultimately convert the pancreas into a thin hard cord.

Effects

Apart from the complications due to cyst rupture, destruction of pancreatic tissue may lead to:

1. Insufficiency of exocrine secretion ⟶ steatorrhoea and wasting.
2. Diabetes mellitus. This is a rare complication due to destruction of islet tissue.

Aetiology

1. The main factor in 75% cases in Western civilisation is alcohol. Patients have generally consumed more than 150 g daily over a long period of time.

2. In 1% of cases there is biliary disease.

3. Some cases may follow recurrent attacks of acute pancreatitis.

4. A peculiar type of chronic pancreatitis occurs in Africa and Southeast Asia. It is related to chronic malnutrition with particular deficiency of protein, from infancy. Extensive calcification of the pancreatic tissues occurs. It has been suggested that there is a genetic predisposition to the disease.

CHRONIC PANCREATITIS

MUCOVISCIDOSIS (Cystic Fibrosis of the Pancreas)

This is a common autosomal recessive inherited disease due to three base deletions on chromosome 7; a high percentage (about 4%) of the population are carriers. All the exocrine secretory tissues are affected to a greater or lesser degree: the pathological results vary according to which organ is mainly affected — pancreas, bronchi, bowel or biliary tree.

The essential change is as follows:

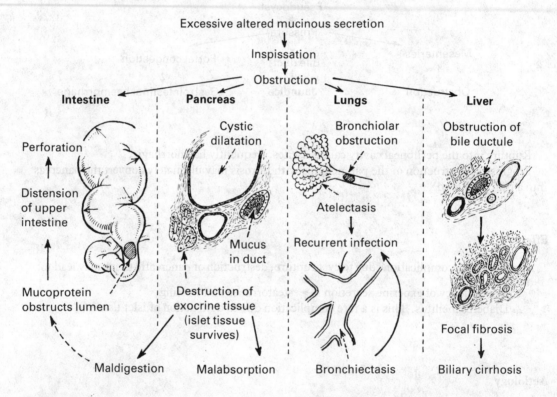

Clinical features

Neonatal

Intestinal obstruction (meconium ileus) may lead to intestinal perforation and fatal peritonitis.

Childhood:

There is failure to thrive due to maldigestion and malabsorption steatorrhea is common — all features of pancreatic insufficiency. If the lungs are affected, there is chronic respiratory difficulty with emphysema and bronchiectasis, usually proving fatal at an early age. Liver lesions are of late development.

There is increase of sodium chloride in the sweat of patients and their heterozygote siblings. This provides a diagnositc test.

TUMOURS OF PANCREAS

Simple tumours of the pancreas are very rare. Occasionally cystadenomas, lipomas and fibromas occur. They may produce symptoms due to pressure on other structures.

CARCINOMA

This is by no means rare, particularly in Western countries and Japan. It is the second commonest gastrointestinal cancer in the U.S.A.

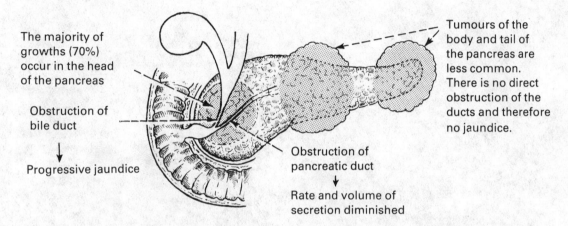

The majority of growths (70%) occur in the head of the pancreas

Obstruction of bile duct
↓
Progressive jaundice

Obstruction of pancreatic duct
↓
Rate and volume of secretion diminished

Tumours of the body and tail of the pancreas are less common. There is no direct obstruction of the ducts and therefore no jaundice.

Regional and/or distant metastases are found in 85% of cases at the time of diagnosis and the 5 year survival rate is 1% — the lowest of all cancers.

The growth arises from the duct epithelium and in almost all cases it is an adenocarcinoma. Papillary cystadenocarcinoma, adenosquamous carcinoma and giant cell carcinoma are forms occasionally encountered.

Tumours in the body and tail are commonly larger than tumours of the head, probably due to later diagnosis in the relative absence of symptoms. Thrombosis of unknown cause and at distant sites, e.g. femoral, is apt to occur when the tumour is in the body or tail.

Aetiology

1. Pancreatic carcinoma is most frequent in males in the 5th – 7th decades.
2. There is a statistical association with alcohol, cigarette smoking and a diet high in fat and carbohydrate.
3. In the U.S.A., the incidence is higher in the black population and a similar situation is true of the Maoris in New Zealand.

Endocrine Tumours

Islet cell tumours are decribed on page 840.

CHAPTER 12

HAEMOPOIETIC AND LYMPHO-RETICULAR TISSUES

HAEMOPOIESIS

The derivation of blood cells

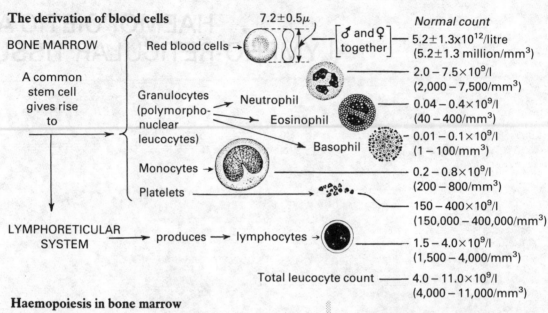

Normal count

BONE MARROW — Red blood cells →
$7.2\pm0.5\mu$

[♂ and ♀ together] — $5.2\pm1.3\times10^{12}$/litre
(5.2 ± 1.3 million/mm^3)

A common stem cell gives rise to

Granulocytes (polymorpho-nuclear leucocytes) → Neutrophil — $2.0-7.5\times10^9$/l
($2,000-7,500$/mm^3)

→ Eosinophil — $0.04-0.4\times10^9$/l
($40-400$/mm^3)

→ Basophil — $0.01-0.1\times10^9$/l
($1-100$/mm^3)

Monocytes → — $0.2-0.8\times10^9$/l
($200-800$/mm^3)

Platelets — $150-400\times10^9$/l
($150,000-400,000$/mm^3)

LYMPHORETICULAR SYSTEM → produces → lymphocytes → — $1.5-4.0\times10^9$/l
($1,500-4,000$/mm^3)

Total leucocyte count — $4.0-11.0\times10^9$/l
($4,000-11,000$/mm^3)

Haemopoiesis in bone marrow

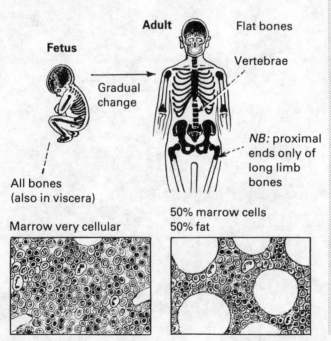

Fetus

Adult   Flat bones

Vertebrae

Gradual change

NB: proximal ends only of long limb bones

All bones (also in viscera)

Marrow very cellular

50% marrow cells
50% fat

When extra blood cells are required MARROW HYPERPLASIA occurs

Extension down long bones

Increased cellularity — obliteration of fat spaces

HAEMOPOIESIS

Mechanisms influencing the production of blood cells

They fall into 2 broad groups: (1) humoral factors and (2) nutrient factors.

Humoral factors with feedback controls

e.g. (a) Erythropoietin stimulates RBC production.

(b) Granulopoiesis is stimulated by crude bacterial and tissue extracts.

Haemopoiesis is also influenced in a non-specific way by hormones, e.g. thyroid deficiency causes anaemia.

Nutrient factors

These are important and some, e.g. vit. B_{12}, folic acid and iron, have a specific effect.

Most blood diseases are conveniently considered under three headings:

1. Increased numbers of cells, e.g. polycythaemia (RBCs)
   leucocytosis and leukaemia (leucocytes)
   thrombocytosis (platelets)

2. Decreased numbers of cells, e.g. anaemia (RBCs)
   leucopenia (leucocytes)
   thrombocytopenia (platelets)
   pancytopenia (all 3 elements)

3. Dysfunction — may occur alone or as a complication of (1) or (2) above.

DISEASES OF THE RED BLOOD CELLS

Diseases of the red cells are reflected in changes in the composition of the blood. The following measurements are useful and provide values of reasonable accuracy:

1. **HAEMOGLOBIN (Hb) concentration**
   Expressed as g/dl whole blood.

   (Normal values: male — 155±25; female — 140±25)

2. **PACKED CELL VOLUME (PCV)**
   PCV is obtained by centrifugating anticoagulated whole blood in a haematocrit tube.

PCV = 0.45 l/l (45%)

Normal ranges:
male — 0.47±0.07 l/l
female — 0.42±0.05 l/l

3. **Red cell count**

   Particle counting machines give reliable measurement

   (Normal values: male — $5.5±1.0×10^{12}$/l; female — $4.8±1.0×10^{12}$/l.)

   From these basic results the ABSOLUTE VALUES may be calculated.

A. *MEAN CELL HAEMOGLOBIN CONCENTRATION (MCHC)*

$$\text{Calculation:} \quad \frac{Hb}{PCV} \quad \text{e.g.} \quad \frac{15}{0.45} = 330\text{g/l (33\%) Range}±20$$

A low MCHC is due to a low average Hb content in the red cell mass and indicates deficient Hb synthesis.

e.g. Blood
film

Pale red cells (hypochromic) associated with low MCHC

High MCHCs do not occur in red cell disorders because the haemoglobin concentration is already near saturation point in normal red cells.

Note that because the MCHC is obtained by easy calculation from two simple and accurate measurements — the PACKED CELL VOLUME and the HAEMOGLOBIN — it is extremely useful and widely employed where sophisticated instrumentation is not available.

DISEASES OF THE RED BLOOD CELLS

B. *MEAN CELL HAEMOGLOBIN (MCH)*

This is the average haemoglobin content of each red cell and is measured in pg (picograms).

Calculation: $\dfrac{\text{Blood haemoglobin (g/dl)}}{\text{Red cell count } (10^{12}/l)}$ Normal range = 29.5±2.5pg

C. *MEAN CELL VOLUME (MCV)*
Measured in fl (femtolitres).

Calculation: $\dfrac{\text{Volume of red cells}}{\text{Number of red cells}}$ Normal range = 85±8 fl

Note: The accuracy of B and C depends on the availability of modern instruments. Where manual methods only are available the MCHC is important.

In addition to changes in the absolute values, valuable information is obtained by examination of blood films stained by a Romanowski method.

Normal blood film (dry)

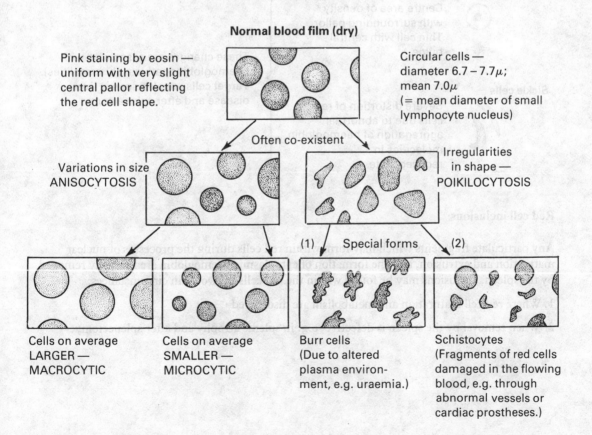

Pink staining by eosin — uniform with very slight central pallor reflecting the red cell shape.

Circular cells — diameter 6.7 – 7.7μ; mean 7.0μ (= mean diameter of small lymphocyte nucleus)

Often co-existent

Variations in size ANISOCYTOSIS

Irregularities in shape — POIKILOCYTOSIS

(1)   Special forms   (2)

Cells on average LARGER — MACROCYTIC

Cells on average SMALLER — MICROCYTIC

Burr cells (Due to altered plasma environment, e.g. uraemia.)

Schistocytes (Fragments of red cells damaged in the flowing blood, e.g. through abnormal vessels or cardiac prostheses.)

503

DISEASES OF THE RED BLOOD CELLS

Variations in colour (staining)

The haemoglobin content is reflected in the red cell staining.

Normal   *Hypochromic*

Ring staining of cells
indicates poor haemoglobinisation.

Other pathological variations are:

Spherocytes

Small dense red cells
reflect the cell shape.
Loss of biconcavity.

These changes are due to cell membrane
abnormalities which may be
congenital or acquired. The cells
show increased fragility in hypotonic
saline.

Target cells

Centre area of density
with surrounding pallor.
Thin cell with central
bulge.

Sickle cells

Severe distortion of red
cells due to abnormal
aggregation of haemoglobin
molecules in
reduced state.

These changes are associated with
haemoglobinopathies (abnormalities).
Target cells are also seen in liver
disease and after splenectomy.

Red cell inclusions

Any particulate fragments which may form within red cells during the processes of nuclear
maturation and extrusion, and the formation of cytoplasmic haemoglobin are normally removed
by the spleen. Inclusions may be found within the red cells in two main circumstances:

1. Where red cell maturation and metabolism are disordered

2. When removal by the spleen is defective, e.g. in splenic atrophy and after splenectomy.

DISEASES OF THE RED BLOOD CELLS

Red cell inclusions (continued)

	Appearance	Staining method	Occurrence
Howell-Jolly bodies Fragments of nuclear chromatin $1 - 2\mu$		Romanowski (eosin-methylene blue)	In anaemias — esp. macrocytic types
Pappenheimer bodies Small fragments containing iron		Prussian blue stain for iron	Especially after splenectomy
Heinz bodies Refractile crystalline bodies — denatured globin		Supravital staining, e.g. brilliant cresyl blue	Esp. associated with chemical poisons
Punctate basophilia Small particles of RNA		Romanowski (eosin-methylene blue)	In various anaemias, esp. lead poisoning

Nucleated red cells (erythroblasts) in the peripheral blood

Normally nucleated red cells are not seen in the peripheral blood. They appear in many blood and marrow disorders.

Normoblasts (see p.507) are seen in several types of anaemia but especially when the marrow is actively responding to any demand for new red cells, e.g. after severe acute haemorrhage or haemolysis.

In seriously ill patients, the appearance of normoblasts in the peripheral blood is a grave prognostic sign preceding death by hours.

Megaloblasts (see. p.507) are seen especially in pernicious anaemia and folic acid deficiency.

The nucleated red cells are found with the leucocytes in the haematocrit.

Buffy coat smears are particularly useful for their detection.

100 — Plasma

50

0 — RBCs

Nucleated RBCs

Polymorph

Lymphocyte

Monocyte

DISEASES OF THE RED BLOOD CELLS

The **physical properties** of red cells change in some disorders. The osmotic fragility is altered when the cell shape is abnormal.

1. Decreased saline concentration

Cell takes in water, enlarges and bursts liberating haemoglobin, i.e. haemolysis.

Normal RBC (in normal 0.9% NaCl)

2. Increased saline concentration

Cell loses water and becomes wrinkled (crenated).

The initial shape of the red cell clearly will influence the amount of water it will take in before it bursts.

In the osmotic fragility test, the lysis of RBCs in varying concentrations of saline is assessed by measuring the haemoglobin liberated. The graph shows typical results.

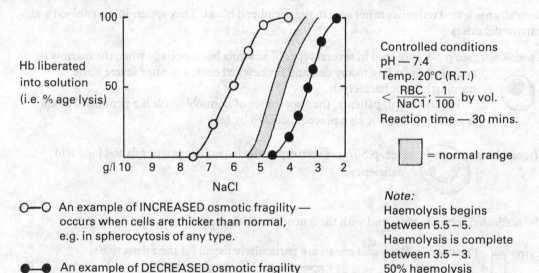

Hb liberated into solution (i.e. % age lysis)

g/l 10 9 8 7 6 5 4 3 2

NaCl

Controlled conditions
pH — 7.4
Temp. 20°C (R.T.)
$< \dfrac{RBC}{NaC1} ; \dfrac{1}{100}$ by vol.
Reaction time — 30 mins.

= normal range

O—O An example of INCREASED osmotic fragility — occurs when cells are thicker than normal, e.g. in spherocytosis of any type.

●—● An example of DECREASED osmotic fragility occurs when cells are unusually thin, e.g. in thalassaemia: iron deficiency anaemia.

Note:
Haemolysis begins between 5.5 – 5.
Haemolysis is complete between 3.5 – 3.
50% haemolysis (i.e. medium corpuscular fragility MCF) at 4 – 4.45.

The fragility to mechanical and chemical damage (including changes in pH) also varies in red cell disorders.

DISEASES OF THE RED BLOOD CELLS

BONE MARROW

Erythropoiesis (production of red cells) takes place in the marrow of the flat bones and vertebrae. The process involves mitotic division along with differentiation and maturation from the primitive stem cell.

Normal marrow erythropoiesis is said to be NORMOBLASTIC.

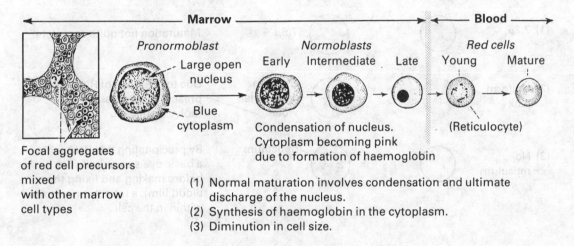

Focal aggregates of red cell precursors mixed with other marrow cell types

(1) Normal maturation involves condensation and ultimate discharge of the nucleus.
(2) Synthesis of haemoglobin in the cytoplasm.
(3) Diminution in cell size.

When the essential factors vit. B_{12} or folic acid are deficient, the red cell precursors show clear morphological changes — erythropoiesis is said to be MEGALOBLASTIC

Greatly increased marrow cellularity

(1) Nucleus remains loose and large.
(2) Haemoglobin synthesis proceeds normally.
(3) Cells remain very large, i.e. the nuclear/cytoplasmic maturation are out of phase.

Abnormal cells in peripheral blood

507

DISEASES OF THE RED BLOOD CELLS

Reticulocytes

These are the red cells very recently (within 2 days) released from the marrow and may be recognised by the following characteristics:

	Mature red cell	Reticulocyte		
(1) 7.2μ	◯	◯ 7.5μ		Maturation not quite complete.
(2) Uniform pink		Uniform light bluish violet		Due to presence of RNA still present in cytoplasm (polychromasia).
(3) No reticulum	◯	Reticulum		By precipitating this RNA with a basic dye supravitally (i.e. before making and fixing the blood film), a reticulum is formed within in the cell.

The reticulocyte count (normal range $0.2 - 2.0\%$, i.e. $25 - 85 \times 10^9/l$) gives an indication of erythropoiesis in the marrow. High counts are seen:

(a) in haemolytic disorders
(b) after severe haemorrhage
(c) when specific therapy is given in megaloblastic anaemias, e.g. vit B_{12} in pernicious anaemia.

Note. When the reticulocyte count is expressed as a percentage of the RBC count, the results may be misinterpreted when that count is low.

ANAEMIA

The most important function of the red cell is the transport of haemoglobin. The most common and important disorder associated with disease of the red cells is ANAEMIA, which is defined as a reduction below normal of the concentration of haemoglobin in the blood.

Normal Hb concentration: 150 g/l (range: men — 155±25; women — 140±25)

Effects of anaemia

Clinical associations

1. Diminished exercise tolerance, *i.e.* dyspnoea on exertion.

2. Rapid, full, bounding pulse: decreased circulation time.

Note: Pallor is not a reliable sign of anaemia — it may be obscured by the circulatory changes.

ANAEMIA

The effects of anaemia are greatly influenced by its severity, duration and rate of development.

In moderate anaemias of slow evolution, symptoms such as dyspnoea only appear on exertion, and even when the haemoglobin falls as low as 67 g/dl, clinical indications may be slight.

Pathological complications of anaemia

1. Effects of degenerative arterial disease are aggravated, e.g. symptoms of ANGINA PECTORIS and lower limb CLAUDICATION are increased.

2. In severe anaemias effects are seen in organs.

Hypoxia

Fatty change in **myocardium**

Fatty change in **liver**

Kidneys sensitive to hypoxia

Erythropoietin, production

Marrow hyperplasia

This change, along with circulatory compensatory changes, weakens the myocardium so that acute CARDIAC FAILURE is easily precipitated.

Note: Therefore blood transfusion used in the treatment of anaemia is given *slowly* and as *packed cells.*

In very rapidly developing anaemias, the compensatory mechanisms cannot adjust adequately — the condition merges into shock (see p. 145)

✓ANAEMIA

Aetiology

Although in the last analysis any anaemia is due to the failure of the bone marrow to produce sufficient red cells in any particular circumstance, an understanding of the role of various aetiological agents and of the four main mechanisms by which anaemia develops depends on a knowledge of the basic facts of the life cycle of the red blood cells.

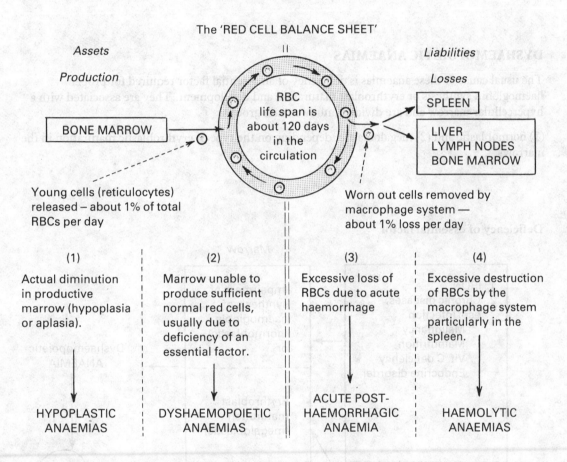

The 'RED CELL BALANCE SHEET'

Note: These are not rigidly exclusive compartments.

e.g. 1. The abnormal cells produced in the hypoplastic and dyshaemopoietic anaemias usually have a shortened life span so that a haemolytic element is superimposed.

2. The anaemia of chronic blood loss is almost wholly dyshaemopoietic in type due to the external loss of iron.

ANAEMIA ✓

HYPOPLASTIC and APLASTIC ANAEMIAS

These are rare conditions and, as the names imply, are due to marrow failure with diminished numbers or absence of haemopoietic cells. Usually all three marrow cell lines are affected, resulting in *pancytopenia* in the peripheral blood.

Marrow failure is dealt with in detail on page 557.

DYSHAEMOPOIETIC ANAEMIAS

The usual cause of these anaemias is deficiency of an essential factor required for proper haemoglobin synthesis or erythroblast maturation and development. They are associated with a hypercellular marrow and are divided into two main groups:

(1) normoblastic and (2) megaloblastic, depending on the type of erythroblastic maturation in the marrow.

Deficiency of essential factor

IRON DEFICIENCY ANAEMIA

Without IRON the haem moiety of the haemoglobin molecule cannot be synthesised.

IRON DEFICIENCY
↓
DEFECTIVE SYNTHESIS OF HAEMOGLOBIN
↓   (see p.517)
ANAEMIA

Haem - - - - →
(see. p.21)

Changes in the blood are mainly in the red cells which become:
MICROCYTIC (cells smaller – mean) diameter $< 6.7\mu$)
HYPOCHROMIC (contain less haemoglobin less well stained).

Normal

Fairly uniform red cells
— size and shape
(mean diameter 7.2μ)

Definite central pallor — ring staining
Variation in size — anisocytosis
Variation in shape — poikilocytosis

MCV (fl) (mean cell volume) is .... LOW (< 80)
MCH (pg) (mean cell haemoglobin) is .... LOW (< 25)
MCHC (mean corpuscular haemoglobin concentration) is .... LOW: 30%
    derived from Hb and haematocrit PCV: $\dfrac{Hb}{PCV} \times 100$. Normal mean = 34%
Serum IRON (normal 13-32 μmol/l) is .... LOW (<10)
Serum IRON BINDING CAPACITY (45-70 μmol/l) is .... RAISED (>70)
                          (2.5 – 4.0 mg/l)

Serum IRON SATURATION $\left(\dfrac{IRON}{Binding\ capacity \times 100} \right)$ (Normal 35%) is LOW (<15%)

The reticulocyte count is NORMAL except following episodes of haemorrhage.

Usually there are no changes in the leucocytes and platelets.

The bone marrow is hypercellular and contains many small poorly haemoglobinised
normoblasts; no stainable iron is present.

513

IRON DEFICIENCY ANAEMIA

IRON METABOLISM

Iron is normally conserved and is recycled so that absorption of iron from the diet, which occurs maximally in the duodenum and upper jejunum, is required to replace only the small inevitable losses. Since the diet contains iron in excess of requirements, the intestinal mucosal apoferritin mechanism exists to control absorption.

The iron (X) in the diet enters the mucosal cell and having combined with apoferritin (O) is retained in the cell as ferritin (⊗)
NB This bound iron is subsequently shed along with the cell into the lumen.

Iron unbound by apoferritin passes through the cell and is transported in the blood to join the iron recycling system.

Note: new haemoglobin formed in the bone marrow contains 95% iron from recycling system, 5% from diet.

The state of the iron stores controls the apoferritin (a form of intracellular transferrin) content of the intestinal mucosal cell by a feed-back mechanism, thus:

APOFERRITIN LOW
∴ Decreased binding (ferritin)
∴ *Increased absorption*

APOFERRITIN HIGH
∴ Increased binding
∴ *Decreased absorption*

ACUTE IRON OVERLOAD

If a large does of medicinal iron preparations is taken (particularly by children in error) the absorption and transport mechanisms are overwhelmed and free iron radicles exert very toxic effects.

IRON DEFICIENCY ANAEMIA

The *iron balance* may be summarised as follows.

INPUT (Adult male)	BODY IRON Total 3 — 6g	OUTPUT
Average: 1 mg/day derived from foods (a) animal muscle (b) vegetables The average diet contains 10 – 20 mg iron, of which about 10% is absorbed. In the adult female, the average daily input is about 2 mg.	(a) *Functional iron* in haemoglobin, myoglobin, enzyme systems, transferrin } 80% at least (b) *Storage iron* in liver, spleen, bone marrow as ferritin, haemosiderin } 20% or less	Average: 1 mg/day Skin desquamation and miscellaneous secretions *Menstruation* This extra loss of about 0.5 to 1 mg requires extra input in the female

Anaemia results when this delicate balance is upset in one of three main ways.

1. *Increased output* This almost always is caused by blood loss — often small in amount and chronic (1ml blood = 0.5 mg iron). In the female, uterine bleeding is a common cause, and in both sexes bleeding from the alimentary tract is important.
2. *Decreased input*
   (a) Poor diet (including diets containing substances antagonistic to iron absorption, e.g. phytates, phosphates)
   (b) Malabsorption — due to bowel disease or post-surgical.
3. *Increased body requirement*
   (a During rapid growth in childhood
   (b) In pregnancy.

Usually anaemia develops slowly (except in cases of serious haemorrhage).

(1) →	(2) →	(3) →	(4)
Iron deficiency	Mobilisation of reserves (first haemosiderin then ferritin)	Exhaustion of reserves Increased absorption if available in diet may postpone (4)	Deficient synthesis of haemoglobin ↓ (5) Anaemia

PREVALENCE of IRON DEFICIENCY ANAEMIA

This is the commonest anaemia on a world basis due to: (a) poor nutrition, (b) intestinal parasites (esp. hookworm) causing bleeding and (c) multiple pregnancies.

In Western countries in the adult male and postmenopausal woman, iron deficiency anaemia is nearly always due to alimentary blood loss and reflects the incidence of the causative diseases, e.g. cancer, peptic ulceration, hiatus hernia, aspirin ingestion, haemorrhoids, etc.

IRON DEFICIENCY ANAEMIA

Associated changes

In addition to the pathological changes due to anaemia per se, the following conditions may be associated with iron deficiency anaemia.

(1) *Angular cheilosis*
    Atrophic glossitis

(2) *Dysphagia* — the Brown-Kelly-Paterson or Plummer-Vinson syndrome

Fissures at angles of mouth

Smooth tongue

Incoordinate movements in pharynx

Sometimes actual web forms

Occasionally carcinoma is a late complication

(3)

Thin mucosa

Hypochlorhydra
↓
Achlorhydria

With gastritis and mucosal atrophy

This aggravates any malabsorption of iron

(4) *Koilonychia*

Brittle spoon-shaped nails

5. *Minimal changes in Peripheral nerves — causing Paraesthesia* (tingling in hands and feet)

These associated changes are in part due to iron deficiency itself, but in many cases are probably the result of deficiencies of other factors in addition, e.g. vitamins and minerals.

THE MEGALOBLASTIC ANAEMIAS

These dyshaemopoietic anaemias are almost always caused by deficiency of either vitamin B_{12} or folic acid which are intracellular co-enzymes, particularly important for the production of nuclear DNA.

The effects of deficiency occur in most organs of the body but are prominent where cell turnover is rapid, e.g. in the marrow.

Normal

Vit B_{12} and folic acid

Rapid DNA synthesis to double nuclear chromatin

↓

Mitosis

Normal daughter cells

Normal blood values

Deficiency

Synthesis of DNA slowed

Nucleus grows but remains 'young', open consistency, delicate chromatin pattern

Cytoplasm continues to grow

Cell division slow

Red cells diminished
Haemoglobin low

Results in organs particularly affected

1. MUCOUS MEMBRANES of alimentary tract and genitalia ⟶ Regenerative activity cannot balance surface losses ⟶ THINNING (atrophy) often with functional deficiencies

2. BONE MARROW ⟶ blood cell precursors of all series affected ⟶ No surface loss: cells not mature enough for release; although many are destroyed locally in the marrow the numbers of abnormal cells increase. ⟶ Hypercellular: megaloblastic

Note:

(a) Vit B_{12} (but not folic acid) has a separate function in the maintenance of the integrity of myelin. Therefore deficiency leads to neuropathies — particularly **subacute combined degeneration** (p. 521).

(b) The marrow and blood appearances are essentially similar in deficiency of vit B_{12} and folic acid from any cause. The classical disease of this type is **pernicious anaemia.**

PERNICIOUS ANAEMIA

This serious and severe anaemia was first described by the English physician Addison in the mid 19th century. At that time it was invariably fatal, but nowadays it can be treated with complete success. It is due to vitamin B_{12} deficiency and is always associated with achlorhydria and gastric mucosal atrophy.

Vitamin B_{12} metabolism and causes of deficiency:

	Deficiency of vitamin B_{12}	
Normal	**In PA**	**Other causes**
Source: Food — vit B_{12} in animal products, e.g. meat, eggs. Daily requirement = 1 μg	Normal	Dietary deficiency, e.g. strict vegans — takes many years to develop
Secretion of intrinsic factor (IF) by gastric mucosa IF: B_{12} complex formed	Gastric atrophy No IF ∴ No IF : B_{12} complex	Surgical operations on stomach
Passage through intestine to terminal ileum	Normal	Loss during passage in intestine, e.g. utilised by tape worms or bacteria (blind loop syndrome).
Absorption site — can only be absorbed if complexed with IF	No absorption	Disease of ileum, e.g. Crohn's disease.
Storage in liver — up to 10 years' supply	Gradual depletion of liver stores over several years	

Released into blood stream to act as important co-enzyme in several intracellular synthetic pathways but particularly of DNA

Especially important to:
(1) Bone marrow
(2) Nervous system
(3) Epithelial coverings

ANAEMIA (MEGALOBLASTIC)
±NERVE CHANGES
±TONGUE & VAGINA } ATROPHY

PERNICIOUS ANAEMIA

Blood changes

There is a pancytopenia, i.e. reduction in RBCs, granulocytes and platelets.

Normal   **RA**

RBCs
Macrocytic
Normochromic

Anisocytosis
Poikilocytosis

Special features

Seen specially in
buffy coat preparations.

Howell-Jolly bodies
(fragments of residual
nuclear material)

Large
hypersegmented
polymorph

Megaloblast

Absolute values

Red cell count ———— LOW (may be very low), e.g. 1.0×10^{12}/litre
Hb ———— LOW
PCV ———— LOW
MCV ———— HIGH, e.g. (average cell is larger than normal)
MCH ———— HIGH (average cell contains more Hb than normal)
MCHC ———— NORMAL (NB average cell contains normal Hb concentration)

Biochemical

Serum vit B_{12} —— LOW < 120 (normal>160 ng/l)
Serum bilirubin —— Slight increase — due to increased haemolysis of fragile cells.

PERNICIOUS ANAEMIA

Marrow changes

Hyperplasia — often complete cellularity in flat bones and extension down length of femur.

Normal   **In PA**

Total cellularity

Megaloblastic change

All marrow elements affected

The gastric lesion – The extreme form of diffuse atrophic gastritis (see p. 382).

Normal

In PA

Note:
Thin mucosa
No specialised cells
No IF and no HCl
(histamine-fast achlorhydria)

Muscle   Muscle

Parietal cells producing both IF and HCl

Increased numbers of lymphocytes in lamina propria

Mechanism of production of gastritis

PA is an autoimmune disease. The gastric atrophy is caused by an immune reaction against parietal cell cytoplasmic constituents and specifically by antibodies to intrinsic factor (IF).

(1) *Anti-parietal cell immune reaction* gradually causes complete mucosal atrophy including destruction of parietal cells.

(2) *Anti IF antibody* secreted in stomach lumen as well as blood. Specifically blocks any residual IF activity.
   (a) Receptor sites for B_{12} complex are blocked.
   (b) Receptor sites for ileal absorption are blocked.

IF

There is an increased familial incidence of PA and other autoimmune disease, e.g. Hashimoto's thyroiditis.

PERNICIOUS ANAEMIA

Associated changes

1. *Nervous system*
   (a) Subacute degeneration of spinal cord

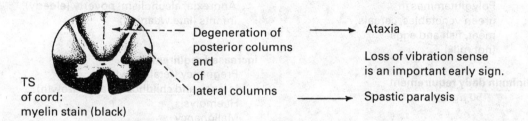

TS
of cord:
myelin stain (black)

Degeneration of
posterior columns
and
of
lateral columns

→ Ataxia

Loss of vibration sense
is an important early sign.

→ Spastic paralysis

NB This serious degeneration may occur before clinical anaemia is present, and is aggravated by the administration of folic acid.

(b) Peripheral neuropathy — both sensory and motor loss.

2. *Epithelial Surfaces*

Atrophy is common especially in the tongue and vagina — where senile atrophy is aggravated

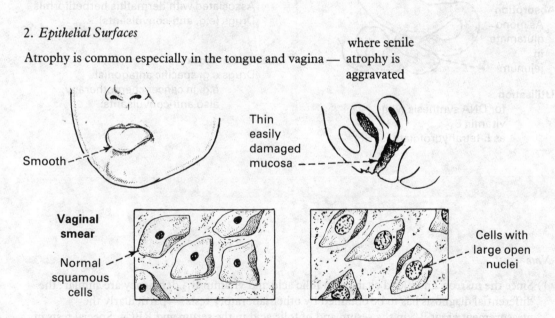

Smooth

Thin
easily
damaged
mucosa

**Vaginal
smear**

Normal
squamous
cells

Cells with
large open
nuclei

3. *Effects of long continued haemolysis*

   The abnormal cells have a shortened life cycle.
   (a) Mild/moderate splenic enlargement.
   (b) Iron deposition in liver, kidney, spleen and marrow.
   (c) Increased bilirubin in blood (mild jaundice).

FOLIC ACID DEFICIENCY

FOLIC ACID (Pteroyl-glutamic acid) DEFICIENCY

Normal metabolism	Deficiency

Source

Polyglutamines in
green vegetables, cereals,
meat, fish and eggs
(not milk)

Dietary

Anorexia, alcoholism, poverty (elderly),
infants (late weaning)

Increased requirements

Pregnancy (fetal growth)
Infancy and childhood (rapid growth)
Haemolysis
Malignancy

Minimun daily requirement

50 μg

Body reserves   50 – 100 days

Absorption

As mono–
glutamate
in
jejunum

Utilisation

for DNA synthesis with
vitamin B_{12}
as 5-tetrahydrofolate (5THF)

Malabsorption

Coeliac disease: sprue
Surgical by-pass
Associated with dermatitis herpetiformis
Drugs (e.g. anti-convulsants)

Utilisation block

Drugs e.g. specific antagonists
e.g. in cancer chemotherapy,
also anti-convulsants.

Note

(1) Since the marrow and blood changes in folic acid and vitamin B_{12} deficiency are similar, the differential diagnosis has to be obtained by other laboratory tests — particularly the measurement of vit B_{12} in the serum and of folic acid in the serum and RBCs. Special tests of absorption of vit B_{12} (e.g. Schilling test) are available.

(2) Since the causes of vit B_{12} and folic acid deficiency are often non-specific and associated with malabsorption, other deficiencies (e.g. iron) may also occur at the same time (see p. 545)

(3) All megaloblastic anaemias are macrocytic, but *not all* macrocytic anaemias are megaloblastic.

ACUTE POST-HAEMORRHAGIC ANAEMIA

ACUTE POSTHAEMORRHAGIC ANAEMIA

The effects of severe acute haemorrhage are considered under two main headings:

1. The adaptive haemodynamic changes which are usually at least partly successful in maintaining perfusion of vital organs — see section on SHOCK (p.147).

2. The changes reflecting the body's reactions to restore the blood constituents.

The rate and volume of the blood loss are important influences on both types of effect.
For example — in a young healthy adult male (assume blood volume = 5000 ml) :

Blood loss		Duration of loss	Effects	
ml	%vol.			
500 e.g. Blood donation	10%	15 min	Nil or negligible	
1700	33%	3 hrs	Shock ↓ usually survival	**Aggravating factors** (a) pre-existing cardiac or debilitating disease
2500	50%	3 hrs	Severe shock ↓ usually death	(b) old age
2500	50%	36 hrs	Shock ↓ usually survival	(c) anxiety associated with vasovagal stimulation — especially if haemorrhage is external and visible

While the bleeding is continuing, the shock syndrome is predominant, and although the marrow begins to react to the anoxia, the full haematological effects — particularly the ANAEMIA — are not seen until the haemorrhage is controlled or stops and the plasma volume begins to be restored.

ACUTE POST-HAEMORRHAGIC ANAEMIA

In the following example the effects of a severe haemorrhage — 2500 ml (50%) in 36 hours — in a healthy young adult male are seen. It is assumed that blood transfusion has not been given — a rare circumstance nowadays.

During the bleeding phase

100 %

45

0

Haematocrit normal —— not anaemic
RBCs normocytic
normochromic

Platelets ↑
e.g. 500 –
1,000×10⁹/l.

Neutrophils ↑
e.g.
15 – 20+10⁹/l.

Peak at 3 – 4 days:
return to normal   5 – 7 days

After bleeding

Restoration of plasma volume by fluid ingestion
↓   (1 – 2 days)

Dilution of remaining RBCs

100 %

22

Haematocrit low —— ANAEMIA at fist
normocytic normochromic...

Blood film

...later slighty macrocytic due to reticulocytes (MCV up to 105 fl)

May be scanty normoblasts

RETICULOCYTES 15 – 20%
Peak 7 – 10 days

Erythropoietin

Mobilisation of iron stores (plasma iron low)

BONE MARROW

Erythropoiesis increased

The plasma proteins and other biochemical constituents are restored rapidly — 2 – 3 days. The full red cell restoration may take up to 6 weeks.

Note: With recurrent less severe haemorrhages the picture merges into that of **iron deficiency anaemia.**

THE HAEMOLYTIC ANAEMIAS

HAEMOLYTIC ANAEMIAS

In all haemolytic anaemias, the basic pathological change is a reduction in the life span of the red cells; another way of expressing this is that there is an increased rate of red cell destruction — haemolysis.

The balance between the increased haemolysis and the consequent increased production of red cells by the bone marrow may be illustrated in three main situations:-

1. Shortened red cell life span — e.g. 1/6 normal (20 days)   Marrow production increased × 6

       Balance maintained - - - - - ∴ - -> No anaemia (compensated erythropoiesis)

2. Shortened red cell life span — e.g. 1/12 normal (10 days)   Marrow production increased maximally × 8 to 10 normal

       Balance not maintained - - - - - ∴ - -> ANAEMIA

3. Shortened red cell life span —

     (a) e.g. 1/6 normal   (b) e.g. 1/12 normal   The hyperplastic marrow is susceptible to deficiency of essential factors; thus infections, pregnancy may limit the marrow response e.g. to × 3

     Compensated haemolysis   Haemolytic anaemia

     Precipitated into haemolytic anaemia   Serious aggravation (crisis)

THE HAEMOLYTIC ANAEMIAS

The pathological changes associated with haemolytic anaemia are conveniently considered under two main headings:

1. Associated with the shortened RBC life span (increased haemolysis).

2. The bone marrow reaction.

1. RBC LIFE SPAN

(1a) Measurement of red cell life span by radioactive sodium chromate

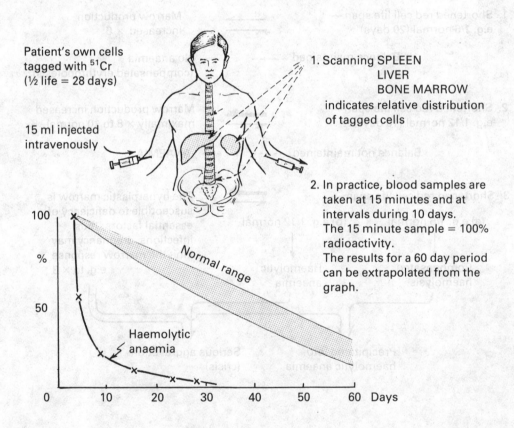

Patient's own cells tagged with ^{51}Cr (½ life = 28 days)

15 ml injected intravenously

1. Scanning SPLEEN
   LIVER
   BONE MARROW
   indicates relative distribution of tagged cells

2. In practice, blood samples are taken at 15 minutes and at intervals during 10 days.
   The 15 minute sample = 100% radioactivity.
   The results for a 60 day period can be extrapolated from the graph.

Normal range

Haemolytic anaemia

Note:

In *normal* curve, gradual loss of radioactivity 50% level at 30 days.
In *haemolytic* anaemia, rapid loss of radioactivity 50% at 3 days.

THE HAEMOLYTIC ANAEMIAS

(1b) Effects of the increased degradation of haemoglobin

In most haemolytic conditions, the red cells are removed and the haemoglobin degraded in the usual way, i.e. by phagocytosis by the macrophage system.

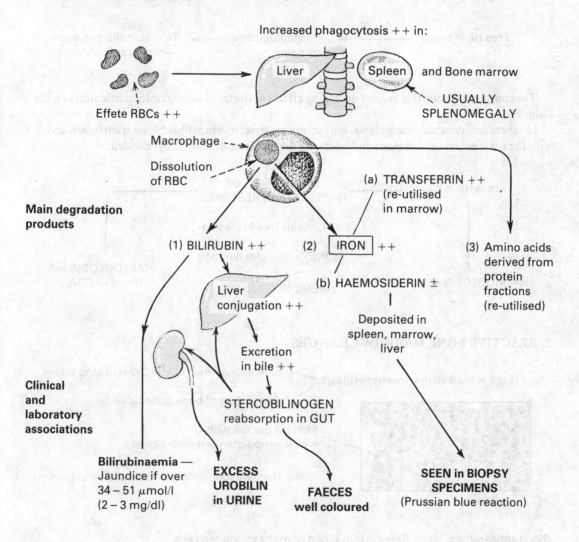

Increased phagocytosis ++ in:

Liver   Spleen   and Bone marrow

USUALLY SPLENOMEGALY

Effete RBCs ++

Macrophage

Dissolution of RBC

Main degradation products

(a) TRANSFERRIN ++ (re-utilised in marrow)

(1) BILIRUBIN ++   (2) IRON ++   (3) Amino acids derived from protein fractions (re-utilised)

(b) HAEMOSIDERIN ±

Liver conjugation ++

Deposited in spleen, marrow, liver

Excretion in bile ++

Clinical and laboratory associations

STERCOBILINOGEN reabsorption in GUT

Bilirubinaemia —
Jaundice if over
34 – 51 μmol/l
(2 – 3 mg/dl)

EXCESS UROBILIN in URINE

FAECES well coloured

SEEN in BIOPSY SPECIMENS (Prussian blue reaction)

Note: 1. The bilirubin is unconjugated and is attached to protein so that renal excretion does not occur — **acholuric jaundice.**

2. Unconjugated bilirubin is toxic to the central nervous system of neonates; **kernicterus** (see p. 535) is a serious complication of haemolytic disease of the newborn.

THE HAEMOLYTIC ANAEMIAS

(1c) Effects of liberation of haemoglobin

In all haemolytic processes, small amounts of haemoglobin are liberated into the blood stream. The free haemoglobin rapidly forms a complex with **haptoglobin** — an α globulin.

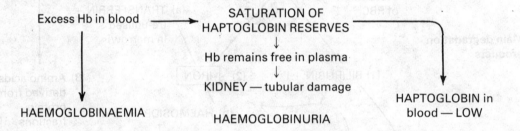

Free Hb in blood $\xrightarrow{\text{Rapid}}$ Hb/Haptoglobin complex $\longrightarrow$ To macrophage system — disposal as above.

The complex is protective against damaging effects of the free haemoglobin, particularly on the kidneys.

In severe intravascular haemolysis, e.g. severe malaria, incompatible blood transfusion and with the toxic action of chemicals and bacteria, the mechanism may be overloaded.

Excess Hb in blood $\longrightarrow$ SATURATION OF HAPTOGLOBIN RESERVES

↓

Hb remains free in plasma

↓

KIDNEY — tubular damage

HAEMOGLOBINAEMIA   HAEMOGLOBINURIA

HAPTOGLOBIN in blood — LOW

2. REACTIVE BONE MARROW CHANGES

There is marked marrow hyperplasia — Extension of RED MARROW into long bones

— Absorption of bone trabeculae

Marrow packed with well haemoglobinised normoblasts

±Haemosiderin depending on rate of iron utilisation

Blood appearances   Release into blood of many young red cells
20 – 30% RETICULOCYTES — occasional normoblasts.
Film — normocytic: may be mild macrocytosis due to young cells.
— normochromic: — may be polychromasia due to young cells.

The blood film may of course reflect the specific red cell abnormality responsible for the anaemia, e.g. spherocytosis.

INTRINSIC HAEMOLYTIC ANAEMIAS

The causes of shortened red cell survival are divided into two main groups:
(1) INTRINSIC (defects of the red cells) and (2) EXTRINSIC (factors outside the red cells).

INTRINSIC DEFECTS —— Usually hereditary.

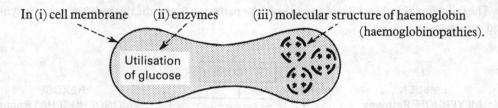

In (i) cell membrane   (ii) enzymes   (iii) molecular structure of haemoglobin
(haemoglobinopathies).

Utilisation
of glucose

(a) Cell membrane defects

1. *Hereditary spherocytosis:* the majority of cases are familial (autosomal dominant).

Na+	Na+		Spleen

The primary defect
allows excessive
permeability of Na+

This is followed
by increased
glycolysis to
maintain the
sodium pump

Membrane
weakened by
secondary loss
of intrinsic lipid
Cell becomes
spheroidal

Premature sequestration
in splenic pulp
Splenomegaly is a
constant association

The severity of the haemolysis is variable; many cases are compensated and not anaemic, but crises are common. Intercurrent infections may precipitate increased red cell destruction with jaundice or temporary bone marrow hypoplasia with severe anaemia.

The laboratory diagnosis depends on:
(1) typical blood film with spherocytes,
(2) high reticulocyte count and
(3) increased osmotic fragility of RBCs.

2. *Hereditary elliptocytosis* is similar to spherocytosis in many respects, but it is usually not severe enough to cause anaemia or jaundice.

3. *Hereditary abetalipoproteinaemia:* a rare disease in which the red cell membranes are abnormal and the cells become spiky (acanthocytes).

4. *Paroxysmal nocturnal haemoglobinuria* — a rare, acquired condition in which the red cell membrane is particularly susceptible to the action of complement (usually activated by the alternative pathway) at low pH.

529

INTRINSIC HAEMOLYTIC ANAEMIAS

INTRINSIC DEFECTS of the RED CELLS (continued)

(b) **Enzyme defects**

Usually hereditary. Glucose is the source of energy with which the red cell metabolism is maintained. Glycolysis is effected by two classical enzyme pathways.

The following simplified diagram outlines the pathways and indicates only the main enzymes and substrates.

G-6PD deficiency shows X-linked inheritance so that in the male the defect is fully expressed, while in the female heterozygote there are two populations of red cells in the blood (1) normal cells and (2) defective cells.

In both these defects and in the rare defects of other enzymes in the pathways which have been described the expression of the abnormal gene is very variable from case to case.

INTRINSIC HAEMOLYTIC ANAEMIAS

INTRINSIC DEFECTS of the RED CELLS (continued)

(c) Haemoglobinopathies

In these hereditary disorders, the molecular structure of haemoglobin is abnormal.

Normal haemoglobin molecule: 4 subunits each consisting of a haem core with a polypeptide chain attached. The haem core is constant while the polypeptide chains occur in pairs.
4 different polypeptide chains occur normally.

▮ α chain	▦ γ chain
▯ ß chain	▨ δ chain

Mol. wt.=68,000

There are 3 types of normal haemoglobin.

97% adult Hb —— Haemoglobin A = 2 α + 2ß chains

3% adult Hb —— Haemoglobin A$_2$ = 2 α + 2δ chains

Fetal Hb —— Haemoglobin F = 2 α + 2γ chains

Fetal haemoglobin is replaced by adult haemoglobin during the first year. Note that the chain occurs in all normal haemoglobins.

531

INTRINSIC HAEMOLYTIC ANAEMIAS

Very many abnormal haemoglobins have now been described. Only a few have serious consequences.

Abnormal haemoglobins may be formed in two ways:

(1) Due to variation in the amino acid content and sequence of one of the chain pairs.

e.g.

Haemoglobin-S
ß chains are abnormal —
SICKLE CELL DISEASE results

(2) By a slowing or failure to synthesise

α *chains*   or   ß *chains*

This leads to an excess of ß chains which form a tetramer called Hb-H.

This leads to an excess of α chains.

These do *not* form tetramers. ∴ No abnormal Hb formed.

The deficiency of Hb A is compensated for by an increase in Hb A_2 and F.

The disease is designated

This disease is termed
α -*THALASSAEMIA*

↓
ß-*THALASSAEMIA*

Sickle cell disease

Hb-S molecules stack abnormally and cause sickling in reduced O_2 state — serious haemolysis.

Sickle cell trait — heterozygote — symptoms mild but trait can be detected by in vitro sickling using a reducing agent or electrophoresis of Hb.

NB: malaria resistant.

Thalassaemia

Major — homozygous.

Serious haemolytic anaemia; 'target cells'; increased osmotic resistance.

Minor — heterozygous — presents as hypochromic microcytic anaemia.

Note. The anaemias resulting from the haemoglobinopathies are usually at the same time *both* dyshaemopoietic and haemolytic in type.

EXTRINSIC HAEMOLYTIC ANAEMIAS

In extrinsic haemolytic anaemias, the premature destruction of red cells is caused by agencies arising outside the cells. They are usually acquired and may be idiopathic (i.e. with no known cause) or secondary to some other disorder (i.e. symptomatic).

They will be considered in five main groups:

1. ANTIBODIES to RBCs
2. INFECTIONS
3. DRUGS and poisonous chemicals
4. TRAUMATIC DAMAGE to RBCs
5. MISCELLANEOUS

(1a) DESTRUCTION of RBCs due to ISO-ANTIBODIES

In these, the antibodies act against antigens which are derived from another individual of the same species.

Incompatible ABO blood transfusion is a classical example.

e.g. **Donor Blood**

   Group A
   i.e. cells contain
   A antigen

Recipient

Group O (cells contain neither A or B antigen)
Plasma contains *Anti-A* (iso-antibody) (and Anti-B)

Agglutination

Haemolysis

Clinical and pathological effects

Rigor: loin pain
Haemoglobinuria
Jaundice (after 12 hours)
SHOCK → maybe DEATH

Perhaps later :
Haemostatic failure → maybe DEATH
Renal failure

Notes

(a) The severity of the effects is influenced by (1) the transfusion rate and (2) the strength (titre) of the antibody.

(b) Only rarely does incompatible donor plasma destroy the recipient red cells because the plasma antibodies are rapidly diluted in the recipient circulation.

EXTRINSIC HAEMOLYTIC ANAEMIAS ✓

DESTRUCTION of RBCs due to ISO-ANTIBODIES (continued)

Incompatibilities within the Rh blood group systems cause haemolytic disorders in two main circumstances: (a) Incompatible blood transfusion and (b) haemolytic disease of the newborn.

1. **Blood transfusion**

Donor
Rh-positive (i.e. RBCs contain Rh antigen)

Recipient (<u>not</u> previously transfused or pregnant)
Rh-negative (i.e. RBCs do not contain Rh antigen)
Plasma contains **no Rh antibodies**
∴ **No agglutination**.

To macrophage system for degradation in usual way but NB Rh-positive cells act as foreign antigens.

Later (months, years)
Transfusion of Rh-positive blood

Formation of ***anti-Rh antibodies*** stimulated.

Agglutination and haemolysis } → Effects as in ABO incompatibility

Note: In Rh-negative males anti/Rh antibodies can only be stimulated by the parental injection of Rh-positive blood. In Rh-negative females pregnancy with an Rh-positive fetus is an additional and more common mechanism.

2. **Haemolytic disease of the newborn (HDN).** This occurs in Rh-positive fetuses conceived by Rh-negative mothers. The usual mechanism is as follows:
   First pregnancy: Rh-positive fetus in Rh-negative mother — no antibodies present;
   ∴ *Healthy Baby*
   But during this pregnancy, iso-immunisation of the mother may occur.
   Towards term and particularly during labour the placental barrier is breached and fetal RBCs enter the maternal circulation.

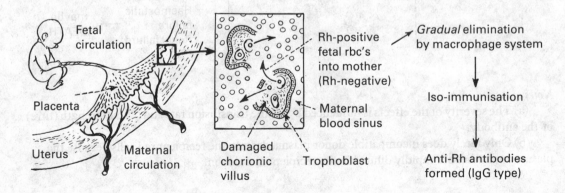

Fetal circulation

Placenta

Uterus

Maternal circulation

Damaged chorionic villus

Trophoblast

Rh-positive fetal rbc's into mother (Rh-negative)

Maternal blood sinus

Gradual elimination by macrophage system

Iso-immunisation

Anti-Rh antibodies formed (IgG type)

534

EXTRINSIC HAEMOLYTIC ANAEMIAS

Haemolytic disease of the newborn (continued)

The basic mechanism is influenced by three important factors:

(a) The maternal immune response tends to be proportional to the number of fetal cells entering the circulation.

(b) The material immune response is boosted in successive Rh incompatible pregnancies — the highest maternal antibody titres are found in the latest of multiple pregnancies.

(c) Fetal/maternal ABO compatibility influences the Rh immune response.

e.g. *ABO compatible*		*ABO incompatible*	
Fetus	*Mother*	*Fetus*	*Mother*
Group O Rh+	Group O Rh-	Group A Rh+	Group O Rh-
Gradual elimination		*Rapid* destruction	
of fetal cells		of fetal cells	
∴ *Maximum* immune response		∴ *Minimum* immune response	

Subsequent pregnancies: All Rh-positive fetuses conceived by a mother who has acquired anti-Rh antibodies either during previous pregnancies or by blood transfusion (in this case the first fetus also) are at risk.

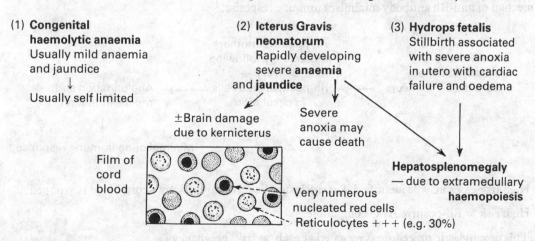

Placenta —— Uterus

Maternal anti-Rh antibodies IgG type
↓
Pass placental barrier
↓
Enter fetal circulation and **destroy fetal red cells** (agglutination and haemolysis)

The effects are graded into three categories of severity:

(1) **Congenital haemolytic anaemia**
Usually mild anaemia and jaundice
↓
Usually self limited

(2) **Icterus Gravis neonatorum**
Rapidly developing severe **anaemia** and **jaundice**

±Brain damage due to kernicterus

Severe anoxia may cause death

(3) **Hydrops fetalis**
Stillbirth associated with severe anoxia in utero with cardiac failure and oedema

Hepatosplenomegaly — due to extramedullary **haemopoiesis**

Film of cord blood

Very numerous nucleated red cells

Reticulocytes +++ (e.g. 30%)

EXTRINSIC HAEMOLYTIC ANAEMIAS

Haemolytic disease of the newborn (continued)

The Paternal 'role' in HDN

The father's genotype influences the risk for the fetus as follows:

HDN is particularly associated with incompatibility at the D locus.
Rh-negative individuals are homozygous — dd.
Rh-positive individuals may be heterozygous Dd or homozygou DD.
If the father is homozygous all his children must be Rh-positive and therefore at risk.
If he is heterozygous the chances of an Rh-negative child is 1 : 1

	Rh-negative mother	Rh-positive father	Offspring
(a)	dd	(homozygous) DD	Dd Dd, all Rh + ∴ all at risk.
(b)	dd	(heterozygous) dD	Dd dd —— 1 Rh-negative 1 Rh-positive

Laboratory tests in HDN

During pregnancy {
1. Blood grouping of pregnant women.
2. Screening of Rh-negative women for antibodies in early pregnancy.
3. Titring antibodies found — gives some indication of riks of affected child.

At birth ... 4. Baby's cord blood — DIRECT COOMB'S TEST: a positive result indicates HDN.
Hb and bilirubin estimations and reticulocyte counts indicate severity.

Modern prophylaxis

Injection of anti-Rh antibody minimises immune response:

Anti-Rh (anti-D) usually obtained from male volunteers ⟶ Rh-negative mother* immediately following delivery — Rh-positive fetal cells in circulation ⟶ Agglutination and *rapid* elimination ↓ Minimal or no immune response

*High risk cases may be identified if anti-Rh supplies are scarce. Baby's cord blood is grouped:

High risk = Rh-positive ABO compatible.

This prophylactic procedure is repeated at each 'at risk' pregnancy.

EXTRINSIC HAEMOLYTIC ANAEMIAS

(1b) DESTRUCTION of RBC's due to AUTO-ANTIBODIES

This is the commonest type of haemolytic anaemia. The great majority of cases are SECONDARY to other diseases, e.g. systemic lypus erythematosis (SLE) or rheumatoid arthritis, lymphomas and other malignant diseases.

The mechanism by which AUTO-ANTIBODIES emerge is not known with certainty. The main possibilities are:

A. Loss of tolerance due to depression of T cell surveillance

The normal surface antigens on red cells are recognised as 'self' and the *tolerance* response is evoked.

In some diseases, e.g. lymphomas and malignant disease, T cell activity is depressed — the tolerance response is bypassed.

B. The tolerance response may be bypassed by changes in the antigen

(i) Surface antigens modified by *drugs* or *viruses*.

Normal

= Modified antigen now recognised as 'foreign'

∴ Antibodies produced (Y)

(ii) Cross-reaction with *bacterial* antibodies. RBC and bacterium sharing antigen determinant ▲.

Bacterium recognised as 'foreign'

∴ Antibodies produced (Y)

Cross-reaction with RBC

EXTRINSIC HAEMOLYTIC ANAEMIAS

The autoimmune haemolytic anaemias are divided into two main groups depending on the temperature at which the reactions occur.

1. *Warm antibody type*
   Reaction at normal temperature (37°C)
   人 = Antibody usually IgG type

Cell
membrane
→
modified

Cell becomes
microspherocyte

● = Antigenic determinant
often of Rh e type

With consequences similar to
hereditary spherocytosis —
early sequestration in spleen etc.

Clinically presents as chronic haemolytic anaemia ± crises.

2. *Cold antibody type*
   Reactions at temperatures usually below 30°C ∴ they occur in peripheral circulation and in cold weather.

Antibody ┄┄┄→ ┄┄┄ Usually of IgM type

Combines
with RBC

● = Antigenic determinant
(usually I or i type)

Reactions

AGGLUTINATION

AMBOCEPTOR EFFECT

Ag/Ab activaties COMPLEMENT cascade.

Acute intravascular RBC lysis.

Clinically presents as painful
hands and feet

Presents as HAEMOGLOBINAEMIA
and HAEMOGLOBINURIA
(Paroxysmal cold haemoglobinuria)

Note: The classical paroxysmal haemoglobinuria associated with syphilitic infection is rare nowadays. It is due to an IgG antibody, and the antigenic determinant on the red cell is usually P type.

EXTRINSIC HAEMOLYTIC ANAEMIAS

2. INFECTIONS

There are three mechanisms by which infections cause haemolysis:

(1) *Induction of autoantibodies* e.g.

Patchy pneumonia due to *Mycoplasma pneumoniae*

↓

Autoantibodies formed

rbc

(2) *Direct damage to RBC membrane by toxin* e.g. *Clostridial* infection

Exotoxin

RBC

HAEMOLYSIS

(3) *Entry into red cell by infecting parasite* e.g. *malaria* (see p.541)

Parasite

Intracellular multiplication

Rupture

3. DRUGS AND CHEMICALS

The three main mechanisms by which drugs and chemicals cause haemolysis are:

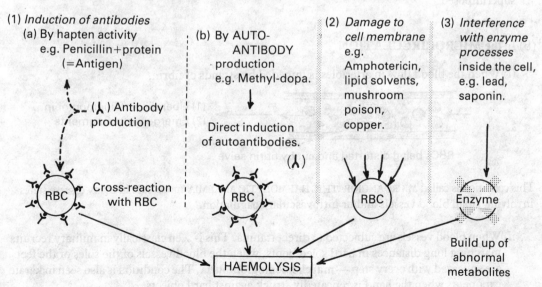

(1) *Induction of antibodies*
  (a) By hapten activity e.g. Penicillin+protein (=Antigen)

(λ) Antibody production

RBC

Cross-reaction with RBC

  (b) By AUTO-ANTIBODY production e.g. Methyl-dopa.

Direct induction of autoantibodies.

(λ)

RBC

(2) *Damage to cell membrane* e.g. Amphotericin, lipid solvents, mushroom poison, copper.

RBC

(3) *Interference with enzyme processes* inside the cell, e.g. lead, saponin.

Enzyme

Build up of abnormal metabolites

HAEMOLYSIS

EXTRINSIC HAEMOLYTIC ANAEMIAS

4. MECHANICAL TRAUMA

The results of damage to red cells within the circulation are:

(1) Intravascular haemolysis

(2) Formation of red cell fragments (schistocytes) seen in blood film as 'burr', 'triangle', 'helmet' cells

Haemoglobinuria

The main circumstances in which red cells are damaged are:

(a) In the **heart and great vessels**

When the blood flow is subjected to undue turbulence or jet effect. An important example nowadays is with prosthetic valves in left side of heart.

RBCs damaged by shearing stresses where valve seating is defective

Other examples are:
Aortic stenosis and regurgitation
Arterio-venous shunts.

Note that in this chronic situation, iron is lost in the urine so that *iron deficiency anaemia* is often superimposed.

(b) In the **MICROCIRCULATION**

(i) When the blood flow in arterioles is impeded by strands of fibrin.

(1) Liberation of haemoglobin
(2) Emergence of fragments

RBCs being distorted and cut by fibrin seive

This condition is called MICROANGIOPATHIC HAEMOLYTIC ANAEMIA and occurs in many disease states involving small blood vessels and/or intravascular coagulation.

(ii) When blood vessels are subjected to direct trauma. This is seen classically in military recruits marching long distances in hard soled boots, when the blood vessels of the soles of the feet are squeezed with every step — **march haemoglobinuria.** The condition is also seen in karate exponents when the hand is repeatedly struck against hard objects.

    The haemolysis is usually not severe enough to be of clinical significance, but haemoglobinuria may cause alarm.

EXTRINSIC HAEMOLYTIC ANAEMIAS — MALARIA

Malaria is an endemic disease in many parts of Africa, Asia, Central and South America. Many millions of cases occur each year and the mortality is at least 1%. The disease is particularly severe in non-immune subjects from temperate climates; in endemic areas where the 'herd' immunity is high, a low grade chronic illness is common.

Female anopheline mosquitos act as intermediate hosts in the life cycle of the parasite, a protozoon (genus *Plasmodium*).

(1) Infected mosquito injects parasites with saliva into capillary before sucking blood

(5) Mosquito sucks infected blood including sexual forms of parasite

Complex cycle in mosquito ends in mature sporozoa in salivary glands, ready to infect a new subject.

Skin →

Capillary

Gametocytes ♂ ♀

Stage 4 characterised by high fever

Invasion of liver cells and maturation of **Schizont**

(2)

Cells rupture
↓
Merozoites into blood

(4)

(3)

Trophozoite — 'ring form' of parasite

RBC entered

Reinfection of RBCs

5 – 16 days depending on species of plasmodium

In some species, schizonts lie dormant in the liver; relapse may occur after long remissions.

Stages (1), (2) and (3) are symptomless.

Pathological changes

1. *Parasitism and destruction of red cells* ⟶ | ANAEMIA | (haemolytic)

   In a few severe cases, massive haemolysis leads to haemoglobinuria with kidney damage – **blackwater fever**.

   Cerebral malaria is due to capillary blockage by parasitised RBC (see p.742).

   Liberation of pigment and red cell debris → very marked macrophage activity
   ↓
   | SPLENOMEGALY |
   ↑
   Macrophage activity

2. *Immune responses:* humoral antibodies
   cellular antibodies } +

3. *Associations:* Burkitt's lymphoma (p.608): Sickle cell resistance (p.532).

EXTRINSIC HAEMOLYTIC ANAEMIAS

5. EXTRINSIC — MISCELLANEOUS

1. Hypersplenism (see P.582).

In enlargement of the spleen from any cause, the sequestration of red cells is increased so that haemolytic anaemia may result.

Normal

RBCs

Effete cells (about 1%) removed in pulp

RBC life span 120 days

Hypersplenism

RBCs

RBCs removed in greater numbers and before they are completely effete

RBC life span reduced

2. Burns

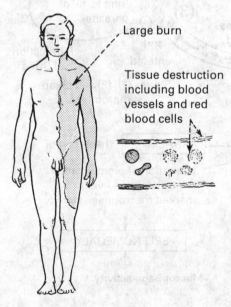

Large burn

Tissue destruction including blood vessels and red blood cells

In severe burns haemolysis is an important component of the acute anaemia which develops.

3. Use of water or hypotonic solutions

Given intravenously by mistake

Blood vessel   RBCs swell and burst

Intravascular haemolysis

ANAEMIAS — MISCELLANEOUS

There remain anaemias of which the causative mechanisms are obscure or complex and the morphological details indeterminate.

This miscellaneous group can be subdivided as follows:

1. Anaemias associated with chronic disease states.

Postulated mechanism:

Blocks iron release from macrophages

The components have varying significance from case to case.

The chronic disease states commonly associated with anaemia of this type are:

(a) Chronic infections and inflammations e.g. tuberculosis: rheumatoid arthritis.
(b) Renal disease — in addition the following factors are often important:

Renal
— RBC survival is inversely proportional to severity of uraemia
— Burr cells (e.g. in renal disease with vascular fibrin deposition)
— Erythropoietin specifically lost.

In dialysis, folate and iron loss.

(c) Liver failure — additional factors are:

Liver
— Bleeding Varices
— Deficiency of coagulation factors
— Hypersplenism
— Alcoholic — other nutritional deficiencies

In addition, malignant tumour growth may cause anaemia by two more specific mechanisms.

(a) Chronic bleeding from the surface of an ulcerated tumour — especially from the alimentary tract.

(b) Actual invasion of the bone marrow by malignant tumour

543

ANAEMIAS — MISCELLANEOUS

2. The sideroblastic anaemias

In these rare anaemias, failure of synthesis of the haem component of the haemoglobin molecule is indicated by the presence of a ring of iron granules around the normoblast nucleus.

Ringed sideroblast

Iron granules (in mitochondria) stained by Prussian blue reaction

In a few cases, pyridoxine allows haem synthesis to proceed normally

The condition arises secondarily in many of the chronic disease states mentioned on previous page, or as a result of drug treatment or chemical poisoning (e.g. lead). A few cases are 'primary'.

The anaemia is usually hypochromic and may be normocytic or macrocytic.

3. Anaemias associated with endocrine deficiencies

These anaemias have no specifically identifying features and their mechanism of production is obscure.

The anaemia of hypothyroidism is often macrocytic.

4. Refractory anaemias

These rare anaemias of unknown aetiology fail to respond to many various treatments. They are usually macrocytic. As the aetiology of anaemias is elucidated, the number of 'refractory' cases diminishes.

5. Leucoerythroblastic anaemia

In this condition, primitive myeloid cells as well as nucleated red cells appear in small numbers in blood film; the cause is usually a serious bone disorder often due to infiltration by malignant tumour or fibrosis.

The foregoing classification is based on the basic aetiological mechanisms, and although in some cases the mechanisms overlap, the classification is fundamental to rational treatment.

ANAEMIA — MORPHOLOGICAL CLASSIFICATION

The initial investigation of any anaemia consists of an examination of blood (and/or marrow) films and determination of absolute values. A morphological classification is therefore very useful.

The three broad divisions which depend on the red cell size may be further subdivided in respect of haemoglobin content of the cell:

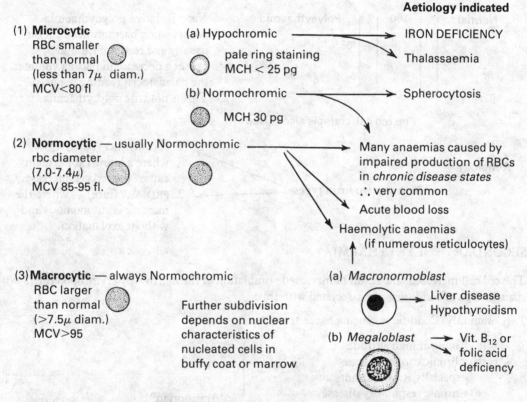

Aetiology indicated

(1) **Microcytic**
RBC smaller than normal (less than 7μ diam.) MCV<80 fl

    (a) Hypochromic   → IRON DEFICIENCY

        pale ring staining MCH < 25 pg → Thalassaemia

    (b) Normochromic → Spherocytosis

        MCH 30 pg

(2) **Normocytic** — usually Normochromic
rbc diameter (7.0-7.4μ) MCV 85-95 fl.

→ Many anaemias caused by impaired production of RBCs in *chronic disease states* ∴ very common

Acute blood loss

Haemolytic anaemias (if numerous reticulocytes)

(3) **Macrocytic** — always Normochromic
RBC larger than normal (>7.5μ diam.) MCV>95

Further subdivision depends on nuclear characteristics of nucleated cells in buffy coat or marrow

    (a) *Macronormoblast* → Liver disease / Hypothyroidism

    (b) *Megaloblast* → Vit. B$_{12}$ or folic acid deficiency

In some cases of anaemia, there are two distinct populations of abnormal red cells (e.g. microcytic/hypochromic and macrocytic/normochromic). These DIMORPHIC anaemias are usually caused by double deficiencies.

The logical use of these classifications in the investigation of anaemia:

ANAEMIA → Examination of blood film Determination of absolute values → Morphological classification → Indication of aetiology

Subtle changes in cell morphology →

Confirmatory tests ↓ Aetiological classification

ANAEMIA Hb – below 12 g

DISEASES OF RED BLOOD CELLS

POLYCYTHAEMIA

Polycythaemia (erythrocytosis) is defined as a sustained increase in red cell mass: the haematocrit is always elevated.

Normal   -100-   **Polycythaemia**

65%

45%

-0-

The red cell count is also raised

Note: **Relative polycythaemia** occurs when haemoconcentration, usually as a result of fluid loss, causes a decrease in plasma volume; the haematocrit reading is raised. This is not true polycythaemia.

Aetiology

There are two main types

1. SECONDARY (reactive) — where a known abnormality causes the red cell increase.
2. PRIMARY (rare) — where the increase is autonomous and without explanation.

SECONDARY POLYCYTHAEMIA

The red cell increase is the result of increased stimulation of the marrow by erythropoietin. Two main groups of conditions are associated with this:

1. (Commonly) Conditions causing tissue HYPOXIA:

    (a) Living at high altitudes
    (b) Chronic cardiac disease
        especially R → L shunts
    (c) Chronic respiratory disease
    (d) Presence of abnormal haemoglobin causing defective release of O_2 to tissue — usually hereditary, sometimes due to drugs.

2. (Rarely) Renal tumours and ischaemia; occasionally tumours of other organs.

'Appropriate'

ERYTHROPOIETIN production

'Inappropriate'

MARROW HYPERPLASIA (RED CELLS)

POLYCYTHAEMIA — increase of red cells only

PRIMARY POLYCYTHAEMIA (*Polycythaemia Rubra Vera*)

The red cell increase in this rare condition is autonomous. It may be associated with an increase in other marrow elements and is grouped within the myeloproliferative disorders (see p. 557). Splenomegaly is always present.

DISEASES OF RED BLOOD CELLS

Effects of polycythaemia
(a) There is usually a distinctly florid complexion.
(b) Increased blood viscosity causes: (i) **hypertension** and (ii) a tendency to **thrombosis.**
(c) Increased marrow activity → increased uric acid metabolism → tendency to gout.

Comparison of SECONDARY and PRIMARY polycythaemias

	Secondary	**Primary**
Prevalence	Lesser degrees COMMON	RARE
Cause	Underlying disease — especially HYPOXIA	Not known (associated with non specific chromosome aberrations)
Erythropoietin	+ +	Not increased; may be decreased
Marrow	Increased cellularity but some fat spaces remain: pure red cell hyperplasia	Total cellularity — including increase in myeloid elements and megakaryocytes → May terminate as acute **myeloid leukaemia** → Marrow fibrosis may follow
Blood	RBC's normal	Leucocyte count often increased Platelet count often raised RBC's may by hypochromic
Splenomegaly	None	+ +
Hypertension	+	+ +
Tendency to thrombosis	+	+ +
Tendency to gout	+	+ +
	Increased cellular breakdown in marrow causes uricaemia	
Progress	Where the erythropoietin excess is 'appropriate' the outcome depends on the progress of the basic disease	Without treatment — **poor** Progressive deterioration over a few years

THE WHITE BLOOD CELLS

NEUTROPHIL Polymorphonuclear Leucocyte (Neutrophil granulocyte)

The essential function of these cells is protection against microbial infection by phagocytosis and killing. They are produced alongside red blood cells, platelets and monocytes from a common stem cell in the marrow.

Marrow Production — stained by a Romanowski method

	Stem cell (Primitive-multipotential)	Myeloblast (committed)	Promyelocyte	Myelocyte	Metamyelocyte	Polymorph in marrow and blood
% age	<1	<5	<15			
Size (Diameter)	$15 - 25\mu$	$10 - 18\mu$	$12 - 18\mu$	$12 - 18\mu$	$12 - 15\mu$	$10 - 15\mu$
Nucleus	Spherical; even dispersal of chromatin	Spherical; even dispersal of chromatin	Spherical; chromatin slightly condensed	Ovoid; condensation of chromatin	'Band' of 'stab' shape; chromatin condensed	2 – 5 lobes; Chromatin condensed
Nucleoli	Several	2 – 4	2 – 4	None	None	None
Cytoplasm	Blue (High RNA content)	Blue (High RNA content)	Blue	Less blue	Less blue Glycogen++	Less blue Glycogen++
Granules	None	None	Scanty large granules; contain *myeloperoxidase* and *hydrolases*	Many small granules; alkaline *phosphatase*, various lytic enzymes		

WHITE BLOOD CELLS IN DISEASE

NEUTROPHIL POLYMORPHONUCLEAR LEUCOCYTOSIS

Normal bone marrow production

Focal aggregation of granulocyte precursors (myeloid series) mixed with other cell types. Myeloid/Erythroid (ME) ration 3 to 8:1

Blood circulation

Life span: 1 – 3 days

Count: $2.5 – 7.5 \times 10^9/l$ ($2,500 – 7,500/mm^3$)

(1) To surface epithelia

(2) To tissues

(3) To local macrophages
To macrophages in spleen and liver

Disposal

e.g. mouth, throat, cervix, resp. tract

An increase in the number of circulating neutrophils reflects an increased activity in the tissues at the site of an acute inflammatory reaction.

Neutrophil activation

TISSUES

INFECTION or NECROSIS — PHAGOCYTOSIS and KILL

CHEMICAL MEDIATORS

COMPLEMENT ACTIVATION

CHEMOTAXIS

Leucocyte releasing factor

Stimulating factor

Blood stream

Marrow

Hyperplastic

Increased number of neutrophils

Normal

Neutrophil leucocytosis (count over $7.5 \times 10^9/l$)

'Stab' cells nucleus not segmented

Neutrophil leucocytosis does not occur in:
(a) some acute bacterial infections, e.g. typhoid fever, brucellosis
(b) many chronic bacterial infections
(c) most virus infections unless acute bacterial infection or necrosis occurs
(d) overwhelming infections with severe toxaemia.

4-lobed nuclei frequent   Fewer nuclear lobes

549

DISORDERS OF NEUTROPHILS

In most disorders, increased susceptibility to infection is the important sequel and clinical presentation.

Absence (agranulocytosis) or diminished numbers — $<2.5\times10^9$/l (2,500/mm³)(neutropenia)
There are two main mechanisms which often co-exist.

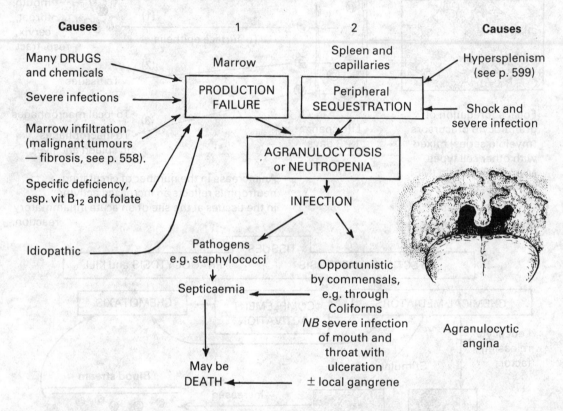

Drugs may act in the following ways:

1. By direct dose related toxic effect, e.g. benzine and, NB, modern chemotherapeutic agents.

2. By an immunological reaction, the drug acting as a **hapten**, e.g. amidopyrine.

Drugs and chemicals may affect the production of all three marrow cell types together or in various combinations.

3. By an idiosyncratic action in sensitive subjects small doses are effective, e.g. chloramphenicol.

DISORDERS OF NEUTROPHILS

Disorders of neutrophil function

Divided into three groups: (1) chemotaxis, (2) microbial phagocytosis and (3) microbial kill.

Chemotaxis and phagocytosis may be defective due to:

(a) an intrinsic defect of the neutrophils e.g. lazy leucocyte syndrome
(b) plasma deficiency of chemotactic factors and opsonins — seen especially when there are deficiencies in the complement cascade.

Microbial kill fails when there is an intracellular enzyme defect e.g. in *chronic granulomatous disease* (CGD) and the Chediak-Higashi syndrome where the neutrophils contain abnormal giant granules.

The normal sequence following phagocytosis is:

(1) Bacterium in phagosome

The act of phagocytosis rapidly triggers a burst of intracellular enzyme activity...

(2) Powerful bactericidal effect

... with rapid production of H_2O_2
+
Myeloperoxidase
+
Halogen (I or Cl)

(3)
(a) Bacterium digested by acid hydrolases and other enzymes
(b) Neutrophil degranulated

In CGD, the rapid production of H_2O_2 is defective (in the neutrophils and also in macrophages — ? due to cytochrome deficiency).

(2a)
The bacteria are not killed and are protected from antibiotics and extracellular defence mechanisms by the cell membrane.

(2b)
Death of neutrophil (1 – 3 days) liberates bacteria.

DISORDERS OF NEUTROPHILS

CHRONIC GRANULOMATOUS DISEASE (CGD)
CGD is a rare hereditary disorder in which the neutrophils have normal phagocytic function but are unable to kill certain bacteria.

Presentation
The disease is fully expressed only in males. It presents as multiple chronic abscesses and granulomas affecting skin, lungs, bones, spleen and liver. The abscesses contain abundant debris derived from tissue breakdown. This is seen as fatty material and pigment within macrophages and illustrates the unimpaired phagocytic capacity.

Bacteriology:
Infection is by a limited range of organisms —
e.g. staphylococci, coliforms (no H_2O_2 production).
Organisms, e.g. streptococci, which naturally produce H_2O_2 contribute this missing factor and are themselves killed and the infection is eliminated.

Inheritance
The disease is X-linked.

($\circledX$ = affected chromosome)

Normal father XY   X$\circledX$ Carrier mother

X X — normal ♀   X$\circledX$ — carrier ♀   X Y — normal ♂ $\circledX$Y — affected ♂

Note 1. Affected males die of chronic infection before the age of sexual maturity.
2. The carrier female may present with minor skin inflammation.
3. The carrier female has two approximately equal populations of neutrophils:
  (a) with normal ability to kill bacteria.
  (b) with defective ability to kill bacteria.

The Lyon hypothesis states that in the female, the XX chromosomes are randomly inactivated during cellular growth and differentiation. The neutrophils of the carrier female support this hypothesis.

(a) If $\circledX$ is inactivated, the normal X remains active and the polymorph has normal ability to kill.

A small drumstick-like projection from the nucleus carries the inactivated sex chromosome.

(b) If X is inactivated, the defective $\circledX$ remains active and the ability to kill is defective.

These are rare defects and usually have a hereditary basis.

Other acquired abnormalities of neutrophil function are more difficult to pin-point but are probably relevant in the increased rate of infection seen in diseases such as diabetes mellitus, rheumatoid arthritis and glomerulonephritis.

EOSINOPHILS

EOSINOPHIL Polymorphonuclear Leucocyte

These cells circulate in the blood (normal count $0.04 - 0.4 \times 10^9$/l or $40 - 400$/mm^3) and are found in the tissues, particularly near points of external environmental contact.

Production is in the bone marrow as a component of myeloid haemopoiesis.

Marrow precursor — Mature cell — 'Spectacle' nucleus (bilobed)

Large crystalline granules (take up eosin, strongly staining bright pink) containing enzymes including a specific peroxidase.

$(10 - 14\mu)$

Myeloblasts → Myelocytes → Eosinophil
(Analogous to neutrophil series)

Although their basic function is similar to that of neutrophils and they are found in small numbers in inflammatory cellular infiltrates, they exhibit specialised functions in certain disorders:

1. They protect against 'foreign' substances — especially the foreign proteins of infesting helminths.
2. They exert a controlling influence on mast cells and the effects of histamine release at the site of Type I antigen-antibody reactions.

There are several specific eosinophil chemotactic agents, particularly those derived from mast cells, which complement activation and T cell lymphokine release.

Eosinophilia (an increased number of eosinophils in the blood) is seen in:

1. Parasitic infestations — e.g. ankylostomiasis, schistosomiasis

2. Hypersensitivity (atopic) reactions — both generalised and local, e.g. asthma and hay fever; food and drug sensitivity

3. Chronic eczema of the skin (probably due to antigen-antibody reaction)

4. Occasionally in association with malignant tumours — but particularly in Hodgkin's disease.

'Allergic' nasal polypi

The typical cellular infiltrate consisting of numerous eosinophils and plasma cells under mucosa in a loose myxomatous stroma.

553

LYMPHOCYTES

The main function of lymphocytes is concerned with the immune responses occurring in the lymphoid organs, and the immune reactions occurring at surfaces and adjacent tissues (see p. 98). Their presence in the blood is only one component of their complex circulation.

NOTE: B and T cells are indistinguishable by routine staining methods.

Lymphocytes in peripheral blood Dense round nucleus and thin rim of blue cytoplasm (8 – 11μ diameter)

Count: 1.5 – 4.0 × 10⁹/l (1,500-4,000/mm³)

In many diseases there may be significant changes in the functional activity of lymphocytes, but these are seldom reflected in lymphocyte counts and lymphocyte morphology. Age has an important effect on blood lymphocyte counts, probably reflecting the amount and activity of the lymphoid tissues which gradually atrophy with age — as exemplified in thymus, tonsils and appendix. In childhood, there are active immune responses to a host of first contact antigens.

Infants: 3.5±1.5×10⁹/l. *Children:* 7.0±1.5×10⁹/l. *Adults:* 1.5 – 4.0× 10⁹/l.

Lymphocytosis — (a) *Relative.* If the neutrophil numbers decrease it is unusual for the lymphocyte numbers to fall also: a differential WBC in these circumstances shows an increased ratio (% age) of lymphocytes. This relative lymphocytosis must not be confused with
(b) an *Absolute* lymphocytosis, i.e. count >4.0× 10⁹/l.
This occurs in many virus infections in children, and in adults in GLANDULAR FEVER and smallpox as well as in typhoid fever and brucellosis. *NB* In the late middle aged and elderly, an absolute lymphocytosis should always raise the suspicion of a *neoplastic proliferation of lymphocytes* (leukaemia, lymphoma, see p. 592).
Lymphopenia (count<1.5×10⁹/l). Apart from rare hereditary diseases seen in childhood, lymphopenia is commonly seen in medical practice during therapy using ionising radiation, cytotoxic drugs and corticosteroids.
Morphological changes are seen in blood film particularly in virus infections.

Normal lymphocyte: dense spherical nucleus with thin rim of cytoplasm.

Larger cell with loose-textured nucleus with clear foamy cytoplasm; can easily be mistaken for monocyte.

Larger cell with dense eccentric nucleus: a type of plasma cell (Turck cell).

The changes in Glandular Fever (infectious mononucleosis) are described on page 68.

MONOCYTES

These cells, derived from stem cells in the bone marrow, are the circulating members of the mononuclear phagocyte system. Their main function is to replace local macrophages (see p.105).

Marrow

Very occassional monocytes derived from stem cells

Blood

$19\mu \pm 3\mu$

Kidney-shaped nucleus
Finely granular cytoplasm
Blood count: $0.2 - 0.8 \times 10^9/l$
(2 – 8%)

To 'top up' tissue macrophage population, especially in lymph nodes and spleen, lungs, mesentery and bowel, liver.

To augment macrophage population at sites of continuing inflammatory and immune reactions.

Although many macrophages may be present at these sites, only occasionally is the monocyte blood count significantly increased. The following are examples of conditions in which there may be a monocytosis.

Infections:			Immunological disease	Chemical poisoning
Bacterial	**Rickettsial**	**Protozoal**		
Subacute bacterial endocarditis	Typhus fever	Malaria Kala-azar Trypanosomiasis	Systemic lupus erythematosus (SLE)	Tetrachlorethylene

Little is known about disease associated with abnormal monocytic function.

Note: The abnormal cells seen in the blood in 'glandular fever' (infectious mononucleosis) are transformed 'T' lymphocytes and not monocytes.

THE LEUKAEMIAS

Increased numbers of any one type of leucocyte or its precursors are seen in most cases of leukaemia — a neoplastic proliferation of white blood cells.

The various types of leukaemia are dealt with on pages 586-593.

BLOOD PLATELETS

These small, non-nucleated discs, derived from the cytoplasm of the bone marrow megakaryocytes, are released into the blood stream by a budding process.

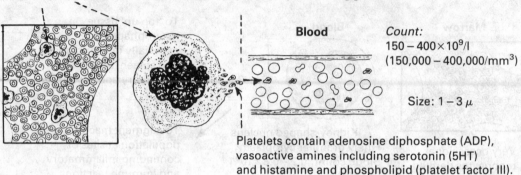

Blood

Count:
$150 - 400 \times 10^9/l$
$(150,000 - 400,000/mm^3)$

Size: $1 - 3\,\mu$

Platelets contain adenosine diphosphate (ADP), vasoactive amines including serotonin (5HT) and histamine and phospholipid (platelet factor III).

Their main role is concerned with haemostasis:

1. By aggregating to form the **haemostatic plug.**

and 2. by activating and augmenting the

Loose aggregation of platelets.

(Release of platelet thromboplastin factor III)

Release of ADP and thromboxane

Further disruption of platelets

Reinforcement of plug

At site of endothelial damage: triggered by contact with *collagen* and mediated by *prostaglandin*

Closer adherence and release of more ADP and *vasoactive amines.*

Prothrombin

THROMBIN

Fibrinogen

FIBRIN

A prostaglandin (prostacyclin) synthesised by endothelium is antagonistic to platelet 'release' and normally prevents intravascular coagulation.

Disorders of the platelets include:

1. (a) deficiencies of number – thrombocytopenia
   (b) defective function leads to **purpura** (see p. 566).

2. Increased *adhesiveness* with or without increased numbers (thrombocytosis) occurs as a reactive state in many conditions — after haemorrhage, trauma and operations, childbirth, myocardial infarction, pulmonary embolism, splenectomy and during the use of the contraceptive pill. This change in platelet function is an important factor in the aetiology of **thrombosis** (see. p. 122).

DISEASES OF THE BONE MARROW

The role of the bone marrow and the reactive changes occurring in it in disorders of the blood cells have been described.

Primary disorders of the bone marrow are also important. There are two main groups: (1) marrow hypoplasia and (2) myeloproliferative disorders.

1. MARROW HYPOPLASIA or APLASIA (diminished or absent haemopoietic cellularity)

The marrow throughout the body has a pale, fatty gelatinous appearance.

Microscopically the haemopoietic cells are reduced or absent.

Sparse foci of lymphocytes or plasma cells remain.

Blood

Pancytopenia
Reduction in red blood cells, granulocytes, platelets

Lymphocytes normal

Congenital and idiopathic forms are rare. Most cases are ACQUIRED as the result of therapy:

(a) marrow toxic drugs and radiations used in the treatment of cancer
(b) idiosyncratic reactions to a wide range of drugs — chloramphenicol is a good example.

The effects of the pancytopenia are serious (severe anaemia, susceptibility to infection and haemorrhage) and usually fatal unless the marrow activity is resumed.

2. MYELOPROLIFERATIVE DISORDERS (increased cellularity)

The various acquired reactive states of the bone marrow already described are specifically excluded from this category which embraces proliferations of the various marrow cellular components in a purposeless way and without known cause. It is important to note that a significant number of cases of myeloproliferative disorder terminate in acute leukaemia. The leukaemias and other primary marrow neoplasms will therefore be described separately in order to avoid confusion in classification.

The disorders included in the group comprise proliferations of:

1. All haemopoietic cells including fibrous tissue
2. Erythroid cells predominantly
3. Megakaryocytic cells.

DISEASES OF THE BONE MARROW

Myeloproliferative Disorders (continued)

MYELOFIBROSIS

In this rare affection of the elderly, the haemopoietic cellular proliferation is overshadowed by progressive FIBROSIS of the marrow; SPLENOMEGALY (often of massive proportions) due to EXTRAMEDULLARY HAEMOPOIESIS (myeloid metaplasia) is an invariable concomitant.

Marrow: ordinary marrow puncture usually results in a 'dry tap', therefore trephine or cutting needle biopsy is required.

At this stage bone changes may be seen on X-ray — OSTEOSCLEROSIS.

Total cellularity
— all types of cell
— very early reticulin increase.

Reticulin ++
— early fibrosis
— cellularity decreasing.

Established fibrosis
— only small foci of haemopoietic cells remaining.

Blood findings

RBC	WBC	Platelets
low	may by increased	may be increased

as marrow cells are replaced

↓

Progress to PANCYTOPENIA (this is exaggerated by enlarged spleen)

Film *Leucoerythroblastic blood picture*

- - - Nucleated reds

Poikilocytosis

- - - 'Tear drop' cells

- - - Abnormally large platelets

- - - Myelocytes

Note: The Philadelphia chromosome is absent (cf. chronic myeloid leukaemia).

POLYCYTHAEMIA VERA

In this condition, erythroid proliferation predominates (see p. 546).

THROMBOCYTHAEMIA (ESSENTIAL)

In this condition, megakaryocytic proliferation is associated with increased circulating platelets. The signs of the disease which range from spontaneous bleedings to thomboses are associated with abnormality of platelet function.

In these chronic myeloproliferative disorders, progress to marrow fibrosis is a common end result.

DISEASES OF THE BONE MARROW

Myeloproliferative Disorders (continued)

EXTRA-MEDULLARY HAEMOPOIESIS (Myeloid metaplasia).

When the blood forming capacity of the bone marrow is impaired, the primitive stem cells, still resident in the extra-medullary sites of haemopoiesis of fetal life, may be stimulated.

Initiating causes

NB Infiltration of marrow
    by metastatic tumour

IMPAIRMENT
of
MARROW
FUNCTION

Also Hodgkin's disease
    Tuberculosis
    Irradiation
    Severe haemolysis
    Marrow poisons,
    e.g. benzene,
        strontium

Extra-medullary haemopoiesis
presents as foci of blood cell
precursors in organs   **Spleen**

Haemic cells
including **Mega-
karyocytes**
in red pulp

Liver

In
sinusoids

Lymph node

In
sinuses
and medulla

In these conditions extra-medullary haemopoiesis is compensatory.

The most extreme forms of splenic enlargement due to extra-medullary haemopoiesis are seen in **MYELOPROLIFERATIVE DISORDERS** at the **MARROW FIBROSIS** stage.

Two factors combine:

1. Compensation for fibrosis of marrow
2. Stimulation of extra-medullary haemopoiesis by the unknown mechanism which is responsible for the myeloproliferation.

NB Hypersplenism due to the enlarged spleen aggravates the pancytopenia.

HAEMOSTASIS

The essential purpose is prevention of blood loss after injury.

(1) Wound in skin

Free flow of blood from vessel

Very rapid activation of the haemostatic mechanisms follows:

(2)

(a) **Contraction** of damaged vessel

(b) **Platelets** adhere together and aggregate to form a plug

(c) **Coagulation** of blood with formation of **fibrin network** reinforces platelet plug

(3) Later, when bleeding has stopped, a complex healing process begins (see p. 81) and includes solution of the fibrin web — fibrinolysis.

COAGULATION MECHANISM

Prothrombin

Thromboplastins (in blood and tissues)

Thrombin

Fibrinogen

FIBRIN

FIBRINOLYTIC MECHANISM

Plasminogen

Activators (in vascular endothelium and tissue)

Plasmin — digests fibrin (fibrinolysis) and other proteins

Inhibitors are also active in both mechanisms

These diagrams indicate the basic mechanisms in a complex enzyme cascade system, the end product of which in **FIBRIN**.

Disorders affecting the contractility of vessels, platelet function and the fibrinolytic system are comparatively rare.

The pathological process involving the formation of a coagulum within the circulation is very common and may cause serious effects — it is called THROMBOSIS.

COAGULATION DEFICIENCY DISEASES

The coagulation of blood is essentially the result of conversion of **FIBRINOGEN** to **FIBRIN,** but the chemical pathway leading to this final phase is complicated.

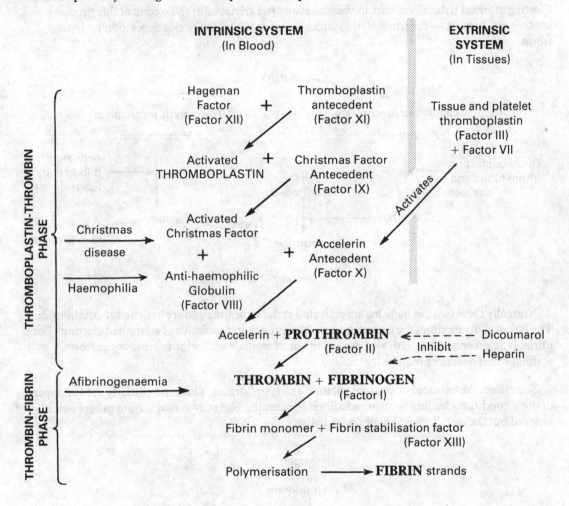

Vitamin K is required for the production of prothrombin, Christmas factor and accelerin (also known as Stuart-Prower factor). CALCIUM ions and phospholipids (mainly derived from platelets) are essential for many of the steps in thrombin production. Once thrombin is formed, it appears to stimulate several of the preceding reactions and also the polymerisation of fibrin.

COAGULATION DEFICIENCY DISEASES

FIBRINOLYSIS

Clotting of blood naturally occurs in vessels, even after trivial injury. To control this process another mechanism — the fibrinolytic system — exists which limits clot deposition by lysing fibrin.

Normally these two mechanisms are activated at the same time and are in dynamic equilibrium. The lytic activity modifies the coagulation process preventing excessive or continued clotting. The fibrinolytic process is also activated during repair of wounds and helps to remove the fibrin scaffold when no longer required.

Sometimes the balance between coagulation and lysis is upset. This is particularly apt to happen in those conditions leading to acquired afibrinogenaemia. Not only is coagulation progressively reduced but the clots formed are of poor quality.

The poorly formed fibrin is more susceptible to fibrinolysis and a vicious circle ensues.

COAGULATION DEFICIENCY DISEASES

FIBRINOLYSIS (continued)

As the lytic activity intensifies, the patient often shows symptoms of stress in a degree quite unrelated to the severity of the causal condition. The mechanism may be as follows:

Kinins are produced by digestion of α_2 globulins. They cause pain, increased permeability of capillaries, contraction of some smooth muscles and relaxation of others.

As a result of these complex interlocking mechanisms, the patient becomes increasingly shocked and the incoagulable condition of the blood is difficult to correct.

ANTI-COAGULANT THERAPY

Dicoumarol has already been mentioned (p.561). Heparin, commonly used therapeutically as an anticoagulant, inhibits the conversion of prothrombin to thrombin and also the action of thrombin on fibrinogen. Overdosage with heparin will result in incoagulability of the blood and possible haemorrhages from mucous membranes.

COAGULATION DEFICIENCY DISEASES

HAEMOPHILIA

This is due to a congenital functional deficiency of factor VIII.

The production of factor VIII is controlled by a gene on the X chromosome. In haemophilia, this gene is defective.

The family history of a case of haemophilia may be visualised as follows:

Carrier Mother X^A X (1 2)   Father X Y (3 4)

Other fertilisations —
XX (chromosomes 2 and 3) and XY (chromosomes 2 and 4) will result in normal offspring.

$X^A X$ $X^A Y$

CARRIER DAUGHTER   AFFECTED SON

The female carriers ($X^A X$ mother and daughter) have one abnormal chromosome (X^A) and one normal X. The normal chromosome will allow for production of normal factor VIII, thus offsetting the influence of the abnormal X^A.

In the affected male there is no normal X and the factor VIII produced under the influence of the abnormal X^A is functionally defective.

The clinical severity of the disease is related to the level of factor VIII in the blood.

Mild = 5 to 15% of normal.   Moderate = 1 to 5% of normal.

Severe = <1% of normal

In the severe condition, persistent bleeding occurs apparently spontaneously or after trivial injury. This may result in death after minor operations, or permanent disablement, e.g. joint ankylosis after injury. Blood coagulation time is greatly lengthened, but bleeding time (depending on vessel contraction and platelet accumulation) after needle prick is normal.

CHRISTMAS DISEASE (HAEMOPHILIA B)

This is due to a deficiency of factor IX (Christmas factor). Clinically the condition is indistinguishable from true haemophilia. The defect is sex linked, inherited in the same fashion as haemophilia and only manifested in males.

Congenital deficiencies of the other factors in the coagulation cascade are very rare causes of bleeding diseases.

COAGULATION DEFICIENCY DISEASES

VITAMIN K DEFICIENCY

Vitamin K is necessary for the production of several factors involved in coagulation, but prothrombin is the most important. Lack of vitamin K results in failure of the blood to clot, but it is also characterised by spontaneous haemorrhages from mucous membranes.

In adults vitamin K deficiency may arise in four situations:

1. Defective synthesis — in liver disease
2. Inhibition of activity — overdosage of vitamin K antagonists (anticoagulants of the coumarol type used in the treatment of thrombotic conditions)
3. Deficiency of absorption — vitamin K is fat soluble, ∴ deficiency may arise where absorption of fat is defective, e.g. obstructive jaundice.
4. Dietary deficiency — a very rare occurrence.

Haemorrhagic disease of the newborn
This is apt to occur in premature infants who have an inadequate supply of vitamin K. There may be gross haemorrhages from the umbilical cord and severe melaena.

AFIBRINOGENAEMIA
This occurs in two forms:

1. *Congenital.* A rare disease in which there is complete absence of fibrinogen in the blood, resulting in an incoagulable state. Slight injury may be fatal due to haemorrhage. The condition is familial.

2. *Acquired.* This is commonly caused by conditions which result in the release of thromboplastins into the circulation, e.g. lung operations, abruptio placentae, amniotic embolus or retention *in utero* of a dead fetus. The thromboplastins cause the formation of multiple fibrin clots in the circulating blood (disseminated intravascular coagulation — DIC). A vicious circle is set up as follows:

These conditions are frequently associated with shock which temporarily disturbs liver function and thus interferes with fibrinogen production. The combination of increased consumption and diminished production of fibrinogen leads to incoagulability of the blood.

THROMBOCYTOPENIA

Although the normal platelet count ranges from $150-400 \times 10^9/l$, a risk of dangerous spontaneous haemorrhage is unusual unless the count falls below $30 \times 10^9/l$.

The causes of thrombocytopenia fall into two main groups:

1. **Deficient marrow production**

   Hypoplasia or aplasia

   Replacement
   (e.g. leukaemia, fibrosis)
   } of marrow

   Dyshaemopoiesis
   (e.g. Vit. B_{12} deficiency)

2. **Increased destruction**

   Platelets damaged by *drugs, immune mechanisms*

   Platelets sequestered in *hypersplenism*

   Platelets utilised in coagulative disorders (e.g. DIC)

NB Marrow examination throws light on the possible mechanism.

In (1) megakaryocytes are reduced in number (except in vit.B_{12} deficiency)

In (2) megakaryocytes are increased and immature in an attempt to make good the platelet loss

Idiopathic thrombocytopenia occurs particularly in children and is usually self limiting; evidence has accumulated that platelet antibodies are responsible. The marrow picture is characteristic with numerous megakaryocytes.

PURPURA

This is the term used for disorders involving bleeding from capillaries, with the production of small petechial spots. In severe cases, more massive bleeding occurs; the subarachnoid space, the alimentary and renal tracts are particularly vulnerable. Thrombocytopenia is the most common cause, but abnormalities of the capillary walls are also due to a variety of agents, e.g. vit C deficiency, allergic immune reactions (Henoch-Schonlein purpura), drugs acting both directly and also as haptens, infections and intoxications and the hereditary condition, haemorrhagic telangiectasis. In the purpuras, the clinical tests for increased capillary fragility are usually positive, while the laboratory tests of coagulation function are normal.

BLOOD TRANSFUSION

Two antigenic group systems, ABO and Rhesus, are of paramount importance, but blood is a complex mixture of many antigenic substances and the increasing use of blood and blood products can give rise to new antibodies with the danger of reactions.

ABO system

One of three alleles, A, B or O, is borne on each of two chromosomes. There are thus six possible genotypes — AA, BB, AB, AO, BO and OO. The O allele is nonantigenic and therefore individuals can be divided into four groups — A, B, AB and O. Plasma contains natural antibodies to the A and B antigens according to the rule: — the particular antibody, anti-A or anti-B, is present in the plasma, provided the red cells do not contain the corresponding antigen. Thus:

Blood group	Antigens on cells	Isoantibodies in plasma
A	AA or AO	Anti-B
B	BB or BO	Anti-A
AB	A + B	none
O	None	Anti-A + Anti-B

AB individuals having no antibodies in their plasma could receive blood of any group and have been termed 'Universal Recipients'. Similarly, group O blood possessing no antigens could be given to any person and is termed 'Universal Donor'. Except in dire emergencies, however, neither of these actions should be taken.

The distribution of these blood groups varies with geography. In Western Scotland, the incidence of the various groups is as follows:

Group O — 53%.   Group A — 33%
Group B — 11%.   Group AB — 3%

The distribution is changing due to population movement and immigration.

Rhesus system

This is another sequence of red cell antigens — first discovered in Rhesus monkeys. There are three pairs of alleles, C or c, D or d, E or e, one of each pair occupying a position on one chromosome, i.e. if C is absent c is present, D absent d present, E absent e present, and vice versa. With any three of the six alleles transmitted by each parent, the genetic make-up is very varied.

BLOOD TRANSFUSION

Rhesus system (continued)

The most frequent groupings of three alleles on one chromosome in the United Kingdom are: CDe, cde, cDE. The most common genotypes are:

| (Abbreviated notation) ----> | CDe/CDe — 17.5% (R R) | cde/cde — 15.0% (r r) | cDE/cde — 5.0% (R r) |
| | CDe/cde — 16.0% (R r) | CDe/cDE — 6.0% (R R) | Other combinations are rare |

The D antigen has the strongest antigenic power and individuals possessing it are termed Rhesus positive. Those who have no D antigen (homozygous for d) are termed Rhesus negative and are at greatest risk of developing antibodies if given Rhesus positive blood. The C antigen also has strong antigenic activity and it is important to test for this antigen and its corresponding antibody.

There are no natural antibodies to Rhesus antigens. They only arise when red cells bearing Rhesus antigens foreign to the patient are introduced into the circulation. They develop in two particular situations:

1. After a Rhesus incompatible transfusion, especially if the transfused cells contain the D antigen and the patient is Rhesus negative.
2. In a proportion of pregnant Rhesus negative women, Rhesus positive (D derived from the father) fetal red cells escape into the maternal circulation inducing antibody formation. The antibody crosses the placenta and causes haemolysis of fetal red cells (see page 534). Rhesus positive blood must never be given to a Rhesus negative patient.

In emergency, where Rhesus grouping is impossible, Rhesus negative ABO compatible blood is given.

Grouping and cross-matching
ABO grouping

1. Standardised anti-A and anti-B sera are used.
2. The test red cells are mixed with the appropriate antiserum.
3. Controls are set up with the individual's RBC versus:
   Group O serum (contains both anti-A and anti-B) and versus:
   Group AB serum (contains no antibodies and should cause no reaction).

The whole set of tests is carries out at room temperature.

Agglutination reaction

	Anti-A	Anti-B	Group O	Group
Patient's RBC	+	−	+	A
or	−	+	+	B
Donor's RBC	+	+	+	AB
	−	−	−	O

BLOOD TRANSFUSION

Rhesus grouping

Anti-C and anti-D are both used. These antisera are collected from sensitised donors and standardised. A mixture of the two antisera previously absorbed to remove anti-A and anti-B is used, and the reactions must be carried out at 37°C.

Two types of antibody may arise in individuals receiving Rh incompatible blood. One, used for Rhesus typing, produces a visible reaction with test red cells suspended in saline. The second type will not do so unless the test cells are suspended in albumin. This is liable to give rise to errors. A more sensitive test has been devised for dealing with this situation.

Coombs' test

The usual test for antibodies is carried out -

A   + Patient's serum = No agglutination

Test cells suspended in saline

Even if there is no reaction, 'albumin' antibodies may be present, attached to the red cells. A further test is now carried out to detect the presence of antibodies (immunoglobulins) on the red cell surface.

B   → Centrifuge →

Tube with test RBC + patient's serum from test A

Discard supernatant fluid. Repeat several times, suspending RBC in fresh saline. This gets rid of patient's serum possibly containing free antibody.

Cells suspended in saline

+ Coombs' reagent (anti-immunoglobulin)

No reaction Coombs' negative = Patient's serum does not contain antibody

Cells agglutinated Coombs' positive = Patient's serum contains antibody

BLOOD TRANSFUSION

Despite tests for ABO and Rhesus groupings, mistakes can still occur due to:

1. Faulty testing — very infrequent
2. Irregular antibodies
3. Clerical errors — wrong identification of patients, donors, specimens, containers, storage.

A final cross-matching test is carried out before transfusion. The red cells of each donor unit of blood are tested against the patient's plasma for the possibility of an antibody reaction against them.

DANGERS of blood transfusion

In addition to incompatibility, other dangers arise in transfusion practice:

1. *Reactions occurring during or very shortly after transfusion*

(a) Fever — may be due to pyrogens in the blood or allergies to degradation products of leucocytes.

(b) Biochemical disturbances — particularly in massive transfusions or if out-dated blood is used.
   (i) Hypocalcaemia (citrate in blood binds Ca^{++}).
   (ii) Hyperkalaemia (lysed RBCs contribute excess K^+).

(c) Circulatory overload — in cases of anaemia or incipient cardiac failure where transfusion is too rapid or excessive.

2. *Delayed infections*

Hepatitis B, AIDS and other infections, e.g. syphilis and malaria are potential risks.

THE LYMPHORETICULAR TISSUES

The basic function of these tissues is FILTRATION of a variety of materials varying from 'foreign' microorganisms and particles to the degradation products of cells and metabolism.

Filtration occurs at the following sites:-

Lymph nodes — tissue fluids
Nasopharynx — tonsils and adenoids
Alimentary tract — submucous lymphoid aggregations
Spleen — blood.
} — surfaces

In the two remaining important lymphoid organs, filtration is not an important function:

Thymus — T lymphocyte processing.
Bone marrow — site of (a) mature lymphoid aggregates
(b) lymphoid stem cells.

In addition, microscopic aggregates of lymphoid cells are scattered throughout the body.

The LYMPH NODES in DISEASE
The basic anatomy reflects the primary function.

Afferent lymphatics conducting lymph from tissues

Efferent lymphatic

FILTER BED — composed of anastomosing sinuses with wide pores and a reticular network

In addition, the presence of special cells reflects functions superimposed on filtration.

(1) Phagocytosis

(2) Immune response

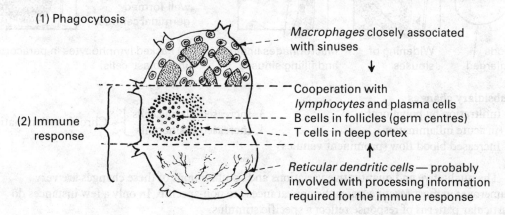

Macrophages closely associated with sinuses

Cooperation with *lymphocytes* and plasma cells
B cells in follicles (germ centres)
T cells in deep cortex

Reticular dendritic cells — probably involved with processing information required for the immune response

DISEASES OF THE LYMPH NODES

The LYMPH NODES in DISEASE (continued)

In physiological conditions, the lymph nodes are small and show minimal evidence of functional activity: the major contribution towards disposal of particles derived from metabolic processes is performed by the spleen.

Very shortly after infection occurs or when the nodes begin to filter noxious particles, **reactive changes** occur — usually causing enlargement of the nodes.

The changes may be **general** ----- or ----- **local** — reflecting disease in the
in systemic INFECTIONS   drainage area, e.g. simple chronic gastric
— bacterial or viral,   ulcer (enlarged reactive nodes in omentum)
e.g. syphilis, measles   — local low grade inflammation;
      ± absorption of foreign particles.

The changes include three basic and several subsidiary:

Normal small inactive lymph node

Small, ill-defined germinal centres

Rather sparse scattering of lymphocytes in reticular framework
Very narrow peripheral sinus

Sinuses *not* prominent

Macrophages *not* prominent

Basic changes

ACTIVATION

(1) Increased flow   (2) Macrophage activation and increase   (3) Lymphocyte activation and increase

(a) Numerous well-formed germinal centres

Node enlarged   Widening of sinuses   Macrophages lining and filling sinuses   (b) Packed lymphocytes in paracortex (incl. 'blast' cells)

Subsidiary changes

1. Infiltration by polymorphs (in acute inflammation)
2. Increased blood flow (prominent venules)

3. Increased plasma cells
4. Increased eosinophils }⟶ Chronic inflammation

The qualitative and quantitative variations and combinations of these changes are very numerous; in most reactive states the appearances are non-specific. In only a few instances do particular patterns of response reflect a specific stimulus.

ACUTE LYMPH NODE ENLARGEMENT

This is usually due to acute infections causing **ACUTE LYMPHADENITIS.**

(a) In many bacterial infections neutrophil infiltration is a feature.

Typhoid fever is an exception — mesenteric node.

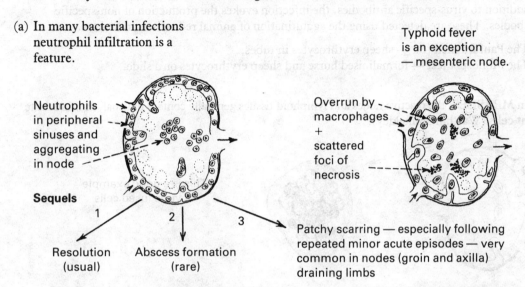

Neutrophils in peripheral sinuses and aggregating in node

Overrun by macrophages + scattered foci of necrosis

Sequels

1
2
3

Resolution (usual)

Abscess formation (rare)

Patchy scarring — especially following repeated minor acute episodes — very common in nodes (groin and axilla) draining limbs

(b) In the majority of acute virus infections, polymorphs are absent and the nonspecific reactive changes previously described are seen.

In **GLANDULAR FEVER** (Infectious mononucleosis), a virus infection (Epstein–Barr virus) of young adults, the cervical lymph nodes are particularly involved.

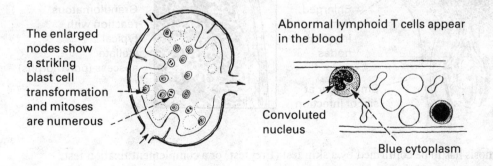

The enlarged nodes show a striking blast cell transformation and mitoses are numerous

Abnormal lymphoid T cells appear in the blood

Convoluted nucleus

Blue cytoplasm

Similar changes are seen in the pharyngeal lymphoid tissues, the spleen and bone marrow.

ACUTE LYMPH NODE ENLARGEMENT

Diagnostic tests

In addition to virus-specific antibodies, the infection evokes the production of non-specific antibodies. These are detected using the agglutination of animal red cells as indicators.

The Paul Bunnell test — sheep erythrocytes in tubes.
The Monospot test — formalinised horse and sheep erythrocytes on a slide.

In **MEASLES,** the reactive nodes and lymphoid tissues generally contain unusual, multinucleate **giant cells** (Warthin-Finkeldey).

This is a good example of virus fused cells

In **LYMPHOGRANULOMA VENEREUM (LGV),** the enlarged lymph nodes show a striking histological appearance.

LGV is an infection by a **chlamydial** organism. The portal of entry is by venereal contact and the disease runs a subacute course.

Enlarged, firm inguinal nodes

Small ulcer at site of infection

Granulomatous reaction with typical stellate abscess (polymorphs)

The diagnosis has to be confirmed by a skin test (Frei test) or a complement fixation test.

In **CAT SCRATCH FEVER,** the nodes draining the scratched area show similar histological changes but the organism has not yet been identified.

CHRONIC LYMPH NODE ENLARGEMENT

This common and important clinical sign may give rise to difficulty in diagnosis in practice.

Aetiology
The many and varied causes are considered under three main headings:

1. **Enlargement due to low grade chronic INFLAMMATION, local or general**
   In most cases, the enlargement is due to reactive hyperplasia and the morphological changes are essentially similar so that the aetiology cannot be deduced from the histological appearance of the node.

   Specific diagnosis depends on identification of the infecting organism (a) by direct staining and/or (b) by culture and/or (c) by serological tests for specific antibodies.

   In only a few conditions do the histological appearances give a clue to the aetiology, e.g. (a) tuberculosis and sarcoidosis and (b) toxoplasmosis.

	TUBERCULOSIS	SARCOIDOSIS
Basic lesion	Follicular granuloma	Essentially similar
Progress	Confluence and caseation	Follicles remain discrete No caseation
Identification of tubercle bacilli (direct staining and/or culture)		No organisms identified
Mantoux test — positive (using tuberculo-protein)		Mantoux text — negative
Kveim test — negative		Kveim test – positive (using sarcoid tissue)

Somewhat similar follicular granulomata occur in other conditions, e.g. Crohn's disease, primary biliary cirrhosis, and other penetrating ulcerations of the alimentay tract.

CHRONIC LYMPH NODE ENLARGEMENT

Low grade infections (continued)

TOXOPLASMOSIS

In toxoplasmosis, a protozoal disease (*Toxoplasma gondii*) which may cause serious damage to the fetus or neonate and present with lymph node enlargement in the adult, the histological appearances in the node may indicate the aetiology. The diagnosis has to be confirmed by a serological dye test.

In addition to the usual reactive changes

↓

A scattering of large clear macrophages

↓

Numerous smaller macrophages in the sinuses

2. **Enlargement due to filtration of surfaces and tissues — NON-INFECTIVE**

In these conditions, particulate matter (and in some cases soluble material) of a non-infective nature is filtered and deposited in excess. In the majority of cases, there is a reactive hyperplasia and the enlargement is accentuated if the particles have an "irritant" effect.

The source of particles may be:
  Exogenous, e.g. exposure to environmental pollutant (lung hilar lymph nodes in SILICOSIS)
  Endogenous, due to breakdown of tissues or abnormal metabolism,
  e.g. (a) In **tumour necrosis**

Particulate and soluble material

Breast carcinoma necrosis

(1) Reactive hyperplasia in axillary nodes

(2) Infiltration by **SECONDARY CARCINOMA** is itself an important and common cause of lymph node enlargement

In tumour cases, the distinction between these two causes of lymph node enlargement can only be made with certainty by histological examination.

CHRONIC LYMPH NODE ENLARGEMENT

Filtration — Non-infective (continued)

(b) In **chronic skin disease** with a considerable component of tissue damage.

In addition to the usual
reactive hyperplasia the
following may be seen
lying free and in macrophages:
    Fat
    Melanin — from damaged skin
    Haemosiderin — from minor
    bleeding in skin

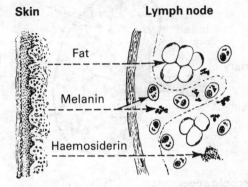

The identification of these substances in the node allows the diagnosis of **DERMATOPATHIC LYMPHADENOPATHY** (lipomelanic 'reticulosis').

In **metabolic diseases** such as haemachromatosis (p. 24) and the storage diseases (p. 27) the lymph nodes are enlarged due to the presence of large quantities of the abnormal deposit (e.g. iron, lipids). The contribution of reactive hyperplasia to the enlargement is usually small.

3. **Enlargement due to PRIMARY LYMPHOID NEOPLASMS** (see p.595)
The main examples are:
    Hodgkin's disease and the non-Hodgkin's lymphomas particularly the follicular lymphomas in which lymph node enlargement may be considerable.
    There is an additional group of conditions involving a proliferation of macrophages, called histiocytosis-X in which lymph node enlargement is often a feature.

SPLEEN

The anatomy of the spleen reflects both its basic function, which is filtration of the blood, and sequential functions of phagocytosis and the immune response. Normal average weight — 150g.

Artery

Vein

Slow circulation through red pulp which forms the bulk of the spleen tissue

The white pulp consists of aggregates of lymphoid tissue just visible to the naked eye

Capsule and supporting trabeculae

Microscopic appearance

Lymphoid aggregate — mediates IMMUNE RESPONSE.

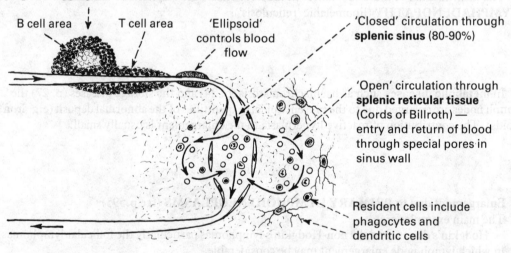

B cell area   T cell area   'Ellipsoid' controls blood flow

'Closed' circulation through **splenic sinus** (80-90%)

'Open' circulation through **splenic reticular tissue** (Cords of Billroth) — entry and return of blood through special pores in sinus wall

Resident cells include phagocytes and dendritic cells

The red pulp is the site of filtration and phagocytosis of the following:

1. Effete cells and cell debris — especially blood cells but also cell debris derived from the body generally

2. Microbes and their toxins

3. Abnormal or excess material derived from metabolic processes.

SPLENOMEGALY

Enlargement of the spleen is an important and common clinical sign. Increase in the red pulp due to increased numbers of phagocytes and/or increased numbers of blood cells is the major component; in chronic infections particularly, hyperplasia of the lymphoid tissue contributes.

An aetiological classification under 5 broad headings is convenient.

Enlargement associated with:

      1. INFECTIONS
      2. CIRCULATORY DISTURBANCES
      3. STORAGE DISEASES and DEGENERATIONS
      4. NEOPLASIA — primary and secondary
      5. DISORDERS OF THE BLOOD.

1. INFECTIONS

In acute systemic bacterial infections the spleen shows slight to moderate enlargement (200 – 400 g).

Cut surface uniform
pink or red — white
pulp obscured due to:
  CONGESTION
  ↑ PHAGOCYTES
  ↑ NEUTROPHILS
      ↓
  After death the enzymes
rapidly digest splenic tissues

'SEPTIC' spleen at autopsy

Soft with
wrinkled
capsule

Red fluid
flows from
cut surface

Sequels

  (a) Resolution as infection resolves.
  (b) Occasionally spreads through capsule (perisplenitis) to adjacent tissues, with or without abscess formation.
  (c) Only extremely rarely does abscess formation occur within the spleen.

In non-pyogenic and chronic infections, there may be moderate enlargement.

Firm

Cut surface shows
lymphoid aggregates

Red pulp contains
increased PHAGOCYTES.
often PLASMA CELLS

Examples: Subacute bacterial endocarditis
              Tuberculosis
              Typhoid fever
              Infectious mononucleosis
              Brucellosis
              Malaria   } protozoal
              Kala-azar } diseases
              – often massive enlargement

SPLENOMEGALY

2. CIRCULATORY DISTURBANCES

Congestive splenomegaly occurs in two main conditions:

(1) Congestive cardiac failure

(2) Hepatic cirrhosis

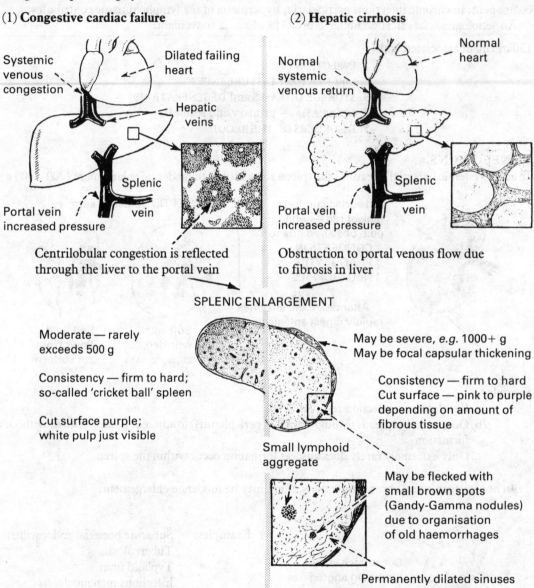

Systemic venous congestion

Dilated failing heart

Hepatic veins

Splenic vein

Portal vein increased pressure

Centrilobular congestion is reflected through the liver to the portal vein

Normal heart

Normal systemic venous return

Splenic vein

Portal vein increased pressure

Obstruction to portal venous flow due to fibrosis in liver

SPLENIC ENLARGEMENT

Moderate — rarely exceeds 500 g

Consistency — firm to hard; so-called 'cricket ball' spleen

Cut surface purple; white pulp just visible

May be severe, *e.g.* 1000+ g
May be focal capsular thickening

Consistency — firm to hard
Cut surface — pink to purple depending on amount of fibrous tissue

Small lymphoid aggregate

May be flecked with small brown spots (Gandy-Gamma nodules) due to organisation of old haemorrhages

Permanently dilated sinuses

The type of splenomegaly associated with portal venous hypertension may have serious haematological effects (see hypersplenism).

SPLENOMEGALY

3. STORAGE DISEASES AND DEGENERATIONS

The diseases associated with this type of enlargement are rare.

Examples are:

Amyloidosis (see pp.15-18)

Lipid storage diseases, (see p.27) including Gaucher's disease,
Neimann Pick disease and Tay-Sachs disease

Some disorders of glycogen storage.

4. NEOPLASIA

(a) PRIMARY — the spleen is rarely the seat of primary tumour growth.

(b) SECONDARY — the spleen is rarely affected by other types of secondary.
tumour, e.g. carcinoma and sarcoma, but it is commonly
affected during the systematised spread of **lymphomas**
and **leukaemias.**

Normal spleen 150 g	Moderate enlargement 500 g	Massive enlargement 1500 g

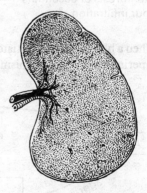

Nodules of white
lymphoma tissue
e.g. Hodgkin's disease

Uniform, beefy, cut surface
in chronic leukaemia

Splenic enlargement may be a feature of histiocytosis-X (see p. 607).

SPLENOMEGALY

5. DISORDERS OF THE BLOOD
Splenic enlargement is associated with blood disorders in two main circumstances:

1. Splenic enlargement causing blood disorders.

ENLARGED SPLEEN from any cause, but particularly in cases of **portal hypertension** → Increased capacity for sequestration of blood cells → Reduction in circulating blood cells, i.e. *anaemia, leucopenia, thrombocytopenia,* separately or together, i.e. **pancytopenia**

Marrow hyperplasia ←

This syndrome is called **hypersplenism** (splenic anaemia)

2. Blood disorder causing splenic enlargement

(a) Production of abnormal blood cells, e.g. in haemolytic anaemias: idiopathic thrombocytopenia (antibody coated platelets) → Increased demand on sequestration function of spleen → Increase in spleen size

(b) In leukaemias and lymphomas → Infiltration of spleen by neoplastic cells / Increased sequestration of abnormal cells → Increase in spleen size

(c) In chronic marrow failure due to fibrosis or secondary tumour infiltration → Resumption by spleen of fetal blood forming role → Increase in spleen size — may be massive (500 — 2,000 g)

Note: When a blood disorder initiates splenic enlargement the disability may be compounded by a superimposed hypersplenism, e.g.

MALARIA (haemolysis of parasitised red cells)

ANAEMIA

SPLENIC ENLARGEMENT

Anaemia aggravated

INCREASED SEQUESTRATION of RBCs (HYPERSPLENISM)

DISEASES OF THE SPLEEN — MISCELLANEOUS

HYPOSPLENISM

Hyposplenism is not usually a cause of major disability. It occurs following splenectomy and in cases of splenic atrophy.

The effects are considered under two main headings:-

1. *On the cells of the blood*

Loss of splenic sequestration function

↓

Deficiency in disposal of abnormal cells

Red cell series:
(a) increased acanthocytes
(b) increased Howell-Jolly bodies
(c) increased number of iron-containing cells

Neutrophils:
may be
leukocytosis

Platelets:
may be
thrombocythaemia

Seen especially after splenectomy
— usually not permanent

2. **On resistance to infection**

Loss of filtration of
bacteria from blood → Occasional cases of **septicaemia** — especially caused by *Diplococcus pneumoniae* — young children are particularly susceptible

CIRCULATORY AND VASCULAR CHANGES

(a) *Infarction*
(i) Embolism causing infarction is not uncommon but usually clinically unimportant.

(ii) Enlarged spleens are particularly susceptible to infarction without embolism.

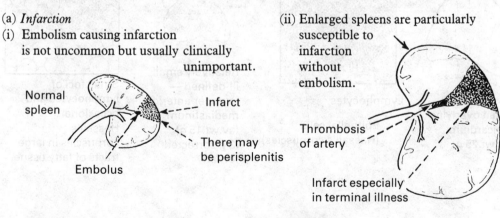

Normal spleen

Infarct

There may be perisplenitis

Embolus

Thrombosis of artery

Infarct especially in terminal illness

(b) *Hyalinisation of splenic arterioles*
This is an almost invariable concomitant of ageing and is not related to systemic arteriosclerosis or hypertension.

Hyaline thickening of arteriolar wall

THYMUS

This 'primary' lymphoid organ is concerned with the development and processing to maturation of the long-lived T lymphocytes which are then contributed to the lymphoid tissues and to the circulating pool of T lymphocytes.

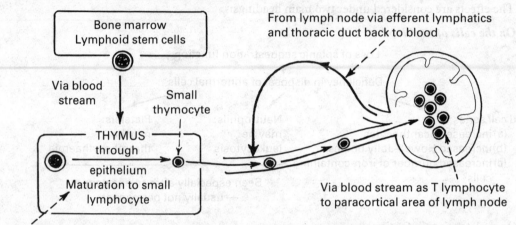

Mechanism — stimulation by hormones formed locally to thymic epithelial cells.

This activity is maximal in the fetal and childhood stages. Involution is rapid after puberty.

Large cellular organ overlying pericardium (av.wt.25 g)

Childhood

Lymphocytes

Epithelial cells (Hassall's corpuscles)

Adult

Relatively small, ill-defined — in upper anterior mediastinum (av.wt.15 g) (3 g corrected for fat)

Small foci of lymphocytes and occasional Hassall's corpuscles in large tracts of fatty tissue.

Congenital thymic aplasia or hypoplasia

The resulting T cell deficiency is associated with disordered cell-mediated immune response.

Note: Thymectomy in adult life has little pathological significance since the T lymphocytes produced in childhood are long enough lived to obviate serious immune deficiency.

THYMUS

Thymic hyperplasia

Assessment by weight alone is unsatisfactory due to the variability of the fat content in adult life. A weight over 35 g probably represents hyperplasia, but the appearance of lymphoid follicles with germinal centres is a more reliable indication of hyperplasia.

Associated conditions:
Auto-immune disorders,
e.g. Systemic lupus erythematosis
Addison's disease
Thyrotoxicosis
Pancytopaenia
and *NB* MYASTHENIA GRAVIS

Thymic tumours

These rare tumours, which are composed of a variable mixture of both lymphocytes and epithelial cells, rarely metastasise. Their pathological effects and associations form two main groups:

(1) By their sheer bulk these lobulated and nodular tumours compress adjacent mediastinal structures

(a) Compression of respiratory passages → dyspnoea and cough.
(b) Oesphagus → dysphagia.
(c) Great veins → cyanosis and suffusion of face.

(2) Associated conditions:

These have an auto-immune component similar to those associated with thymic hyperplasia. *NB* MYASTHENIA GRAVIS.

The thymus in myasthenia gravis (MG)

MG is a disease of voluntary muscles in which weakness is the main feature. The association with the thymus is striking in that 4/5 of all cases of MG have either thymic hyperplasia or thymoma.

Follicular hyperplasia (80%) — seen especially in young females.
Thymoma (20%) — seen especially in middle aged males.
The results of thymectomy in MG patients are very unpredictable.

The detailed pathological changes in MG and the mechanisms by which the thymus is linked with the disease are described on page 784.

585

LEUKAEMIA

Primary neoplasia of the bone marrow and lymphoreticular tissues

Since all these tissues are the sites of blood cell production or important staging posts in the complex circulation of the blood cells, it is convenient to consider their tumours together.

1. Neoplastic proliferation in the bone marrow usually leads to an increased number of circulating white blood cells — the condition is called LEUKAEMIA.

   In some cases there is no spill over into the blood, and the white cell count is low or normal — this condition is called ALEUKAEMIC LEUKAEMIA.

Neoplastic leucocytes filling marrow including long bones.

Total marrow cellularity (no fat spaces)

(a) Spill over into blood

LEUKAEMIA

Increased WBC, e.g. 20,000 to 250,000/ml

(b) No spill over

ALEUKAEMIC LEUKAEMIA

WBC normal or low

2. Neoplastic proliferation within the lymphoid tissues results in solid tumours — called LYMPHOMAS, but in some cases spill over into the blood occurs (leukaemic phase).

Neoplastic proliferation of lymphoid cells

(a) Begins in local lymphoid tissue – (enlarged lymp nodes)

(b) Spread to other lymphoid tissues including spleen and bone marrow

} LYMPHOMA

(c) May overflow to peripheral blood — LEUKAEMIC phase

LEUKAEMIA

In all leukaemias, the marrow is eventually over-run by functionally abnormal neoplastic cells.

CELL KINETICS

Cell longevity beyond the normal (due to failure of response to mechanisms controlling ageing and destruction) is as important as proliferative rates in increasing the marrow cell population.

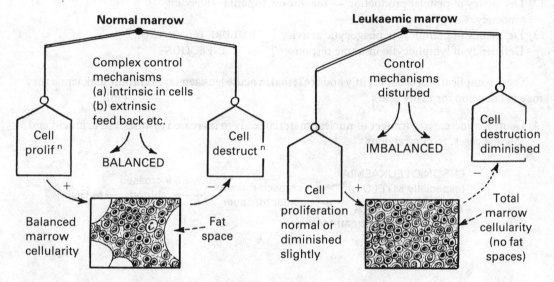

The rate at which marrow overcrowding occurs influences the rate of progress of the disease and allows classification into two broad groups: (1) the ACUTE and (2) the CHRONIC LEUKAEMIAS.

Cell differentiation

The ability of the leukaemic cells to differentiate also reflects the rate of progress.

Acute leukaemia	*Chronic leukaemia*
Numerous 'blast' cells.	Few blast cells — numerous cells on differentiation pathway to granulocytes or lymphocytes.

Considerations of cell kinetics and differentiations are important in treatment.

Further classification in two main groups depends on the neoplastic cell types.

(a) MYELOID LEUKAEMIA
  — cells of the granulocytic series.

(b) LYMPHOCYTIC LEUKAEMIA
  — cells of the lymphoid series.

Rarer leukaemias are of monocytic and plasma cell types. Similar proliferative conditions can affect red cells and megakaryocytes.

LEUKAEMIA

The marrow overcrowding and, more important, the functional abnormalities of the neoplastic cells lead to functional marrow failure and the complications which cause the major clinical signs.

Complications

(1) Deficiency of red cell production — **anaemia**
(2) Deficiency of platelet production — **thrombocytopenia** – bleeding tendency.
(3) Deficiency of granulocyte phagocytic activity ⎫ FAILURE TO CONTROL
     Deficiency of lymphocytic immune response ⎭ INFECTION

These complications occur rapidly and are lethal in acute leukaemia; in chronic leukaemia they may not develop for many years.

(4) Gout: the increased turnover of nuclear material leads to increased synthesis of uric acid and, in some cases, to clinical gout.

CHRONIC LEUKAEMIA
(especially MYELOID) ⟶ Increased marrow cellular turnover ⟶ Increased blood uric acid ⟶ GOUT
ACUTE LEUKAEMIA ⟋
(especially during treatment)

Metastases

Since leukaemic cells have a natural tendency to circulate in the blood and/or lymph, it is theoretically possible for metastasis to occur anywhere in the body. Nodular deposits in the body generally are rare however.

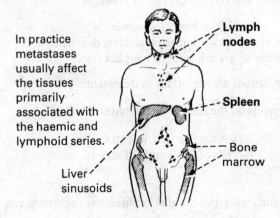

In practice metastases usually affect the tissues primarily associated with the haemic and lymphoid series.

Lymph nodes

Spleen

Bone marrow

Liver sinusoids

NB: after initially successful treatment, leukaemia infiltration may recur especially in the CNS (meninges) and the testis.

THE ACUTE LEUKAEMIAS

The marrow

Over-run by *blast cells*

The blood

⅔ cases: WBC
20,000 – 50,000
blast cells
⅓ cases: **aleukaemic**

Decreased
platelet count: **thrombocytopenia**

Other organs+splenomegaly+hepatomegaly+lymph node enlargement

Since modern chemotherapy is geared to the neoplastic cell type, it is important, if possible, to establish an accurate diagnosis. The most primitive blast cells are truly undifferentiated. However in most cases the cells go a short way towards differentiation. Cytochemical tests, particularly with, enzyme markers, are used.

The modern classification (FAB) of the acute myeloid leukaemia includes the relatively rare monocytic or promyelocytic types.

Monocytic leukaemia

There are two morphological types:

1. The Naegeli (myelomonocytic) type
   the cells have "myeloid" features
2. The Schilling type
   the cells closely resemble monocytes.

   The serum contains an increased amount of
   lysozyme (muramidase) produced by the tumour cells.

Promyelocytic leukaemia

In this subtype maturation arrest occurs at the promyelocyte stage.

Primitive cell
with primary
myeloid
granules

The destruction of effete cells releases
1. *Vit B₁₂ binding protein*
   High serum vit B₁₂
2. *Thromboplastic substances*
   ↓
   Coagulation and bleeding
   complications (compounding
   effects of thrombocytopenia)

589

THE ACUTE LEUKAEMIAS

The following table gives an indication of the methods used to differentiate the acute leukaemias.

	Acute myeloid (AML)	Acute lymphoblastic leukaemias (ALL)
Age	Adults mainly	Children mainly
Associated cells	May be recognisable granulocyte precursors	May be recognisable lymphocytic types
Blast cell: nucleoli	Multiple	Single
Cytoplasmic features PAS (glycogen)	+ Fine granules	++ Coarse granules
Peroxidase and Sudan Black B	++	–
Auer rods (crystalline — staining red)	+	
Acid phosphatase	–	Lumps

In addition, monoclonal antibodies to lymphoid antigens are useful in differentiating the acute lymphoblastic leukaemias.

THE CHRONIC LEUKAEMIAS

These disorders occurring in middle and late adult life probably are present in latent form long before clinical presentation, and continue to evolve slowly over years. The basic pathological features are:

TOTAL MARROW CELLULARITY
well differentiated cells → HIGH LEUCOCYTE COUNT in BLOOD

INFILTRATION OF ORGANS
especially SPLENOMEGALY and HEPATOMEGALY
± lymph node enlargement

The two distinct types of chronic leukaemias — **myeloid** and **lymphocytic** will be described separately.

THE CHRONIC LEUKAEMIAS

CHRONIC MYELOID LEUKAEMIA (CML)

Marrow

Total cellularity:
cells of granulocyte
series — late forms
numerous (including
eosinophil and
basophil types).

Often increase in megakaryocytes;
may be increased fibrosis

Increased pressure in bones may cause
clinical tenderness and pain.

Blood

(a) WBC: 75,000 – 250,000/mm^3
Differential WBC
Blasts
Promyelocytes $\Big\}$ <5%

Majority of cells are
late myelocytes and
mature granulocytes

(b) ANAEMIA

(c) THROMBOCYTOPENIA
(sometimes thrombocytosis)

Splenomegaly

Firm, may be
massive, e.g. 3kg

May be
infarction
± perisplenitis

↓

Clinically painful

Lymphoid
follicles
inconspicuous

Red pulp
with cells of
granulocyte series ± megakaryocytes
± red cell precursors

Complications

1. Bleeding and thrombotic tendency.
2. Gout.

Progress

1. The majority of cases terminate in a **'blast cell crisis'** — the marrow is overrun by primitive
   myeloid cells and the course is that of acute leukaemia.
2. A small minority end with marrow failure due to **FIBROSIS**.

Specific chromosomal abnormalities — the Philadelphia chromosome (Ph')

About 90 per cent of cases show deletion of a short arm of chromosome 22 in the granulocyte
precursors (red cell precursors and megakaryocytes are also affected).

591

CHRONIC LYMPHOCYTIC LEUKAEMIA (CLL)

This is the commonest leukaemia (30% of all cases); it is best considered as the leukaemic form of DIFFUSE LYMPHOMA — well differentiated lymphocytic type (see p. 602).

The disease is found in late middle and old age and in many cases it has probably been present for many years before clinical symptoms appear: an increasing number of cases are discovered by blood examination during routine health checks.

The disease begins and spreads in the lymphoid tissues, and in the established case there is generalised moderate lymph node enlargement and splenomegaly.

Lymph node

Spleen

The lymph node and splenic architecture is obscured by closely packed small lymphocytes
Mitotic activity is minimal, but very small foci of larger active cells (proliferation centres) are the source of new neoplastic cells.

Germinal centres destroyed by infiltrating lymphocytes

In some cases the lymphoid enlargement precedes the leukaemic phase.

The marrow

The blood picture

Early

Scattered foci of small lymphocytes in otherwise normal marrow

At this stage the lymphocyte count may be only slightly raised, e.g. 20,000; other blood cells normal

Later

Marrow packed with monotonous population of small lymphocytes

Lymphocyte count up to 100,000 — smear cells in film

Neutropenia, thrombocytopenia, anaemia

CHRONIC LYMPHOCYTIC LEUKAEMIA (CLL)

The LYMPHOCYTE in CLL

The disease is the result of the very slow **MONOCLONAL** proliferation of B lymphocytes which differentiate to the small **LONG-LIVED** type.

Although the cells can be recognised as B cells with typical surface markers, they are usually functionally incompetent so that IMMUNOLOGICAL DEFICIENCY is an important complication.

The immunological deficiency allows opportunistic infections and occasionally *autoimmune haemolytic anaemia*.

Other complications are:
Hypersplenism – aggravating the anaemia,
                 neutropenia and
                 thrombocytopenia
                 mentioned on previous page

and
Skin rashes with pruritus.

THE LEUKAEMIAS

LEUKAEMOID REACTIONS

Mimicking chronic myeloid leukaemia

In these rare reactions, the blood changes resemble leukaemia. CML may be mimicked by the reactive leucocytosis of pyogenic infections, in miliary tuberculosis and following treatment with folic acid in macrocytic anaemia of pregnancy.

The following points may be useful in diagnosis:

	CML	Leukaemoid reactions
Splenomegaly	+++	±
Blood film **shift to left** **myelocytes** **basophils**	+ + +	+ ± +
Alkaline Phosphatase **(in neutrophils)**	↓	↑
Serum vit. B$_{12}$	↑	Normal or ↓
Philadelphia **chromosome**	+	—

Mimicking lymphoid leukaemias

In childhood infections, e.g. whooping cough and chicken pox, and in glandular fever the peripheral blood picture with increased numbers of abnormal lymphocytes may cause diagnostic difficulty. The neoplastic lymphocytes are usually much more homogeneous in contrast to the range of morphological atypia seen in 'virocytes'.

THE LYMPHOMAS

These solid tumours which arise in the peripheral lymphoreticular tissues are divided into two main groups: (1) HODGKIN'S DISEASE (HD) and (2) The NON-HODGKIN LYMPHOMAS (NHL).

Paradoxically although the histogenesis of the neoplastic cell in HD is still not known, a histological classification of world-wide acceptance has been established and clearly linked with clinical progress and therapy. In contrast, the classification of NHL is confused due to differences in nomenclature and difficulty in relating the histological appearances to the rapidly growing knowledge of lymphocyte function.

HODGKIN'S DISEASE

Incidence

The disease, which is the commonest type of lymphoma, may occur at any age but there are two peaks of incidence.

Natural course

1. The majority of cases evolve slowly — several years }   Ultimately
2. A minority progress rapidly — months   }   fatal.

NB Modern therapy has completely changed the outcome in this disease — a majority of cases are now cured.

Presentation on spread

The disease begins in a single lymph node, followed by spread to adjacent nodes and then to other organs in a fairly consistent pattern. It often presents clinically as enlargement of accessible nodes (e.g. cervical) without other symptoms, but if the disease has begun in deep nodes considerable spread may have occurred and there are then clinical symptoms referrable to the complications.

HODGKIN'S DISEASE

Presentation and spread (continued)

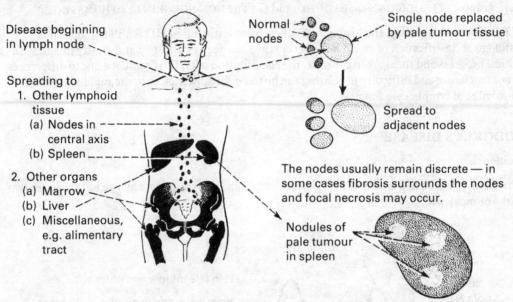

Disease beginning in lymph node

Spreading to
1. Other lymphoid tissue
   (a) Nodes in central axis
   (b) Spleen

2. Other organs
   (a) Marrow
   (b) Liver
   (c) Miscellaneous, e.g. alimentary tract

Normal nodes

Single node replaced by pale tumour tissue

Spread to adjacent nodes

The nodes usually remain discrete — in some cases fibrosis surrounds the nodes and focal necrosis may occur.

Nodules of pale tumour in spleen

The amount of spread which has already occured at first clinical presentation influences prognosis and the therapeutic attack so that the 'staging' of the disease in the individual case is of great importance.

Staging

Stage I	Disease involving single node or group of nodes
Stage II	Disease in more than one site — all lesions either below or above the diaphragm
Stage III	Disease on both sides of diaphragm
Stage IV	Widespread involvement of extralymphoid sites ± lymph node involvement

The suffix (E) indicates an extralymphoid site.
The suffix (S) indicates splenic disease,
e.g. Stage III SE means disease in nodes on both sides of diaphragm with splenic and extralymphoid involvement.
The absence (A) or presence (B) of systemic clinical symptoms also relate to prognosis.

HODGKIN'S DISEASE

The diagnosis of Hodgkin's disease and the presence or absence of spread can only be made with certainty by microscopic examination of tissues.

The disease presents a considerable variety of histological patterns, but the one constant feature is the presence of Reed-Sternberg (RS) cells.

Typical RS cell

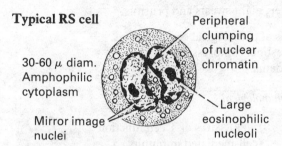

30-60 μ diam. Amphophilic cytoplasm

Peripheral clumping of nuclear chromatin

Large eosinophilic nucleoli

Mirror image nuclei

The further histological classification of Hodgkin's disease depends on the recognition of histological patterns.

The RYE classification

1. *Lymphocyte — predominant (15%)*

Scanty RS cells

Very numerous Lymphocytes

2. *Nodular sclerosing (20 – 30%)*

Thick bands of collagen separating Hodgkin's tissue

Lacunar cells often numerous

Often mediastinal presentation

3. *Mixed cellularity (40 – 50%)*

Plasma cells and eosinophils present in addition to RS cells and lymphocytes

Cells closely related to the RS cell:

1. **The lacunar cell**

Shrinkage of cell cytoplasm towards cell wall and nucleus, leaving a clear space

2. **Mononuclear Hodgkin's cell**

Nuclear characteristic similar to RS cell but smaller

These cells are not specifically diagnostic of Hodgkin's disease.

4. *Lymphocyte — depleted (15%)*

Very numerous RS and mononuclear Hodgkin's cells — few lymphocytes ± diffuse fibrosis

Transition from better to worse prognosis type occurs 1 → 3 → 4 but nodular sclerosing usually remains true to type.

HODGKIN'S DISEASE

Symptomatology and complications

The symptoms can be divided into two main groups:

1. Symptoms for which the mechanisms are obscure — include
   variable fatigue, weight loss, intermittent fever, night sweats and pruritus.

2. Symptoms associated with three broad groups of pathological complications.
   (a) *Lymph node enlargement* causing mediastinal compression
   and lymphoedema.

(b) *Haematological*

ANAEMIA
    ESR elevated
    Occasionally eosinophilia
    Occasional myeloid
       leukaemoid reactions
    Occasionally lymphopenia

(c) *Immunological*

DEPRESSION of T cell function
(cell-mediated immunity)

Susceptibility to infection (esp. opportunistic)

Skin tests modified, e.g. tuberculin test becomes negative

NB MODERN THERAPY
may aggravate these complications

The nature of the disease

The essential nature is not clear — the aetiology is not known. The disease presents some of the features of a neoplasm, but inflammatory changes are also an intrinsic component so that the possibility of an infective origin still remains.

The current, most widely held view is that it is a malignant neoplasm — the neoplastic cells being the Hodgkin's mononuclear cells of which the RS cells are a special type; the inflammatory and immunological changes are interpreted as being secondary to the neoplastic proliferation.

THE NON-HODGKIN LYMPHOMAS

The non-Hodgkin lymphomas are solid tumours arising in the peripheral lymphoreticular tissues, particularly of the LYMPH NODES but also of the oropharynx, the gut, skin and other sites.

Aggregate of enlarged cervical nodes affected by lymphoma

By tradition the lymphoid neoplasms arising in the bone marrow and thymus are considered separately, but this separation is essentially artificial.

The relationship to leukaemia has also been referred to (see p. 586).

Spread   The spread reflects the natural circulation of lymphocytes.

(a) Tumours arising in lymph nodes

Spread to:

Other nodes

Bone marrow

Spleen

(b) Tumours arising in extranodal sites

e.g. Orbit

Breast

Intestine

Testis

May show 'ecotaxis' i.e. a homing instinct and spread first to the contralateral organ.

Eventually spread can be generalised and many organs may be infiltrated, e.g. heart, CNS, kidney, liver and lungs.

CLASSIFICATION

The traditional classifications are purely morphological and were established when knowledge of the development and functional activities of lymphoid cells was minimal.

Modern classifications incorporating the new knowledge in various ways and using varying nomenclatures have been proposed and used by some authorities.

THE NON-HODGKIN LYMPHOMAS

CLASSIFICATION (continued)

Most modern classifications incorporate three basic components with varying emphasis on each: (1) morphological considerations, (2) degree of malignancy (i.e. the rate of progress) and (3) functional cell types.

1. Morphological considerations

(a) *Architectural*

A striking architectural feature distinguishes two main groups:

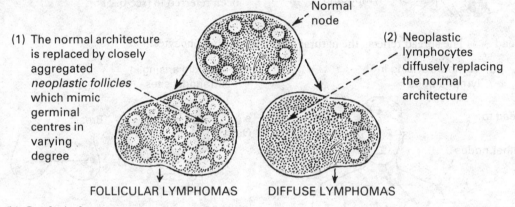

(1) The normal architecture is replaced by closely aggregated *neoplastic follicles* which mimic germinal centres in varying degree

Normal node

(2) Neoplastic lymphocytes diffusely replacing the normal architecture

FOLLICULAR LYMPHOMAS   DIFFUSE LYMPHOMAS

(b) *Cytological*

The cellular morphology of lymphomas can be related to some of the cell types seen in lymph nodes.

(1) Small round lymphocyte

(2) Cells of the germinal centre (follicular centre cells, FCC)

Small   Large FCC

The counterparts are easily recognised in lymphomas.

(3) Cells showing differentiation towards plasma cells. (lymphoplasmacytoid)

(4) Blast cells

    (a) large transformed cells (immunoblasts) seen in reactive nodes

Large nucleolus

Cytoplasm full of RNA

    (b) smaller blast cells (lymphoblasts) identified with difficulty in reactive nodes

Identification of blast cell types and histiocytes may give rise to difficulty in lymphomas.

(5) Macrophages (histiocytes)

THE NON-HODGKIN LYMPHOMAS

DEGREE OF MALIGNANCY

The natural history tends to separate lymphomas into two main groups which have links with the morphological appearances.

1. *Low grade malignancy* associated with well differentiated relatively inactive cell types, — progress of years.

2. *High grade malignancy* associated with primitive actively proliferating cells, — progress over weeks or months.

FUNCTIONAL CELL TYPES

Using special techniques, the lymphomas can be classified in terms of the broad functional groups of normal lymphocytes (B, T and 'null' cell types) and of macrophages.

Technique

Histological Sections (PAP technique)   *Cells identified*

(a) The demonstration of monoclonal immunoglobulin (Ig) synthesis. —— Some B cell lymphomas, all lymphoplasmacytoid and plasma cell tumours

(b) The demonstration of muramidase (lysozyme) —— Histiocytic tumours

Cell preparations

Surface markers

(a) Ig —————————————— B cells
(b) Rosettes with sheep erythrocytes ———— T cells
(c) (a) and (b) negative ———————— 'null' cells

Notes: 1. Monoclonal antibodies are now used in both histological sections and cell preparation to identify an increasing number of antigen surface markers (particularly useful in T cell identification).
2. The great majority of lymphomas are of B cell type. They include all follicular and lymphoplasmacytoid types and most cases of chronic lymphocytic leukaemia (CLL).
3. The more primitive the cells the less likely are markers demonstrable, therefore many primitive tumours are of 'null' cell type.

The rapid advances which are now being made in the discrimination of lymphocyte subsets are superimposed on a basic morphological classification.

THE NON-HODGKIN LYMPHOMAS

CLASSIFICATION (continued)

In the meantime a practical classification has still to be based on the morphological appearances using light microscopy.

The following classification is used in Britain by the National Lymphoma Investigation.

Degree of malignancy	Morphological type	Functional cell type
		—
Low	**FOLLICULAR LYMPHOMA** 1. (a) Follicle cells predominantly small (b) Follicle cells mixed small and large (c) Follicle cells predominantly large	B
	DIFFUSE LYMPHOMA 2. Lymphocytic, well differentiated (CLL) (Small round lymphocytes)	B or T
	3. Lymphocytic, intermediate differentiated (small follicle lymphocyte and lymphoplasmacytic types)	B
High	4. Lymphocytic, poorly differentiated (lymphoblastic) (a) non-Burkitt (includes ALL)	T (or B) or 'null'
	(b) Burkitt	B
	(c) convoluted cell mediastinal tumour (Sternberg)	T
	5. Lymphocytic, mixed small and large cell (mixed follicle cells)	B
	6. 'Undifferentiated' large cell (large lymphoid cell)	B or 'null'
	7. Histiocytic cell	Mononuclear phagocytic cell
Variable	8. Plasma cell (extramedullary)	B
	9. Unclassified	—

THE NON-HODGKIN LYMPHOMAS

Pathological complications

These are very similar to those of Hodgkin's disease.

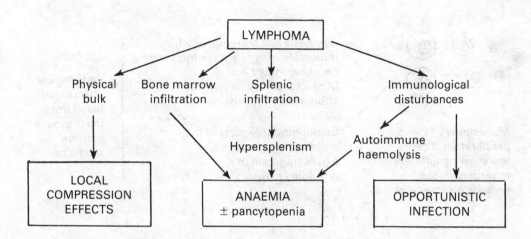

Progress of disease

Low grade malignancy

Often widespread especially to marrow → may be minimal clinical effects.

Follicular lymphomas particularly, may change at any time to blast cell type with serious deterioration.

High grade malignancy
Local nodes initially affected ⟶ rapid spread with extensive
formation of tumour nodules.
may be leukaemia (ALL).

Staging

Unlike Hodgkin's disease, there is no clear-cut relationship between the pathological staging and the clinical progress.

Five particular types of tumour are worthy of more detailed description since they present special features of interest.

1. The lymphoplasmacytic tumours
2. The plasma cell tumours
3. Macrophage (histiocytic) tumours
4. Lymphomas of the alimentary tract
5. Burkitt's lymphoma.

THE NON-HODGKIN LYMPHOMAS

The LYMPHOPLASMACYTIC TUMOURS

These low grade tumours, arising particularly in lymph nodes, but sometimes in the alimentary tract, synthesise and may secrete monoclonal immunoglobin (Ig) into the plasma.

Monoclonal proliferation of cell line showing differentiation to various stages towards plasma cells.

Synthesis and secretion of whole molecules of Ig — always monoclonal, i.e. either IgG or A or M or (D or E very rarely) with either K or L light chains

Sometimes only parts of the molecule are produced, e.g. Fc fragment or K or L light chains

Pathological effects may result from the presence of these products

WALDENSTRÖM'S MACROGLOBULINAEMIA is the classic example. It affects the lymph nodes in the late middle aged and elderly with a preponderance of males. In addition to the usual pathological complications of low grade lymphomas, the production of IgM in large quantity produces special complications.

MONOCLONAL IgM

Polymerises in cold (cryoglobulin)

Increased blood viscosity

Coats surface of platelets and interferes with fibrin polymerisation

Capillary stasis

Red cell agglutination and haemolysis

Visual and CNS disturbances

Haemorrhages

PLASMA CELL TUMOURS

SOLITARY PLASMACYTOMA

A very small number of plasma cell tumours present as solitary growths, e.g. in the nasopharynx, a lymph node, alimentary tract or in a long bone. It is likely that these slow growing tumours have been present for long periods before they present clinically. In many cases, dissemination particularly to the bone marrow ensues. Elevation of the ESR or the presence of M proteins in the serum are indications of latent dissemination at the time of first clinical presentation.

MULTIPLE MYELOMA (MYELOMATOSIS)

The great majority of plasma cell tumours present as widespread deposits in the
bone marrow. Classically the lesions are seen as punched out defects in the bones —

the skull showing this appearance particularly
well. These focal proliferations of
plasma cells usually occur against a background
of more diffuse infiltration throughout
the marrow.

Binucleate cell - - - -

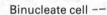

The disease is not common, having an incidence similar to
Hodgkin's disease, with an age peak in the 5th and 6th decades.
After initial presentation, the progress is usually fairly rapid
leading to death in 2 to 4 years.

Pathological effects are considered under two main headings:

1. Tumour growth and its effects

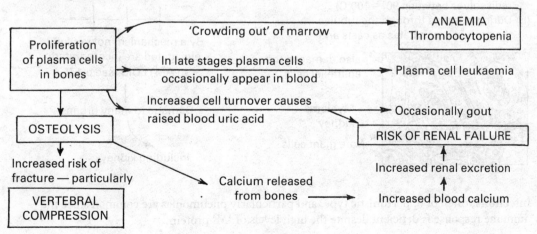

PLASMA CELL TUMOURS

Pathological effects (continued)

2. Synthesis of immunoglobulin and its effects

Myelomatosis, being a monoclonal tumour (see p.604), will produce a single Ig, but the type of Ig varies from case to case, unlike Waldenström's macroglobinaemia where the immunoglobulin is always IgM. The common heavy chains are G(60%) and A(20%). Light chains of K type are encountered more frequently than λ reflecting the normal K: λ ratio, i.e. 65:35. This myeloma of IgGK is the most frequent.

The presence of a single type of Ig is reflected in the electrophoretic pattern

Note: 'M' stands for myeloma and it does not signify IgM

Spike of 'M'yeloma protein

In most cases high levels of 'M' protein cause:
1. High ESR
2. Marked rouleaux formation,
3. Depending on type of Ig — increased blood viscosity.

Release of light chains

In many myelomas, some of the Ig molecules are incompletely formed, and unattached light chains are released with important effects. Because of their low molecular weight the light chains:

(1) Pass through the glomerular filtrate,
(a) appearing *in the urine* as Bence-Jones protein (precipitates during heating — redissolves between 90° – 100°C).
(b) During passage through the tubules the protein precipitates as casts and

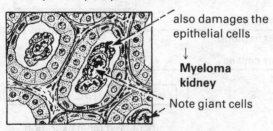

also damages the epithelial cells

↓

Myeloma kidney

Note giant cells

(2) Pass through capillaries

Light chains

By a mechanism not yet fully elucidated are incorporated in AMYLOID (see p.17)

↓

Damage to many organs

↓

Including kidneys

Infections, often of opportunistic type, and particularly pneumonias are common since the immune response is deficient despite the high levels of 'M' protein.

MACROPHAGE TUMOURS

The large cell lymphomas form a mixed group consisting of histiocytic (macrophage) tumours as well as tumours of lymphoid origin. Identification of the histiocytic tumours is possible by testing for the presence of the enzymes muramidase and alpha-1 antitrypsin, while in the lymphatic tumours immunoglobulins are found in the cell cytoplasm. In the connective tissues, tumours considered to be of histiocytic origin are described. They range from benign neoplasms in the dermis (histiocytomacutis) to aggressive sarcomas.

Histiocytosis-X

This term encompasses a spectrum of diseases of unknown aetiology which have not with certainty been proved to be neoplastic, but in all of which proliferation of a special type of macrophage (histiocyte) is an essential feature. This is the Langhan's cell, best recognised by electron microscopy which reveals the diagnostic 'Birbeck granules'.

Benign end of spectrum

Eosinophilic granuloma of bone (see p.807)

(a) *Solitary*

Histology: Eosinophils +++
                  Mononuclear cells ++
                  (Histiocytic) giant cells +
                  Fibrosis +

Progress: slow.

Hand-Schuller-Christian disease

(b) *Multifocal* →If skull bones affected there may be
- DIABETES INSIPIDUS
- EXOPHTHALMOS
- DEAFNESS

There may also be HEPATO-SPLENOMEGALY

Age range: children usually; occasionally adults.

Malignant end of spectrum

Letterer-Siwe disease: An acute febrile illness with widespread organ and tissue involvement, particularly lymph nodes, spleen, liver, bones and skin.

Histology: Mononuclear cells (histiocytic) +++
              Lymphocytes and plasma cells +
              Eosinophils ±
              Polymorphs +
              Necrosis ++

Progress: Rapid → death.

Age: Infants only.

LYMPHOMAS — MISCELLANEOUS

ALIMENTARY TRACT

Primary lymphomas of the alimentary tract are rare tumours (in the small intestine the incidence is about the same as that of adenocarcinoma). They may be solitary or multifocal. Histologically, the various types of lymphoma already described are encountered, but diffuse lymphomas of B cell and histiocytic origin predominate.

There are two main points of interest:

1. Solitary tumours of the small bowel may perforate early, ensuring detection and successful removal in some cases.
2. There is an increased incidence of lymphoma of the small intestine in cases of long-standing gluten enteropathy.

BURKITT'S LYMPHOMA

This tumour is of particular interest because there are strong indications that environmental factors are of great importance in its aetiology. It is encountered in particular terrains with similar climatic characteristics in East Africa, Nigeria, New Guinea and South America where malaria is endemic; where malaria has been eradicated the incidence of the tumour falls. The relationship with the Epstein-Barr (EB) virus has already been described (pp.68, 198). Only very rare cases have been recorded in Europe and North America.

The histological appearance is typical and striking.

Diffuse proliferation of LYMPHOBLASTS (B cell type) – – –

Cells medium-sized and uniform

Scattering of macrophages containing debris derived from very rapid cell turnover – contributing 'starry sky' appearance.

Mitoses frequent

Progress: The disease usually first appears in the jaw (60%) or ovaries (retroperitoneal tissues in males) (30%), but grows extremely rapidly and spreads extensively, leading quickly to complications.

(a) The physical effects of sheer tumour bulk destroy and distort organs and tissues.
(b) The very rapid tumour cell turnover releases metabolites in excess, e.g. lactic acid → acidosis.

The tumour responds dramatically to treatment. *NB* sudden extensive necrosis may have serious effects, e.g. release of cellular potassium → hyperkalaemia.

LYMPHOMAS — DIAGNOSIS

Lymph node enlargement is a common condition. Three broad groupings are considered.

Enlargement due to:

1. REACTIVE CHANGES infection is the common cause — Common
2. SECONDARY TUMOURS —————————————————————— Common
3. PRIMARY LYMPH NODE NEOPLASIA —————————————— Rare

Since the prognosis of group (1) is so different from (2) and (3), accurate diagnosis is essential. In the majority of cases, it is easily reached by a synthesis of all the clinical information. In a minority, laboratory tests are required.

Biopsy

The basis of an accurate diagnosis usually rests on LYMPH NODE BIOPSY.

The tissue has to be removed and processed with particular care since artefact can easily obscure the histological details so essential for accurate diagnosis.

Procedure: (1) A **whole** node is taken with minimal trauma.
(2) Preparation of routine and special histology.

(a) Fixation in 10% formalin — 48 hr., then routine processing.
(b) Frozen sections for surface markers — especially T cell identification.
(c) Imprints on slides. Special plastic section. Small blocks for EM (glutaraldehyde fixation).

Using a sharp blade, two thin slices of the face of the cut surface are obtained.

Microscopic diagnosis

1. May be extremely easy, e.g. SECONDARY CARCINOMA stands out against the lymphoid tissues — but establishing the source of origin of the carcinoma from the histological appearances may be difficult.

2. Great difficulty may arise in distinguishing reactive conditions from primary neoplasia (e.g. follicular lymphoma).

In these circumstances, other laboratory tests may be useful, e.g. to search for infecting organisms and to identify 'foreign' materials.

Full haematological examination, plasma protein analysis and assessment of the immune status may all make important contributions.

CHAPTER 13

GENITOURINARY SYSTEM

KIDNEY — ANATOMY AND PHYSIOLOGY

The kidney is essentially a lobulated organ and its blood supply is arranged in a regular pattern which frequently determines the extent of pathological lesions.

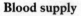

Arteries:

- Renal
- Interlobar
- Arcuate
- Straight

Blood supply

The renal artery divides into anterior and posterior branches which subdivide in a regular manner to supply the lobules.

From the straight arteries small branches (afferent arterioles) supply the functional unit of the kidney — the nephron.

The arteries and afferent arterioles are end vessels.
Anastomoses unite the peritubular capillaries of one nephron unit with another, but where the blockage of the arteriolar supply occurs, these anastomoses are insufficient to maintain a proper circulation.

Peritubular capillaries

- Efferent arteriole
- Afferent arteriole
- Straight artery
- Arcuate artery

THE NEPHRON

Glomerulus

Distal convoluted tubule

Proximal convoluted tubule

Collecting tubule

Loop of Henle

Excretory duct

Each part of the nephron has its own special structure and function, its own peculiar blood supply and control mechanism — partly hormonal.

THE GLOMERULUS is a bulbous structure, the end of which is invaginated by a capillary network derived from the afferent arteriole.

The large surface area of the capillaries makes this an efficient filtration unit. The filtration is precisely controlled by the unique structure of the glomerulus.

KIDNEY — ANATOMY AND PHYSIOLOGY

Ultrastructure

The barrier separating
blood from the lumen of the
nephron consists of three layers:

Mesangial matrix

Capillary

1. Endothelium (fenestrated)
2. Basement membrane - - - - -
3. Epithelium - - - - - - - - -

Mesangial nucleus

These layers form a complicated sieve controlling glomerular permeability.
Wide pores in the endothelium allow passage to all chemical
components of the plasma, including the largest protein
molecules.

750Å

The basement membrane has a dense layer offering
resistance to large molecules.

The epithelial cells are attached to the basement membrane
by foot processes, leaving pores 300 – 400 Å in width
between. These pores are covered by a thin membrane which
has slits 50×120Å in size, slightly smaller than a molecule of
albumin (37×140Å).

The main barriers to filtration of large molecules are the lamina densa of the basement
membrane and the slit diaphragm covering the epithelial pores.

Filtration

The glomerular filtrate is
virtually protein free plasma.
Its rate of production is
dependent upon: ————

① Afferent
arteriolar
hydrostatic
pressure

Blood

② Plasma
protein
osmotic
pressure

③ Pressure
within
the renal
tubule

Filtrate

Variation in any of these factors
affects the output of urine. Diminished
urinary output results from a reduction
in renal blood flow as in shock, from
an increase in osmotic pressure as in
haemoconcentration, or from obstruction
to the outflow of urine.

KIDNEY — ANATOMY AND PHYSIOLOGY

Glomerular damage

The usual consequences of this are threefold:

       1. Reduction in urinary output

       2. Proteinuria

       3. Haematuria

The mechanism underlying these changes is probably as follows:

THE TUBULE

During passage along the tubule, the glomerular filtrate, initially isotonic and neutral, becomes hypertonic and quite strongly acid. Within 24 hours, 180 litres of filtrate are reduced to 1.5 litres of urine. The main functions of this process are:

    (a) to get rid of waste products, particularly those of protein metabolism

    (b) to aid in maintaining the normal acid-base balance

    (c) to conserve fluid, electrolytes and other essential substances.

Three mechanisms are involved:

1. Active absorption of substances from the filtrate by the tubular epithelium

2. Passive interchange between the filtrate and the interstitial tissues to maintain osmotic equilibrium

3. Secretion by the tubular epithelium

KIDNEY — ANATOMY AND PHYSIOLOGY

PROXIMAL TUBULE

The main function is active reabsorption of sodium, potassium, glucose, amino acids, phosphate, calcium and uric acid.

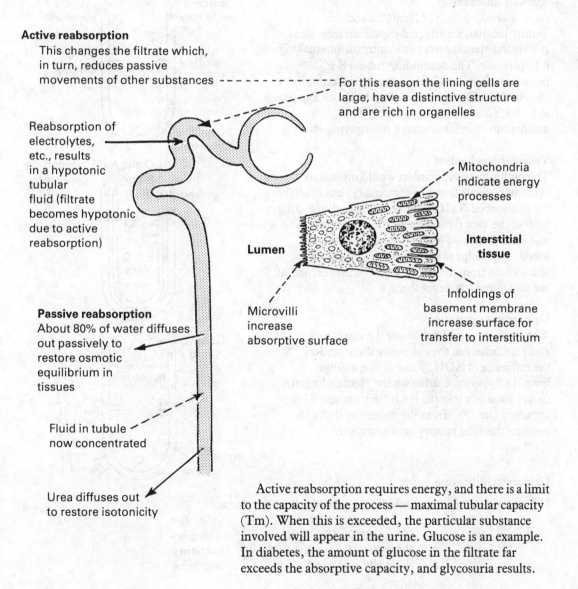

Active reabsorption
This changes the filtrate which, in turn, reduces passive movements of other substances - - - - - - - - - - - - For this reason the lining cells are large, have a distinctive structure and are rich in organelles

Reabsorption of electrolytes, etc., results in a hypotonic tubular fluid (filtrate becomes hypotonic due to active reabsorption)

Mitochondria indicate energy processes

Lumen

Interstitial tissue

Microvilli increase absorptive surface

Infoldings of basement membrane increase surface for transfer to interstitium

Passive reabsorption
About 80% of water diffuses out passively to restore osmotic equilibrium in tissues

Fluid in tubule now concentrated

Urea diffuses out to restore isotonicity

Active reabsorption requires energy, and there is a limit to the capacity of the process — maximal tubular capacity (Tm). When this is exceeded, the particular substance involved will appear in the urine. Glucose is an example. In diabetes, the amount of glucose in the filtrate far exceeds the absorptive capacity, and glycosuria results.

KIDNEY — ANATOMY AND PHYSIOLOGY

LOOP OF HENLE AND ASCENDING TUBULE
In this zone, there is active reabsorption of Na^+Cl^- and passive reabsorption of water. This is augmented by a counter current mechanism due to proximity of tubules and blood vessels. The changes are as follows:

Tubular mechanism
At A (ascending limb of Henle), a sodium 'pump' mechanism effected by aldosterone (see p.844) transfers the ion to the interstitium making it hypertonic. The descending tubule B is permeable to water which is attracted from it by the Na^+Cl^-. The urine therefore becomes hypertonic at C (Na^+Cl^- concentration high). This mechanism therefore exerts a multiplying effect.

Vascular mechanism
The multiplying mechanism would ultimately cause impossible tissue hypertonicity, but much of the reabsorbed Na^+Cl^- passes into the descending limb of the vasa recta (D). As the vessel turns and ascends (E), water is attracted into the blood. This helps to maintain the flow of water and sodium from the tubule into the tissues, and at the same time conserves them.

Urinary concentration
Water absorption occurs along the distal tubule and particularly in the collecting ducts under the influence of ADH. Some of the sodium from the hypertonic urine. in the Henle's loop (C) moves passively into the medullary tissues. This attracts water (5%) from the collecting ducts to produce the final urinary concentration.

Urinary acidification
H ions, excreted by distal tubule, take part in three reactions:

$$
\begin{aligned}
1.\quad & H^+ + HCO_3 = H_2CO_3 \\
2.\quad & H^+ + NH_3Cl = NH_4Cl \\
3.\quad & H^+ + HPO_4 + Na = NaH_2PO_4
\end{aligned}
\left.\right\}
\begin{aligned}
&\text{Urinary} \\
&\text{excretory} \\
&\text{products}
\end{aligned}
$$

KIDNEY — ANATOMY AND PHYSIOLOGY

Variations in nephrons

There are variations in the size of glomeruli, and therefore variation in the filtration surface, but the most striking difference is between the tubules of the cortical glomeruli and those of the juxtamedullary glomeruli.

The rate of blood flow through the medulla is only one-fifth of the cortical rate. This, together with the long loops of Henle of the juxtamedullary nephrons which allow reabsorption of large quantites of water, suggests a mechanism for conservation of fluid and electrolytes which may operate when the circulating volume of blood is low and cortical flow is reduced as in shock.

Effects of tubular damage

It is obvious that damage to the tubules will result in gross biochemical changes.

1. Loss of mechanisms controlling balance of electrolytes, water and urea.

2. Upset in acid-base balance.

3. Loss of substances in urine normally completely or almost completely reabsorbed — glucose, potassium, amino acids.

4. Proteinuria due to damage to associated capillaries.

It must also be apparent that glomerular lesions and pathological changes in the renal pelvis will upset tubular function by interfering with blood supply.

617

RENAL FUNCTION

INVESTIGATION

Numerous tests of renal function have been formulated, some simple, others sophisticated. It must be emphasised that the simple tests are, in their own context, important. Tests can be divided into three groups:

1. **Simple diagnostic tests indicating renal damge**

   (a) Tests for the presence of protein, red cells, haemoglobin and polymorphs in the urine. Estimation of specific gravity and measurement of urinary output.

   (b) Urinary casts. These are composed of foreign elements of various types which are moulded into cylindical form by passage along tubules.

Protein casts (also called hyaline or colloid) composed of precipitated protein are usually not of pathological significance

Red cell casts

Epithelial casts consisting of desquamated tubular epithelium

Granular casts; the remains of necrotic tubular cells

In jaundice, casts of bile-stained debris are found.

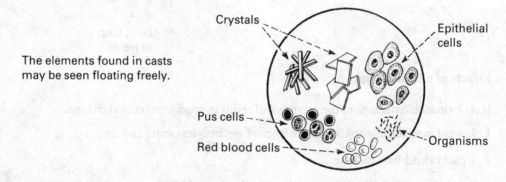

The elements found in casts may be seen floating freely.

Crystals

Epithelial cells

Pus cells

Red blood cells

Organisms

2. Blood chemistry

Many substance will show altered values in renal failure, but the following are always elevated and are commonly used in estimating the progress of the disease.

Urea ———— normal range ---- 2.5 – 7.0 mmol/l (20 – 40 mg/100 ml).

Creatinine ——— normal range ---- 50 – 100 μmol/l (0.6 – 1.2 mg/100 ml).

CO$_2$ content —— normal range ---- 22 – 28 mmol/l.

RENAL FUNCTION

3.Clearance tests

These are employed to determine the degree of renal damage and the residual function. The principle underlying all of these tests is similar — an estimation of the rate of extraction of a particular substance from the blood by the kidney in unit time. The simple formula UV/P is used to calculate the amount of blood so cleared.

U = the urinary concentration.
V = the volume of urine per minute.
P = the plasma concentration.

A loading dose of the test substance is administered intravenously followed by an infusion to sustain a constant blood level.

Glomerular filtration rate

Inulin is the ideal substance for this purpose. It is filtered at the glomerulus and is excreted unchanged in the urine. The amount appearing in the urine is proportional to the amount of blood being 'cleared' of inulin per unit time.

Following infusion of the inulin, a timed urine specimen is collected and a plasma sample is obtained halfway through the collection. The formula VU/P is applied to the values obtained. The normal filtration rate is around 125 ml/min.

Frequently in practice creatinine, which is a normal constituent of urine and blood and therefore eliminates the need for infusions, is used instead of inulin. It is also easier to estimate. The value obtained is not quite as accurate since creatinine is partly secreted by the renal tubules.

Renal plasma flow

Para-amino hippuric acid is both filtered at the glomerulus and secreted by the tubular epithelium so that 90% is extracted from the arterial blood. This gives an approximate idea of the renal plasma flow. The procedure is exactly the same as that employed for inulin. The same formula (UV/P) is used to calculate the clearance rate of PAH.

Average result is 630 ml/min. Since only 90% of PAH is cleared, the actual renal plasma flow will be:

$$\frac{\text{Clearance}}{\text{Extraction ratio}} = \frac{630}{0.9} = 700\text{ml/min}$$

Other substances, such as urea, can be used to give an indication of renal function. Since urea is normally present in the blood and urine, it eliminates the need for intravenous infusions.

NEPHRITIS

The pathological changes and clinical syndromes may be divided into 3 main groups, but two other less common and ill-defined conditions are described.

1. **Acute glomerulonephritis**

This condition is characterised by moderate proteinuria, haematuria, oedema, oliguria and a degree of renal failure.

2. **Nephrotic syndrome**

Affected individuals suffer a long continued illness with widespread oedema, effusions in serous cavities and susceptibility to infections. There is gross proteinuria and raised blood lipid. Nitrogen retention occurs late in the disease process.

3. **Serious renal failure**

This may occur:

(a) Early — within a few weeks or months. Uraemia is the main manifestation and it may end in death.
(b) Late — after several years. Hypertension develops and death may be due to vascular complications or uraemia.

Unfortunately, these syndromes are not disease entities. The aetiology of the three syndromes is very mixed, and the clinical features of all three may be exhibitied at different times by the same patient. Different pathological processes may produce the same clinical condition. This is particularly true of the nephrotic syndrome. The clinical syndromes provide little indication of pathogenesis, nor are they a guide to prognosis. In addition, any one of these renal syndromes may be a manifestation of a number of systemic diseases.

It has been found that diagnosis and an estimate of prognosis are best achieved by a study of the histological changes using renal biopsies. In the following account, primary renal lesions will be described, beginning with the acute glomerulonephritic conditions. Subsequently, consideration will be given to renal dysfunction associated with systemic disease.

ACUTE DIFFUSE GLOMERULONEPHRITIS

This condition in its classical form follows 2 – 3 weeks after an infection, usually a pharyngitis due to group A haemolytic streptococci. It is commonest in children and young adults.

Kidney enlarged

Cortex broad, pale, without markings

Medullary rays congested

Glomeruli just visible as grey avascular dots

The lesion is essentially acute inflammation of the glomerulus

Glomerulus large, fills capsular space: solid and cellular

Projects into tubule

Normal

Cells flat and inconspicuous

Endothelial cells swollen and more numerous

Capillary lumen narrowed

Polymorphs sometimes present

Oedema, basement membrane swollen

Necrosis of individual endothelial and epithelial cells occurs

In some cases, the epithelial cells of Bowman's capsule and covering the glomerulus proliferate and adhere to produce crescents

621

ACUTE DIFFUSE GLOMERULONEPHRITIS

Other changes

Proximal tubules
Protein droplets
appear in cytoplasm

Distal tubules

Cells swollen,
cytoplasm granular
(cloudy swelling)

Interstitial tissue
Round cell
infiltration common:
lymphocytes,
a few polymorphs

Some distal tubules
contain
casts

Clinical features

These may be relatively slight. Malaise with some facial oedema (periorbital), oliguria, the urine being smoky and dark, and a moderate increase in blood pressure are the most constant features.

The relationship of clinical findings to pathological changes can be visualised as follows:

ACUTE DIFFUSE GLOMERULONEPHRITIS

Electron microscope studies
These studies reveal deposits of granular material in the glomerulus.

Small granules constantly seen in subepithelial position (occasionally larger subendothelial granules may be seen)

Capillary lumen

Endothelial cell

Basement membrane

Epithelial cells

In addition to these deposits, the electron microscope shows focal fusion of the foot processes of the epithelial cells (podocytes).

Immunofluorescence staining reveals that the granular material in the subendothelial position consists of IgG, sometimes IgA, C3 factor of the complement complex and fibrin.

The proteins show as a granular, irregular deposit in the glomerular capillary walls.

White indicates the presence of reacting protein.

Progress
This tends to vary with the age of the patient. Children almost always recover (95%) completely. Endothelial and epithelial changes are reversed. The protein deposits are either excreted in the urine or are phagocytosed by mesangial cells. Capillary patency is restored.

Complications arise in more than one third of adults

Acute diffuse glomerulonephritis

Cardiac failure or uraemia

Mild proteinuria persisting for month or two

Persisting proteinuria and haematuria

Rapidly progressive glomerulonephritis

Death in acute phase

Recovery

Chronic nephritis

Death years later

623

RAPIDLY PROGRESSIVE GLOMERULONEPHRITIS

Initially, this condition is clinically and pathologically indistinguishable from acute diffuse glomerulonephritis, but subsequently additional changes take place.

Adhesions between tuft and capsule are common

Thrombosis may be seen in tuft capillaries

Strands of fibrin are prominent in the crescents

Crescent formation occurs in almost all glomeruli

Crescents enlarge, compressing the tufts and obliterating capillaries.

The tuft collapses and collagen fibres appear in crescents and tuft.

Ultimately, glomerulus becomes a mass of hyaline fibrous tissue.

The tubules present the same appearances as in acute diffuse glomerulonephritis, but focal necrosis is more common, probably due to ischaemia caused by the glomerular lesion. Epithelial atrophy takes place and the interstitial tissue increases in amount. These changes take place over a period of a few weeks and are progressive.

Clinical effects

These are similar to those found in acute diffuse glomerulonephritis but are much more evident and increase in severity. Death, due to hypertension and uraemia, is almost inevitable within a matter of weeks or a year, depending upon the progress of the pathological changes and the occurrence of complications.

The complications are those of uraemia — superadded infection, fibrinous pericarditis and anaemia. In addition, malignant hypertension may supervene, intensifying the renal changes and also causing cardiac hypertrophy.

RAPIDLY PROGRESSIVE GLOMERULONEPHRITIS

Electron microscope findings

Subendothelial and subepithelial granular
deposits may be found in the tuft capillaries
as in acute diffuse glomerulonephritis. In
addition, as the lesion progresses, changes
occur in the basement membrane.

Lumen

Basement membrane
swollen, crinkled
and shows numerous
breaks

Aetiology

Rapidly progressive glomerulonephritis appears to arise mainly in two circumstances:

1. It may follow a streptococcal infection, and in the early stages is indistinguishable from acute
   diffuse glomerulonephritis (see p.621).

2. Associated with lung disease. This usually takes the form of Goodpasture's syndrome, a
   condition almost exclusively confined to young adult males. There are repeated episodes of
   pulmonary haemorrhage causing severe anaemia. This is followed by renal changes. Death can
   be due to pulmonary or renal insufficiency. Autoantibodies to basement membranes are present
   in the blood and are thought to be responsible for the renal damage.

Immunofluorescence studies differentiate between these two aetiological forms of the nephritic
process.

Post-streptococcal

Granular
deposits of
IgG, IgM
and C3

Goodpasture's syndrome

Linear
deposits of
IgG, IgM
and C3 in
the capillary
basement
membranes

The prognosis is somewhat better in the post-streptococcal condition.

FOCAL GLOMERULONEPHRITIS

In this condition the changes may occur in almost all glomeruli, or in only a small number. In addition, the lesion is usually only seen in one or two lobules of each affected glomerulus.

Major portion of glomerulus normal

Affected lobule hypercellular

Thrombosis of capillary loops common

Adhesions to capsule develop

Red cells in capsular space

The hypercellularity is due to proliferation of mesangial cells. The capillaries are often thrombosed and necrotic.

The reason for the focal nature appears to be due to the variation in size of the immune complexes. These reach all glomeruli, but the majority are small and pass through to the urinary space and are excreted. Others, larger, are held in the glomerular sieve and cause an acute reaction.

Immunofluorescence reveals deposits of immunoglobulins IgG and IgA in the ground substance (mesangium) of the affected lobule. The IgA molecule appears to be of particular significance.

No deposits in capillaries

Clinical features

Haematuria, sometimes severe, and proteinuria are the only signs. Usually they last only a few days and there is no sign of subsequent renal impairment, but the condition can recur repeatedly and may end in chronic renal failure.

Aetiology

1. It is an uncommon condition mainly found in male children.
2. The cause is unknown, but in most cases it follows a few days after a vague flu-like respiratory infection.

A similar lesion may be found as a complication in other diseases (see p.634).

NEPHROTIC SYNDROME

Renal lesions associated with nephrotic syndrome

In fatal cases, the kidneys may show striking changes to the naked eye, but this gives little indication of the pathological process involved.

Enlargement and general pallor due to oedema

Yellow streaks of lipid

Histological changes

Several distinct conditions become apparent on microscopic examination:

MEMBRANOUS GLOMERULONEPHRITIS

In this form there are generalised changes in the glomerular capillary basement membranes. Several stages can be recognised:

Early stage

Tuft enlarges

— Diffuse hyaline thickening of capillary

Glomeruli not hypercellular

Specific silver staining of the basement membrane shows a typical pattern.

Basement membrane material is increased and shows spikes

Immunofluorescence reveals deposition of IgG and IgM in the capillary walls.

Electron microscope findings explain this appearance.

Loss of foot processes

Basement membrane material between deposit ≡ spikes

Subepithelial deposits

Single layer of basement membrane

NEPHROTIC SYNDROME

Membranous Glomerulonephritis (continued)

Late stage

Capillaries narrowed

Massive increase in basement membrane

Adhesions to capsule

Intervening spikes of basement membrane

Silver staining

Basement membrane shows a double contouring with joining spikes (rail track)

Electron microscope findings

Two layers of basement membrane

Deposits

Capillary lumen

Tubular changes

In the early stages, protein droplets and lipid globules appear in the tubular epithelium. Lipid is also found in the interstitial tissue. Foamy macrophages and giant cells form granulomas in association with cholesterol deposits. With progress of the disease, narrowing of the glomerular capillaries causes ischaemic atrophy of the tubules and interstitial fibrosis.

Clinical features

The disease is commonest in males and occurs more often in adults.

It presents with the usual features of the nephrotic syndrome — gross proteinuria and generalised oedema. Fluid accumulates in the serous cavities.

Biochemical changes include hypoproteinaemia due to loss of protein in the urine and hyperlipidaemia which accounts for the lipid deposits in the kidneys.

Serious infections can be troublesome. The disease is only slowly progressive, but ultimately glomerular destruction leads to uraemia. At this stage, proteinuria may disappear.

Aetiology

This is vague. In some cases, the disease is associated with infections such as quartan malaria, syphilis and Hep B infection.

MINIMAL CHANGE GLOMERULONEPHRITIS

This occurs mainly in children but is occasionally seen in adults. It is the commonest cause of the nephrotic condition in children.

The macroscopic appearance of the kidneys is the same as that in all examples of the nephrotic syndrome, but the apparent lack of glomerular change gave rise to the term 'lipoid nephrosis'.

Capillary loops widely patent

Occasional area of mesangial increase

Basement membrane not thickened

Immunofluorescence fails to demonstrate immunoglobulins or complement.

Fusion of foot processes

Basement membrane

Endothelial cell

Capillary lumen

No evidence of deposits in or around basement membrane.

Tubular changes, common to all nephrotic states, consist of lipid and protein droplets in the epithelial cells.

Clinical features

These are the same as in any nephrotic process — gross oedema and proteinuria with hyperlipidaemia. Infection is no longer a problem, due to the use of antibiotics.

Glomerular filtration appears to be normal. The proteinuria is highly selective, only albumin being found in the urine, and is apparently due to increased permeability of the glomerular capillaries. Lipid-rich protein casts appear in the urine.

Aetiology and progress

This is unknown. Occasionally it may follow a respiratory infection but is not related to any particular type.

The condition in children responds to steroid therapy. It tends to recur, and the prognosis depends on the frequency of recurrence and the duration of the interval between attacks. The response to steroids suggests an immunological reaction. The lack of evidence of immunoglobulin in the glomerulus may be due to elimination.

In adults, the prognosis is not so clear and some patients may subsequently develop renal failure.

FOCAL GLOMERULOSCLEROSIS (HYALINOSIS)

The clinical features of this condition are the same as those of minimal change glomerulonephritis, but the prognosis is quite different. In the early phase, the microscopic appearance of the glomeruli is almost the same as in the minimal change lesion, but it is a progressive lesion.

Early change

Focal thickening of capsular basement membrane

Focal basement membrane thickening

Focal prominence of mesangium

Increasing hyalinosis

Mesangial increase — often vacuolated and showing hyalinised areas

Disappearance of capillaries

Adhesions to tuft capsule

Immunofluorescence reveals deposits of IgM in basement membranes.

Electron microscope appearance

Early   *Late*

Fusion of foot processes

Deposits in basement membrane

Lumen

Lumen

Large amount of material deposited in basement membrane

Ultimately, the glomerulus becomes completely sclerosed. The process starts in juxtamedullary glomeruli but spreads peripherally to outer cortical glomeruli. Associated tubules undergo atrophy. Proteinuria is unselective and haematuria may occur. The condition is unresponsive to steroids and ends in renal failure.

Aetiology

The true aetiology is unknown. It could be a variant of minimal change glomerulonephritis, accounting for those cases of the latter condition which recur frequently and end in renal failure.

MEMBRANOPROLIFERATIVE GLOMERULONEPHRITIS

In many ways this lesion is a bridge between acute diffuse glomerulonephritis and membranous glomerulonephritis, showing some of the features of each of these conditions.

Tufts are lobulated and hypercellular

Capillaries narrow

Increase of mesangium between capillaries; sometimes areas of hyalinosis

Epithelial cells swollen; occasionally crescents form

Silver staining of basement membrane

Duplication of basement membrane as in membranous glomerulonephritis, but without spikes

Electron microscopy

Findings explain the basement membrane duplication

Outer basement membrane

Mesangium interposed

Epithelial cell

Foot processes show some fusion

Inner layer of basement membrane

Swollen endothelial cell

Subendothelial and mesangial deposits are found, and immunofluorescence shows that they are immunoglobulins IgG, IgA or IgM, C3 and granular fibrin.

The glomeruli usually show increasing hyalinisation until they are completely sclerosed. Tubules undergo atrophy with increasing interstitial fibrosis.

Clinical features

This condition usually affects older children. It may have an acute onset, but with no symptoms apart from proteinuria, progressing to a nephrotic syndrome. Some patients may recover, but most develop chronic renal failure. Hypertension may be a prominent feature. The blood level of C3 is always low.

Aetiology

This is unknown. In some cases there has been a preceding streptococcal infection, but other factors in the plasma, as yet not well defined, may activate the complement system in the glomerular tuft.

GLOMERULONEPHRITIS

Mechanisms of damage

The essential mechanism is the effect of immune complex deposition.

The glomerulus is the ideal site for the deposition of immune complexes because of its microstructure. The most important factor is the size of the complex, and this will vary with the stage and intensity of the immune reaction, e.g.:

(1) Antibody in low concentration (e.g. early in reaction)

Very small soluble molecule — causes no trouble.

(2) Antibody equivalent to antigen (immune reaction fully mounted)

A very large insoluble molecule excites a macrophage reaction resulting in phagocytosis and digestion in the circulation, and causing no renal damage.

(3) Intermediate amounts of antibody

Molecules of intermediate size.

Deposition of immune complex

The third type of molecule is important. All are able to pass through the fenestrations of the capillary endothelium. Thereafter their migration will depend mainly on their size and the degree of permeability of the basement membrane. The smallest molecules will reach a subepithelial position.

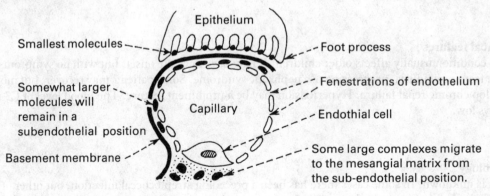

GLOMERULONEPHRITIS

Subsequently, fixation of complement by these immune complexes takes place:

Factors modifying the pathological changes in the kidney

1. The amount of antigen and its persistence.
2. The intensity of the immune reaction and the rate of production of antibody; the type of antibody formed may also be important.
3. The availability of complement and the degree of its 'fixation'.

Factors (1) and (2) will determine the amount and rate of deposition of the immune complexes, and the interplay between all three factors can account for the variations in the pathological changes and clinical manifestations of glomerulonephritis, e.g. a short-lived infection (e.g. scarlet fever) may produce an acute nephritis, but the antigen disappears rapidly and the nephritis resolves. A more chronic condition with persisting antigens can result in a slower but ultimately more destructive process in the kidneys. Equally, a poor immunological reaction in a chronic disease can cause a similar picture.

RENAL MANIFESTATIONS OF SYSTEMIC DISEASE

In a number of diseases, the kidneys are sometimes severely affected, and the renal manifestations may dominate the clinical picture. According to their pathogenesis the renal lesions fall into two main groups.

GROUP A. Diseases associated with immune complex deposition.

Systemic lupus erythematosus. Two forms of renal disease may be found.

	EM and immuno-fluorescence	Serum complement	Clinical features
1. Membranous glomerulonephritis	Deposits of IgG, IgM and IgA	Low	Nephrotic syndrome
2. Glomerulonephritis, focal or general	Deposits of IgG, IgM, IgA, C1, C3	Low	Proteinuria, haematuria may proceed to nephrotic syndrome
Henoch Schonlein purpura Glomerulonephritis, focal or general	Mesangial deposits of IgA, IgG, fibrin	Normal	Proteinuria, haematuria

Group B. Diseases associated with thrombotic phenomena.

	EM and immuno-fluorescence	Serum complement	Clinical features
Vasculitis of various forms e.g. periarteritis nodosa Glomerulonephritis, focal or general	Intracapillary fibrin and mesangial proliferation	Normal	Proteinuria, haematuria, azotaemia
Disseminated intravascular coagulation e.g. thrombocytopenic purpura, malignant hypertension	Capillary and subendothelial fibrin	Normal	Acute renal failure or progressive renal failure

This is by no means an exhaustive list. Many other systemic diseases can have signs of kidney damage, but in most instances the renal component is a minor manifestation of the clinical syndrome.

CHRONIC GLOMERULONEPHRITIS

CHRONIC GLOMERULONEPHRITIS is the final stage of glomerulonephritis when sclerosis has eliminated many glomeruli and their associated tubules.

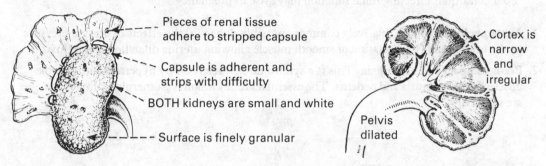

Pieces of renal tissue adhere to stripped capsule

Capsule is adherent and strips with difficulty

BOTH kidneys are small and white

Surface is finely granular

Cortex is narrow and irregular

Pelvis dilated

This is often the late result of membranous or membranoproliferative glomerulonephritis, less commonly postinfectious acute nephritis. Many cases have a 'silent' onset and some may be of viral origin. At the end stage, it is difficult to determine the aetiology of the pathological lesion.

Uraemia is the main clinical feature, but hypertensive cardiac failure or cerebral haemorrhage may cause death.

URAEMIA

This is due to a failure to excrete the products of protein breakdown. It occurs in acute renal failure with anuria after 5 – 7 days. The patient is lethargic. Anorexia, nausea and vomiting are usual, followed by mental confusion, muscle twitchings, convulsions and death if the condition is not alleviated. More commonly, a milder but inevitably progressive condition exists. An acute phase may be precipitated by intercurrent disease or further deterioration in the renal condition.

Since uraemia can be brought about by changes outwith the kidneys it is sometimes classified in three groups:

1. *Pre-renal.* Commonly due to conditions inducing shock, including haemorrhage, burns, severe infection, obstetric accidents, extensive surgery, etc.
2. *Renal.* Including glomerulonephritis, pyelonephritis, tubular necrosis due to poisons, toxins etc., transplant rejection.
3. *Post-renal.* Uraemia in this instance is due to obstructive lesions in the urinary tract, e.g. calculi, fibrosis, tumour, papillary necrosis and damage by trauma.

It is doubtful if such a classification is really useful, since in most cases the causes of a uraemic state are multiple. More important is to remember that the blood urea may rise in the absence of a renal lesion e.g. due to breakdown and absorption of the products of a large haematoma.

INTERCURRENT RENAL CONDITIONS

RENAL FUNCTION AND PREGNANCY

Four conditions affecting renal function may arise in pregnancy.

1. **Acute pyelonephritis** is relatively common, possibly due to (a) the effects of uterine pressure on the ureters and (b) relaxation of smooth muscle allowing uterine dilatation and reflux.

2. **Pre-eclampsia and eclampsia.** This is a syndrome characterised by hypertension, variable unselective proteinuria and oedema. The essential kidney lesion is glomerular; tubular changes are secondary.

Glomerulus enlarged

Basement membrane normal

Endothelial cells swollen

Mesangial cell proliferation and ground substance increased

Subendothelial fibrinoid in afferent arteriole

EM examination shows mesangial deposits of fibrin, fibrinogen, IgM and complement.

The appearances resemble minimal change or membranous glomerulonephritis plus hypertensive changes.

The lesion appears to resolve rapidly after parturition. So far as kidney function is concerned, the danger of eclampsia lies in the occasional development of the third lesion.

3. **Bilateral cortical necrosis.** This hitherto fatal condition is now considered as a variation of the 'haemolytic-uraemic' syndrome. It may also follow abruptio placentae and abortion.

4. **Acute tubular necrosis.** This is associated with complications of pregnancy causing shock i.e. septic abortion, retroplacental haemorrhage and postpartum haemorrhage.

INTERCURRENT RENAL CONDITIONS

DIABETES

Renal complications are common in diabetes. Ten per cent of all diabetics die of renal failure. In juvenile diabetics, the figure is fifty per cent. In most cases the kidneys show typical changes.

Diabetic glomerulosclerosis   This takes one of two forms:

Diffuse

Capsular hyaline deposits

Capsule thickened

Capillary basement membranes thickened

Hyaline material is deposited in the mesangium in a diffuse or nodular manner

Afferent and efferent arterioles both show hyaline thickening

Nodular

Tubular atrophy

Deposited material is PAS-positive and resembles amyloid. The nodular form is often termed the Kimmelstiel-Wilson lesion. Progressive closure of capillaries can occur together with fibrous obliteration of the capsular space and the whole glomerulus. The changes in the afferent arterioles are an important factor in this process. Secondary tubular atrophy follows.

Clinical effects

Proteinuria is usually present and may produce a nephrotic syndrome. Chronic renal failure with uraemia and hypertension may ensue.

The cause is unknown, but poor control of diabetes and the development of antibodies to insulin may be contributory.

Pyelonephritis

This is common in diabetes and may be complicated by papillary necrosis.

Atheroma

This disease is uncommon in the renal arteries and their branches except in diabetes. It increases the renal ischaemia.

INTERCURRENT RENAL CONDITIONS

AMYLOID DISEASE

The general features of amyloidosis have already been described (p.16). Amyloid is deposited around the capillary basement membranes of the glomeruli.

Early

Thickening
of capillary
basement
membranes

Late

Progressive
obliteration
of capillaries

Gross proteinuria leading to a nephrotic syndrome is common. Interstitial fibrosis results from tubular degeneration and ischaemia due to glomerular and arteriolar lesions. Chronic renal failure results. Renal vein thrombosis can occur in amyloidosis causing acute renal failure.

DRUGS AND THE KIDNEYS

Three types of renal damage may be induced by drugs.

1. **Interstitial nephritis.** A hypersensitivity reaction induces a peritubular inflammation and tubular necrosis. Acute renal failure results.

2. **Acute tubular necrosis.** Mercurial diuretics and sulfonamide drugs can damage the tubular epithelium during concentration of the urine. The same mechanism may operate when using cytotoxic drugs and antibiotics, especially if renal function is already deficient.

3. **Chronic papillary necrosis.** This is the result of long-continued use of analgesics (aspirin, phenacetin) in large doses. The pathological picture is complicated by secondary changes.

ACUTE TUBULAR NECROSIS

This arises in two circumstances:

1. During a state of shock, e.g. due to haemorrhage, burns, trauma, acute intestinal obstruction, incompatible transfusion and abdominal operations.
2. Following administration of toxic substances, e.g. carbon tetrachloride, trilene, ethylene glycol, compounds of mercury, uranium, chromic acid and various drugs.

The gross appearance of the kidneys is the same in both groups, although there is some difference in the type and distribution of the lesions.

Kidney is enlarged

Cortex is broad and pale; markings absent

Pyramids grossly congested

Cut surface bulges due to oedema

Shock cases

The lesions are the result of ischaemia, and this determines the part of the kidney affected and the portion of the tubule damaged.

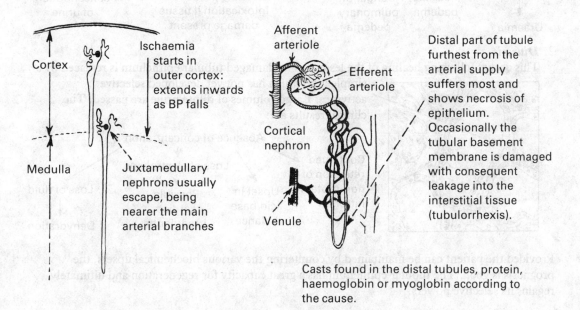

Cortex

Ischaemia starts in outer cortex: extends inwards as BP falls

Medulla

Juxtamedullary nephrons usually escape, being nearer the main arterial branches

Afferent arteriole

Efferent arteriole

Cortical nephron

Venule

Distal part of tubule furthest from the arterial supply suffers most and shows necrosis of epithelium. Occasionally the tubular basement membrane is damaged with consequent leakage into the interstitial tissue (tubulorrhexis).

Casts found in the distal tubules, protein, haemoglobin or myoglobin according to the cause.

ACUTE TUBULAR NECROSIS

Toxic cases

The lesions are evenly distributed, affecting all nephrons. They are maximal in the proximal tubules and are the direct result of the poison, the action of which is intensified by the concentrating activity of the tubule.

    The lesion is typified by carbon tetrachloride poisoning.

Degenerate
proximal tubules
containing debris

Normal distal tubule

Clinical effects

There are two clinical phases:

1. *Oliguria*

The glomerular filtration rate is greatly reduced. Unselective reabsorption of the filtrate occurs through the damaged tubule. The effects are:

Reduced GFR

Tubular damage

Retention of non-protein nitrogen

Retention of fluid

Upset in electrolyte balance

Acidosis due to inability to control hydrogen ion concentration of urine

Possible oedema

Danger of pulmonary oedema

Possible potassium intoxication if tissue damage present

Uraemia

2. *Diuresis*

This occurs following healing of the lesions. The damaged tubular epithelium is replaced by a simple type which has not yet developed selective activities. Large volumes of dilute urine are passed. The clinical results are:

Absence of concentration

Loss of electrolytes

Continued retention of non-protein nitrogen

Upset in acid/base balance

Possible cardiac irregularity

Loss of fluid

Dehydration

Provided the patient can be maintained by countering the various biochemical upsets, the prognosis is good. The tubular epithelium has a great capacity for regeneration and ultimately regains its selective powers.

HAEMOLYTIC URAEMIC SYNDROME

This is a rare complication of many apparently dissimilar conditions. The mechanism appears to be as follows:

Activation of clotting mechanism

↓

Disseminated intravascular coagulation

Haemolysis (typical burr cells in blood) ← ↓ → Ischaemic lesions in organs, especially the kidney

Fibrin emboli

The renal lesions are similar to those seen in malignant hypertension. There is fibrinoid necrosis of the afferent arterioles and capillaries of the glomeruli, and resulting areas of tubular necrosis. In the most extreme cases, bilateral cortical necrosis of the kidneys may occur. The underlying pathology is sometimes termed thrombotic microangiopathy. Clinical manifestations are varied. Renal failure, haemolytic anaemia, hypertension, and sometimes purpura with thrombocytopenia are the main features, but lesions in other organs and the symptoms of the initiating disease produce a complicated picture.

Pale necrotic cortex

Congested haemorrhagic margins

Aetiology

Activation of the clotting system can occur in many differing circumstances:

1. Antigen-antibody reactions, e.g. associated with infections. Respiratory and alimentary infections are important in children.

2. Shock conditions, e.g. following abruptio placentae in pregnancy, endotoxic shock.

3. Malignant hypertension. This can be a sequel to the syndrome and equally can predispose the patient to it.

TUBULAR LESIONS OF METABOLIC ORIGIN

This type of lesion is brought about by a metabolic defect which may arise outside the kidney (primary) or be the result of renal dysfunction (secondary).

The basic pathological mechanism is very similar in many of the conditions:

The following are some examples:

Hyperparathyroidism

Primary form. Hypersecretion of parathormone results in calcium deposition in and around the renal tubules.

Secondary form. Retention of phosphate due to renal failure causes parathyroid stimulation and withdrawal of calcium from bones. Before puberty this causes a condition like osteitis fibrosa cystica (renal rickets). Renal deposition of calcium further affects the renal condition producing a vicious cycle.

Hypervitaminosis D

This rare condition, like hyperparathyroidism, produces a high plasma calcium with deposition in the kidney leading to fibrosis and calculus formation.

Gout

The deposition of urates in the renal pyramids causes tubular degeneration and interstitial inflammation progressing to fibrosis.

Fanconi syndrome

This is one example of a number of rare genetic defects causing aminoaciduria.

Cystinuria, glycosuria and phosphaturia are associated with acidosis resulting in renal deposition of calcium and cystine. Fibrosing interstitial nephritis follows, and the tubules show degeneration and cystic dilatations.

PYELONEPHRITIS

Pyelonephritis is the commonest type of renal disease and probably also the commonest single cause of renal failure. Two phases of the disease can be clearly defined, acute and chronic, but there is a spectrum of change and the division into phases is arbitrary.

ACUTE PYELONEPHRITIS

This is an acute pyogenic infection and the patient exhibitis the usual general features of pyrexia, nausea, vomiting, headaches, rigors, etc., plus localising signs, e.g. frequency, dysuria, loin pain and sometimes haematuria.

Pale streaks with surrounding congestion in medullary rays

Pelvis and parenchyma acutely congested and swollen

Streaks and wedges of suppuration in cortex

Some tubules destroyed: abscesses formed

Patches of suppuration in cortex and medulla

Inflammation is mainly interstitial

Glomeruli usually unaffected

Other tubules filled by pus cells

Urine

1. **Microscopy**

Bacteria

Red cell

Cast of pus cells

Pus cells

2. **Chemical** — protein, blood

3. **Bacteriology.**

Large numbers of bacteria are found in the urine, several hundred thousand per ml in the acute phase.

The commonest infecting organism is *Escherichia coli,* but other faecal bacteria may also be found, e.g. pseudomonas, *Streptococcus faecalis.*

643

ACUTE PYELONEPHRITIS

Routes of infection

In the majority of cases, the condition is an ascending infection from the lower urinary tract, frequently associated with obstruction. Both sexes may be affected.

The condition is more common in females, possibly due to the short wide urethra, moist conditions in the perineum and proximity to the anus. In the male, obstruction is almost always present; in the female it may be absent. The condition occurs at an earlier age in the female.

Male	Female
Calculi or tumours in renal pelvis	
Tumours pressing on ureter	
Calculi in ureters	
Tumours of bladder	
Prostatic enlargement	Pregnancy or tumour of uterus or ovaries

Influence of urinary tract obstruction

Obstruction of the urinary tract acts in three ways to promote infection:

1. The urine tends to stagnate and encourages growth of bacteria.
2. A tendency to vesicoureteral reflux during micturition develops especially when cystitis occurs.
3. Catheterisation is commonly carried out in these cases and can introduce infection. In this case the infection is likely to be mixed.

Progress The possibilities are as follows:

Perinephric abscess and papillary necrosis are now rare due to specific antibiotic therapy.

Papillary necrosis (maximal at the kidney poles) is most apt to occur in cases associated with urinary obstruction.

Line of demarcation

Inflammation spreads into renal papilla → Intense interstitial inflammation ↓ Thrombosis of vessels and necrosis of renal tissue ↓ Destruction of collecting ducts and calyces

This can lead rapidly to renal failure.

ACUTE PYELONEPHRITIS

Healing stage
Involvement of the interstitial tissue and destruction of the tubules make resolution impossible and healing by a form of granulation tissue is inevitable.

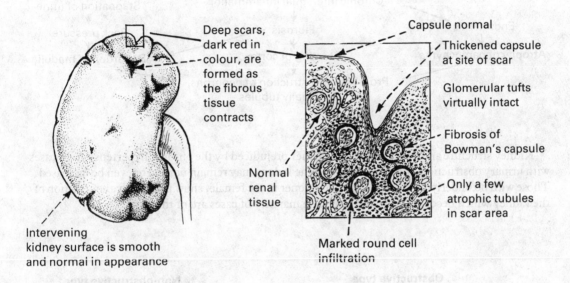

Deep scars, dark red in colour, are formed as the fibrous tissue contracts

Intervening kidney surface is smooth and normal in appearance

Normal renal tissue

Capsule normal

Thickened capsule at site of scar

Glomerular tufts virtually intact

Fibrosis of Bowman's capsule

Only a few atrophic tubules in scar area

Marked round cell infiltration

The lesions are very patchy, and the remaining kidney substance is normal. Eventually the whole area of the lesion is converted into fibrous tissue containing a few glomeruli showing progressive obliteration and sprinkling of round cells.

Danger lies in recurrence of infection, which is prone to happen especially in 'obstruction' cases. This causes a progressive destruction of the renal tissue leading to clinical chronic pyelonephritis.

Bacteriuria

Bacteria are commonly found in the urethra and are constantly flushed away by the urine. It becomes difficult therefore to assess the importance of their presence in a patient who may be ill and febrile but has no localising signs. It is now considered that a count of more than 100,000 bacteria per ml in a mid-stream specimen indicates urinary tract infection.

Significant bacterial counts may be found in patients with no signs or symptoms. This is not uncommon in female children and may account for those cases of chronic pyelonephritis where there has been no evidence of an acute phase.

CHRONIC PYELONEPHRITIS

Chronic pyelonephritis is essentially the result of repeated attacks of inflammation and healing. The process can be visualized as follows:

Kidney structure and function may be further prejudiced by the onset of hypertension. In cases with urinary obstruction, the external size of the kidney may remain normal or even be increased. Those with no underlying abnormality, commoner in the female, show progressive contraction of the kidney which becomes greyish white. The majority of cases are of this type.

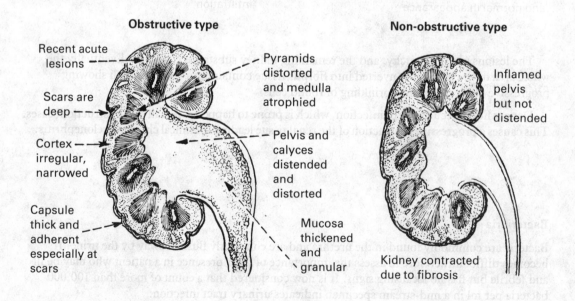

Depending on the cause, only one or both kidneys may be affected to variable degrees (c.f. chronic glomerulonephritis, p.635).

CHRONIC PYELONEPHRITIS

Microscopically, three types of lesion are seen in most cases:

1. Changes similar to those seen in the healing stage, but more advanced and extensive.

2. Occasionally acute suppurative lesions due to recent infection.

Periglomerular fibrosis

Heavy round cell infiltration
Absence of tubules

Endarteritis obliterans

3. Foci of dilated tubules in the cortex. This is due to destruction of the collecting tubules so that they end blindly. Upper tubules dilate, develop colloid casts and come to resemble thyroid tissue.

   The patchy inflammation results in fibrosis and atrophy irregularly distributed throughout the cortex and medulla.

Flattened or cuboidal epithelium

Dense colloid (protein)

Clinical effects

These are due to destruction of tubules and distortion of the anatomy of the renal medulla.

1. There is a progressive loss of the renal concentrating power.

2. The sodium pump effect of the counter-current mechanism is upset; base is lost thus causing acidosis. In children this can interfere with calcium metabolism.

   Renal failure with uraemia develops, although the patient may still be passing relatively large quantities of dilute urine. Chronic pyelonephritis is probably the commonest cause of fatal uraemia. Where unilateral obstruction is the cause only one kidney is affected and uraemia is not a feature.

3. Hypertension is common. This may be partly coincidence since pyelonephritis is more frequent in males over 50, but it does not explain the association of hypertension with pyelonephritis in women and children. Ninety per cent of patients are hypertensive when renal failure occurs. Equally striking, malignant hypertension develops in at least 15% of cases of severe chronic pyelonephritis. Where the inflammation is confined to one kidney, its removal has relieved the hypertension in some cases.

TUBERCULOUS PYELONEPHRITIS

This is now uncommon in many Western countries, due to population screening for tuberculosis and the effect of specific treatment. It is due to blood spread of infection from another site, e.g. the lungs. Alternatively, but much less commonly, there may be an ascending infection from some other part of the genitourinary system, e.g. epididymis or fallopian tubes. As usual, the tuberculous process develops slowly and lesions in the lungs which are the source of infection may have healed and disappeared by the time pyelonephritis is clinically apparent. The disease is commonly unilateral.

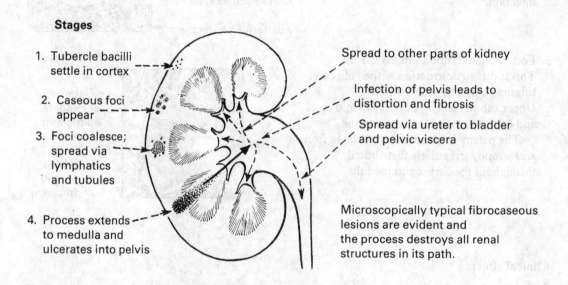

Stages

1. Tubercle bacilli settle in cortex

2. Caseous foci appear

3. Foci coalesce; spread via lymphatics and tubules

4. Process extends to medulla and ulcerates into pelvis

Spread to other parts of kidney

Infection of pelvis leads to distortion and fibrosis

Spread via ureter to bladder and pelvic viscera

Microscopically typical fibrocaseous lesions are evident and the process destroys all renal structures in its path.

Clinical features

There may be no localising features, the patient merely showing the general features of tuberculous infection — fever, night sweats and loss of weight. Lumbar discomfort or pain, dysuria and haematuria can develop. Secondary pyogenic infection is common leading to pyuria. Tubercle bacilli can usually be demonstrated in the urine either on direct microscopic examination or by guinea-pig inoculation. If, however, the ureter is blocked by caseous material, the urine, now coming solely from the uninfected kidney, may be sterile.

The danger is that infection may spread to the unaffected kidney and lead to renal failure.

THE KIDNEY AND ESSENTIAL HYPERTENSION

Two types of essential hypertension, benign and malignant, are recognised, and these have grossly different effects on the kidney function.

BENIGN ESSENTIAL HYPERTENSION

This is a chronic condition which may continue for 20 – 30 years. The anatomical changes in the kidney are due to progressive but patchy occlusion of the interlobular arteries and afferent arterioles.

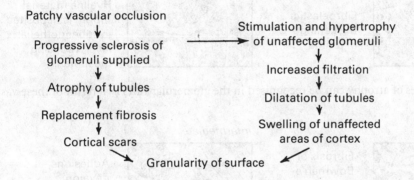

Patchy vascular occlusion
↓
Progressive sclerosis of glomeruli supplied → Stimulation and hypertrophy of unaffected glomeruli
↓ ↓
Atrophy of tubules Increased filtration
↓ ↓
Replacement fibrosis Dilatation of tubules
↓ ↓
Cortical scars Swelling of unaffected areas of cortex
↓ ↓
Granularity of surface

Kidney may be slightly smaller

Surface granular with depressed dark red scars

Dilated tubules

Depressed scar

Sclerosed glomeruli

Hypertrophied glomerulus

Tubules absent

Fibrous tissue infiltrated by lymphocytes and plasma cells

BENIGN ESSENTIAL HYPERTENSION

Where the changes are advanced, a contracted kidney is produced.
The vascular changes are of two types:

Interlobular arteries

Afferent arterioles

Fibrosis of media

Fibroelastic thickening of intima

Intimal thickening due to plasmatic vasculosis

Hyaline material (fibrin) is deposited in subendothelial layer, reducing the lumen.

Various stages of atrophy can be recognised in the glomerular tufts as a result of these vascular changes.

Early

Intermediate

Fibrosis of Bowman's capsule

Wrinkling of capillary basement membrane

Adhesions develop

Increasing fibrosis of capsule

Capillaries collapse and disappear

Late

Due to the patchy nature of the lesion, there is little clinical evidence of renal involvement and only rarely does renal failure develop in the uncomplicated case.

Usually patients die from one of three causes:

Glomerulus completely sclerosed

1. Cerebrovascular accident
2. Congestive cardiac failure
3. Coronary insufficiency.

MALIGNANT HYPERTENSION

In this acute clinical condition, which ends in fatal uraemia in a matter of months if untreated, the blood pressure rises very rapidly to a high level. While the pathological lesions are patchy, they are rapidly progressive both in the degree of change in individual glomeruli and the number of glomeruli affected. As a primary condition, it is a disease of the 3rd and 4th decades in males. In most cases it is secondary to a pre-existing kidney lesion. The significant vascular lesions are to be seen in the afferent arterioles and interlobular arteries.

Interlobular arteries

Afferent arterioles. Some of these will show intimal thickening due to plasmatic vasculosis, but in many this proceeds to fibrinoid necrosis.

Lumen reduced

Increase in medial layer

Concentric fibrous layers (onion skin) in intima

Escape of red cells into capsular space

Crescent formation stimulated by haemorrhage and fibrin formation

Thrombosis extending into tuft

Fibrinoid necrosis of arteriole

Fibrinoid necrosis may also affect some of the interlobular arteries.

Related tubules of affected glomeruli show eosinophilic and red cell casts and necrosis of epithelium where the lesion is recent. This is followed by tubular atrophy. The gross appearance of the kidney is striking:

Blotchy haemorrhages shine through capsule ('Flea bitten' kidney)

Surface smooth

Kidney normal size

Cortical haemorrhages

Occasional tiny infarct

MALIGNANT HYPERTENSION

Clinical features

The main sign is high and rapidly increasing blood pressure. Proteinuria and haematuria are present intermittently. Oliguria eventually becomes progressive and symptoms and signs of uraemia supervene.

    The same vascular changes occur in other viscera e.g. intestines, and may cause symptoms. Headache is common and blurring of vision is caused by papilloedema and retinal haemorrhages, and the cerebral lesions of hypertensive encephalopathy may supervene.

HYPERTENSION AND THE KIDNEY

There is an obvious inter-relationship between renal disease and hypertension. Essential (primary) hypertension occasionally causes serious renal dysfunction, and the vascular changes are most marked in the kidneys. Primary renal disease on the other hand is almost always associated with hypertension (secondary). In cases of chronic renal failure, it is sometimes difficult to disentangle the factors involved. There is a spectrum of pathological change in which the contribution of each of the two factors — renal disease and hypertension — varies greatly. The causes of primary and secondary hypertension are unknown, but the opinion of many is that the kidney plays a central role in both and the search for a common factor continues. At the present moment, the following diagram provides a general idea of a possible mechanism.

In this diagram the common factor is renal ischaemia, and it is thought that this stimulates the renin-hypertensin mechanism. Experimentally, hypertension can be produced by restricting the blood flow to one kidney, and in the human situation hypertension has followed partial obstruction of one renal artery by atheroma or due to looping round a ureter. Removal of the affected kidney has allowed a return to normal blood pressure.

PROGRESSIVE RENAL FAILURE — END-STAGE KIDNEY

In any pathological condition in which there is significant loss of functioning renal tissue, compensating mechanisms are seen. The surviving nephrons show (1) COMPENSATORY HYPERTROPHY and are (2) CONTINUALLY ACTIVE with no 'down time'. (In the normal kidney, the nephrons do not all function simultaneously.)

The postulated mechanism of progressive renal failure is due to failure of the compensatory mechanism and is illustrated diagrammatically in a single glomerulus:

Wear and tear effects:

1. Endothelial cell damage
   ↓
2. Platelet thrombosis
   ↓
3. Hyalinisation
   ↓
4. Fibrosis (sclerosis)

The clinical state is eventually reached when the functional renal tissue has been reduced to a level where life cannot be maintained.

The major pathological causes are chronic pyelonephritis and chronic glomerulonephritis.

The progressive effects of this functional failure are *uraemia* and its complications.

URAEMIA

This is a syndrome encompassing a group of clinical and biochemical signs derived essentially from the retention of waste products and the failure to control fluid and electrolyte balance.

Classically, blood urea levels were measured to assess the degree of waste product retention; nowadays creatinine levels are more commonly measured. (Note that the retention of urea itself is not damaging.)

The following associations and complications are important (see p.654):

PROGRESSIVE RENAL FAILURE — END-STAGE KIDNEY

(1) **Polyuria.** Despite the reduced glomerular filtration rate there is an increased volume of diluted urine. The mechanism is complicated but is presented in simplified form as follows:

	Normal kidney	End-stage kidney
Glomerular function	GFR — 125 ml/mm ≡ 180 litres/day	Many glomeruli sclerosed. ∴ GFR — say 10 ml/min ≡ 14 litres/day
Tubular function	99% reabsorption of water *Urine output:* 1 ml/min ≡ 1.4 litres/day	Many tubules damaged ∴ great reduction in reabsorption *Urine output:* 7 ml/min ≡ 10 litres/day

The inability to deal with water will lead to dehydration and rise in blood nonprotein nitrogen if the intake is reduced.

If intake is increased it may cause water intoxication and rise in blood oedema.

2. **Urine of fixed specific gravity** — usually 1010. This follows from the inability to concentrate the urine and the failure of the selective reabsorptive mechanisms, including the counter-current sodium pump. Urea, creatinine, uric acid, sulphate, chloride and phosphate are retained.

3. **Acidosis.** Difficulty in dealing with phosphates and the inability of the damaged tubules to form ammonia means that the hydrogen ion concentration of urine cannot be varied to suit body needs, and retention acidosis results. Retention of phosphate causes a fall in plasma calcium leading to stimulation of the parathyroids. Bone lesions may result — renal osteo-dystrophy.

Complications

1. **Hypertension.** This is almost inevitable and several consequences are possible.

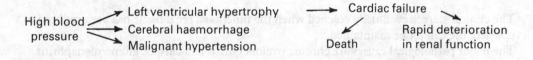

2. **Fibrinous exudates,** e.g. fibrinous pericarditis, 'uraemic pneumonitis' with pleural exudate, (pseudo)membranous colitis.

3. **Haemorrhagic ulcers** of the gastro-intestinal tract.
   The lesions noted in 2 and 3 will cause further difficulty in maintaining biochemical equilibrium by causing changes in fluid balance and acid-base interchange.

4. **Anaemia.** This is due largely to depression of the bone marrow. It has been suggested that it is due to lack of erythropoietin production in the kidney.

5. **Depression of immunological reaction.** Infections are common and will in turn affect renal function. Claims are made that the lack of reaction is beneficial in that there may be less likelihood of a renal transplant rejection.

CONGENITAL DISORDERS

Malpositions and malformations of the kidney
are relatively common and the variations are numerous.
Some of the commoner are:

1. **Ectopic kidney (pelvic kidney)**
   One or both kidneys fail to reach the
   normal adult position. The condition causes
   difficulty:

   (a) During parturition
   (b) In differential diagnosis of pelvic neoplasms
   and infections
   (c) When the renal artery may originate at the normal
   level and the long vessel creates
   problems in arterial supply.

2. **Fusion of kidneys**

This is usually partial, producing
the so-called 'horse-shoe' kidney.
The ureters may be partially
obstructed leading to hydronephrosis,
infection and calculus formation.
Frequently the kidneys are also
ectopic, adding another hazard.

3. **Single kidney**

   This may be a form of fusion and there
   may be two ureters. In other cases, there is
   absence (agenesis) of one kidney, usually
   the left. There is no interference with
   renal function unless, of course, the single
   kidney becomes diseased.

CONGENITAL CYSTIC DISEASE

This occurs in two main forms:

1. **Adult polycystic disease** *autosomal dominant*

   This is relatively common, and varying degrees of the change may be seen from single cysts up to the classical type where the kidneys (rarely only one) are converted into a mass of cysts.

weighs up to 4 kg

Kidney greatly enlarged:
(often exceeds 1 kg)

Cysts vary in size
(largest 5 or 6 cm)

Many are brownish
(fluid serous or mucoid)

Cystic collecting tubule

Normal nephrons

The defect is in the branching of some of the collecting tubules, causing a mixture of normal and abnormal nephrons. Cystic change develops after birth and is progressive, resulting in atrophy of normal nephrons by pressure. The cystic change may not be primarily due to obstruction, but opinion varies.

Intrahepatic cysts are often present but rarely numerous. Death from cerebral haemorrhage is more frequent than expected, partly due to the hypertension secondary to the kidney disorder and perhaps to aneurysms of cerebral arteries.

Clinical Findings

(a) Usually discovered during 3rd and 4th decades, rarely in childhood.

(b) Atrophy of the normal nephrons leads to chronic renal failure, uraemia and hypertension. Progress varies with the number of normal nephrons.

2. **Infantile polycystic disease (Polycystic kidney of the newborn: sponge kidney)**

   This is a rare condition.

Fetal lobulation preserved

Cystic change extends from medulla to cortex

Uniform spongy appearance

The nephrons are said to be normal in number and formation. Cystic dilatation is situated in the terminal branches of the collecting tubules. The disease is incompatible with life, and death occurs shortly after birth. It is said to be related to an autosomal recessive trait. Small liver cysts and multiplication of the intrahepatic bile channels are often present.

TUMOURS OF THE KIDNEY

BENIGN GROWTHS

1. **Fibroma.** This is the commonest simple tumour. It is found incidentally at autopsy in the medulla as a tiny round white nodule, usually less than 1 cm in diameter.

2. **Adenoma.** This is a relatively rare, small nodular proliferation of tubular type epithelium.

MALIGNANT TUMOURS

Two are of importance: renal cell carcinoma and nephroblastoma.

Renal cell carcinoma (Grawitz tumour: hypernephroma)
This is the commonest primary malignant renal tumour. It usually has a typical appearance.

Bands of mucoid connective tissue

Tumour commonly large when diagnosis made

Areas of haemorrhage and necrosis

Circumscribed and apparently encapsulated

Local extension

Through capsule

Into pelvis

Cells usually rather uniform in appearance; large with clear cytoplasm and small round nuclei

Venous invasion is common

Carcinomatous thrombus extends into the inferior vena cava

Secondaries in lungs and bones

Forms solid masses or acini. Sometimes intra-acinar papillary structures are present

Cytoplasm contains glycogen and double refractile lipid.

Stroma is fine and lace-like

TUMOURS OF THE KIDNEY

Malignant (continued)

Nephroblastoma (Wilm's tumour)
This is one of the commonest malignant tumours of childhood. It is an embryonic type of tumour derived from kidney rudiments, and forms a large well-circumscribed growth which rapidly invades blood vessels, giving rise to pulmonary secondaries.

Much of the growth consists of spindle cells resembling sarcoma

This merges with tubules and acini

Occasionally there are primitive glomerular structures

There may be masses of striped muscle.

Secondary carcinoma
Secondary deposits of carcinoma are not uncommon in the kidney.

DISEASES OF URINARY TRACT

The urinary tract is essentially a collecting and discharge system. There are four main pathological processes affecting its function: (1) obstruction (2) infections, (3) calculus formation and (4) neoplastic disease.

Congenital anomalies, which are relatively rare, produce their effects by one or other of these processes.

Obstruction
Acute obstruction, if complete, causes rapid cessation of urine production. If both kidneys are involved, renal failure quickly follows. Chronic obstruction is more common and leads to anatomical changes, with sequels.

Hydronephrosis
This is a dilatation of the renal pelvis and calyces, due to chronic incomplete or intermittent obstruction.

1st stage
Hypertrophy of muscle to overcome obstruction
Obstruction incomplete

2nd stage
Increasing pressure
Kidney substance not reduced
Wall stretches and thins

3rd stage
Pelvis greatly distended
Kidney compressed
Very thin wall
Cortex thin and renal tissue reduced

DISEASES OF URINARY TRACT

Hydronephrosis (continued)

Microscopically, the kidney shows atrophy of tubules in the third stage. This is followed by obliteration of glomeruli. Both changes are the result of pressure directly on the tubules and on the intrarenal vessels. Urine formation is upset and may eventually cease.

Sequels

1. **Infection.** This is almost inevitable and usually takes the form of a chronic pyelonephritis. It exacerbates the whole process and a vicious cycle is set up.

The effects on kidney function have already been considered (p.646 et seq.).

2. **Calculus formation.** The combination of stasis and infection causes precipitation of phosphates and a stone is produced. The mechanism may be:

Aetiology

The condition may affect one or both kidneys. This is related to the site of obstruction.

Unilateral obstruction:
above the bladder

Common sites:
1. Pelvi-ureteric junction.
2. At pelvic brim.
3. At entrance to bladder.

Causes:
1. Calculus.
2. Tumour growth.
3. Inflammatory stricture.
4. Congenital abnormality.

Gross hydronephrosis is more commonly unilateral.

Bilateral obstruction:
in or around bladder or urethra. The ureters are also affected and become dilated and tortuous.

Causes:
1. Prostatic enlargement.
2. Tumour of bladder.
3. Urethral stricture.
4. Pelvic neoplasm.

659

URINARY TRACT INFECTION

Pyelonephritis has already been considered. Inflammation of the ureters is due to extension upwards from an infection of the bladder and urethra.

Acute cystitis

The bladder shows the usual signs of inflammation. Small haemorrhages are common in the oedematous mucosa. The following points are important:

1. It is common in females, especially frequent in pregnancy.
2. In males it is usually secondary to obstruction, e.g. due to enlarged prostate or a urethral stricture.
3. Obstruction encourages infection, enhances its effects and prolongs the inflammatory process.
4. In non-obstructive cases, infection is usually due to *E.coli*. Mixed infections, proteus and staphylococcus, are common in obstructive cases.
5. Vesicoureteric reflux is very important allowing retrograde spread of infection to the kidneys. It occurs as a congenital defect in children but also may be secondary to cystitis.

Chronic cystitis

This is the result of repeated attacks of acute cystitis, but it is usually associated with obstruction of the urethra causing stasis of urine and is commonest in males.

Mixed infection including proteus is common and, together with urea-splitting organisms forming ammonia, result in an alkaline urine. Phosphates precipitate and can form crumbling whitish calculi. A rare granulomatous cystitis is caused by malakoplakia.

Tuberculous cystitis

This is always secondary to a tuberculous infection elsewhere, usually in the kidney. Less commonly, the epididymis is the source of infection. Small tubercles form in the submucous layer, usually at the bladder base. These ulcerate and secondary infection is common.

Urethritis

Acute inflammation of the urethra is commonly due to the gonococcus, but another form is now more common in Western countries — non-specific urethritis. The actual cause is unknown: suggestions include virus, mycoplasma and allergy.

Urethritis may also occur in trichomonal infection and Reiter's disease in which arthritis and conjunctivitis are also present.

RENAL CALCULI

Three basic types of renal calculi are recognised.

(1) **Calcium oxalate** — Surface is rough; colour brown, probably due to old blood pigment

(2) **Uric acid and urates** — Smooth light brown colour

(3) **Phosphate (calcium apatite)** — Flaking surface, greyish white

Commonly the stones are mixed.

1. Urate stones frequently have a rough covering of oxalate.
2. Both oxalate and urate stones tend to develop a covering of phosphates.

Sites of formation. Two suggestions have been made.

1. Precipitates form in the collecting tubules and pass into the renal pelvis where they enlarge.
2. Deposits are formed in the lymphatics of the renal papillae and are extruded into the renal pelvis.

Mode of formation. This is unknown, but the following is one modern theory:

Excess excretion of stone subtance (e.g. oxalate) + Calcium

Lack of urinary fibrinolysis

Supersaturated solution of salt

Lack of substances keeping calcium salts in solution (magnesium, phosphates, etc.)

Lack of inhibitors of crystal formation

Protein nidus → Precipitation and stone formation

Predisposing factors

1. **Urinary pH.** Urate and oxalate stones form in an acid urine; phosphate stone in alkaline urine.
2. **Dehydration** — causing increased urinary concentration.
3. **Stasis.** Obstruction to urine flow encourages salt precipitation.
4. **Renal disease.** The pH of the urine is frequently disturbed, and the composition of the urine is always altered.
   (a) Renal infection is one of the most important factors. In many cases of renal sepsis, the urine becomes alkaline, favouring phosphate precipatation. Ischaemia causing degeneration and necrosis induces calcification in many chronic renal diseases, and this may lead to stone formation.
   (b) Renal tumours encourage stone formation. Areas of tumour necrosis may calcify, and tumours tend to cause urinary stasis.

RENAL CALCULI

Predisposing factors (continued)

5. **Metabolic factors.** These can operate by altering the pH of the urine and especially by increasing the output of substances e.g:

    (a) Hypercalcuria and hyperphosphaturia. These may be caused by:

        Hyperparathyroidism, primary or secondary to renal failure

        Vitamin D overdosage

        Diet, e.g. excessive milk and alkalies over years in peptic ulcer cases

        Immobilisation leading to loss of calcium from bones.

    (b) Oxaluria. Due to:

        Congenital metabolic defect

        Poisoning by ethylene glycol.

    (c) Urate excess is found in:

        Gout

        Excess intake of purines

        Following ileostomy.

    (d) Rare stones, e.g. cystine, xanthine, are related to inborn metabolic defects.

Effects and complications

These are related to passage of the stone and develop in two situations.

(1) Passage of small stone → Injury to ureter → Stricture → Subsequent impaction of stone

    Passage of small stone ↓ Colic

(2) Passage of larger stone → Impaction (at upper and lower ends of ureter, or at brim of pelvis) → Stasis → Hydronephrosis / Infection

    With the development of stasis and infection, further stone formation is encouraged. This can lead to some peculiar results, e.g:

Staghorn calculus

This large single stone is associated with suppuration and ulceration of the pelvis and calyces. It is composed mainly of phosphates.

    Stones and infection in the pelvis can lead to squamous metaplasia of the epithelium. In a few instances this may develop into squamous carcinoma.

BLADDER CALCULI

These may have passed down the ureter. In the bladder they can increase greatly in size. Cystitis is common and the enlargement is due to deposit they can increase greatly in size. Cystitis is common and the enlargement is due to deposit of phosphates. Stones may actually form in the bladder when there is urethral obstruction and chronic cystitis.

TUMOURS OF THE URINARY TRACT

These occur in two sites: (1) the renal pelvis and (2) the bladder (the commoner site).

They arise from the stratified transitional epithelium lining the tract. While it is customary to divide them into benign and malignant types, they form a spectrum of change and it is frequently difficult to exclude malignancy. Two main forms exist.

Papillary tumours

Benign tumours have a uniform, well-differentiated epithelial covering showing no mitotic activity. They have a slender stalk and delicate branching fronds. With this structure, and their fine vascular connective tissue, haemorrhage is common and infection is usually present.

In malignant forms, the stalk of the tumour is broader and the epithelial cells show mitoses and variability. Invasion may be absent but, despite this, recurrence is common.

Sessile solid tumours

These are broad-based, raised plagues. All are in some degree malignant. The more malignant show necrosis and ulceration with anaplastic changes in the epithelium. Invasion of the muscle and lymphatics occurs early. Squamous carcinoma and adenocarcinoma are occasionally seen.

Aetiology

Bladder tumours are an industrial hazard:

painless hematuria 50-70 years

   (a) in aniline dye manufacture due to beta-naphthylamine

   (b) in the rubber industry

   (c) in manufacturing processes involving benzidine

   (d) in chronic analgesic abuse.

No known factor, however, has been incriminated in the majority of cases. In Egypt, schistosomiasis is an important factor.

FEMALE GENITAL TRACT — ANATOMY AND PHYSIOLOGY

The ovaries, fallopian tubes, uterus, vagina and vulva form an integrated system which is unique in that full function is limited to a period of roughly 40 years from puberty to menopause. A two-tier system of hormonal control operates. Secretion of steroids by the ovary prepares the uterus for pregnancy, and the ovarian secretion is controlled by the anterior pituitary and hypothalamus.

Ovarian cycle

(Day 14) Ovulation

(Day 1) Primordial follicle

Developing follicle

Corpus luteum

Regressing corpus luteum *(Day 22)*

(Day 28) Early corpus albicans

Follicular development

Primordial follicle

Nucleus

Pregranulosa cells

Zona pellucida

Fat globules

Granulosa cells

Zona pellucida

Theca { interna / externa

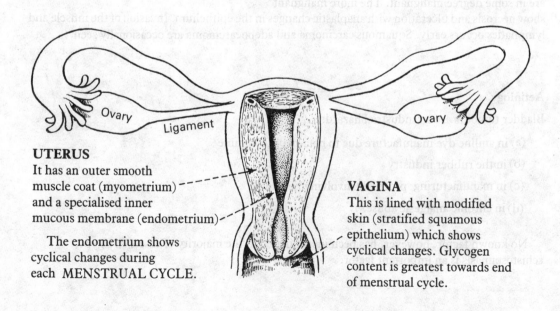

Ovary

Ligament

Ovary

UTERUS

It has an outer smooth muscle coat (myometrium) and a specialised inner mucous membrane (endometrium)

The endometrium shows cyclical changes during each MENSTRUAL CYCLE.

VAGINA

This is lined with modified skin (stratified squamous epithelium) which shows cyclical changes. Glycogen content is greatest towards end of menstrual cycle.

CYCLICAL ENDOMETRIAL CHANGES

Menstruation

Proliferation   Secretion   Regression

Day 0 1 3 4   14   23   28

ASSOCIATED OVARIAN STEROID SECRETION

Oestrogen

Progesterone

Day 1   14   28

Proliferative phase

This is induced by oestrogen produced by developing ovarian follicles.

Stromal cells narrow spindles to begin with, become plump

Epithelium is cuboidal, growing taller as ovulation is approached

Glands are simple, narrow tubes dilating prior to ovulation

Secretory phase

Progesterone produced by the corpus luteum stimulates secretion by the glands. Oestrogen is also produced. The stromal cells enlarge, oedema is present and vascularity greatly increased.

Glands dilated and tortuous

Cells tall, cytoplasm clear, nuclei basal

Premenstrual regressive phase

Endometrial growth ceases 5 – 6 days before menstruation. Prior to menstruation, it shrinks due to decreased blood flow and discharge of secretion. This increases the tortuosity of glands and blood vessels.

665

CYCLICAL ENDOMETRIAL CHANGES

CONTROL MECHANISM
The control of these events
is two-way, involving both
steroids and gonadotrophins.
The time relationship between
these two classes of hormone
may be represented thus:

Feed back systems are involved in stimulating and controlling the hormones secreted.

1. At the end of a menstrual cycle,
   the plasma oestrogen is low.
   This is a signal to the pituitary
   to secrete FSH (positive stimulation)
   which stimulates follicular growth.

2. As follicles grow, they secrete
   oestrogen which damps down the
   secretion of FSH (negative feedback).
   Only the larger follicles
   possessing sufficient receptors for
   FSH continue to grow.

3. The blood oestrogen goes on
   rising as a result of secretion
   from these large follicles. When
   it reaches a sufficiently high
   level, it stimulates the centre in
   the median eminence which secretes
   gonadotrophin releasing
   factor (positive feedback). This
   causes a surge of secretion of
   FSH and LH which induce ovulation

Morphological cyclical changes also take place in the fallopian tubes, cervix, vagina and vulva.

DISEASES OF UTERINE BODY

ENDOMETRIUM

Acute inflammation

This is almost confined to infection associated with parturition and abortion. The usual acute inflammatory changes take place. Infection at the time of parturition is commonly associated with retention of products of conception. In the case of abortion, another factor is the introduction of infection by criminal interference. A mixed bacterial flora, pyococci, coliform organisms and proteus is usual. Occasionally *Cl. welchii* is present. Gonococcal infection does not commonly extend beyond the cervix, but occasionally the endometrium and myometrium are affected. Untreated, the condition may become chronic. Complications may follow endometritis:

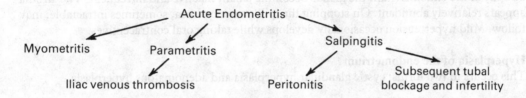

Septicaemia was a common problem as a result of puerperal infection by haemolytic streptococci prior to the introduction of antibiotics.

Chronic endometritis

This is a rare lesion as a primary condition. It can follow an acute endometritis which may be mild. The uterine changes occur in two phases:

The normal cyclical changes fail to take place.

DISEASES OF UTERINE BODY

Tuberculous endometritis
This is now uncommon in the British Isles. It is the result of infection spreading from the fallopian tubes. If the patient is still menstruating, the tubercles are shed each month. In some cases, menstruation ceases and caseation occurs.

Intrauterine anti-fertility devices
A mild chronic inflammation may be associated with the use of these devices. There may be focal atrophy with mild plasma cell infiltration. Irregular bleeding may result.

Oral contraceptives
These are commonly a combination of an oestrogen with a progestogen. They tend to induce atrophy of the endometrium, the glands becoming small, inactive and infrequent. The stroma appears relatively abundant. On stopping the 'pill', amenorrhoea, sometimes intractable, may follow. Mild hypertension occasionally develops while taking oral contraceptives.

Hyperplasia of the endometrium
This occurs in two forms: cystic glandular hyperplasia and adenomatous hyperplasia.

Cystic glandular hyperplasia
This may occur around puberty, during reproductive life or in the postmenopausal period. It is commonest in the premenopausal years.

Myometrium thickened

Uterus enlarged

Endometrium thick and sometimes polypoidal

Stroma cellular with plump cells

Thrombosis of superficial vessels

Epithelial cells taller and basophilic

Glands dilated sometimes irregularly

Areas of haemorrhage

Clinically, there is irregular, frequent and heavy bleeding.

Pathogenesis
The uterine changes suggest excessive oestrogen stimulation. Bleeding and endometrial necrosis indicate that the high oestrogen production falls from time to time.

DISEASES OF UTERINE BODY

Cystic glandular hyperplasia (continued)

Aetiology

This endometrial pattern is associated with lack of ovulation. Persisting large cystic Graafian follicles, producing oestrogen, may be found in the ovary. Endometrial haemorrhage and necrosis are thought to follow involution of the cystic follicles. There is obviously an upset in the hormonal control of the ovary, but the cause is unknown.

A similar endometrial change may be brought about by:

      1. Injudicious use of oestrogens in therapy
      2. Granulosa cell tumour
      3. Thecoma.

These conditions occur most commonly in post-menopausal patients.

Adenomatous hyperplasia

In this condition the hyperplasia is focal and more intense, and mitotic figures are common.

Normal endometrium

Epithelium tall, sometimes stratified

Stroma reduced in adenomatous areas.

Glands focally more plentiful.

Variation in size of glands.

Intervening endometrium may show cystic glandular hyperplasia. The importance of adenomatous hyperplasia is its possible relationship to the development of adenocarcinoma.

DISEASES OF UTERINE BODY

ADENOMATOUS POLYP
This is a localised proliferation of endometrial glands which becomes pedunculated.

Sometimes polyps are associated with general endometrial hyperplasia. Progressive elongation of the pedicle jeopardises the blood supply. Compression by the uterine muscle results in venous congestion at the tip leading to bleeding and necrosis.

CARCINOMA
This growth may form a *localised* plaque or polyp.

In some cases, however, it appears as a *diffuse* change involving much of the endometrium. It grows initially within the endometrial layer, bulging into the uterine cavity. Surface necrosis occurs at an early date.

Most growths are well-differentiated adenocarcinomas

but anaplastic growths are not uncommon

Areas of squamous metaplasia are relatively common (adeno-acanthoma); they have no prognostic implication

The endometrium possesses no lymphatics and invasion of the myometrium takes place slowly.

Local extension: this may take place in several directions.

Spread towards tube

Penetration of uterus and growth in the parametrium

Spread to cervix and vagina

Direct invasion of the bladder

DISEASES OF UTERINE BODY

CARCINOMA (continued)
Metastases

1. **Via lymphatics**

Para-aortic nodes

Internal iliac nodes

By local lymphatic channels to vagina

2. **Via blood vessels**
Secondary deposits in the vagina and ovaries may be due to this mode of spread

3. **Via fallopian tube**

Ovary

Peritoneal spread

4. **Distant metastases.** At a late date, secondaries may appear in the liver, lungs and bones. These may be the result of lymphatic or blood spread.

Prognosis
The occurrence of bleeding early in the disease leads to early diagnosis. Lack of lymphatics in the endometrium limits extension for a considerable time. There is a 5 year survival rate of at least 80%.

Aetiology
The cause is unknown. Adenocarcinoma is uncommon before the 5th decade. There is some evidence that oestrogen may be an aetiological factor. An increased incidence occurs in association with oestrogen-secreting tumours of the ovary and in obese, diabetic and hypertensive women who tend to have a high level of blood oestrogen. Oestrogen therapy is associated with an increased incidence.

STROMATOSIS (Stormal endometriosis)
This is a rare condition in which there is an overgrowth of endometrial stroma which may form foci in the myometrium and can grow along lymphatics.

ENDOMETRIAL SARCOMA
Another rare tumour which arises from the endometrial stroma. It is extremely malignant.

MIXED MESODERMAL TUMOUR
This also arises from the endometrium, but it consists of epithelial and stromal elements forming varying proportions of carcinoma and sarcoma. The stromal elements may differentiate forming osteoid, cartilaginous or even rhabdomyosarcoma.

DISEASES OF UTERINE BODY

HYDATIDIFORM MOLE
This occurs in two forms:

1. **Complete.** This is a pregnancy lacking a fetus. It starts early in pregnancy and the uterus is filled by cysts of varying size.

Weeks
16
12
8

Normal   Hydatidiform
mole

Uterus filled by cysts of varying size

Cysts are greatly enlarged chorionic villi.

Hyperplasia of cytotrophoblast and of syncytiotrophoblast.

Oedematous connective tissue containing cisterns

Absence of vessels

Blood and urine levels of chorionic gonadotrophin are high. (TSH also increased — possible hyperthyroidism.) Chorionic epithelium may invade the uterus but regresses after hysterectomy. Hydatid mole is uncommon in the West (1 in 2000 pregnancies) but common in the East (1 in 120 pregnancies).

2. **Partial.** Sometimes only part of the placenta shows hydatid change and a fetus, usually malformed, is present.

Genetics: The genetic sex of the complete form is XX, but both chromosomes are paternal. The female pronucleus disappears and the male pronucleus duplicates.

In the partial form there is triploidy — XYY or XXY — due to polyspermy or an error in meiotic division.

CHORIOCARCINOMA
This usually follows hydatid mole. Pleomorphic cytotrophoblast and syncytium, showing

Clot

numerous mitoses, invade blood vessels causing haemorrhage and early lung metastases either as a single large 'cannon-ball' haemorrhagic mass or multiple small emboli ('snow-storm' lung). The high blood and urine concentrations of chorionic gonadotrophin are used to monitor progress and treatment.

The myometrium is invaded by masses of malignant chorionic epithelium and blood vessels are eroded.

DISEASES OF UTERINE BODY

MYOMETRIUM

The myometrium is never a primary site of inflammation, acute or chronic. It is involved secondary to lesions in the endometrium or peritoneum. Tumours however are quite common.

LEIOMYOMA (Myoma, fibromyoma, fibroid)

This is a circumscribed growth derived from uterine muscle.

Tumour is hard, round, white with a whorled structure

The cells are typical long spindle muscle cells, arranged in interlacing bundles

They vary in size from tiny (mm) growths to several cm in diameter and are frequently multiple. Apparent encapsulation is due to compression by adjacent muscle.

Fibroids may be found in any part of the uterus.

Tumours beneath the endometrium tend to bulge into the cavity and may eventually develop to form a fibroid polyp.

Similarly subserous polyps may form

Complications

Infertility ← Fibroid → Sarcoma (very rare)

Degeneration → Submucous polyp   Subserous polyp

Hyaline   Mucoid   Necrosis and haemorrhage   Torsion

Calcification

Leiomyoma is one of the commonest tumours, occurring in 15 – 20 per cent of women over the age of 35. Growth ceases at the menopause. There is an association with endometrial carcinoma.

SARCOMA

This is a rare tumour. It may arise from a preceding leiomyoma, but this is not certain. Usually it is extremely malignant.

DISEASES OF UTERINE BODY

ENDOMETRIOSIS

This consists of deposits
of endometrium outside of
the uterine cavity.

In almost all cases,
the disease is confined
to the pelvis and the
genital tract.

Other sites: Caecum and appendix,
bladder, rectum,
laparotomy scar.

Sites:

Fallopian tube

Ovary

Broad
ligament

Surface of uterus

These deposits react to the stimulus of ovarian steroids and show cyclical changes. The result is haemorrhage into the local tissues at the time of menstruation. Adhesions develop.

Aetiology

In some instances deposits are formed in laparotomy scars after uterine operations, but in most cases there has been no surgical interference. Three theories have been proposed.

    1. Retrograde spill of menstrual debris.
    2. Metaplasia of tissues into Mullerian duct elements.
    3. Lymphatic and blood borne emboli of endometrial tissue.

ADENOMYOSIS

This is a condition of ectopic endometrial deposits in the myometrium. There is an accompanying overgrowth of muscle and connective tissue. Two macroscopic forms occur:

1. **Diffuse**
Deposits are confined
to inner part of
myometrium
Foci of endometrium
often brownish in colour

2. **Localised**
Resembling
fibroid
but with
brownish
foci

The endometrial deposits are said to communicate with the uterine cavity, but despite this they often contain altered blood in the glands which become cystic. The diffuse type is commoner.

674

DISEASES OF CERVIX

The cervix constitutes the lower one third of the uterine body.

It is in two parts: endocervical and vaginal or ectocervical. The dividing line is quite sharp and is determined by the character of the lining epithelium.

Internal os

5cm

External os

2.5cm

Tall mucus-secreting epithelium

Stratified squamous epithelium, non-keratinised

Branching glands

Ectocervix

Endocervix

The remainder of the cervical wall consists of circular smooth muscle lying in abundant fibroelastic tissue.

At the internal os, the structure gradually merges with that of the uterus proper, the branching glands giving place to the simple tubules of the endometrium, and the proportion of muscle increases greatly.

CERVICAL EROSION. This is a misnomer. There is no erosion until infection supervenes. It is a simple replacement of the ectocervical squamosa by columnar mucus-secreting epithelium.

Red colour; soft velvety texture

Aetiology
1. Related in part to hormonal stimulation.
2. Common in pregnancy.
3. Sometimes associated with taking contraceptive pills.
4. May be a persistence of normal infantile structures.

CERVICAL POLYP. This is a local proliferation of endocervical mucosa which becomes pedunculated and may protrude through the cervix.

Cystic glands are common due to obstruction by chronic inflammation

The above two conditions, together with cervical injury at parturition, are probably the main causes of **cervicitis**.

DISEASES OF CERVIX

CERVICITIS

This is usually a mild, chronic condition
and in most cases the bacterial flora is mixed,
but in a small number of cases acute inflammation
may result from gonococcal infection or infection
with other pyogenic organisms particularly
during childbirth with lacerations of cervix.

In chronic cervicitis, the mucus-secreting
endocervical epithelium undergoes squamous
metaplasia. This is a simple condition, the result
of chronic irritation. In some instances, this
squamous epithelium is 'restless', showing proliferative
activity and cellular abnormalities,
termed dysplasia. Dysplasia, intraepithelial
carcinoma (carcinoma in situ) and invasive carcinoma
are thought to be stages in a continuing process. Dysplasia was considered in three stages — mild,
moderate and severe — but each stage merges with the next and the differentiation between severe
dysplasia and carcinoma in situ is difficult. A new pragmatic classification has been adopted which
provides a practical guide for the surgeon.

Again three stages are defined: cervical intraepithelial neoplasia (CIN) (1), (2) and (3).

Benign squamous metaplasia
Stratification well defined with:

Squames at
surface

Oval polygonal
cells form
several layers

Basal cells usually
a single layer
at right angles
to the surface.

CIN 1 ≡ mild dysplasia

Upper two thirds
stratified

Cells of basal third
have high nucleocytoplasmic
ratio; pleomorphic nuclei
at all levels

CIN 2 ≡ moderate dysplasia

Upper half of
epithelium shows
stratification and
maturation

Basal cells
occupy
lower half

Although a clear distinction is made in these illustrations between CIN 1 and CIN 2, in practice
all degress of change are seen and the grading depends on the individual pathologist.

DISEASES OF CERVIX

Cervical intra-epithelial neoplasia (continued)

CIN 3: Severe dysplasia and carcinoma in situ are included in this grade. The differentiation between them is even more subjective. By adopting the CIN grading, this subjective problem is eliminated since no attempt is made to separate the two conditions, and the clinician understands that CIN is a dangerous lesion.

Examples are:

CIN 3 ≡ severe dysplasia or Ca in situ

(1) There may be one or two layers of stratified epithelium on surface.

(2) Remainder is immature with large nuclei.

(3) Mitoses are common.

Classical Ca in situ

(1) Almost complete loss of stratification.
(2) Loss of polarity of the cells, the majority being at right angles to the surface; the remainder irregularly arranged.
(3) Variation in nuclear size with increase in nuclear/cytoplasmic ratio.
(4) Cells lose their squamous appearance.
(5) Mitotic figures found at all levels.

The lesion develops at the squamocolumnar junction, i.e. where endocervix and ectocervix meet. Less than 20% occur within the cervical canal. The epithelium is loosely attached to the underlying stroma, especially type 3 and may be removed by swabbing, thus leading to misdiagnosis.

This preinvasive stage may last for many years before invasion develops, but in many cases does not progress to the invasive stage. Most are diagnosed in the 4th decade but very occasionally as early as the 2nd decade and as late as the 7th. Unfortunately, it is obviously impossible to say how soon invasion will occur.

DISEASES OF CERVIX

CARCINOMA

This is said to be the most common malignant tumour of the female genital tract, but the incidence varies from country to country and appears to be significantly reduced where there is a vigorous campaign for early diagnosis and eradication of carcinoma in situ.

The growth is a squamous cell carcinoma in 95% of cases, the remaining 5% being adenocarcinomas. The site of the growth has no relationship to the histological type. It usually arises at the squamocolumnar junction. Twenty per cent of squamous carcinomas are found within the cervical canal, and occasionally an adenocarcinoma originates in the glands near the external os.

The cervix becomes very indurated; necrosis and ulceration commonly follow quickly.

Later, a large fungating mass is produced. Sloughing may leave an excavated crater.

Spread

Until a very late stage, the disease is confined to the pelvic cavity. The patient commonly dies before distant metastases appear.

Local spread takes place in several directions:

1. **Downward extension.**

2. **Lateral extension.** The anatomy of this region is important.

Uterus

Trigone of bladder

(a) The growth encircles the external os. In some cases, it causes obstruction of the cervical canal and pyometra may develop.
(b) Extension to the vagina takes place by direct continuity.

The ureters come very close to the cervix in their travel to the bladder, and are apt to be involved in extension of the growth to the parametrium. The ureters may be obstructed by pressure or invasion. Renal infection and failure follow.

DISEASES OF CERVIX

Spread of carcinoma (continued)

3. **Anterior and posterior extension**

Direct invasion of the bladder or rectum results in fistulous communications. Spread along the uterosacral ligaments involves the sacral nerves, causing intractable pain.

4. **Lymphatic spread**

This occurs early and involves the chains of lymph nodes in the pelvis.

Aortic

Common iliac

Internal iliac

Sacral

External iliac

Obturator

Paracervical

Histology

Squamous cell carcinoma

The appearances are typical, but cell nests are absent and keratinisation is rarely seen.

Central cells ovoid and obviously of squamous type

Peripheral cells cuboidal

Adenocarcinoma

Solid masses invading the stroma

Isolated gland structures and cystic spaces lined by tall mucus-secreting epithelial cells

Progress

The prognosis is poor in invasive cervical cancer. Overall five year survival rate is 40% but much depends on the extent of the disease.

Death is commonly due to a combination of renal failure and sepsis. Fatal haemorrhage from eroded vessels may occur.

DISEASES OF CERVIX

CYTOLOGY and UTERINE CANCER

Cells from endometrial and cervical cancers are exfoliated and appear in the vagina. These can be collected by aspirating the posterior vaginal fornix, fixed smears made and stained by Papanicolau's method. Malignant cells from cervical cancers will be found in 80% of cases by this method, but only in 10% of cases of endometrial carcinoma. Scraping the squamocolumnar junction and examination of the cells obtained will increase the figure for cervical cancer to 90%.

The main use of cytodiagnosis, however, lies in the detection of suspicious cells in smears from healthy women, leading to further examination and possible detection of dysplasia or carcinoma in situ.

Aetiology

1. *Epidemiological facts*
   (a) The disease is rare in virgins (in a community of nuns, no cases were seen) and the incidence is highest in prostitutes. The disease is rare in strictly orthodox Jewish women and significantly increased in less strict Jewish communities.
   (b) Historically the disease was seen most commonly in the 4th and 5th decades. Nowadays, in Western Societies, dysplasia and carcinoma are seen in young women (2nd and 3rd decades) and the prevalence has greatly increased. These changes are statistically related to sexual promiscuity and early age of first coitus.
   All of these facts strongly indicate a *carcinogenic agent* transmitted by *sexual intercourse*.

2. *Virus infection*
   It has now been shown that a **human papilloma virus** is present in all cases of carcinoma and also in preceding warty dysplasias.

3. Possible promoters (co-factors) have not yet been defined.

DISEASES OF VAGINA AND VULVA

Trichomonas vaginalis

Vaginal discharge is a common complaint especially in parous women. In many cases it is related to chronic cervicitis. There are however a number inflammatory conditions which arise primarily in the vagina.

Gonococcal infection may produce an acute inflammation with purulent discharge but it is often asymptomatic.

Purulent discharge is also associated with infection by a protozoon, Trichomonas vaginalis. The discharge tends to be frothy. It is commonly transmitted during sexual intercourse. The male can also be infected.

DISEASES OF VAGINA AND VULVA

Candida albicans infection is common in pregnancy and in patients undergoing antibotic or immunosuppressive therapy.

Primary tumours of the vagina are rare. Squamous carcinoma occurs in the upper vagina of old women and leads to fistula formation between the vagina and the bladder and rectum.

Adenocarcinoma is sometimes found in adolescent girls. It has been traced to the effect on the fetus of administration of diethylstilboestrol to the patient's mother during early pregnancy.

Vulval inflammation is common in postmenopausal women. It is related to atrophy of the skin, which has very thin epithelial covering at this phase of life and is easily abraded. Inflammation at other periods of life frequently involves Bartholin's gland.

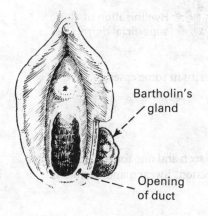

Bartholin's gland

Opening of duct

The duct which opens into the vagina in front of the hymen is apt to become blocked. If the inflammation subsides a simple cyst of the duct arises but an abscess may form.

Two conditions which mainly occur in the tropics but may make their appearance in temperate countries are:

1. **Lymphogranuloma venereum.** This is a chlamydial infection which starts as an ulcer on the vulva or in the vagina. It heals in a short time, only to be followed by a chronic suppurative reaction in the inguinal and sometimes pelvic lymph nodes. This leads to extensive scarring and sometimes fistulous openings in the pelvic viscera.

2. **Granuloma inguinale.** This begins as a papule on the vulva, perineum or vagina. It ulcerates and can spread widely, causing extensive destruction of tissue. Histologically, it is a granuloma and the infecting organism (Donovan bodies) can be seen in macrophages.

DISEASES OF VAGINA AND VULVA

LEUKOPLAKIA AND PREMALIGNANCY

Leukoplakia is a descriptive term meaning white patches. These are common on the vulval and perineal regions in almost any chronic inflammatory skin condition due to the local moist conditions, e.g. neurodermatitis, fungal infection and in atrophic lesions, e.g. senile keratosis and lichen sclerosis et atrophicus.

There is however one type of lesion appearing as white patches in this region which shows epithelial dysplasia and is premalignant.

Hyperkeratosis and Parakeratosis

Epithelial hyperplasia with mitotic activity and abnormal cells

Hyalinisation of superficial dermis

Chronic inflammatory reaction

The degree of dysplasia varies, amounting to carcinoma in situ in some cases.

TUMOURS OF THE VULVA

Simple tumours are uncommon. Papillomata are occasionally seen and one form, condylomata acuminata, consists of multiple papillomata due to a viral infection. Sweat gland tumours (hidradenomas) may also occur.

Carcinoma of vulva

This is a rare condition found in women in the 6th and 7th decades of life.

Starting as an indurated plaque it becomes ulcerated

Atrophic postmenopausal vulva

The inguinal glands on both sides are invaded at an early date.
The growth is usually a squamous carcinoma but adenocarcinoma and basal cell carcinoma also occur.

DISEASES OF FALLOPIAN TUBE

Apart from ectopic pregnancy, the fallopian tubes are rarely the site of primary disease.

Acute salpingitis. Two types of lesion are recognised.

1. **Endosalpingitis.** The inflammation spreads in the mucosa, involving the plicae of the tube. This type follows acute endometritis due to pyogenic infections such as gonorrhoea. Occasionally the infection is the result of spread from an acute peritonitis.

2. **Interstitial salpingitis.** In this case, the inflammation involves the whole wall of the tube including the mesosalpinx, but excluding the mucosa. The tube is greatly swollen. Usually the primary lesion is an acute endometritis and metritis associated with abortion or puerperal infection.

Complications are more common with endosalpingitis:

Tuberculous salpingitis.
Tuberculous infection of the female genital tract, for some unexplained reason, almost always starts in the fallopian tube. It is usually due to blood spread from some other site: only very occasionally it is secondary to tuberculous peritonitis.

The complications are these expected of a chronic salpingitis with the added element of caseation.

Tumours of the fallopian tube.
Benign tumours such as fibroma and myoma occasionally occur. Small cysts of congenital origin are common around the fimbrial ends of the tubes.

Carcinoma, usually a papillary adenocarcinoma, is extremely rare.

ECTOPIC PREGNANCY

This means implantation of the fertilised ovum outside the uterine cavity.

Sites of implantation

Ampullary implantation
This is the commonest.

Interstitial implantation (rare)

Lumen of tube

Broad ligament

Ovum implants in tubal wall

There is no decidua and it burrows into the muscular wall.

Uterine changes

Uterus enlarges

Decidua develops

Erosion of the tubal tissues by the ovum results in **rupture**. This is the commonest finding. The direction of rupture varies:

(1)

Rupture into the lumen of the tube and leakage into peritoneal cavity.

(2)

Rupture directly into the peritoneal cavity. If the implantation is interstitial, there may be a further complication — damage to the uterine arteries with arterial bleeding.

Very occasionally the whole pregnancy — ovum and placental tissue — abort into the peritoneal cavity where it reimplants. Usually development is limited and the fetus dies, but continuation of the pregnancy almost to term has been reported.

Aetiology. Most commonly the tube has been previously damaged by salpingitis, leading to partial blockage of the tube. Recently there has been an increased incidence of ectopic pregnancy in women fitted with intrauterine contraceptive devices.

(3)

Rupture into the broad ligament
↓
Extraperitoneal haematoma

DISEASES OF OVARIES

Oophoritis

Inflammation of the ovaries is always secondary to disease of the fallopian tubes or peritoneum. In the case of the tube, the inflamed fimbrial end becomes adherent to the ovary and direct spread of infection occurs. Extensive changes take place despite treatment.

Swollen tube — Tubo-ovarian inflammation

Inflammation subsides

Adhesion of fimbrial end of tube to ovary

Possible development of tubo-ovarian abscess or peritonitis

Extensive adhesions result.

The ovary may be similarly involved in tuberculous salpingitis, and caseating lesions can occur.

If bilateral, which is frequent, sterility results.

Ovarian changes of functional origin

The control mechanisms of ovarian function frequently develop faults resulting in abnormalities of structure:

Follicular cysts

These may be single or multiple. The maximum diameter of a normal Graafian follicle is 1.5 – 2 cm. Single follicular cysts may be several centimetres in diameter. Amenorrhoea is common in such instances. Multiple follicular cysts, usually small, are associated with endometrial hyperplasia.

Theca lutein cysts

These are cysts from which the granulosa cells have disappeared, leaving cysts surrounded by luteinised thecal tissue. Bilateral, multiple small cysts of this nature occur in polycystic ovarian disease and are associated with obesity, hirsutes and oligomenorrhoea.

Granulosa cells lining cyst

DISEASES OF OVARIES

A multiplicity of types of ovarian tumours exist. Various classifications have been suggested; none satisfactory. The following is a simple working classification:

> 1. Epithelial tumours.
> 2. Sex Cord/Stromal tumours.
> 3. Germ cell tumours.
> 4. Secondary (metastatic) tumours.

1. COMMON EPITHELIAL TUMOURS

These are found in adult life, very rarely in children.

Papillary cystadenoma

Twenty-five per cent of all ovarian tumours are of this variety. In a third of cases they are bilateral, but they almost never reach the large size of the mucinous growths.

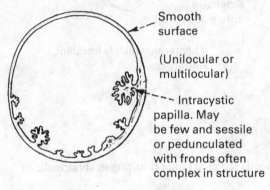

Smooth surface

(Unilocular or multilocular)

Intracystic papilla. May be few and sessile or pedunculated with fronds often complex in structure

Some tumours have small loculi with papillary formations making them appear solid.

Epithelium cuboidal with central nuclei. Fluid is watery.

Torsion may occur as in the mucinous type.

Complications

> 1. Torsion may occur as in the mucinous variety of cyst.
> 2. Malignant transformation is common and 30% of malignant tumours are bilateral.

Histogenesis of common epithelial tumours

1. Histochemical studies of mucinous tumours and analysis of their mucinous content suggest that they are probably derived from two sources.

    (a) **Type 1,** the commonest, show argyrophil cells and contain intestinal type mucin and are therefore of enteric origin.
    (b) **Type 2,** lack argyrophil cells and contain urogenital type mucin. They also contain albumin and globulin, hence the alternative name — serous cystadenoma. The cells are therefore thought to be similar to those of the endocervix.

2. Papillary cystadenoma is almost certainly derived from the coelomic epithelium, and therefore in many instances the cells may resemble those of the fallopian tube or epithelium which have a similar origin.

DISEASES OF OVARIES

Common epithelial tumours (continued)

Mucinous cystadenoma

This accounts for 20% of all ovarian tumours. It can reach a very large size and is typically multilocular. Twenty three per cent are bilateral.

Slightly nodular
due to loculi

The cut surface shows the
multilocular mosaic pattern

Gelatinous glycoprotein
secretion

Smooth peritoneal
covering

The tumour is usually
unilateral

Nuclei
basal

Tall
columnar
epithelium
(septa from the
capsule support cyst)

Complications

1. **Torsion of the pedicle.** This is not uncommon with a large ovarian tumour of any type.

2. **Rupture.** This may lead to seeding of the mucin-secreting epithelium on the peritoneum. It continues to secrete, leading to the condition 'pseudomyxoma peritonei', with a peritoneal cavity filled with mucin.

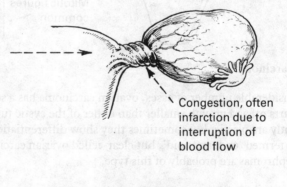

Congestion, often
infarction due to
interruption of
blood flow

3. **Malignant transformation**
Cells large, with large irregular nuclei. Mitoses common. Slight secretion present. Stroma minimal.

DISEASES OF OVARIES

Common epithelial tumours (continued)

Mucinous cystadenocarcinoma

This accounts for 20% of all cases of primary carcinoma of the ovary. It almost always arises as a malignant transformation of a benign cystadenoma.

Areas of solid growth appear in the cyst wall.

Frequently in the malignant areas, florid papillary structures are formed and where the change is widespread it may be difficult to differentiate it from the malignant form of papillary cystadenoma.

Papillary (serous) cystadenocarcinoma

This is the commonest malignant tumour of the ovary — responsible for 60% of the toal. Usually it takes the form of exuberant papillomatous growths extending over the surface and obliterating the ovarian structure.

Mitotic figures common

Invasion of capsular tissues

Solid carcinoma

In a considerable number of cases, ovarian carcinoma has a solid or semi-solid appearance and as such starts off as a growth smaller than either of the cystic tumours. Microscopically, they are frequently anaplastic, but sometimes they show differentiation towards an endometrial pattern and are termed 'endometrioid', but clear-celled ovarian carcinomas previously termed mesonephromas are probably of this type.

Progress in ovarian carcinoma

Spread of ovarian cancer in the early stages is by direct extension to the pelvic peritoneum.

The papillary serous cancer seeds widely in the peritoneal cavity and only later are lymphatics invaded and metastases appear.

The mucinous variety rarely spreads by lumphatics.

The overall 5-year survival rate for ovarian cancer is only 30% and death often takes place within 2 – 3 years due to cachexia and interference with intestinal and renal function.

DISEASES OF OVARIES

2. SEX CORD and STROMAL TUMOURS

These may be divided into two broad groups:

1. Those tending to produce excess oestrogen: granulosa cell tumours and thecomas.
2. Those producing androgens and virilization: Sertoli-Leydig cell tumours, hilus cell tumours and lipid cell tumours.

Granulosa cell tumour

This is composed of cells resembling the granulosa cells lining Graafian follicles. They vary in size from a few mm to large cystic structures. Commonly, the smaller varieties are found deep in the ovarian substance.

— Rosettes of cells with nuclei radially arranged are common

This tumour may be found at any age:

5% occur in children; 60% in the child-bearing years; 30% postmenopausally.

Occasionally these tumours recur — sometimes many years after removal.

Thecoma

This is a growth consisting of spindle cells and often resembles a fibroma. It has been suggested that fibromas found in ovaries are thecomas which have undergone fibrous degeneration. They are found mainly during the 3rd, 4th and 5th decades of life. They are of simple nature and rarely recur.

Function of these tumours varies widely. Oestrogen manifestations consist of:

1. Precocious puberty in children
2. Hyperplasia of endometrium. This may be atypical and carcinoma is said to develop in 14%
3. Enlargement of breasts.

Sertoli-Leydig cell tumours (androblastoma, arrhenoblastoma)

Tubules lined by cells, sometimes pyramidal with clear cytoplasm.

Leydig cells occasionally with Reinke crystalloids in their cytoplasm

This typifies the virilizing tumour group. It is a rare tumour. The degree of virilization varies. Usually a small yellow tumour within the ovarian substance, it has a characteristic microscopical structure.

The presence of Sertoli and Leydig cells in the ovary is unexplained. Some of these tumours are malignant and consist of poorly differentiated spindle cells with occasional tubule formations.

The androgens, if secreted, result in:

1. atrophy of breasts and external genitalia
2. deepening of voice, temporal recession of hair
3. growth of facial and body hair
4. enlargement of clitoris

DISEASES OF OVARIES

3. GERM CELL TUMOURS

These arise from primitive germ cells capable of differentiating in many ways. The following diagram indicates the main varieties of tumour produced.

Dysgerminoma

This is a solid tumour of characteristic appearance. It is usually ovoid with a smooth capsule, greyish colour and rubbery consistence. Like all germ cell tumours it is commoner in younger age groups and is often bilateral. Some cases are found in association with intersex.

    Microscopically, it consists of large clear round cells with large nuclei resembling germ cells. These are arranged in alveoli separated by fine connective tissue infiltrated by lymphocytes.

    Most dysgerminomas are of benign nature and do not recur after removal.

Lymphocytes

Teratomas

These are of two main varieties: (1) cystic and (2) solid.

Cystic teratoma (*dermoid*)

Hairs

Eminence

Tooth

Hairs

Sebaceous glands

This is one of the commonest ovarian tumours and it occurs at all ages. It is largely a mono-dermal structure, i.e. the elements are derived from only one of the embryonic layers.

    It is unilocular with an eminence on one aspect from which hairs grow. Teeth may be present on this eminence. It is lined by stratified squamous epithelium. Sebaceous glands, nervous tissue, respiratory, intestinal epithelium and thyroid tissue may also be present.

    Very occasionally the squamous epithelium may undergo malignant change.

DISEASES OF OVARIES

Teratomas (continued)

Solid teratoma
This consists of a mixture of all types of tissue arranged in no set order. The variation in histological appearance is so great, no adequate description can be given. This type of tumour is more common in younger age groups, and one or more of the tissue components frequently shows malignant change.

Monodermal solid tumours are occasionally seen consisting of thyroid tissue (struma ovarii) or carcinoid tumour cells. Some of the common epithelial cystic tumours may also be examples of monodermal teratomas.

Extra-embryonic tumours (embryonal carcinoma, yolk sac tumour, choriocarcinoma)
These are very rare. The main feature in all of them is their extreme malignancy.

4. SECONDARY TUMOURS
The ovaries are often the site of metastatic growths from the breast, lung, intestinal system, etc. They are commonest during the child-bearing years.

Krukenberg tumour
This is a very characteristic secondary tumour due to metastatic deposits from an undiscovered stomach carcinoma in a pre-menopausal woman. Both ovaries are involved. They are firm and fibrous, of equal size, smooth and slightly lobulated. No adhesions are present.

Histologically they may be mistaken for a spindle cell sarcoma, but among the undifferentiated cells are large cells with eccentric nuclei and clear cytoplasm containing mucin (signet ring cells).

Other tumours.
Certain tumours are thought to arise from mesonephric elements — mesonephroma and the Brenner tumour. Fibromas are not uncommon, some being fibrotic thecomas. They are sometimes associated with serous effusions in the peritoneal and pleural cavities (Meig's syndrome).

DISEASES OF BREAST

Acute inflammation
Clinically, two forms of breast inflammation are recognised:

1. **Associated with lactation.** This appears to be due to failure to establish lactation and may be hormonal in origin. Although there is congestion, oedema and frequently pyrexia, there appears to be no infection.
2. **Pyogenic mastitis.** This also occurs most frequently in the lactating breast. Fissures or abrasions of the nipple predispose to the condition. Infection is transmitted by the suckling neonate who is carrying hospital staphylococci. Abscesses may form in the lobules of the breast leading to scarring during healing.

Chronic mastitis
This generally follows acute mastitis and is a localised granulomatous reaction.

Another chronic inflammatory reaction is associated with ectasia of the ducts (cystic dilatation).

Hyperplasia of elastic tissue around cystic ducts

Lipid laden fluid with fatty macrophages

Lymphocytes and plasma cells

Infection of the dilated ducts allows escape of contents into the tissues resulting in granulomatous reaction. Clinically it may raise suspicion of duct carcinoma.

Non-neoplastic hyperplasia of the breast (cystic mastopathy, hyperplastic cystic disease).
In this condition there are four characteristic features, and the form which the disease takes varies according to the relative proportions of these features:

1. **Fibrosis.** This is mainly an increase in the amount of collagen rather than a true growth of fibrous tissue.
2. **Cyst formation.** Obstruction of ducts leads to dilatations of the ducts and acini. The lining epithelium may show apocrine metaplasia.
3. (a) **Adenosis.** This is an increase in the number of lobules and in the size of existing lobules.

Normal lobule

Hyperplastic lobules

(b) **Sclerosing adenosis**

This is a localised condition which may simulate carcinoma. There is proliferation of acini and stroma, and mitotic activity can be marked but there is no danger of malignancy.

DISEASES OF BREAST

Non-neoplastic hyperplasia (continued)

4. **Epitheliosis** is a term used to indicate epithelial hyperplasia within the ducts and acini. Three forms are described:

(a) Solid

Ducts are filled in varying degrees by the heaped up cells

(b) Cribriform

Intra-acinar acini without stroma

(c) Papillary

Cystic mastopathy is very common, and the various changes are ascribed to abnormal and exaggerated responses of the breast tissues to the cyclical physiological menstrual hormonal stimuli; they are essentially benign, but a link with carcinoma has been established when the component of EPITHELIOSIS shows ATYPICAL CELLULARITY (DYSPLASIA). In these circumstances, particularly if the changes are widespread, the risks of carcinoma developing are increased.

TUMOURS OF BREAST

Fibroadenoma
Two forms of this growth exist. Both are usually small tumours of similar naked eye appearance.

Well circumscribed, rounded and elastic in consistency

(1) **Peri-canalicular form**

(2) **Intra-canalicular form**

Small acinar and duct structures resembling normal breast

Greyish colour

Epithelium forms clefts; these are due to pressure from the projecting fibrous tissue

Fibrous tissue arranged around acini

DISEASES OF BREAST

Fibroadenoma (continued)

Commonly both peri- and intracanalicular forms of growth are seen in the same tumour. These growths occur mainly in young women and are of simple nature, but if any part is left behind at operation recurrence may take place.

Phyllodes tumour ← A giant form of intracanalicular fibroadenoma is found in older women. It tends to recur repeatedly after removal and ultimately the stroma may show sarcomatous transformation.

Cystadenoma (papillary cystadenoma)

This is an uncommon tumour. It consists of multiple cysts in which the epithelium may be heaped up to form papillary structures, but without the connective tissue core of true papillomata. They can grow to a large size and by pressure may ulcerate through the skin. Occasionally a cystadenocarcinoma develops.

Duct papilloma *(intraductal)*

This tumour may develop in any part of the duct system of the breast, but is most common in the lacteal sinuses at the nipple. Two forms exist:

1. **Solitary papilloma.** These are almost always near the nipple.

Complex branching pedunculated tumour filling lacteal sinus

Columnar epithelium

Connective tissue core

Often there is a double layer of epithelial cells which have an apocrine appearance. (This may be related to the fact that developmentally the breast is a modified sweat gland.) → *signals benign*

2. **Multiple papillomata**
   These may be distributed throughout the duct system. In this form, multicentric carcinoma occasionally develops.

In both forms, there is frequently a discharge from the nipple which may be haemorrhagic. Examination of the discharge will reveal the tumour epithelial cells which are benign.

DISEASES OF BREAST

PRE-CANCEROUS LESIONS

Intra-duct carcinoma

This is a carcinoma in situ of the ducts and sometimes of the acini. It may be visible as greyish-white material filling the dilated ducts, and the epithelial cylinders may be squeezed out of the ducts (comedocarcinoma).

Solid or cribriform cylinders of cells showing the usual features of malignancy — variation in size and shape of both cell and nucleus, relatively greater size of nuclei, mitotic figures, etc.,

The condition has to be differentiated from simple epitheliosis occurring in cystic mastopathy, especially when the carcinoma-in-situ lesions occur in acini.

The natural history is unknown, but it seems likely that it may exist for several years prior to invasion. Whether regression of the lesion ever occurs is not known. When the acinar lesion becomes invasive the prognosis is poor.

Paget's disease of the nipple

This represents intraepithelial spread from an underlying cancer.

Nipple is red, swollen and inflamed with crusts on the surface.

Fluid exudes from surface

Microscopic examination reveals:

Pockets of pale cells in the basal epithelium

Marked inflammatory reaction in dermis with plasma cells.

Paget cells (nuclei large with prominent nucleoli: cytoplasm clear)

Occasional mitosis

Basal epithelial cells are compressed and atrophic

These malignant cells infiltrate the epidermis and do not invade the dermis.

This condition is always associated with an intraduct carcinoma deeper in the nipple, and the Paget's appearance is due to growth the intraduct carcinoma component upwards to the nipple, followed by lateral spread within the epidermis.

695

DISEASES OF BREAST

INVASIVE CARCINOMA

This is the commonest form of malignancy in the female and presents in two main forms: scirrhous and encephaloid carcinoma.

1. Scirrhous carcinoma

This is by far the commoner. It may be found in any part of the breast, but most frequently it is in the upper and outer quandrant.

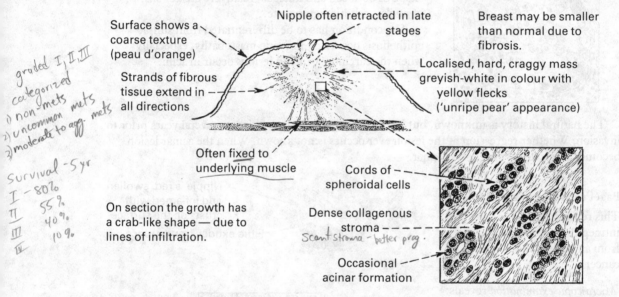

graded I, II, III
categorized
1) non-mets
2) uncommon mets
3) moderate to agg. mets

Survival - 5 yr
I - 80%
II   55%
III   40%
IV   10%

Surface shows a coarse texture (peau d'orange)

Strands of fibrous tissue extend in all directions

Nipple often retracted in late stages

Breast may be smaller than normal due to fibrosis.

Localised, hard, craggy mass greyish-white in colour with yellow flecks ('unripe pear' appearance)

Often fixed to underlying muscle

On section the growth has a crab-like shape — due to lines of infiltration.

Cords of spheroidal cells

Dense collagenous stroma

Scant stroma - better prog.

Occasional acinar formation

Some areas show degeneration of the tumour cells. These are responsible for the yellow flecks seen by the naked eye. The increased collagen is said to be produced by the tumour cells. Although inrease in size of the primary growth is slow, metastases appear early.

2. Encephaloid carcinoma

This is much less common. It forms a large soft tumour, particularly liable to undergo necrosis. The necrosis may involve the skin, producing a fungating growth. It has ill-defined margins.

Large spheroidal cells

Fine stroma often heavily infiltrated by lymphocytes

DISEASES OF BREAST

Invasive carcinoma (continued)

Spread

This is mainly by local lymphatics:

1. To axillary lymphatics at early stage.
2. To internal mammary lymphatics.
3. Through pectoral fascia and muscle to pleural cavity.
4. At a late date, skin lymphatics may be invaded causing:
   (a) local lesion
   (b) widespread lesion — skin becomes stiff and board-like: cancer-en-cuirasse
   (c) blockage of lymphatics, $\longrightarrow$ oedema of the skin; except where hair follicles exist — fine mammillated appearance; 'peau d'orange'.
5. Ultimately, secondaries may appear in many viscera and in bones, especially the thoracic and lumbar spine.

Spread is equally rapid in both varieties of growth. Where there is marked lymphocytic reaction, indicating a possible immune reaction, the five year survival rate is improved, but the ultimate prognosis is not good.

Aetiology

Breast cancer is uncommon below the age of 30 years. The risk increases with age, the maximal incidence being in the later decades.

The important risk factors are:

1. *Genetic.* There is a strong familial association. Recently, abnormalities in chromosomes 11 and 17 involving amplification of oncogenes and deletion of tumour suppressor genes have been identified. *autosomal dominant*
2. *Sex hormone associations:*
   (a) Commoner in nulliparous women
   (b) Early menarche and late menopause increase risk — ? prolonged cyclical exposure to sex hormones.
   (c) Breast feeding reduces risk.
   Note: Some breast carcinomas are hormone (oestrogen) dependent and slowing of the growth can be achieved by minimising oestrogenic stimulation. The cells of such tumours show surface oestrogen receptors.
3. *Virus infection.* No virus has yet been incriminated, although possible virus material has been identified in a few breast cancers.

THE MALE BREAST

The breast is seldom the seat of disease in males. Abnormal enlargement — gynaecomastia — may occur in a temporary form at puberty or as a permanent feature in intersex states, e.g. Klinefelter's syndrome (XXY). Oestrogen metabolic upsets (e.g. in liver disease) or excess intake (e.g. treatment of prostatic cancer) are other causes. All tumours are rare.

INFERTILITY

The causes of infertility are multiple and can affect both male and female. The main pathological findings may be grouped in the following manner, but the list does not indicate any form of priority or incidence.

A. Lack of germ cells — due to failure of fetal germ cell migration to the genital ridge. It may be associated with chromosomal abnormalities.

B. Chromosomal defects
1. *Klinefelter's syndrome*. Phenotype male. Genotype XXY or XXXY. No germ cells are present. Testes become atrophic. Usually mental retardation.
2. *Turner's syndrome*. Phenotype female. XO genotype. Genitalia are infantile. The ovaries, lacking germ cells, consist of fibrous tissue.
3. *Super-female*. Extra X chromosome present, e.g. XXX. Fertility reduced.
4. *True hermaphroditism*. XX and XY cells are present. Phenotype usually male. Internally there is a testis and epididymis on one side and an ovary, fallopian tube and uterus on the other.

C. Hormonal abnormalities
1. *Prolactinoma*. The presence of a pituitary adenoma (see p.851)
2. *Adrenal virilism*. This is due to an enzyme defect in cortisol production. Androgens are produced instead, causing virilisation of female infants.
3. *Testicular feminisation*. An abnormality in androgen activity prevents descent of the testes with complete feminisation. It is due to a defective gene on the X chromosome transmitted by a female carrier.
4. Administration of oestrogen or its accumulation due to liver disease causes defective testicular function.

D. Anatomical abnormalities. Maldescent of the testes is the most common. Abnormal external genitalia are an obvious cause of infertility.

E. Infections, X-irradiation, tumours and poisons interfere with fertility. Venereal disease and tuberculosis affect both sexes. Septic abortion in the female and mumps in the male are other causes.

F. Functional defects. In a number of cases, no physical cause for infertility can be found. In the female, alterations in pituitary function upset the normal cyclical ovulation rhythm. In the male, oligospermia and abnormal sperm may be found.

DISEASES OF MALE GENITALIA

The male genital tract consists of a number of structures connected by ducts opening into one another. These interconnections are important in the spread of infection.

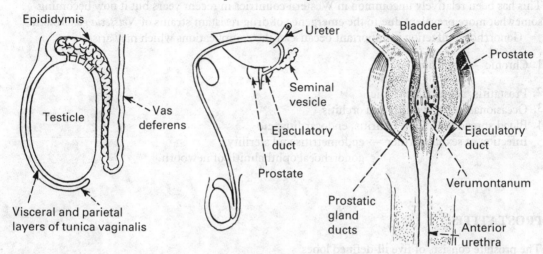

Inflammation of the genital tract in most cases starts in the posterior urethra and spreads to other structures.

The condition in these instances is secondary to urinary infection associated with urethral obstruction caused by an enlarged prostate or urethral stricture. This is indicated by the fact that in 80% of cases of prostatitis, the infecting bacterium is *E.coli*. In the remaining 20%, various organisms may be isolated — staphylococci, streptococci, pseudomonas and proteus. Frequent catheterisation is an aetiological factor.

Anterior urethritis is almost always a sexually transmitted disease. Gonococci, trichomonads, mycoplasma and chlamydia are the usual agents. In the case of gonorrhoea, infection may spread back to the posterior urethra and thence to other structures.

DISEASES OF MALE GENITALIA

GONORRHOEA

This has been relatively uncommon in Western countries in recent years but it now becoming somewhat more prevalent due to the emergence of drug resistant strains of *Neisseria gonorrhoea*.

Gonorrhoeal infection is important because of the complications which may arise:

1. Chronic → urethritis
   urethral stricture
2. Prostatitis, acute and chronic
3. Occasionally epididymitis and orchitis
4. Blood spread leading to arthritis, endocarditis, etc
5. Infection of sexual partner → endometritis and sterility
   ↘ gonorrhoeal ophthalmitis of newborn.

PROSTATITIS

The prostate consists of five ill-defined lobes

Anterior — Median

Posterior

Lateral (two)

Main glands

Periurethral glands

Its internal structure is a series of branching glands in a fibromuscular stroma.

Urethra

Inflammation of the prostate always involves the posterior urethra and seminal vesicles. The usual congestion, exudation and polymorph infiltration take place and may proceed to abscess formation. These abscesses are usually small, but if they coalesce and extend they may rupture in several directions.

(1) Into urethra

(4) Into the rectum

(3) Into the ischiorectal fossa

(2) Through the perineum

Chronic prostatitis may follow an acute episode, but it is often of insidious onset. Subsequent fibrosis may cause urethral obstruction.

Abscesses may also form in the seminal vesicels. These can extend to the ischiorectal fossa.

DISEASES OF MALE GENITALIA

EPIDIDYMITIS AND ORCHITIS

Acute inflammations due to bacteria are less common in these organs, but spread via the vas deferens does occasionally take place and may result in destructive suppuration.

In 20% of adult cases of mumps, the epididymis and testes become acutely inflamed. The condition is usually unilateral, but if bilateral there is a distinct danger of subsequent infertility.

Acute inflammation of the testis may be confused with torsion. Torsion generally occurs within the tunica vaginalis and leads to obstruction of the testicular vessels. Infarction results, with destruction of the tissue. Recurrent minor degrees of torsion can cause atrophy.

Chronic inflammations are important, although rare, in this region.

Chronic granulomatous orchitis

This is a condition of unknown origin. The testis is infiltrated by plasma cells, lymphocytes and eosinophils. Atrophy of the germinal epithelium occurs and the testis becomes fibrotic.

TUBERCULOSIS

In this disease, the epididymis is usually the first part of the genital tract to be affected.

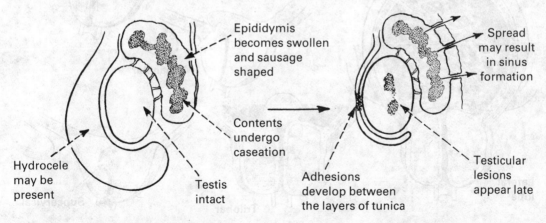

Infection is almost always haematogenous from some other focus in the body. Subsequently the process may spread along the vas deferens to the seminal vesicles, prostate and bladder. In rare cases the infection is in the opposite direction — kidney → bladder → prostate → vas → epididymis.

701

DISEASES OF MALE GENITALIA

SYPHILIS

Apart from the primary sore which appears on the penis, the only other site of syphilitic lesions is the testis. These are common in the tertiary stage, their incidence being only second to those in the aorta at this phase. Two types of lesion are found:

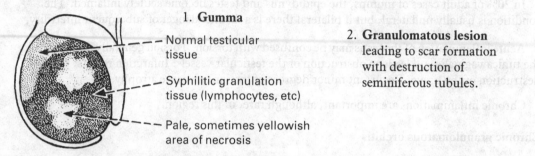

1. **Gumma**

Normal testicular tissue

Syphilitic granulation tissue (lymphocytes, etc)

Pale, sometimes yellowish area of necrosis

2. **Granulomatous lesion** leading to scar formation with destruction of seminiferous tubules.

The primary lesion of lymphogranuloma venereum (see p. 681) appears on the penis and, as in the female, it spreads and causes chronic suppuration in the inguinal lymph nodes. But late complications are less drastic in their effects.

BENIGN PROSTATIC HYPERPLASIA

Several different forms are described:

Dilated bladder with hypertrophic muscle bands (trabeculae)

Median

Lateral lobe

Median bar

Trilobar

Subcervical

DISEASES OF MALE GENITALIA

Benign prostatic hyperplasia (continued)

In practice, the appearances are very variable and can include two or more of the forms illustrated on previous page.

There is a hyperplasia of both the glandular tissue and fibromuscular stroma, the relative proportions varying greatly. Section of the prostate reveals:

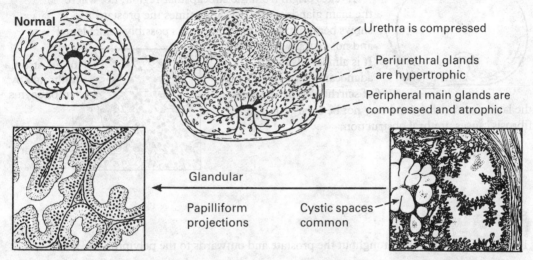

Normal

Urethra is compressed

Periurethral glands are hypertrophic

Peripheral main glands are compressed and atrophic

Glandular

Papilliform projections

Cystic spaces common

The atrophic compressed peripheral tissue forms a false capsule from which the hypertrophied mass can be shelled out.

Aetiology

This is obscure. It is a disease of the elderly and there is often asymptomatic prostatic enlargement in old age. The periurethral glands are said to predominate at this period and hyperplasia may be an exaggeration of this process. It has also been claimed that the central glands are sensitive to oestrogen and hence the hyperplasia may be related to the normal drop in androgens in old age, leaving the action of oestrogen, normally present, unopposed. On the other hand, it has been noted that prostatic enlargement is never seen after castration and does not occur in patients suffering from hepatic cirrhosis (oestrogens are not inactivated).

Complications

1. Chronic retention of urine.
2. Attacks of acute retention are common, probably related to the accompanying urinary infection causing oedema and congestion of the prostatic urethra.
3. Cystitis and pyelonephritis.
4. Hydronephrosis.
5. Bladder stone.

703

DISEASES OF MALE GENITALIA

CARCINOMA OF THE PROSTATE

This is a common cancer and is the fifth most common cause of male death.

It takes origin from the subcapsular region, i.e. where the main glands are found. Sometimes the prostate also shows benign hyperplasia, but this is possibly coincidental and not causally related.

It is almost always an adenocarcinoma, frequently of scirrhous type. Because of the latter feature the gland may not be enlarge but the fibrosis causes urethral obstruction.

Fibrous stroma infiltrated by lymphocytes

Small irregular acini

Spread   *Direct extension*

1. Direct spread occurs throughout the prostate and outwards to the pelviprostatic tissue.

2. Lymphatic spread is the main mode of extension. There is a rich lymphatic plexus and the perineural lymphatics are particularly affected. The pelvic nodes are invaded and subsequently the abdominal chain.

3. Bone metastases tend to be common, especially in the vertebrae. This may be due to retrograde spread from the prostatic venous plexus to the vertebral veins. These secondaries are characterised by the formation of new dense bone around them (osteosclerosis).

Biochemical tests

These tumours produce acid phosphatase and, when matastases are present, an increased level may be found in the blood. When bones are invaded, blood alkaline phosphatase may also rise.

Latent carcinoma

Small subcapsular foci with the histological features of carcinoma may be found in a prostate showing benign hyperplasia. They are particularly common in the very elderly. Invasion of local perineal spaces occurs without further spread.

DISEASES OF MALE GENITALIA

TUMOURS OF THE PENIS

Papillomata may arise in the coronal sulcus. Usually they are greyish and sessile. Viral infection results very often in luxuriant papillomatous growths. These are the so-called condylomata acuminata and are sexually transmitted. Similar lesions occur on the vulva in the female. Peyronie's disease is a cellular fibromatous lesion.

Precancerous lesions

Leukoplakia and Bowen's disease are occasionally found on the penis. Another condition involving epithelial hyperplasia is Queyrat's erythroplasia. The histological appearances vary in these lesions, but all tend to show epithelial dysplasia and may at some stage resemble carcinoma in situ.

Carcinoma of the penis

This is the second most common type of malignancy of the male genital tract, but it accounts for less than 2% of all male malignancy. The site of growth is always in the preputial area, often in the coronal sulcus, but it extends to involve the glans penis. Two forms of growth occur:

Ulcer with sloughing base and hard rolled edges; usually it is adherent to the underlying tissues

Soft cauliflower growth

The growth spreads by the lymphatics to the regional nodes. Distant metastases occur late. The prognosis is reasonably good, the 5 year survival rate being greater than 50%. These squamous cell carcinoma spread by lymphatics.

Aetiology

1. Early circumcision virtually confers immunity against carcinoma; the risk is greatly increased in the presence of poor penile hygiene.

2. There is evidence that a human papilloma virus is the initiating carcinogen. Inspissated smegma trapped behind the foreskin may be an important promotor (co-factor).

DISEASES OF MALE GENITALIA

CANCER OF THE SCROTUM
This is a lesion which is rarely seen nowadays. Previously it was an occupational disease due to exposure to carcinogenic agents, e.g. soot, industrial oils, arsenic, etc.,

TUMOURS OF THE TESTICLE
These are rare, the incidence being 2 – 3 per 100,000 males in Western countries. Their importance is related to the fact that most are malignant and they occur in children and young adults. In this group of the population they account for 1/7th of all cancer deaths. Tumours are more common in undescended testicles.

    A large number of types of tumour have been described, but only two can be considered in any degree common:

painless enlargement

Seminoma
This corresponds to the dysgerminoma in the female. It accounts for 40% of all testicular tumours.

The testis is uniformly enlarged; the surface is smooth.
On section it has a faint lobular appearance and is often described as the 'potato' tumour because of its white solid appearance.

Fine stroma infiltrated by lymphocytes

Large germ cells sometimes in mitosis

    Spread is via the lymphatics along the spermatic cord.
    The prognosis is good, probably because of early diagnosis. It appears to be better if lymphocytic reaction in the tumour is strong.
The growth is extremely radiosensitive. The 5 year survival rate is 90%.

Teratoma
This type of growth is found in 32% of testicular growths. It takes origin from totipotent cells capable of differentiating into derivatives of ectoderm, endoderm and mesoderm. It is therefore impossible to provide an adequate description of the histology of these tumours. It has become customary to classify them according to the degree of differentiation exhibited. The lack of differentiation indicates the malignancy of the tumour.

DISEASES OF MALE GENITALIA

Teratoma (continued)

The tumours form a spectrum from completely simple growth to the most malignant.

Unlike the seminoma, the teratoma produces an irregular, nodular growth.

Differentiated teratoma (*extremely rare*)

All the cells are well differentiated and form recognisable tissues, e.g. intestinal glands, squamous epithelium, cartilage, etc. No signs of malignancy are present and the prognosis is good.

On section there are usually cysts

Malignant teratoma anaplastic

In this type of growth, the cells show no sign of differentiation and are pleomorphic. Mitoses are frequent and necrosis and haemorrhage are common. The prognosis is extremely bad.

Between these two extremes are other tumours showing varying degrees of differentiation on the one hand (MTIA) and pleomorphism on the other (MTIB).

The overall 5 year survival rate for teratoma is 60%, but this drops dramatically in the case of malignant teratoma anaplastic.

Malignant teratoma trophoblastic

Parts of this growth show differentiation to trophoblast tissue — syncytiotrophoblast and cytotrophoblast. Chorionic gonadotrophin is produced and can be used to monitor progress and the response to treatment. Prognosis is poor.

Combined germ-cell tumours

A small number of these tumours are mixed, being part teratoma and part seminoma.

The following miscellaneous tumours are rare — Sertoli cell tumours, Leydig cell tumours, lymphoma and carcinoid.

CHAPTER 14

NERVOUS SYSTEM

NERVOUS SYSTEM — ANATOMY AND PHYSIOLOGY

Considerations of anatomy and physiology have important applications to diseases of the central nervous system (CNS), particularly their effects and spread.

The anatomy of the various coverings is important.

The skull and vertebrae form a rigid compartment protecting the delicate CNS tissues.

This rigidity has serious disadvantages when pressure inside the skull increases, e.g. an expanding lesion soon takes up the small reserves of space available and the delicate brain tissues are progressively compressed, with very serious results.

Meninges and cerebrospinal fluid (CSF)

The CSF circulating freely in the subarachnoid space over the whole CNS surface and in the ventricular system acts as a protective water bath.

Diseases (particularly infections) at this site are usually *widespread* over the whole brain and cord surfaces, e.g. meningitis. Impediment to the flow of CSF causes serious effects — hydrocephalus.

The detailed arrangement of the meninges is important.

The thick **dura,** closely applied to the skull, acts as the periosteum — its rigid reflections (falx cerebri and tentorium cerebelli) complicate the effects of increased intracranial pressure.

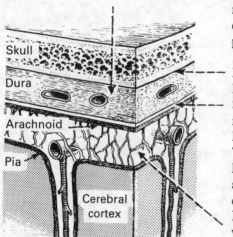

Skull

Dura

Arachnoid

Pia

Cerebral cortex

Extradural lesions tend to be localised; they have to strip the dura from the bone.

Subdural lesions remain local but can spread more widely since the arachnoid and dura are loosely attached.

The **arachnoid,** a delicate membrane, is loosely attached to the dura and sends trabeculae across the subarachnoid space which contains the cerebral blood vessels and the CSF.

Disease in the **subarachnoid** space can spread widely over the whole surface of the brain and spinal cord but is prevented from penetrating into the brain tissue by the **pia.**

NERVOUS SYSTEM — ANATOMY AND PHYSIOLOGY

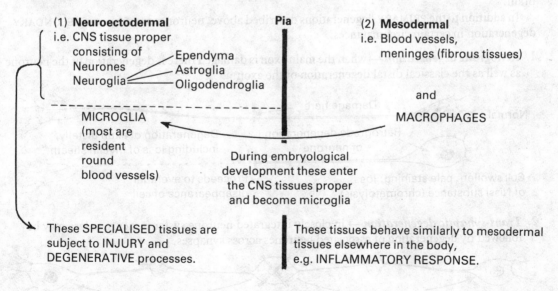

The **pia** is invaginated into the brain substance along with the small penetrating vessels.

The dura, arachnoid and pia act as barriers which selectively separate the CSF and the blood from the CNS tissues.

It is important to understand that, although the CSF is very similar in composition to the extracellular fluid of the brain, changes in the CSF only very indirectly reflect changes in the CNS in disease.

The Pia's barrier function is reinforced by the membrane formed by the foot processes of astrocytes:
1. on the brain surface
2. around the penetrating vessels. The potential space between the vessel wall and the pia is called the Virchow Robin space and is analogous to the subarachnoid space
3. at capillary level the pia is not present, but the foot processes along with the capillary endothelium and basement membrane form a specialised and selective 'blood-brain barrier'.

Thus the PIA and the membrane formed by the foot processes of the astrocytes separate types of tissue derived from two embryological layers.

(1) **Neuroectodermal**
i.e. CNS tissue proper consisting of
Neurones
Neuroglia ── Ependyma
           Astroglia
           Oligodendroglia

Pia

(2) **Mesodermal**
i.e. Blood vessels, meninges (fibrous tissues)

and

MACROPHAGES

MICROGLIA (most are resident round blood vessels)

During embryological development these enter the CNS tissues proper and become microglia

These SPECIALISED tissues are subject to INJURY and DEGENERATIVE processes.

These tissues behave similarly to mesodermal tissues elsewhere in the body, e.g. INFLAMMATORY RESPONSE.

NEURONAL DAMAGE

NEURONES are sensitive to damage by a wide variety of agents including anoxia, hypoglycaemia, virus infections and intracellular metabolic disturbances (e.g. associated with vitamin B deficiencies).

There are two main types, depending on the rapidity of the changes.

1. *Rapid NECROSIS* — associated with acute failure of function.

Healthy cell   Damaging agent   Nuclear pyknosis, cytoplasmic shrinkage   Dissolution of cell with phagocytosis of debris

2. *Slow ATROPHIC CHANGES* — associated with gradual loss of function.

Healthy cell   Damaging agent   Cells usually smaller — but may be distended with abnormal metabolites   Eventual dissolution

The process of ageing involves cumulative atrophy and disappearance of neurones; in some individuals the process is speeded up resulting in *presenile dementia.*
NB There is *no* regeneration of destroyed neurones. A large group of disorders of cerebral function seen in psychiatric practice have (as yet) no morphological evidence of nerve cell damage. They are probably caused by disturbances of poorly understood biochemical control mechanisms within the brain.

In addition to the PRIMARY degenerations described above, neurones are subject to SECONDARY degeneration in certain circumstances.

1. **Retrograde degeneration** — when the main axon is damaged there is degeneration of the neurone as well as the classical distal degeneration of the axon.

Normal   Damage here

Retrograde degeneration of neurone   Degeneration of axon distally, including loss of myelin sheath

Cell swollen; pale staining; loss of Nissl substance (chromatolysis)   Proceeds to eventual disappearance of cell

2. **Trans-synaptic degeneration** — in closely integrated neurone systems, neurone loss may be followed by degeneration of associated neurones across synapses.

Degeneration   Damage   Degeneration

GLIAL REACTIONS

The glial cells react vigorously in many diseases of the CNS.

1. The **NEUROGLIAL** cells have supportive and nutritive functions.

   (a) The **astrocytes** with their numerous fibrillary processes give structural support. They are less susceptible to damage than neurones.

Normal

Damage not sufficient to kill the cell → Cells multiply, and enlarge / Increase in fibril production → Later, cells atrophy leaving dense meshwork of fibres

   This process is called GLIOSIS. It is a feature of many diseases and is analogous to scar tissue.

   Note: Collagenous scar tissue is only formed in the CNS when mesodermal structures such as large blood vessels and their sheaths are damaged.

   (b) The oligodendrocytes — small cells with short processes — have a nutritive function in respect of neurones and especially myelin. This reaction is best seen when neurones are damaged.

Neurone

Normal

Oligodendrocytes

Swollen neurone showing chromatolysis

Increased numbers of larger oligodendrocytes — this process is called **SATELLITOSIS**.

2. The **MICROGLIAL** cells are members of the mononuclear-phagocytic system. Reaction is best seen when there is necrosis of tissues.

Normal

Necrosis

Microglial cells resident near blood vessels

Activated microglia phagocytose degradation products, e.g. lipids, haemosiderin.
Blood monocytes augment resident cells.

Microglical cells are well seen in and around infarcts; the activated cells which have ingested lipids are strikingly different from the small inactive microglia.

Eccentric nucleus

Foamy cytoplasm

These cells have been given a variety of names: compound granular corpuscles or 'gitter' cells, or lipophages.

DEMYELINATION

Loss of the myelin sheath may occur in two main circumstances:

1. **Primary** specific destruction of myelin. Demyelination precedes any axon damage. It is usually not related to specific nerve tracts.

   The mechanism is not clear; it may be autoimmune reaction or virus infection, or both.

   This type, although rare, occurs in an important group of diseases – the DEMYELINATING DISEASES (p.746).

2. **Secondary** loss following nerve cell and axon destruction. This type usually affects nerve tracts in an anatomically predicatable way.

   The mechanism is similar to that described in peripheral nerves (Wallerian degeneration, p.86).

   This type occurs in many disease processes, e.g. the nerve tract degeneration following regional infarction (p. 756).

The pathological sequels which are influenced by time factors are similar in both types.

Myelin degradation

Recent lesions (months)

Demyelinated area filled with lipid particles ± phagocytes

Chronic long-standing or slowly evolving lesions

Surrounding gliosis — lipids previously removed

Demonstration of demyelination

Because routine histological stains are unsuitable, special methods are required. The following example showing descending degeneration (and demyelination) of the corticospinal tract in the cord following infarction of the internal capsule in the brain illustrates the two main methods.

1. *'POSITIVE'* method used in **recent** (months) lesions. The lipid particles are stained, e.g. Marchi's method or Sudan black stain.

2. *'NEGATIVE'* method — used in lesions of **any duration.** Absence of staining using stains for normal myelin, e.g. Weigert-Pal or Loyez methods.

Lateral corticospinal tract (crossed fibres)

Normal myelin

Unstained

Anterior corticospinal tract (uncrossed fibres)

Stained black

Demyelinated tracts stained BLACK

Demyelinated tracts NOT STAINED

CEREBRAL OEDEMA

Swelling of the brain, of which oedema is the major component, is an important complication of many brain diseases because the enlargement either initiates or aggravates increased intracranial pressure.

The process may be localised or generalised depending on the type of initiating disorder.

Localised conditions
Examples:
Infarcts, and local ischaemia
Haematomas (due to vessel rupture and injury)
Tumours

Generalised conditions
Examples: Intoxications
Metabolic disturbances, e.g. hypoglycaemia
Generalised hypoxia
Severe head trauma
Malignant hypertension

The pathological mechanism is as follows:

Notes

    (a) Components (1) and (2) overlap.
    (b) The oedema fluid tends to spread in the white matter.
    (c) The severity of oedema formation is very variable and unpredictable clinically.
    (d) In clinical practice, therapy has two aspects:
        1. Treatment of the initiating disorder by any appropriate means.
        2. Minimising the formation of oedema by the use of
            (i) osmotic agents, e.g. urea or mannitol
            (ii) steroids (the mechanism is not known).

INCREASED INTRACRANIAL PRESSURE

INCREASED INTRACRANIAL PRESSURE occurs in two main circumstances:

1. Due to the presence of an EXPANDING LESION
2. Due to obstruction of the free flow of the CSF — this causes hydrocephalus and is dealt with on page 765.

INTRACRANIAL EXPANDING LESIONS

These lesions may occur within the brain substance or in the meninges. Important examples are:

INTRACEREBRAL

Haemorrhages and haematomas ⟶ Traumatic or Spontaneous

Infarction

Tumours ⟶ Primary cerebral or secondary

MENINGEAL

Haemorrhages and haematomas ⟶ Usually traumatic
(a) Extradural
(b) Subdural
(c) Subarachnoid
Very occasionally meningioma.

The situation is often aggravated by cerebral OEDEMA.

The severity of the effects is modified by two important factors:
(1) the size of the lesion and (2) the rapidity of expansion.

There are three stages in the progress of increased intracranial pressure ICP.

(1) The stage of **Compensation**

Expanding lesion
↓
Potential ICP ↑

↑ CSF absorption
↓ CSF formation

Vasoconstriction

↓ CSF VOLUME

↓ Intracranial BLOOD VOLUME

Allows brain to expand without serious effects

(2) Stage of **Decompensation**

At this stage there are herniations and distortions of the brain with their associated complications. The systemic blood pressure is raised and the pulse slow ('Cushing' effect).

(3) A vicious circle is established leading to the stage of **vasomotor paralysis**.

ICP ↑ → Cerebral perfusion pressure ↓

VASODILATATION

VASOMOTOR PARALYSIS

Cerebral tissue HYPOXIA (also increased PCO_2)

Progressive neuronal damage

INCREASED INTRACRANIAL PRESSURE

Effects

DISTORTIONS and DISLOCATIONS of the brain substance

These are to some extent dependent on the site of the initiating lesion; the effects of a unilateral expanding lesion are illustrated.

(1) Flattened cerebral convolutions (diminished subarachnoid space)

(2) Herniation of cingulate gyrus under the falx

(3) Movement of interventricular septum across the mid-line with distortion of ventricles

(4) Herniation of parahippocampal gyrus past the free edge of the tentorium cerebelli

(5) Midbrain pushed against tentorium of opposite side (Kernohan notch); may give rise to paradoxical signs

(6) Cerebellar tonsils and medulla pushed down into foramen magnum

Falx

Skull

Dura

Expanding lesion (extradural haemorrhage)

Tentorium cerebelli

Foramen magnum

NB The sudden removal of even small amounts of CSF by **LUMBAR PUNCTURE** may precipitate medullary 'coning' with fatal results due to damage to the 'vital centres'.

717

INCREASED INTRACRANIAL PRESSURE

SECONDARY COMPLICATIONS

1. **Vascular damage**

   (a) Compression of the
   central retinal vein
   causes PAPILLOEDEMA,
   an important clinical
   sign of raised ICP.

Oedema of
optic disc

Swelling and blurring
of disc margin

   (b) Stretching and compression of blood vessels may cause haemorrhage and infarction quite
   remote from the initiating lesion — secondary midbrain and calcarine infarction and
   haemorrhage are common.

2. **Intracranial nerve damage**
   Oculomotor (III) and abducens (VI) nerves
   are particularly prone to damage, giving rise
   to paralysis of ocular movements in varying
   combinations.
   The VIth nerve is specially vulnerable due
   to its long subarachnoid course. It is often
   the nerve on the side opposite the lesion
   which is stretched giving rise to paradoxical
   signs.

Vessels compressed

III

3. **Obstruction of flow of CSF**

Expanding
lesion

Lat.vent.
dilated

III vent.
dilated

Aqueduct
of Sylvius compressed

↑ ICP

Compression of
midbrain

CSF dammed back
in IIIrd and lateral
ventricles

Narrowing or
closure of aqueduct

Compression here causes obstruction of CSF
and aggravates the increased ICP

4. **Changes in the skull bones**
   Long continued ICP causes bone erosion and thinning visible on X-ray.

   (a) Erosion of posterior clinoid processes of sphenoid bone.
   (b) In children, before the skull is fully ossified, the inner table is thinned at the sites of
   convolutional pressure giving a striking X-ray appearance.

CIRCULATORY DISTURBANCES

(1) Hypoxia and ischaemia and (2) Intracranial haemorrhage are the important and common mechanisms causing brain damage.

ACUTE HYPOXIC DISORDERS

Blood supply:
20% of cardiac output is delivered via carotid and vertebral arteries

When the cardiac output falls, an autoregulatory vascular control mechanism protects the cerebral blood supply — the arterial BP must be kept above 50 mmHg.

Neuronal aerobic metabolism of glucose

O_2 → Metabolic products, especially lactate
Glucose →

There are no reserves of O_2 or glucose in the brain, therefore a constant delivery via arterial blood is necessary.
Neurones are very susceptible to hypoxia (and hypoglycaemia); with complete O_2 deprivation neuronal **necrosis** occurs in 5 – 7 minutes.
(at normal temperatures)

The following flow diagram illustrates the factors which influence availability of O_2 and the conditions giving rise to hypoxia.

Available O_2

Proportional to

BLOOD FLOW ---- X ---- O_2 CONTENT OF BLOOD

Proportional to ... Proportional to

Cerebral perfusion pressure (arterial pressure less ICP) --X-- Diameter of blood vessel ... Hb concentration --X-- Oxygen tension

Hypotension (e.g. cardiac arrest and shock)

Increased ICP (expanding lesion)

Arterial constriction (e.g. severe atheroma, malig. hypertension)

Anaemia (e.g. acute haemorrhage)

Ventilation failure (e.g. lung disease, chest injury)

These conditions, singly or together, can be responsible for cerebral hypoxia.

719

HYPOXIA

GENERALISED (diffuse) brain damage results when delivery of oxygen to the brain as a whole is severly deficient, e.g. in cardiac arrest. *Note:* A similar type of neuronal damage occurs in severe acute hypoglycaemia, acute carbon monoxide and barbiturate poisoning.

LOCALISED (focal) damage occurs in less severe O_2 deficiency and under the influence of modifying factors.

(a) **Anatomical arterial distribution** — Watershed infarcts occur at sites of arterial boundary zones (see p.153)

(b) **Selective anatomical sites** — where neurones are particularly sensitive to hypoxia, e.g. the hippocampus, layers III, V and VI of the cortex, in the sulci, the Purkinje cells of the cerebellum.

(c) **Pre-existing pathological changes** — in the cerebral arterial system, e.g. the random distribution of atheroma.

These focal lesions are to some extent predictable.

These lesions are not predictable.

The variable operation of these three factors potentiates very variable severity and distribution of damage from case to case.

Pathological appearances

Modern ventilators allow maintenance of respiratory and circulatory functions in the presence of total brain necrosis — in such cases there is liquefaction of the whole brain with no vital reaction.

In cases of focal brain damage, the duration of survival after the damage modifies the pathological appearances.

	Up to 12 hours	Over 12 hours	2 – 7 days	Weeks
Gross	No changes seen	May be cerebral oedema	Focal softenings	Shrinking and scarring of brain
Microscopic	Early neuronal damage seen	Neuronal damage obvious	Loss of cells in selective areas, e.g. Purkinje cells; reactive changes	Reactive gliosis established

CEREBRAL INFARCTION (SOFTENING)

This common condition, one of the two main types of stroke (the other is spontaneous intracerebral haemorrhage), is caused by failure of the supply of oxygen (and glucose) to maintain the viability of the tissues in the territory of a cerebral arterial branch. This is not always due to simple local arterial occlusion, and very often a component of central circulatory deficiency is contributory. The lesion is essentially necrosis of all the tissues in the affected territory.

Mechanism

Precipitating condition → Perfusion failure → INFARCTION (ischaemic|necrosis)
LOCAL ARTERIAL DISEASE (particularly ATHEROMA) and its complications, are the most common.

1. Arterial occlusions

(a)
THROMBOSIS on atheromatous plaque in

Intracerebral artery

Internal carotid artery

(b)
EMBOLISM commonly derived from heart
(i) atrial fibrillation;
(ii) mural thrombus complicating myocardial infarction;
(iii) endocarditis.

Very small emboli derived from ulcerated atheroma in carotid artery may cause small infarcts

2. Arterial stenosis

ATHEROMA – the widespread loss of arterial lumen potentiates cerebral perfusion deficiency in two ways: (1) by disturbing the normal arterial flow and (2) by prejudicing anastomotic communications.

Atheromatous stenosis alone is not usually a cause of infarction, but when central circulatory deficiency is added, infarction is common, e.g. this may vary from the slight fall in BP during sleep to the severe hypotension of shock or myocardial infarction.

Other rarer causes of arterial stenosis are dissecting aneurysm, arteritis. Arterial spasm is a rare cause.

CEREBRAL INFARCTION

SITES

While infarcts may occur anywhere in the brain, depending on the vagaries of the precipitating arterial lesions, certain sites are more commonly affected.

1. In cases of local arterial occlusion, **internal structures supplied by 'end' arterial branches** are particularly vulnerable. The cortex is often protected in variable degree by anastomoses of other cerebral arteries. This is illustrated in the territory of the middle cerebral artery.

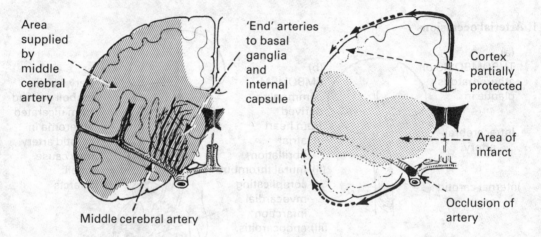

Area supplied by middle cerebral artery

'End' arteries to basal ganglia and internal capsule

Middle cerebral artery

Cortex partially protected

Area of infarct

Occlusion of artery

2. **Boundary zones** (see p.153)

   The cortex is damaged particularly in boundary zone infarction. In these cases, central circulatory deficiency is an important component, e.g. hypotension.

3. **Ischaemic (arteriopathic) cerebral atrophy**

   In cases of widespread severe atheroma of the cerebral arteries, a diffuse form of cerebral atrophy with neuronal loss and reactive gliosis occurs. There may be microinfarction, and the changes seen in the ageing brain may also be present. In Western societies, this type of cerebral atrophy is one of the causes of senile dementia.

CEREBRAL INFARCTION

The diagram below illustrates the evolution of an infarct, e.g. in the territory of the middle cerebral artery. Up to 24 hours there is virtually no visible change.

18-24 hr	After 24 hours	After a few days	After weeks/months

Gross appearances

Very difficult to see	Less difficult to see	Line of demarcation seen	Demolition + scarring

	Slight swelling	Blurring of white/grey junction	Necrotic tissue. Soft to touch; usually pale but may be congested if blood has permeated in	Cyst with pale or yellowish fluid	Shrinkage of scarred area: compensatory dilatation of ventricle

Microscopic appearances

Early neuronal damage	Early neuronal damage ↓ Necrosis of neurones	Organisation of infarct begins Macrophages appear; capillary sprouting; oedema diminishing	Organisation well established; neurones disappear; numerous macrophages; gliosis

Clinical associations

FUNCTIONAL LOSS

Effects are maximal in the early stages when oedema and circulatory disturbance in the adjacent tissues augment the functional loss caused by infarct. Larger infarcts may be associated with loss of consciousness.

The prognostic assessment of final functional loss cannot be made until the changes have subsided and any possible functional compensations have been established. This may take several weeks. Complete clinical recovery may follow small infarcts.

723

INTRACRANIAL HAEMORRHAGE

Spontaneous intracranial bleeding is the second main type of stroke. In the great majority of cases there is localised arterial disease aggravated by hypertension. A small number are associated with cerebral tumours, systemic bleeding diathesis or arteriovenous malformations.

Haemorrhages are divided into two main anatomical groups: (1) **intracerebral** and (2) **subarachnoid.**

INTRACEREBRAL HAEMORRHAGE

In most hypertensives over middle age, **microaneurysms** are found in the very small cerebral arteries. It is believed that rupture of one of these aneurysms is the immediate cause of intracerebral haemorrhage.

Rupture

Thin-walled microaneurysm

Haematoma forms. Commonest site is branches of middle cerebral artery to basal ganglia and internal capsule; also occurs in pons and cerebellum.

Progress

The onset is usually sudden with headache and, because of the high blood pressure, progress is rapid and the haemorrhage large.

↓

Associated raised ICP effects

↓

Death in many cases

When the bleeding is limited, there is survival with varying residual paralysis.

Final outcome
Cystic space containing yellow-brown fluid walled off by gliosis.

Apoplectic cyst

N.B. Intracerebral bleeding may track irregularly and often reaches the subarachnoid space and ventricles.

INTRACRANIAL HAEMORRHAGE

SUBARACHNOID HAEMORRHAGE

This is commonly but not exclusively the result of rupture of a 'berry' aneurysm at or near the circle of Willis. The basic abnormality is a congenital weakness of the elastic tissues in the arterial wall; only rarely is an aneurysm present at birth, and while subarachnoid haemorrhage does occur in young people, the incidence increases with age.

Sites

Often multiple, near arterial junctions.

Circle of Willis

Thin walled aneurysm developing at site of deficiency in arterial wall

Size:
From 1 – 2 mm up to 1 – 2 cm

Not all aneurysms rupture; they are found incidentally at autopsy.
Massive haemorrhage may be preceded by one or more small leaks — marked by headache and no functional loss.

Progress

Haemorrhage spreading throughout subarachnoid space — generalised ICP increased; blood-stained CSF.

Local infarction may be a complication

Irritant effect of haemorrhage causes local arterial spasm

NB The aneurysm may rupture directly into the brain and mimic an intracerebral haemorrhage.

CSF findings

1 – 24 hours — blood stained; blood content constant in sequential samples
(distinguishes blood derived from a traumatic tap)
— centrifuge supernatant — may be pink due to haemolysis.
24 hours onwards — supernatant shows xanthochromia (yellow colour due to presence of blood degradation products).

Other causes of cerebral haemorrhage of either type are vascular malformations and coagulation disorders.

HYPERTENSION

The incidence of strokes in hypertensive subjects is very significantly increased.
1. **Intracranial haemorrhage** — risk increased × 7.

Mechanism

Increased pressure in SMALL arteries → Accelerated degeneration of vessel wall → Microaneurysms form → RUPTURE → HAEMORRHAGE

Hard tortuous pulsatile vessel excavates surrounding cerebral tissue

Space (lacune) formed around vessel

2. **Cerebral infarction** — risk increased indirectly.

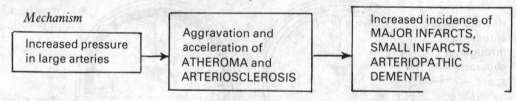

Mechanism

Increased pressure in large arteries → Aggravation and acceleration of ATHEROMA and ARTERIOSCLEROSIS → Increased incidence of MAJOR INFARCTS, SMALL INFARCTS, ARTERIOPATHIC DEMENTIA

In MALIGNANT HYPERTENSION, an additional dimension, HYPERTENSIVE ENCEPHALOPATHY, is added.

Mechanism

Very rapid increase of pressure to high levels → Loss of autoregulatory control

Focal dilatation of small vessels — 'sausage-string' appearance

In dilated segments loss of endothelial integrity → Leak of proteinous fluid (± red cells) → CEREBRAL OEDEMA

Clinically, signs of cerebral 'irritation' including convulsions progress through stupor to coma. Papilloedema, evidence of increased intracranial pressure, is always present.

HEAD INJURY

Head injuries of varying severity are common nowadays, particularly as a consequence of road traffic accidents. Immediate damage is caused by two main mechanisms which overcome the protection of the vulnerable cerebral tissues provided by the skull and the CSF 'water cushion'.

1. **Direct blows to the head**

   usually cause injury to
   the soft tissues of the scalp
   and often fracture of the
   skull with contusion or
   laceration of the
   underlying brain.

Scalp — laceration
± haematoma

Skull — fracture often
comminuted
± depressed
fragments

Brain — contusion, laceration or haematoma

2. Since the head is usually freely moveable on the neck, the sudden application of forces derived from **acceleration, deceleration** and, particularly, **rotation** of the head often cause serious injury.

   (a) **Acceleration/deceleration**

   (i) *Skull damage*

   Skull accelerating rapidly

   Sudden deceleration

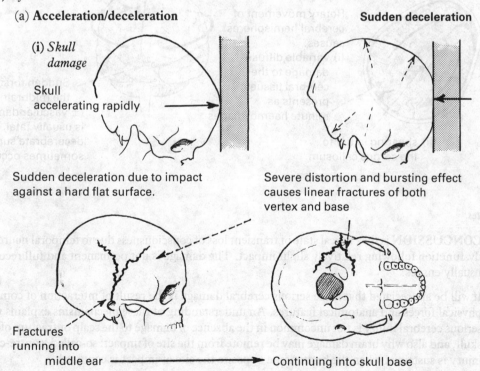

Sudden deceleration due to impact against a hard flat surface.

Severe distortion and bursting effect causes linear fractures of both vertex and base

Fractures running into middle ear ⟶ Continuing into skull base

HEAD INJURY

Acceleration/deceleration injury (continued)

(ii) *Brain damage*

The brain continues to move forward and is contused by the rough surface of the middle fossa and orbital plate

Frontal contusion

Temporal contusion

The damage is characteristically on the surface of gyri, the sulci being spared

Rotation

Rotary movement of cerebral hemispheres causes:
(i) variable diffuse damage to the cerebral tissues; presents as minute haemorrhages

(ii) shearing injury to the corpus callosum

Sudden torsion of the midbrain (± vascular damage) is usually fatal, but decerebrate survival sometimes occurs

Notes:

1. **CONCUSSION** is the clinical state of transient loss of consciousness due to temporal neuronal dysfunction following relatively slight impact. The damage is not permanent and full recovery usually ensues.

2. It will be appreciated that more serious cerebral damage is the result of interaction of complex physical forces and anatomical features. An understanding of these mechanisms explains why serious cerebral injury is not uncommon in the absence of damage to the scalp or fracture of the skull, and also why brain damage may be remote from the site of impact: so-called 'contre-coup' injury is sustained when the brain tissue opposite the site of impact is contused.

HEAD INJURY

DELAYED COMPLICATIONS

In addition to damage sustained immediately at the time of impact, certain serious complications may supervene over the next hours or few days.

1. Haemorrhages

(a) Extradural haematoma

This type of haemorrhage classically occurs as a complication of linear fracture of the skull vault when the middle meningeal artery is torn.

Artery torn at site of fracture   Haemorrhage gradually strips dura from bone   A large, saucer-shaped haematoma forms

The classical clinical association is a direct blow to the head from which recovery is rapid. After a lucid interval of varying duration up to several hours, signs of increased intracranial pressure supervene. This chain of events is explained by the time taken for the haemorrhage to accumulate by stripping the dura from the skull.

(b) Subdural haematoma.

This may occur at any site and is often extensive because of the loose attachment of the dura and arachnoid membranes. It is usually due to rupture of small bridging veins.

Skull

Venous sinus in dura

Dura

Bridging vein

Rupture of vein at entry into dura;

Blood spreads in subdural space

These acute subdural haematomas are often associated with subarachroid haemorrhage and cerebral contusions.

(c) Intracerebral haematomas

occur in association with the cortical contusions particularly in the temporal and frontal lobes, but also at random deep within the hemispheres due to shearing at the time of impact. Large haematomas are uncommon.

HEAD INJURY

Delayed complications (continued)

2. **Cerebral oedema** is an important complication.

    ↓

    Increased intracranial pressure → Cerebral hypoxia.

3. **External leakage of CSF** (and blood) from the ear and nose may complicate fractures of the skull base. This complication may be of long duration and is always a potential entry for infection.

4. **Local infection** may complicate compound fractures and proceed to meningitis.

LATE COMPLICATIONS

1. **Scarring and Epilepsy**

    During the healing process, resorption of necrotic tissues and blood degradation products is gradually effected, leaving pigmented scars. These may act as trigger foci for epilepsy, particularly if the meninges are adherent to the underlying brain.

2. **Chronic subdural haematoma**

    This occurs in the elderly and alcoholics. A thick layer of fluid and partially clotted blood gradually accumulates between the dura and arachnoid membranes which show considerable reactive thickening.

Thickened dura and arachnoid

Skull

Mixture of fluid, clotted blood and blood degradation products

'Atrophic' compressed brain

The precise cause is not known; most cases occur in alcoholics or in elderly people already suffering from cerebral atrophy, and it is possible that the small bridging veins are unduly stretched and become more susceptible to damage.

The clinical signs are usually insidious in onset and progressive, and in nearly all cases there is a history of either none or only very trivial injury.

AGEING AND ATROPHY

It has long been established that progressive atrophy of the brain begins in the 3rd decade and definite morphological changes are associated with simple ageing.

The mean loss of cerebral volume is at the rate of 2 – 3% per decade from age 20 years and the mean loss of brain weight in old age is 100 g from the weight in the 3rd decade.

However it is very important to understand that these figures are means derived from individual measurements covering a wide range and that the individual variation in respect of rate and degree of ageing change is very wide indeed, as is the maintenance of mental and intellectual capacities in old age. Also our ability to link functional loss with morphological change is limited at the present time.

Nevertheless, where dementia occurs in the elderly it is usually associated with obvious degenerative or atrophic changes in the brain.

Changes in old age

1. **Gross** as seen naked-eye at autopsy

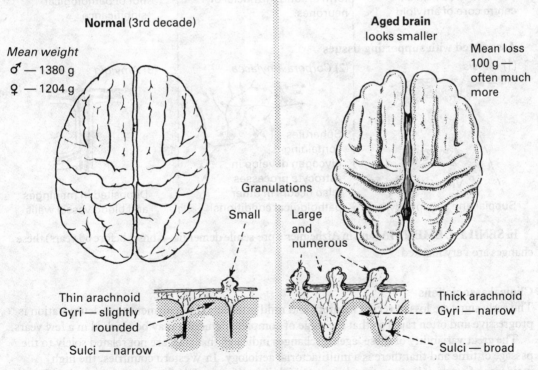

Normal (3rd decade)

Mean weight
♂ — 1380 g
♀ — 1204 g

Thin arachnoid
Gyri — slightly rounded
Sulci — narrow

Aged brain
looks smaller

Mean loss 100 g — often much more

Granulations

Small

Large and numerous

Thick arachnoid
Gyri — narrow
Sulci — broad

AGEING AND ATROPHY

Changes in old age (continued)

2. *Microscopic* changes. The most important change is degeneration and loss of neurones particularly in the neocortex, the Purkinje layer of the cerebellum and the motor cells in the spinal cord. This loss is accompanied by the following lesions:

Associated with neurones

(1) *Senile plaques* (Silver stain)

Tangled aggregates of distended neurites presenting as black dots and rods with a centre core of amyloid

(2) *Alzheimer's neurofibrillary degeneration*

Helical strands of neuroprotein form around the nuclei of neurones.

(3) *Lipofuscin deposition*

(Light microscopy)

Aggregation of yellow wear-tear pigment not of pathological significance

Associated with supporting tissues

(1) *Gliosis*
Pia - -

Ventricle
Subpial and subependymal

(2) *Corpora amylacea*

Spherules containing glycogen develop in astrocyte processes (also occurs in other pathological conditions)

(3) *Amyloid*

Deposited in meninges and blood vessel walls

In **SENILE DEMENTIA** (and in Alzheimer's pre-senile dementia — onset before 60 years) these changes are very marked.

Clinical associations

The early signs are loss of recent memory and mild intellectual impairment, but deterioration is progressive and often rapid so that the stage of complete dementia may be reached in a few years.

The great variability of these 'ageing' changes indicates that they are not related solely to the passage of time and that there is a multifactorial aetiology. In Western countries, the high incidence of arterial degenerative disease (which is itself age-related) may contribute significantly to the loss of brain tissue (p. 722). No doubt hereditary and environmental factors not yet properly identified are also contributory.

INFECTIONS

Compared with the high incidence of infection generally, infection of the central nervous system is uncommon. The pathological effects may be slight and wholly recoverable as in some virus infections, or severe, leading to permanent damage or death.

Anatomically, infections fall into 2 main groups which tend to remain separated due to the intervention of the **pial** barrier (see p.711).

Infection ⟶ Inflammation of

MENINGES (meningitis; empyema; abscess)

PIA

BRAIN SUBSTANCE (encephalitis; abscess)

Infections will be considered in three broad aetiological groups:
(1) Bacterial, (2) Viral and (3) Miscellaneous types.

BACTERIAL INFECTIONS

1. Most commonly by the blood stream

Bacteria settling in subarachnoid space

⟶

Meningitis

(a) Purulent types,
   e.g. meningococcus,
   pneumococcus,
   haemophilus
(b) Granulomatous types,
   e.g. tubercle bacillus,
   treponema pallidum.

Bacteria settling in brain substance

⟶

Brain abscess

(a) Pyogenic type
   — miscellaneous organisms
   NB Staphylococcal pyaemia
(b) Granulomatous type
   — tubercle bacillus

2. From an adjacent local infected site — these are pyogenic infections.

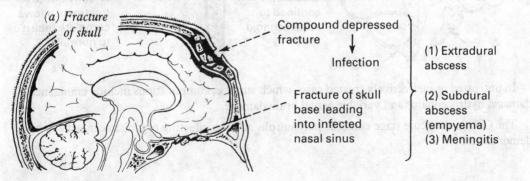

(a) Fracture of skull

Compound depressed fracture

⟶

Infection

Fracture of skull base leading into infected nasal sinus

(1) Extradural abscess

(2) Subdural abscess (empyema)
(3) Meningitis

733

BACTERIAL INFECTION

Bacterial infections from an adjacent local infected site (continued)

(b) *Middle ear and mastoid disease*

In untreated purulent otitis media, three serious complications may arise from spread of the inflammation.

PURULENT MENINGITIS

The whole subarachnoid space contains purulent exudate which is maximal in sulci and around the brain base cisternae.

In untreated or ineffectively treated cases which survive, complications include cranial nerve damage, hydrocephalus and variable actual brain damage.

The CSF in the acute stage contains polymorphs and the infecting organism can usually be demonstrated.

BACTERIAL INFECTION

PURULENT BRAIN ABSCESS

The abscesses resulting from direct spread of adjacent infection or by blood borne infection — as seen particularly in bronchiectasis — are often well circumscribed by a pyogenic membrane.

Clinical note: An abscess is often silent early in its evolution, and the infection at the site of entry may have healed before the onset of serious complications causes clinical signs.

Multiple small abscesses occur in staphylococcal pyaemia and microabscesses may complicate bacterial endocarditis. The cerebral pathology in these circumstances is only one facet of serious systemic infection.

TUBERCULOSIS

Meningitis is the result of blood borne spread, usually from a primary complex and is often the important component of generalised miliary tuberculosis (see p.59). Although the incidence has fallen sharply in Western countries, it remains a serious disease in many parts of the world.

735

TUBERCULOUS MENINGITIS

Evolution

Before the advent of antibiotic and chemotherapy, tuberculous meningitis was invariably fatal after an illness lasting from several days to a few weeks.

Early

Exudate of polymorphs, lymphocytes and fibrin

Several days

Tubercles appearing round vessels

Exudate of lymphocytes and fibrin

Weeks

Dense fibrinous exudate with caseation

↓

Spread into brain

Destruction of vessel wall

Endarteritis

Microinfarction

HEALING at this stage is normally followed by COMPLETE RECOVERY.

CEREBRAL DAMAGE
Complete recovery prevented by
(a) permanent meningeal adhesions
(b) focal cortical scarring

The CSF characteristically contains lymphocytes and fibrinogen which forms a delicate fibrin web on standing. Tubercle bacilli can be demonstrated or cultured.

At autopsy, the brain usually shows a diagnostic appearance:

Numerous small white tubercles close to vessels

Creamy exudate obscuring anatomy of vessels and nerves at base of brain

TUBERCULOMA: These localised tuberculous cerebral abscesses are now very rare.

SYPHILIS: Neurological syphilis is rare nowadays. The main pathological lesions are described on page 63.

VIRUS INFECTIONS

Compared with the incidence of virus infections in general, affection of the central nervous system is rare, even with viruses having an affinity for the CNS —
NEUROTROPIC VIRUSES

There are three broad groups:-

1. Acute
Cell lysis occurs towards the end of the viraemic phase of infection. This is the common type of disease.

2. Persistent
Viruses which usually cause damage outside the CNS behave uncharacteristically and cause continuing and active disease of the CNS over a long period (months — years)

3. Slow
In these diseases the agents have not yet been fully categorised. After a very long (years) incubation period, unremitting and fatal disease ensues.

Latent virus infection is seen in herpes zoster and possibly plays a role in the demyelinating diseases.
Virus infection also has a possible role in oncogenesis within the CNS.

Routes of infection
Most viruses arrive at the CNS via the blood, but the factors which potentiate the establishment of disease within the CNS are poorly understood.

Primary portal of entry

In rabies, the virus travels from the wound up the peripheral nerves to the CNS.

VIRUS INFECTIONS

BASIC PATHOLOGICAL EFFECTS

(a) Commonly the disease is mild and only the meninges are affected — **ASEPTIC MENINGITIS**. Recovery is usually complete.

(b) In more severe cases, the brain substance is also damaged in varying degree — **ENCEPHALITIS** (meningoencephalitis).

The meninges (CSF) contain increased protein, normal sugar and a mononuclear cellular infiltrate (particularly **lymphocytes,** plasma cells and large mononuclears).

In the brain the characteristic changes are:

1. PERIVASCULAR CUFFING (same infiltrate as meninges)
2. ACUTE NEURONAL DAMAGE up to complete lysis with accompanying neuronophagia and inflammatory changes. In some conditions, surviving neurones contain cytoplasmic and/or nuclear inclusions.

To these basic changes, damage to myelin and glial tissue may be added, and small focal haemorrhages may be seen. The damage is effected in two ways:

1. **Certainly** by the direct effects of virus on cells
2. **Possibly** in some cases indirectly due to virus-antibody complexes initiating a vascular inflammatory response.

Diagnosis

Examination of the CSF is helpful in establishing a diagnosis of aseptic meningitis or meningoencephalitis (see p. 778).

NB The findings in tuberculous meningitis are very similar except that in tubercular meningitis the CSF **sugar is low.**

The specific virus aetiology is more difficult to establish and in severe cases brain biopsy may be required.

Clinical associations and progress

In aseptic meningitis, the illness is mild with fever, headache and neck stiffness the main signs. Recovery is almost always complete.

In meningoencephalitis, signs of cerebral 'irritation' and neuronal damage are seen, e.g. mental confusion, delusion, stupor, convulsions and coma, and there may be localising signs. In mild cases, recovery is complete, but in more severe cases, residual paralyses and other signs indicative of permanent brain damage may follow. Death in coma with respiratory failure occurs in very severe cases.

VIRUS INFECTIONS

ENTEROVIRUSES

These are small RNA viruses (picornavirus group) and include POLIOVIRUSES, COXSACKIE VIRUSES and ECHOVIRUSES.

Infection is acquired by ingestion of faecally contaminated material followed by proliferation in the intestine. In only a small minority of infected cases does the virus pass the blood-brain barrier and cause disease of the CNS.

In addition to aseptic meningitis, the POLIOVIRUSES (and very occasionally Coxsackie and Echo viruses) cause the classical paralytic disease, **ANTERIOR POLIOMYELITIS**.

Pathological changes
The pathological changes are reflected in three clinical stages: (1) acute, (2) recovery and (3) permanent residual disability.

(1) **Acute** (up to 2 weeks)

Febrile illness ------------------------- Viraemia

The virus shows tropism for motor nerve cells, particularly in spinal cord

Aseptic meningitis

Perivascular cuffing

Partially damaged neurone

Damage to anterior horn is often localised and unilateral

Dead neurone (neuronophagia)

Normal neurone

Sometimes RESPIRATORY paralysis ----------------- Damage to bulbar motor nuclei

(2) **Recovery**
(Several weeks/months)
Paralyses improve — in mild cases functional recovery may be complete

Damaged neurone recovers

Dead neurone does not recover — gliosis

Inflammation has subsided

(3) **Permanent residual disability**
Wasting of muscles (neuropathic atrophy), varying deformities due to unopposed action of non-paralysed muscle

Shrunken anterior horn

Thin anterior nerve roots

VIRUS INFECTIONS

The HERPES GROUP
HERPES ZOSTER (See also p.67).

This is a disease of adults, presenting as a painful vesicular rash, usually unilateral and affecting one or a few adjacent dermatomes only. It is due to recurrence of a latent varicella (chickenpox) infection.

Mechanism
Virus lying latent from infection in childhood.

Posterior root ganglion

Activation— local trauma;
radiotherapy;
immunological deficit

INTENSE GANGLIONITIS

Epidermal vesicle — virus can be isolated from contents

Virus travels along sensory nerve fibres to skin, conjunctiva or buccal mucosa where virus multiplies.

Minor secondary degenerative changes in cord

Sequels

1. An occasional sequel is intense pain with varying paraesthesia and anaesthesia long after the acute phase has healed.

2. In cases of Vth nerve herpes, serious damage to the eye may result.

HERPES SIMPLEX

In addition to encephalitis seen in infants suffering from disseminated herpes simplex infection and cases of mild aseptic meningitis, herpes simplex virus on rare occasions causes a severe ACUTE NECROTISING ENCEPHALITIS affecting particularly the temporal lobes. A few cases arise against a background of immune deficit, but the majority are unexplained.

VIRUS INFECTIONS

RABIES
The rabies virus shows marked neurotropism and can infect most mammals. Various wild carnivores (fox, jackal, skunk, vampire bats) are the natural reservoir. Many human cases are contracted from dogs.

Mechanism

An unremitting encephalitis particularly affecting the grey matter is established. Diagnostic Negri bodies (virus inclusions) are found at autopsy in the pyramidal cells of the hippocampus and the Purkinje cells of the cerebellum.

Clinically, the encephalitis presents with extreme excitation of the sensory system. The classical hydrophobia (fear of water) is due to serious disturbance of the swallowing mechanism with muscular spasm.

Death invariably occurs and is due to respiratory muscle spasm or paralysis.

ARTHROPOD BORNE VIRUSES (ARBOVIRUSES)
These cause encephalitis in many parts of the world. Biting insects transmit the viruses from animal reservoirs.

ENCEPHALITIS LETHARGICA — Postencephalitic Parkinsonism
This disease occurred in epidemic form in temperate countries during the 1920's and then died out. Although the agent was never identified, it is considered to have been a virus encephalitis. Its importance is due to the postencephalitic damage to the substantia nigra and related nuclei causing Parkinsonism (see p.754).

PERSISTENT VIRUS INFECTION
An example is subacute sclerosing panencephalitis, a rare invariably fatal disease which affects children and young adults. There is progressive widespread destruction of neurones with reactive inflammatory changes giving the white matter a firm consistency.

The infecting agent is thought to be a reactivated but modified measles virus: high titres of measles antibodies are present in the blood.

VIRUS INFECTIONS

SLOW VIRUS INFECTION

KURU is an example of a subacute spongiform encephalopathy. It occurs in the eastern highlands of New Guinea and is associated with cannibalism. The disease presents as a progressive cerebellar ataxia and is invariably fatal.

The pathological changes are neuronal degeneration and loss with astroglial proliferation presenting as small cystic areas in the grey matter (spongiosis). It is noteworthy that there is no inflammation.

The importance of the disease is that it has been shown to be due to an as yet not identified transmissible agent which resists the usual physico-chemical agents capable of killing viruses.

Creutzfeldt-Jacob disease in man and scrapie in sheep are similar diseases.

MISCELLANEOUS INFECTIONS AND INFESTATIONS

FUNGAL INFECTIONS

1. **Primary infections.** In healthy adults, fungal infections are rare. Occasionally in the presence of heavy exposure to fungus localised infection, often clinically insignificant, may occur and in very rare cases, CNS infection is a complication. In CRYPTOCOCCOSIS (*C. neoformans*), the fungus exhibits neurotropism and occasionally causes meningitis in otherwise healthy subjects.

2. **Opportunistic infections** are becoming more common nowadays due to the use of immunosuppressive therapy. Various fungi including *Candida, Aspergillus nocardia* may cause serious cerebral damage due to abscess formation.

2. PROTOZOAL INFECTIONS

(a) CEREBRAL MALARIA

Cerebral complications may occur in the severe acute malaria (falciparum type) which affects non-immune adults. Clinically, coma rapidly proceeds to death.

Mechanism

MISCELLANEOUS INFECTIONS AND INFESTATIONS

Protozoal infections (continued)

Cerebral Malaria (continued)

At autopsy the brain is swollen (oedema) and there may be petechial haemorrhages. Histologically, the capillaries are congested and malarial parasites and pigment easily seen.

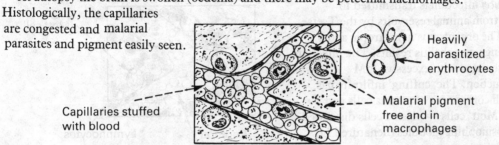

Capillaries stuffed with blood

Heavily parasitized erythrocytes

Malarial pigment free and in macrophages

(b) **TOXOPLASMOSIS.**

Although infection by *T.gondii* is common, serious nervous tissue damage is rare and is seen in two main circumstance. In both, it occurs as part of a systemic infection.

(i) In **congenital toxoplasmosis,** the infection is acquired by the fetus during a primary maternal infection.

Primary infection in pregnant woman ± clinical signs, e.g. lymph node enlargement, mild fever

Placental infection

FETAL INFECTION (esp. brain, eye)

Depending on dose of organism and maturation of fetus

1 ABORTION or STILLBIRTH

2. Severe damage to brain and other organs — early death

3. Moderate CEREBRAL DAMAGE and CHORIORETINITIS

Compatible with life but with permanent disability

(ii) **Opportunistic infection** in adult.

Mechanism

Primary infection when healthy — usually no clinical disease

Organisms encysted and dormant

Reactivation

Acquired immune deficiency, e.g. Hodgkin's disease: immunosuppressive therapy

Systematised infection

Localised meningoencephalitis

743

MISCELLANEOUS INFECTIONS AND INFESTATIONS

Protozoal infections (continued)

(c) TRYPANOSOMIASIS (AFRICAN SLEEPING SICKNESS)

T. brucei infection is transmitted to man from animal reservoirs by the Tsetse fly. The organism is neurotropic and a meningoencephalitis results. The infection is associated with excessive IgM production. The 'cuffing' infiltrate has a high component of plasma cells and also 'Mott' cells — plasma cells distended by eosinophilic globules (denatured Ig).

Mott cell

Cerebral Capillary

Lymphocytes and plasma cells

Amoebiasis

Amoebae are only very rarely the cause of disease. There are two quite distinct types of infection:
1. **Cerebral abscess** very occasionally complicates the colitis and hepatitis caused by *E. histolytica*.
2. **Meningoencephalitis** is caused by amoebae which are free living and not normally pathogenic to man — (*Naegleria* and *Hartmannella* varieties).

Mechanism

Natural water with high content of amoebae → Diving, swimming, water-skiing

Amoebae forced through cribriform plate

Intracranial infection — usually fatal

3. METAZOAL INFESTATION

CRYTICERCOSIS

The larvae of *Taenia solium* may encyst in the brain and can be the cause of epilepsy.

HYDATID CYST —

also occurs in the brain (see p.474).

(see p.474)

DEMYELINATING DISEASES

ACUTE DISSEMINATED ENCEPHALOMYELITIS

An acute encephalitis in which demyelination is a prominent and characteristic feature is a very rare sequel to many natural viral diseases and to vaccination, particularly against smallpox and rabies.

Clinically, there is fever, headache, vomiting and drowsiness followed by coma. There may be clinical evidence of focal neurological damage. Pathological changes are widespread in the brain and cord and rapidly progressive.

Distribution throughout brain or

cord, especially **deep white matter** and pons

Minimal cellular infiltration of meninges

Perivenular cellular infiltrate (lymphocytes: plasma cells and macrophages)

(Normal myelin of white matter stained black)

Perivenular **demyelination** (unstained)

In **ACUTE HAEMORRHAGIC LEUKOENCEPHALITIS,** to these are added actual petechial haemorrhages from damaged vessels, particularly in the white matter; not all cases follow virus infection.

Mechanism. It is thought that in these disorders (particularly encephalitis following anti-rabies inoculation) the damage to the myelin is not the result of direct virus attack but is an *autoimmune* reaction in which the antigen is a component of myelin and the virus in some unknown way acts as a trigger.

| VIRUS INFECTION | ?Trigger mechanism | Release of antigen (myelin component) | AUTOIMMUNE RESPONSE | ENCEPHALITIS |

Experimental allergic encephalomyelitis (EAE) in animals closely mimics the human disease.

ANTIGEN

FREUND'S ADJUVANT

Injected

ANIMAL

Development of cell-mediated immune response — destroys myelin and (?) causes vascular damage

ENCEPHALITIS

Encephalitogenic factor (EF) — a peptide derived from myelin – not species specific

The importance of these rare diseases is that they form a link between virus infections and the chronic DEMYELINATING DISEASES.

DEMYELINATING DISEASES

In the demyelinating diseases, the breakdown of myelin occurs as an almost random patchy process in the white matter; at the same time, neurones and axons usually remain healthy. There are two main types:

1. The **'myelinoclastic'** type.
The myelin is apparently normal until adult life and then breaks down.

2. The **'dysmyelinative'** type.
The myelin is structurally abnormal usually from an early age.

1. MULTIPLE SCLEROSIS (MS)

This is a chronic disease of young adults.

The basic pathological change is an almost random scattering of 'plaques' of demyelination in the white matter.

The fibres of the optic nerve are often affected — retrobulbar neuritis

(Normal myelin stained black)

In the early stages, there may be round cell infiltrate, but in the usually seen late lesions inflammation is absent

Pons

Medulla

Black staining normal myelin

Spinal cord

Plaque — no myelin; axons remain; glial fibres increased; few oligodendrocytes

Clinical associations
The neurological signs reflect *white matter damage* — upper motor neurone weakness and paralysis; incoordination; visual disturbances; paraesthesia.
('Grey matter' signs, e.g. aphasia, fits and muscle atrophy are rare.)

Course of Disease

Onset

Often acute; may be unnoticed.

Progress over many years
Remission...Relapse...Remission →
Incremental deterioration → Death

Variants are: 1. acute severe disease — rapid progress to death
2. chronic progression without remission
3. minimal signs with very long remissions.

DEMYELINATING DISEASES

MULTIPLE SCLEROSIS (continued)
Aetiology

The cause remains unknown and the basic mechanisms poorly defined.

1. The geographical pattern is of interest, but does not as yet contribute to our understanding of the aetiology. The disease is common (60 cases per 100,000 population) throughout temperate Europe and North America and small pockets of much higher incidence do occur. The incidence is low in the tropics.

2. The three most plausible current theories which are not mutually exclusive are based on as yet inconclusive evidence:

(1) MS is a **slow virus** infection — Direct attack →

NORMAL MYELIN + OLIGODEN-DROGLIA | ABNORMAL MYELIN (susceptible to damage)

(3) The apparently normal myelin of MS is really abnormal and contains less unsaturated fatty acids (UFA). It is not known whether this condition is genetic or acquired.

(2) MS is an **autoimmune disease** — Cell-mediated attack ?+ vascular component → Demyelination

2. DYSMYELINATING DISEASES

In this group of 'leukodystrophies', the molecular structure of myelin is abnormal due usually to abnormal or deficient enzyme action. Most cases are genetically determined, present in early life and progress fairly rapidly.

Abnormal metabolites which can be specifically identified accumulate in macrophages, glial cells and sometimes neurones.

> e.g. 1. In **metachromatic leukodystrophy,** the accumulation of a *sulphatide* gives a metachromatic staining reaction and a characteristic EM appearance.
>
> 2. In **Krabbe's disease** there are typical multinucleated histocytes (called globoid cells) containing *cerebroside*.

In some disorders, when the loss of myelin is associated with marked gliosis, the name 'diffuse cerebral sclerosis' is applied.

MISCELLANEOUS DISORDERS

NUTRITIONAL, TOXIC AND METABOLIC DISORDERS (ENCEPHALOPATHIES)

In the last analysis, all disorders in this group are mediated by disturbed neuronal metabolism, so that exact classification may present some difficulty. However, it is convenient to consider them in three broad groups.

1. NUTRITIONAL DEFICIENCY

The vitamins of the B group are important coenzymes in several intracellular oxidative pathways. Deficiency, which may arise from primary malnutrition but more commonly in association with alcohol abuse, is the cause of degenerations of the brain, spinal cord and peripheral nerves.

Wernicke's encephalopathy

Clinically, this condition presents with disturbances of consciousness, ataxia and visual disturbances, and without prompt treatment progresses to death in coma.

In Western countries, chronic alcoholism is usually present; often a particularly heavy bout of drinking precipitates the condition.

Chronic alcoholism ⟶ Poor diet ⟶ NUTRITIONAL DEFICIENCY of vit B complex, esp. THIAMIN.

Accentuates

Bout of heavy drinking ⟶ Vomiting

The blood PYRUVATE level is raised.

The lesions, which are focal, consist of glial proliferations with varying neurone loss. Petechial haemorrhages may be seen.

The lesions have a characteristic anatomical distribution:

Around walls of IIIrd ventricle,

Mamillary bodies

Around aqueduct

Floor of IVth ventricle

Prompt treatment with thiamin minimises the damage, but if treatment is omitted or delayed, permanent damage results. At autopsy, there is visible shrinkage of the mamillary bodies.

MISCELLANEOUS DISORDERS

2. EXOGENOUS TOXIC DISORDERS

The nervous system is affected by a wide range of poisons, many of which are used in medical treatment, including particularly hypnotics and narcotics.

In many acute cases, neuronal metabolism is seriously depressed and may result in death. Very often the effects of cerebral hypoxia as well as the metabolic disturbances caused by damage to other organs are superimposed so that it may be difficult to define neurological damage specifically caused by the poison.

The diagram shows the effects of acute poisoning.

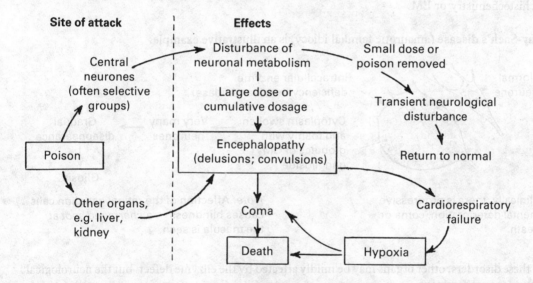

These disorders are the result of biochemical changes in the first place and minimal or no morphological damage is caused. However, at autopsy there are non-specific oedematous and hypoxic changes: specific toxic effects are usually not identifiable.

In some cases, the peripheral nerves are damaged — neuropathy.

Chronic alcoholic intoxication exemplifies this scheme. Specific toxic effects on neurones are difficult to identify, but the brain is damaged by nutritional deficits and as a result of liver disturbance.

Metallic poisons

In the case of heavy metals and arsenic, there is a build up of the poison within the nervous system and encephalopathy with morphological damage results.

749

MISCELLANEOUS DISORDERS

3. METABOLIC DISORDERS

Disorders due to inborn errors of metabolism

These are often due to lysozomal enzyme deficiency.

(a) The *dysmyelinating diseases* (leukodystrophies) in which abnormal central nervous cellular metabolism, especially in glial cells, produces abnormal myelin have already been mentioned.

(b) In the *neuronal storage diseases,* which usually present during the first decade, deficiency of lysozomal enzymes leads to accumulation of intermediate metabolites in the neurones. The diagnosis of the condition often depends on the identification of the abnormal metabolite by histochemistry or EM.

Tay-Sach's disease (amaurotic familial idiocy) is an illustrative example.

Normal neurone

Intracellular enzyme deficiency (hexosaminidase)

Cytoplasm swollen and foamy with globules of GM_2 ganglioside $\longrightarrow$ Very many neurones $\longrightarrow$ Gradual disappearance $\downarrow$ Gliosis

Clinically, there is progressive mental deterioration, coma or death.

Note: Affection of the retinal ganglion cells causes blindness — a *cherry red spot* at the macula is seen.

In these disorders, other organs may be mildly affected by the enzyme defect but the neurological effects are predominant.

(c) In the following examples, the metabolic defect causes neurological disorder, but in addition, other organs are seriously disturbed.

(i) **Aminoacidopathies**

A wide variety of hepatic enzyme defects in the complex metabolism of amino acids have now been described. When neurological damage occurs, it is essentially non-specific and developing in the immediate postnatal period, a critical time in the development of the brain which leads to *mental retardation.*

Phenylketonuria is an example.

The importance of this disease is that the effects can be prevented by dietary restriction of phenylalanine-containing substances, provided the treatment is begun within 60 days of birth.

MISCELLANEOUS DISORDERS

Phenylketonuria (continued)

Mechanism

Liver

Primary defect: ABSENCE of PHENYLALANINE HYDROXYLASE

Blood ↓

Increased PHENYLALANINE and its derivatives

Kidney

PHENYLPYRUVIC ACID in URINE ——— **'PHENYLKETONURIA'**

Brain

Non-specific damage: spongiosis, gliosis, demyelination ——— Mental retardation

(ii) *Hepatolenticular degeneration (Wilson's disease)*

In this rare inherited disorder (autosomal recessive: parental consanguinity in one third of cases) accumulation of COPPER causes serious toxic effects.

The primary lysozomal defect is in the liver cells: in many cases there are also low levels of caeruloplasmin (glycoprotein which normally transports Cu).

Basic mechanism

Copper absorbed from intestine

Liver

Lysozomal defect ↓ Inability to excrete Cu ↓ Cu accumulates in liver

Effects

1. Damage to liver: 'hepatitis' → cirrhosis

2. Release of Cu loosely bound to albumin

BRAIN

Progressive toxic damage to neurones of extrapyramidal system and cortex: gliosis with large astrocytes.

Clinically: tremor, ataxia, choreiform movements, dementia

Possible subsidiary mechanism: Although the relationship of the caeruloplasmin deficit to the primary liver enzyme deficiency is not yet clarified it is possible that it aggravates the condition.

CORNEA

Deposited at limbus of cornea as brown Kayser-Fleischer rings

Intestinal lumen

Cu   Cu

Cu

Mucosal barrier

KIDNEY

Selective tubular damage aminoaciduria, glycosuria etc.

Low Cu/caeruloplasmin level ↓ Failure of feed back control of Cu absorption ↓ Increase Cu → Liver

MISCELLANEOUS DISORDERS

METABOLIC (continued)

Secondary

The metabolism of the nervous system may be seriously affected by disease elsewhere in the body.

Acute hypoxia and **hypoglycaemia**
cause disturbance of the basic neuronal metabolism and serious damage results if these conditions are not corrected quickly.

    In many other disorders, the neuronal disturbances are usually reversible even in cases of fairly long duration, and permanent damage is seen only in late or severe disease.

    Clinically, the condition progresses from delirium through the stuporose state to coma and death.

    The mechanisms are complex, often indirect and not certainly defined. They include particularly:

1. disturbances of water and electrolyte (especially Na^+ and K^+) balance, and also pH affecting neuronal environment.

2. the activity of abnormal 'toxic' metabolites, e.g. ketones; organic acids (including amino acids) directly affecting neuronal metabolism.

3. (1) and (2) combined influence chemical transmission

The following common and important disorders are illustrative:

(a) Diabetes mellitus — the important derangements which act in various combinations are: hypovolaemia (due to dehydration); hyperosmolarity (due to hyperglycaemia); Na^+ and K^+ depletion; ketonaemia and lactic acidosis.

(b) Liver failure — complex disturbances of NH_3 and amino acid metabolism (see p.468).

(c) Renal failure (uraemia) — complex disturbances involving water, electrolyte and nitrogenous waste products (see p.653).

    In addition, in some cases of renal failure, malignant hypertension contributes to the neurological disturbance (see p.726).

EXTRAPYRAMIDAL DISORDERS

The extrapyramidal system is interposed between the higher motor centres (cortical) and the effector motor cells of the anterior horn of the spinal cord.

It consists of the basal ganglia nuclei in the midbrain and pons, and complex interconnections between the nuclei and other parts of the cerebrum, cerebellum and cord.

Its function, which is to integrate motor and sensory impulses so that muscle tone reflexes and movements are smooth and coordinated, is finally effected by facilitation and restraint of anterior horn neurone activity.

Important neurotransmitters within the system are DOPAMINE (also catecholamines and 5-hydroxytryptamine), acetylcholine and γ-aminobutyric acid (GABA).

Disorders of the system result in:

    1. muscular rigidity
    2. tremors
    3. incoordinated and abnormal muscle movements
    4. disturbances of postural reflexes.

Theoretically, damage to any part of the system may be associated with all or any of these derangements.
The following two disorders are illustrative:

PARKINSONISM (Paralysis agitans)

Aetiology: The disease occurs in two main circumstances:
(a) **Idiopathic:** occurring in people over 50; nowadays not infrequent in an ageing population.
(b) **Secondary:** 1. **Postencephalitic,** i.e. as a sequel to encephalitis lethargica which occurred in epidemic form in the 1920s. The number of such cases now surviving is rapidly diminishing.
        2. **Drug induced.** The use of neuroleptic drugs may induce the syndrome temporarily (occasionally permanently), presumably by disturbing the balance of the chemical transmitters.
        3. **Arteriopathy.**
        4. **Heavy metal poisoning.**

EXTRAPYRAMIDAL DISORDERS

Clinically, **Parkinsonism** illustrates the classical features of extrapyramidal damage.

Mask-like expressionless face, often with drooling due to change of muscle tone and reflexes

Bent posture — 'chasing' centre of gravity

'Pill-rolling' tremor of hands

Stiff shuffling gait

Pathological mechanism
In all cases of long-standing Parkinsonism of any type, degenerative changes are seen in the extrapyramidal nuclei. In particular, there is depigmentation of the substantia nigra.

Normal

Also there is a deficiency of DOPAMINE in affected nuclei.

In the idiopathic type, it is possible that the dopamine deficiency is an acquired metabolic disorder which leads to the neuronal degeneration, but this has not yet been established.

THE CHOREAS

These are extrapyramidal disorders in which the presenting sign is involuntary incoordinate movements. There are 2 main types which, apart from both presenting with choreiform movements, differ in many respects.

	INFECTIOUS	HUNTINGTON'S
Age of onset	Childhood	35 – 50 years
Progress	Recovery — complete (may be recurrences)	Deterioration and cerebral cortical degeneration (dementia)
Pathogenesis	Associated with infections, esp. rheumatic fever. *NB* often associated with endocarditis	Hereditary (autosomal dominant) — associated with reduction of neurotransmitter GABA
Pathology	Essentially inflammatory: mild encephalitis (? arteritis) affecting basal ganglia	Essentially neuronal degeneration in caudate nucleus, putamen and cortex

DISEASES OF SPINAL CORD

In purely spinal lesions, basic disease processes have important anatomical and functional implications. Lack of space for expansion produces important compression effects. Examples are:

Fracture/
dislocation
of vertebra

Tumour (usually
secondary) in vertebrae
growing into canal

Prolapse of
intervertebral
disc

Tumour of
meninges or
nerve sheath

Effects

Normal

Cord, nerve roots and
blood vessels loosely
suspended in CSF
'water bath'

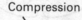

Compression

(3) *Damage to nerve roots*
(radiculitis); a common
complication of spondylosis

(1) *Damage to neurones and
nerve tracts*
May be focal but is often
transverse and complete

(2) *Vascular compression*
Impairment of circulation
may be actual infarction;
this is important particularly
in traumatic cases

At the level of the lesion, there is loss of the sensory and motor connections which constitute the spinal reflex.

In addition, severance of the longitudinal tracts cuts off the cerebral connections to all parts below the lesion.

Sensory impulses stop here

Motor impulses from higher centres
stop here

∴ LOSS OF SENSORY
APPRECIATION
below lesion

∴ PARALYSIS below lesion

Note: The spinal reflexes
remain intact below the lesion.

DISEASES OF SPINAL CORD

ASCENDING AND DESCENDING DEGENERATIONS
The long tract fibres which are cut off from their neurones progressively degenerate.

Ascending degeneration
in gracile and cuneate tracts above the lesion extends as far as their nuclei in the medulla

Sensory neurone in root ganglion

Cortical motor neurone

Level of lesion

Descending degeneration
in lateral corticospinal tracts (pyramidal) below the lesion

Note: In transverse lesions of the cord, all the long tracts degenerate either upwards (sensory) or downwards (motor). These particular tracts are shown for illustrative convenience.

The commonest example of **descending degeneration** is seen following cerebral infarction involving the internal capsule; the degeneration extends from the lesion along the corticospinal axons to their terminations in the anterior horn.

Cortical motor neurones

Internal capsule (infarction)

Direct corticospinal tract

Crossed corticospinal (pyramidal) tract

Degeneration

In cases of recent (months) strokes the degeneration is seen as demyelination, e.g. in cervical cord

Direct corticospinal tract

Pyramidal tract (opposite side)

In cases of long-standing, gliosis and shrinkage occur: well seen at the level of the *cerebral peduncles* and the *pyramids*.

Shrinkage of peduncle (same side as lesion)

Shrinkage of pyramid (opposite side)

DISORDERS OF MOTOR PATHWAYS

The concept of upper and lower motor neuronal activity, based on anatomical and physiological evidence, has great clinical value in diagnosis.

The **upper motor neurones** (UMN) synapse with the **lower motor neurones** (LMN)

consist of

consist of

Cortical motor neurones
(pre-central gyrus)

Motor tracts in cerebrum
(internal capsule)

Motor tracts in brain stem
— fibres crossing to
cranial nerves in opposite
side

Decussation of pyramids

Small direct corticospinal
tract (anterior)

Large crossed pyramidal
tract (anterolateral)

Cranial nerve nuclei
(motor) and their axons
in the cranial nerves

Anterior horn cells
and their axons in
the spinal nerves

It will be appreciated that in its long course from the cerebral cortex to the anterior horn, the upper motor neurone is susceptible to damage from a variety of disease processes acting at various sites. The lower motor neurone may be damaged in the cord or in the peripheral nerve. Important illustrative examples are:

Upper motor neurone damage

Stroke

damaging
internal
capsule

**Multiple
sclerosis**

— random
demyelination
damaging motor
tracts at several
sites.

Lower motor neurone damage

Poliomyelitis – anterior
horn cell damage

Peripheral neuropathy —
damage to axon and
sheath.

757

DISORDERS OF MOTOR PATHWAYS

Clinical points

PARALYSIS occurs in disorders of both systems but the reflexes show important differences.

Upper motor neurone damage	Lower motor neurone damage
↓	↓
Lower motor neurone released from cortical control ∴ muscle tone increased, tendon jerks (and other spinal reflexes) increased, plantar reflex extensor	Loss of final effector mechanism ∴ reflexes absent, also muscle atrophy

MOTOR NEURONE DISEASE

In contrast to these motor disorders, secondary to known diseases, motor neurone disease is of unknown aetiology occuring in adults with a predominant incidence in males.

The basic lesion is a specific progressive degeneration of both cortical and spinal motor neurones with its accompanying pathological effects. There are variations depending on the relative involvement of the upper and lower motor neurone components and the sites of initial damage. Even in the early stages when differentiating features are best seen, there may be considerable overlap and usually in the later stages the distinctions are blurred due to the inexorable progression with severe and widespread motor neuronal degeneration.

1. **In progressive muscular atrophy,** as the name implies, the main signs are of neurogenic atrophy due to degeneration of the anterior horn cells (LMN).

Predilection for cervical cord

Gradual (several years) degeneration of anterior horn cells
↓
Gliosis
↓
Shrinkage

Sites particularly affected are:
1. Small muscles of hand — wasting ('Simian hand')

Note: While degeneration of neurones is proceeding spontaneous irregular discharges cause muscle twitching — **FASCICULATION**

2. Muscles of arm and shoulder girdle.
3. Spread towards medulla.
4. Later leg weakness and paralysis reflect both LMN and UMN damage.

DISORDERS OF MOTOR PATHWAYS

MOTOR NEURONE DISEASE (continued)

2. In **Amyotrophic lateral sclerosis** the main damage is the UMN: 'lateral sclerosis' indicates the degeneration of the pyramidal tracts.

The degeneration affects the *cortical motor cells* — particularly those supplying the lower limbs but spreading over a few years to involve the neck and head centres. Voluntary movements of the face, jaw and tongue muscles are defective.

Corticospinal tracts showing degeneration and later, gliosis.

The lesions are very rarely pure UMN type even initially, and with progression, the LMN lesions increase.

3. **Progressive bulbar palsy** and **pseudobulbar palsy**

In a few cases, the disease begins with signs of cranial nerve dysfunction — swallowing and facial movements are impaired.

In progressive bulbar palsy, the LMN is affected (cranial nerve nuclei); muscle atrophy and fasciculation occur.

In pseudobulbar palsy the lesion is in the UMN and no muscle atrophy is seen.

Overlap of varying amount is again not unusual.

The following diagram illustrates the overlap of UMN and LMN components in motor neurone disease.

Progress

In motor neurone disease after a long progressive illness, the stage is reached when the bulbar degeneration is severe enough to prevent elimination of secretions from the respiratory tract. Death is usually due to aspiration bronchopneumonia but occasionally to acute asphyxia.

759

DISORDERS OF SENSORY PATHWAYS

In **HERPES ZOSTER,** where there is inflammation of the posterior root ganglia in one or two spinal segments on one side only, the damage is not sufficient to affect the ascending spinal tracts.

In **TABES DORSALIS,** a tertiary manifestation of syphilis in which the lumbar cord is commonly affected, there is degeneration of the posterior nerve roots and columns.

Skin-touch: *Joints and muscles* – proprioception

Clinically
Loss of vibration sense and reflexes
Ataxia
Trophic skin ulcers
Severe joint derangement (Charcot)

Additional features
Cranial and sympathetic nerve involvement — disturbance of pupillary reflex
Painful visceral crises

MIXED MOTOR AND SENSORY DISORDERS

SUBACUTE COMBINED DEGENERATION OF CORD
Due specifically to vit B$_{12}$ deficiency. If replacement therapy is begun early enough, there is restoration to normal.

Degenerated tracts
1. Posterior columns →
2. Corticospinal tracts →

Effects
Sensory loss (vibration and proprioception): ataxia

Upper motor neurone damage — spastic paralysis

SYRINGOMYELIA
In this condition, a glial-lined cystic space gradually expands within the cord, usually in the cervical region. The pathogenesis is not certain, but it is suggested that the lesion is essentially an expansion of the central canal associated with a mild developmental abnormality of the distal end of the IV ventricle.

Effects
Damage to sensory fibres decussating in the cord.
Loss of temperature and touch in local segments
(**dissociated anaesthesia**).

Early

Late

Destruction of grey matter and gradual affection of long tracts
Loss of local reflexes.
Severe sensory loss.
Spastic paralysis.

MIXED MOTOR AND SENSORY DISORDERS

Friedreich's ataxia

In this disease, which has a strong familial basis, there is progressive degeneration of sensory (spinocerebellar tracts and posterior columns) and motor tracts. It begins in childhood and progresses to death in a few years. Postural and skeletal deformities complicate the progressive ataxia and paralysis. In some cases there is a cardiomyopathy with arrhythmia.

This disease is mentioned to illustrate the spinocerebellar degenerations, a large group of related disorders, usually familial, in which there is neuronal and tract degeneration particularly affecting gait, posture, equilibrium and movement. There is sometimes optic nerve and retinal damage and intellectual disturbance.

THE PERIPHERAL NERVES

The nerves are a mixture of different types of fibre, myelinated and non-myelinated of varying thickness and length, subserving sensory and motor functions. In most disorders, both functions are disturbed, but in the early stages, selective damage to particular fibre types is often seen.

In affection of one or other nerve roots pure motor or sensory disturbance may be seen separately.

THE NEUROPATHIES

The term neuropathy is preferred to neuritis since most disorders are not essentially inflammatory.

There are two broad groups:

Normal

1. *Parenchymatous*
   The axon and its closely associated Schwann cells and myelin sheath are affected primarily; note that myelin is produced and maintained by Schwann cells. Most disorders of this type are due to toxic or metabolic disturbances and affect many nerves — POLYNEUROPATHY.

2. **Interstitial**
   The damage is primarily in the blood vessels or supporting tissues (epi-, peri- and endoneurium). In this type, single nerves or several nerves may be affected, depending on the nature of the interstitial damage.

THE NEUROPATHIES

The **POLYNEUROPATHIES** occur in a wide range of conditions.

Toxic — diphtheria; lead; arsenic; drugs used in medicine.
Deficiency states — particularly vit B complex deficiency causing Beri-Beri.
Metabolic disorders — diabetes mellitus, porphyria, metachromatic leukodystrophy,
    associated with malignant tumours, in uraemia treated by dialysis.

There are two main mechanisms of degeneration.

1. Degeneration of the axon with concomitant demyelination. This is closely allied to Wallerian
   degeneration following nerve transection.

Ovoids of lipid indicating degenerating myelin

Degenerate axons

2. Primary degeneration occurs patchily in Schwann cells; axon degeneration follows slowly.

Segmental myelin degeneration between nodes of Ranvier indicating individual Schwann cell damage

Normal segments

Since in many polyneuropathies the long large fibres degenerate first, the early clinical effects
are referable to the distal ends of the nerves. Also damage may affect particular nerves and nerve
groups selectively.

INTERSTITIAL NEUROPATHY

Mononeuropathy

Single nerves are subject to damage by compression. The nerve structures may be damaged
directly or more usually as a result of ischaemia. Examples are the carpal tunnel syndrome in which
the median nerve is compressed between the carpal bones and ligaments, and following drunken
stupor where abnormal postures have compressed nerves. The cranial nerves within the skull are
subject to such distortions leading to degeneration where intracranial pressure is increased.

THE NEUROPATHIES

Ischaemic neuropathy
Nerve degeneration may be seen in cases of acute arteritis.

Inflammation of vasa nervorum with thrombosis → The effects are seen *distally*

Severe damage
Degenerate fibres

Focal damage

(Nerves may be normal at site of arteritis)

Vessels may be healthy at site of degeneration

Since the vascular lesions are usually patchy and random, several individual nerves are variously damaged — the condition is called mononeuritis multiplex.

NEURITIS
Nerve damage due to inflammation occurs in three main circumstances.

1. The Landry-Guillain-Barré and related syndromes. The onset is acute, often following 7 – 21 days after a mild non-specific febrile illness. There are peripheral neurological signs with usually a motor (LMN) deficit predominant, beginning in the lumbar nerves and ascending fairly rapidly (ascending paralysis) so that respiratory failure, requiring supportive treatment, is a serious complication.

The interstitial tissues are infiltrated with lymphocytes and plasma cells

There is variable axonal and myelin degeneration

The nerve roots are predominantly affected.

The CSF usually contains excessive protein but few cells.

The disease probably has an immunological basis and is allied to experimental allergic encephalitis (see p.745).

Progress: usually recovery is complete.

2. In **leprosy,** a low grade chronic inflammation of the nerve sheaths is associated with fibrosis and fibre degeneration.

3. Peripheral nerves may be damaged by direct spread of inflammation from adjacent tissues.

THE NEUROPATHIES

1. **Bell's palsy**
   This is a unilateral facial weakness of sudden onset. The cause is not known with certainty, but some cases are associated with draughts and chilling.

   The mechanism is thought to be inflammation with swelling and compression of the facial nerve in its course in the bone adjacent to the internal auditory meatus.

   Note drooping and loss of facial expression on paralysed side. Facial muscles pull across the mid line — mouth is distorted.

   Progress In 75% of cases, there is recovery in about 4 – 8 weeks.

2. Distal neuropathy may occur in long-standing cases of lower limb ischaemia → nerve sheath fibrosis → nerve degeneration.
   This mechanism is a component of ......
3. **Diabetic neuropathy** where there is narrowing of the small vessels but a metabolic component with consequent segmental Schwann cell degeneration also contributes.
4. In **amyloid disease** of the hereditary type particularly, neuropathy due to compression of nerve fibres by amyloid material may occur.
5. **Segmental neuropathy** is exemplified in diphtheria and lead poisoning. Because the functional effects in particular paralyses are essentially due to demyelination without axon degeneration, recovery is usually more rapid than in many other neuropathies.

PORPHYRIAS

These are diseases due to partial deficiencies of liver or marrow enzymes engaged in haem synthesis. The individual is usually healthy; precipitating factors aggravate the defects and increase porphyrin precursors causing symptoms. Two forms exist:

1. **Acute** porphyrias with abdominal pain, neuropathies, psychotic symptoms and often hypertension. Respiratory paralysis may occur. All are due to an autosomal dominant hepatic enzyme defect.

2. **Chronic** porphyrias cause skin blistering and scarring. Most are due to autosomal recessive or dominant marrow enzyme defects. Precipitating factors in both: alcohol, barbiturates, analgesics, tranquillisers, oral contraceptives, hepatic poisons. Ultraviolet light is important in chronic forms.

HYDROCEPHALUS

In hydrocephalus, the volume of the CSF is increased and the ventricles are dilated. In the majority of cases, there is an increase in intracranial pressure. Three possible theoretical **mechanisms** are considered.

1. **Overproduction of CSF**
   The choroid plexus will secrete more CSF to compensate for any external leak, but overproduction is *not* a cause of hydrocephalus.

2. **Obstruction to the flow of CSF is the common mechanism.**

INTRACEREBRAL FLOW

Production (choroid plexuses)

Lateral vent.

Via foramen of Munro

III vent

Via aqueduct of Sylvius

IV vent

Via foramina of Magendie and Luschka

Sites of narrowing particularly vulnerable to obstruction
(1) Aqueduct of Sylvius
(2) Foramina of Magendie and Luschka
(3) The subarachnoid space between the midbrain and forebrain (interposition of tentorium cerebelli)

EXTRACEREBRAL FLOW

SUBARACHNOID SPACE

In cases of obstruction up to the IV ventricular foramina, the CSF cannot reach the subarachnoid space; e.g. sites 1 and 2. The hydrocephalus is NON-COMMUNICATING.

When the obstruction is beyond the foramina, e.g. site 3, the hydrocephalus is **COMMUNICATING.**

3. **Defective absorption of CSF is a rare mechanism.**

Normal: Absorption of CSF into venous sinus via arachnoid granulation

Abnormal: Disease process, e.g. scarring following inflammation or haemorrhage obliterating absorption sites.

Dura

Subarachnoid space

Pia

Brain

Scarring

HYDROCEPHALUS

CAUSES

The diseases causing hydrocephalus fall into two groups:

1. **Congenital (developmental) abnormalities**
   The common conditions are:

(a) *The Arnold-Chiari malformation*

Prolongation of cerebellum and medulla bulging through the foramen magnum

Obstruction to flow of CSF in posterior fossa

Associated with spina bifida, usually *meningomyelocele*

Dura deficient

Arachnoid and nervous tissue lying under bulging skin

(b) *Congenital stenosis or atresia of aqueduct of Sylvius*

Leads to dilatation of IIIrd and lateral ventricles

Stenosis

(c) *Atresia of foramina of Magendie and Luschka*

Leads to dilatation of IVth, IIIrd and lateral ventricles

Atresia

2. **Acquired hydrocephalus**

Of the many possible conditions causing hydrocephalus, the following are most common: (a) cerebral tumour (primary or secondary) and (b) scarring of the meninges following meningitis or subarachnoid haemorrhage.

As already explained, whether any particular disease produces hydrocephalus depends largely on the site affected.

HYDROCEPHALUS

EFFECTS

In the infant and young child, the pliable skull expands to accommodate the enlarging brain.

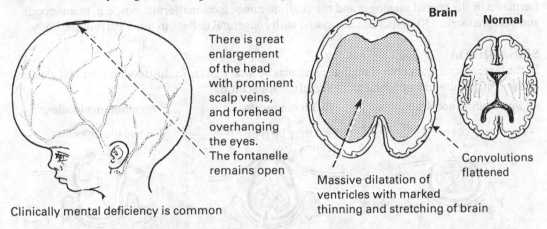

There is great enlargement of the head with prominent scalp veins, and forehead overhanging the eyes. The fontanelle remains open

Brain

Normal

Clinically mental deficiency is common

Massive dilatation of ventricles with marked thinning and stretching of brain

Convolutions flattened

In **the older child and adult,** enlargement of the brain is prevented by the inability of the skull to expand. The main change is dilatation of the ventricles associated with the effects on the brain of increased intracranial pressure.

SPECIAL TYPES OF HYDROCEPHALUS

1. In cases of generalised cerebral atrophy, the ventricular system enlarges to compensate for the loss of cerebral tissue. This also happens locally when cerebral tissue is lost, e.g following infarction.

Primary atrophy of brain (deepened sulci, thinned convolutions)

Secondary dilatation

Local dilatation of ventricle

Old infarct

No increase in pressure is involved and the pathological and clinical effects wholly reflect the primary loss of cerebral tissue. The condition is sometimes called **secondary hydrocephalus.**

2. Normal pressure hydrocephalus.

In this rare condition, progressive mental and neurological deterioration is associated with ventricular dilatation due to no apparent cause. The diagnosis of this condition has assumed importance because in some cases surgical CSF shunting procedures have arrested the progress.

DEVELOPMENTAL ABNORMALITIES

Developmental abnormalities of the brain and cranium are relatively common, varying from virtually complete absence of cerebral substance (anencephaly), with associated failure of formation of the cranial meninges and the skull, to minor local malformations, e.g. meningocele and encephalocele. Often they are associated with congenital defects in other parts of the body.

SPINA BIFIDA

In the lumbosacral and cervical regions particularly, local defects in the development and closure of the neutral tube and vertebral arches result in spina bifida.

(a) Spina bifida occulta

Normal skin covering

Vertebral arches and dura deficient — may be associated with minor nerve defects — particularly affecting bladder function

(b) Meningocele

Skin may be thin at apex

Rounded sac containing CSF

Cord in normal position

(c) Meningomyelocele

Skin usually defective

Cord displaced into sac: often adherent and distorted

May be associated with serious nervous deficit — especially in legs, bladder.

Infection through the deficient skin is a serious complication.

The cause of these defects is not yet known. In some cases there are heredito-familial influences; in others, teratogens are possibly involved and, recently, circumstantial evidence implicates nutritional deficiency (particularly of vitamins) as a cause.

Diagnosis in utero

α-fetoprotein leaks through the defective skin covering and increased amounts are found in the amniotic fluid.

Complications.

In addition to severe neurological deficits which are aggravated by infection, an important complication even in minor defects is **HYDROCEPHALUS**.

TUMOURS OF THE NERVOUS SYSTEM

The following scheme illustrates the various non-specific clinicopathological effects of a tumour within the skull.

An important factor which materially influences the relative importance of each of these effects is the rate of tumour growth.

Tumours will be considered in more detail under the following broad headings:

1 Neoplasms of neuroectodermal origin.

2 Neoplasms arising in supporting tissue (mesodermal)

3 Neoplasms and swellings of developmental origin.

4 Neoplasms of nerve sheaths.

5 Secondary neoplasms.

769

TUMOURS OF THE NERVOUS SYSTEM

1. GLIOMAS

Derived from astrocytes, these are the commonest primary neurological tumours. They vary in growth rate and differentiation over a wide spectrum.

Astrocytoma, at the benign end, is slow growing and the cells well differentiated forming many fibres.

The tumour which has ill-defined margins grows irregularly into the surrounding brain tissues and only latterly causes increased ICP

Note enlargement of hemisphere by ill defined growth.

Glioblastoma multiforme, in contrast, is highly malignant. The cells are pleomorphic, unlike astrocytes, rapidly growing and showing poor fibre formation.

Tumour looks well defined, contrasting with the compressed adjacent cerebral tissue

Necrosis and haemorrhage are common

Tumours derived from oligodendroglia and ependyma occur rarely.

Note: Since none of these tumours ever metastasise outside the nervous system, the terms 'benign' and 'malignant' are relative. Tumours are malignant in respect of their rapid growth and progress to death. Because they often have ill-defined margins, 'benign' tumours are difficult to eradicate and slowly but inexorably they grow and eventually cause death.

2. TUMOURS of NEURONE TYPE CELLS

Fully differentiated neurones can neither multiply nor give rise to neoplasms. Tumours of this type, derived from primitive nerve cell precursors (blast cells), are seen in infancy and childhood before completion of differentiation.

TUMOURS OF THE NERVOUS SYSTEM

TUMOURS OF NEURONE TYPE CELLS (continued)

They display a basic histological pattern.

Closely aggregated small cells with hyperchromatic round or oval nuclei and scanty cytoplasm

Rosettes, the centres of which are formed by rudimentary nerve fibres, are often seen and represent a step towards differentiation

Depending on the site of origin, specific names are given:

Cerebellum:
MEDULLOBLASTOMA

Retina:
RETINOBLASTOMA

Sympathetic ganglia (including adrenal medulla):
NEUROBLASTOMA and GANGLIONEUROMA

Medulloblastoma

This highly malignant tumour arises in and spreads over the surface of the cerebellum, often invading the IVth ventricle. Diffuse tumour nodules may develop on surfaces bathed by CSF.

Retinoblastoma

These tumours which arise in the retina and cause blindness spread into the optic nerves. They often have a hereditary basis (autosomal dominant with variable penetrance).

Neuroblastoma

These are not tumours of the CNS but are derived from the precursor cells of the autonomic system; the majority occur in the adrenal medulla. They grow rapidly to become large, soft, haemorrhagic and necrotic retroperitoneal masses soon metastasising to lymph nodes, liver and bones (esp. skull).

Ganglioneuroma

In some cases, neuronal differentiation proceeds, and mature ganglion cells appear and nerve fibres are formed. In some instances, differentiation is complete; such tumours are found in adult life particularly in the mediastinum where they may grow slowly, eventually causing signs due to their size, but never metastasising. Poorly differentiated forms are termed ganglioblastoma, while with intermediate degrees of differentiation the name ganglioneuroblastoma is used.

   The chemical neurotransmitters noradrenaline and dopamine, which are secreted in varying amounts by these tumours, are useful diagnostic markers as are their urinary degradation products, including vanillyl mandelic acid (VMA) and homovanillic acid respectively.

TUMOURS OF THE NERVOUS SYSTEM

Meningiomas

These are thought to arise from arachnoid granulations and so are found most commonly adjacent to venous sinuses. They are slow growing and essentially 'benign'.

A smooth firm lobulated tumour arising from a broad base adjacent to the sagittal sinus

The effects are due to local compression of nervous tissues.

The skull may be eroded.

Growth to large size is usually slow so that the compensating mechanisms prevent increased intracranial pressure.

The histological appearances are variable depending on the relative amount of cells and collagen, and they mimic in varying degree the arachnoid granulations.

Normal arachnoid granulation projecting into lumen

Venous sinus

Sinus wall

Arachnoid membrane

Whorls of fibrous tissue and spindle cells

Calcified psammoma bodies

Other mesodermol tumours

True vascular neoplasms are rare, but vascular HAMARTOMAS are fairly common and are a cause of intracranial haemorrhage and epilepsy. These lesions show great variation in site, size and complexity.

Occasionally such tumours as lipomas and osteomas cause compression effects.

Primary microglial and lymphoid tumours are rare; the latter may be intrinsic to the CNS or be metastatic from a primary tumour outside the CNS.

The incidence of CNS lymphomas is apparently increasing. This may be due to better diagnosis and/or to the more common use of therapeutic immunosuppression.

TUMOURS OF THE NERVOUS SYSTEM

The fairly common vascular hamartomas and the several developmental defects involving closure of the skull, spinal arches and meninges have already been mentioned.

Small vestigial foci of misplaced epithelial cells are not uncommon around the skull base, particularly in relation to the pituitary. Rarely these give rise to slowly enlarging cysts or tumours which cause compression effects.

Suprasellar cyst

Solid craniopharyngioma

Compression of pituitary and optic nerves

Sella turcica

Teratoma of pineal

Dermoid cyst containing hairs and desquamated debris.

TUMOURS OF PERIPHERAL NERVES

These are essentially collagenous tumours arising in nerve roots within the skull and spine, or in the peripheral nerves. Nomenclature is based on the tissue of origin.

Neurofibroma
Derived from epi-and endoneurium

Schwannoma
Derived from Schwann cells intimately surrounding axons.

Whorls and fascicles of fine collagen fibres; nerve fibres can be found

Note nuclear pallisading in addition to whorls and fascicles of collagen

Note: 1. In many cases, histological distinctions are blurred and are not of importance in diagnostic histology.
2. Since neurones do not give rise to neoplasm, the term neuroma is not used. Traumatic neuroma indicates proliferating nerve endings following injury and is not a true neoplasm (see p.87).

Nerve sheath tumours may be single or multiple; their effects are due to compression of adjacent nervous tissue and are seen best within the skull or spinal cord.

TUMOURS OF PERIPHERAL NERVES

Single tumours

Accoustic Schwannoma is good example of the single type.

This tumour arises from the VIIIth nerve in the cerebellopontine angle. Although this tumour is 'benign', it grows around adjacent structures and has an irregular surface so that it may be difficult to remove.

The tumour exerts its effects by compression — distortion of the VIIIth nerve (tinnitus → deafness) and adjacent nerves. Pressure on IVth ventricle → hydrocephalus → increased intracranial pressure.

VIIIth nerve

Multiple tumours

These may affect peripheral nerves over a wide area or occupy a single group of nerves. They either form rounded nodules or fusiform swellings and may be cosmetically disfiguring.

These conditions occupy the borderland between neoplasms and hamartomas; very occasionally true neoplasia is superimposed with the development of neurofibrosarcoma.

In **Von Recklinghausen's disease** (neurofibromatosis), small nodules which may be very numerous form particularly in subcutaneous nerves.

In **plexiform neurofibroma,** the proliferation slowly proceeds along a group of nerves forming complex thickenings. Growth within the spinal canal causes serious complications.

Pigmentation

The presence of melanin in some of these tumours and the occurrence of skin pigmentation (café au lait spots) in some cases of Von Recklinghausen's disease is a reminder of the common neuroectodermal origin of nerve sheath cells and melanocytes.

SECONDARY TUMOURS

In the general population the incidence of metastatic cerebral tumour is higher than that of primary cerebral neoplasm. The two most common primary sites are lung and breast, but any malignant tumour can metastasise to the brain.

The common presentation is in the form of multiple, well-delineated spherical nodules, randomly distributed

Only occasionally is there a single nodule.

A less common distribution is by permeation of the subarachnoid space — **meningeal carcinomatosis**.

Brain surface covered by a layer of tumour tissue - - - - - - →

Carcinoma, leukaemia and lymphoreticular neoplasms may spread in this way (malignant cells may be seen in the CSF).

Secondary tumours may cause serious spinal damage by destroying the integrity of the vertebrae. The prostate and cervix, in addition to lung, breast and kidney, are usual primary sites.

In contrast to tumours causing neurological damage by their physical presence and growth, less commonly *non-metastatic effects of cancer* are seen.

The tumours cover a wide range of disorders which are conveniently divided into two groups:

1. Neurological disorders in which the mechanism and association with cancer are known:

Examples	**Mechanism caused by cancer**
Opportunistic infections ———————	Immune depression
Metabolic and hormonal imbalance	Destruction of organs, e.g. liver, kidney Inappropriate secretion
Vascular accidents ———————	Coagulation disorders

2. A group of conditions in which the mechanism is not known. This includes dementia, encephalopathy, cerebellar degeneration, neuropathies and a syndrome mimicking myasthenia gravis.

HEADACHE

The symptom of headache can be caused by a wide variety of pathological conditions of which only a minority are intracranial.

Intracranial	Extracranial

Intracranial

Only certain tissues are 'pain sensitive' — particularly to stretching.

Dural sinuses and emissary veins

Arteries and dura at skull base

Painful impulses are conveyed by cranial nerves
V
Above ——— Tentorium——
Below
VII
IX
X
and C1, 2, 3

Extracranial

All tissues are pain sensitive and pain referred to the head via these nerves is very common.

Pathological conditions
in distribution of these nerves.

1. Any inflammatory disease, e.g. sinuses, teeth, ears, eyes.

2. Prolonged muscle contraction — particularly back of neck and jaws.

Pathological conditions

1. Conditions distorting and stretching pain sensitive areas, e.g. brain tumour.
2. Conditions associated with arterial dilatation, e.g. in fevers, intoxications, ? hypertension.
3. Meningeal inflammation and haemorrhage.

3. Vascular distension, e.g. migraine — the extracranial arteries in the neck and head show episodic constriction followed by dilatation due to an as yet unknown mechanism.

COMA

Coma is a clinical state in which there is loss of consciousness and unresponsiveness to stimuli. Various pathological conditions have been seen to proceed to coma.

Basic mechanisms

Consciousness depends on the integrity of the interplay between the cortex and brain stem nuclei on both sides.

Cortex

Brain stem nuclei (particularly reticular nuclei)

Pathological conditions:

which destroy these connections:

(1) **Supratentorial lesions**
   e.g. large haemorrhage, tumours.

(2) **Subtentorial lesions**
   e.g. haemorrhage, infarct, tumour, abscess.

(3) **Metabolic and diffuse lesions** e.g. anoxia, hypoglycaemia, drugs, posions, meningitis, concussion.

EPILEPSY

Organic brain disease is a significant factor in only a proportion of epilepsies which are essentially disorders of cerebral function associated with recurrent episodic excessive and abnormal neuronal discharges. The classical signs of generalised convulsions and loss of consciousness are not seen in all epilepsies.

Note: The common single seizures associated with febrile illnesses in children are not epilepsy, although the basic mechanism is similar.

Incidence: Epilepsy occurs in about 1% of the population.

Mechanism

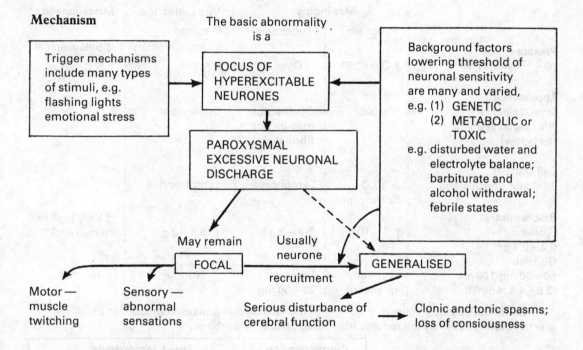

The neurones of the motor cortex, limbic system and the temporal lobe are particularly epileptogenic.

Aetiology

Acquired epilepsy. About 25% of cases are associated with known disease. The hyperexcitable neuronal focus may be due to established brain disease of which congenital abnormalities, post-traumatic scarring and ischaemic change are the most common.

Idiopathic epilepsy. In the remaining 75% of cases, although there is no known cause, genetic influences are important. A hyperexcitable focus is often present deep in the brain substance associated with the reticular system.

CEREBROSPINAL FLUID

Although the CSF and extracellular fluid of the central nervous system are essentially similar in composition, changes in the CSF are not reliable indicators of disease within the brain parenchyma.

However, since the CSF reflects conditions in the subarachnoid space, in clinical practice detailed examination and analysis are important and are mandatory in suspected meningitis. The important observations using CSF obtained by lumbar puncture are grouped under headings as follows.

NORMAL	IN DISEASE			
	Meningitis		Virus infection	Miscellaneous
	Pyogenic	*Tuberculous*	Meningo-*encephalitis*	
Pressure 60 – 180 mm H$_2$0	↑ Over 200	↑ Over 200	↑	↓ Below spinal block
Appearance Crystal clear *(for blood staining see below)	Turbid	Opalescent: may be fine fibrin web	Opalescent	–
Cell content 0 – 4 mononuclears/μl	+ + + > 1000 Polymorphs	+ + + Lymphocytes	± + Lymphocytes	–
Biochemistry Protein 0.2 – 0.4 g/l	↑ 1 – 10 g/l	↑ 1 – 3 g/l	↑ 0.5 – 2 g/l	↑ Very high in spinal block
Glucose 50 – 80 mg/100 ml (2.8 – 4.4 mmol/l)	↓ greatly or absent	Low 20 – 30 mg	Normal	Normal

* When the CSF is blood-stained, it is important to distinguish between contamination due to trauma caused by the tap and true intracranial haemorrhage.

	Contamination	True haemorrhage
Supernatant after centrifugation	Clear	Yellow due to bilirubin (red cell degeneration)
Cell count — leucocyte/RBC ratio	Normal	Increased

Microbiology. Identification of organisms is very important.

(1) Deposit and/or fibrin web — stained ⟨ Gram — pyogenic bacteria and fungi
ZN — tubercle bacilli

(2) Culture: virus isolation

(3) Tests for microbial antigens ⟨ Wassermann reaction for syphilis
Immunoelectrophoresis for other antigens

CHAPTER 15

MUSCULO-SKELETAL SYSTEM

SKELETAL MUSCLE

It is useful to consider the anatomy at various levels of magnification.

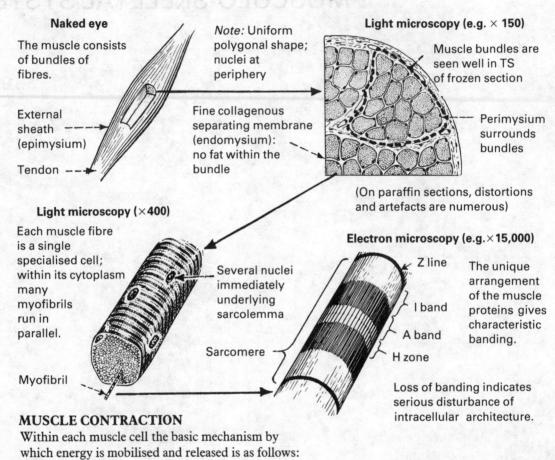

Naked eye

The muscle consists of bundles of fibres.

External sheath (epimysium)

Tendon

Note: Uniform polygonal shape; nuclei at periphery

Fine collagenous separating membrane (endomysium): no fat within the bundle

Light microscopy (e.g. × 150)

Muscle bundles are seen well in TS of frozen section

Perimysium surrounds bundles

(On paraffin sections, distortions and artefacts are numerous)

Light microscopy (×400)

Each muscle fibre is a single specialised cell; within its cytoplasm many myofibrils run in parallel.

Several nuclei immediately underlying sarcolemma

Sarcomere

Myofibril

Electron microscopy (e.g. ×15,000)

Z line

I band

A band

H zone

The unique arrangement of the muscle proteins gives characteristic banding.

Loss of banding indicates serious disturbance of intracellular architecture.

MUSCLE CONTRACTION

Within each muscle cell the basic mechanism by which energy is mobilised and released is as follows:

In mitochondrion

Glucose
Amino acids + O_2
Fat

ATP

ADP + P + ENERGY

Complex enzyme systems including particularly creatine kinase (CK) and aldolase (ALS)

At myofibril

Contraction

SKELETAL MUSCLE

The existence of two types of muscle fibre is related to differences in functional activity.

	Mito-chondria	Oxidative enzymes	ATPase	Myoglobin and lipid	Glycogen	Type of contraction
Type I (red muscle)	+++	+++	+	+++	+	SLOW Sustained
Type II (white muscle)	+	+	+++	+	+++	FAST short duration

In sections, the two fibre types, which are indistinguishable by routine stains, can be identified using histochemical methods.

Normal muscle stained H & E

Normal muscle — stained for oxidative enzyme

Type I fibres stain black

Note: random mosaic of two types.

It is of interest that the muscle fibre function is not intrinsic but is conditioned by its type of nerve supply: any single anterior horn cell innervates fibres only of one or other type.

MUSCLE INNERVATION

The **motor unit** consists of:
a single lower motor neurone and **LMN**

the muscle fibres it supplies.

Disease in any part of the LMN leads to **atrophy** of the fibres supplied.

Muscle fibres — a few to hundreds

Thinner. Shorter. Nuclei more crowded. Round cross-section.

Anterior horn cell

Nerve root

Peripheral nerve

Normal fibre

Atrophic fibre

NB: striations retained

781

DEGENERATION ATROPHY

The distribution of nerve fibres within the muscle is important and is represented diagrammatically in respect of two motor units: A and B.

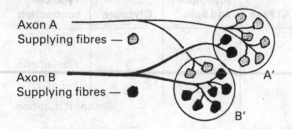

Axon A
Supplying fibres —

Axon B
Supplying fibres —

A'

B'

Note that while A and B respectively innervate the majority of fibres in bundles A' and B', there is overlap between bundles. Since many axons supply a muscle the overlap is considerable

Apart from complete traumatic section of a peripheral nerve, it is unusual for all motor fibres to a muscle to be destroyed. Both the basic pattern of innervation and the variations in nerve fibre damage are reflected in the histological appearances in the denervated muscle.

1. Pattern of atrophy

Groups of atrophic denervated fibres with adjacent groups of normal fibres.

Note the overlap — atrophic fibres among normal, and vice versa.

This is the striking basic pattern seen in most diseases of the LMN.

2. Re-innervation

In an area of denervation, the terminal axonal branches of intact neurones sprout and can re-innervate the atrophic fibres.

(i) Normal

A

B

This muscle bundle is predominantly innervated by axon A, but axon B is also represented

(ii) Denervation of A

A

B

Fibres supplied by A atrophy

Fibres supplied by B remain normal.

(iii) Re-innervation

(a)   (b)

B   B

Terminal filaments sprout and make contact with atrophic fibres.

(iv) Restoration of fibre size

B

Fibres restored to normal —
terminal filaments of B now innervate several fibres.

DEGENERATION ATROPHY

3. Change in muscle type

Since the type (fast or slow) of each muscle fibre is conditioned by its nerve supply, the pattern of distribution of fast and slow fibres within a muscle may be changed by re-innervation.

Normal mosaic pattern of slow (black) and fast (white) fibres

Following re-innervation by a 'slow' type neurone 'slow' fibres now predominate
Mosaic pattern is lost

Thus, although a muscle may be restored to normal in terms of routine histological assessment, slight changes in functional activity may be present.

MUSCLE SPINDLES AND INNERVATION

The crude muscle contraction effected by the motor unit is controlled and refined by neurological connections through the muscle spindles which are situated in the middle of the muscle. Each spindle consists of a delicate, cigar-shaped envelope containing 2 – 15 specialised muscle cells

which are intimately connected to a complex of motor and sensory nerve filaments.

The spindles are connected to the cord by a special nervous circuit; the diagram shows how the cerebellum influences function of the LMN via the muscle spindle.

Because the muscle spindles have a separate innervation in motor neurone disease they may be spared.

Note: surviving normal spindles. There is a spurious impression of increased number owing to the severe atrophy of the surrounding muscle fibres.

POST. ROOT NEURONE

MOTOR CORTEX

CEREBELLUM

α-motor neurone
— large cell in ant. horn (LMN)

γ-motor neurone
— small cell in anterior horn

MUSCLE FIBRES

γ-efferent fibres

Afferent fibre

MUSCLE SPINDLE
CONTRACTION ← EXCITATION

783

MYASTHENIA GRAVIS

The **MOTOR END-PLATE** is the specialised neuromuscular junction situated at the middle of each muscle fibre.

The nervous impulse causes release of **ACETYLCHOLINE** at the specialised nerve endings — depolarisation at this site is the stimulus to contraction. The sarcolemma at this site contains abundant **CHOLINESTERASE**.

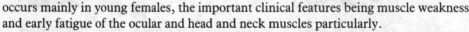

In MYASTHENIA GRAVIS, the essential disorder is at the motor end-plate where there is a defect in the production or release of acetylcholine. This rare disease occurs mainly in young females, the important clinical features being muscle weakness and early fatigue of the ocular and head and neck muscles particularly.

Aetiology and mechanism

There is strong evidence that autoimmunity is the basic abnormality (see p.117).

1. Antibodies to various muscle constituents, including motor end-plate components are found in many cases.
2. In 90% of cases there are THYMIC abnormalities, including **THYMOMA** in 15% and thymic germinal centre hyperplasia in the remainder.
3. There is an association with hyperthyroidism (this has an autoimmune basis).

In the affected muscles, aggregates of lymphocytes with occasional single necrotic fibres may be seen.

ATROPHY AND HYPERTROPHY

Generalised disuse atrophy occurs as a result of prolonged immobilisation in bed. Local atrophy follows immobilisation due to joint disease or often bone fractures.

Hypertrophy of muscle tissue in response to increased work load is well seen in heavy event athletes. Localised hypertrophy can compensate for damage to adjacent muscular tissues.

Normal

Smaller fibres

Fat

Fewer fibrils

Larger fibres (same number)

More numerous fibrils

Note: Atrophy may be partially masked by increased fat in the septal tissues.

MUSCLE DAMAGE

Having dealt with the effects on muscle of denervation and of motor end-plate disorder, muscle disease will be dealt with further under two main headings:

1. Muscle damage which is clearly secondary
2. Disorders in which the abnormality is in the muscle fibres — the myopathies.

1. DISORDERS SECONDARY to TRAUMA, ISCHAEMIA and INFLAMMATION and INFECTION

(a) Trauma and ischaemia

In severe cases where trauma and ischaemia combine to cause necrosis of a considerable mass of muscle, the effects may be serious.

The latter situation is well exemplified in the CRUSH SYNDROME — classically seen in building collapse.

Repair of massive muscle damage

The basic inflammatory response is followed by organisation with removal of the dead muscle. There are two possible results:

(i) If the gap is not too great, regeneration effects restoration to normal.

(ii) If the gap is too great, scar tissue prevents the regeneration.

Occasionally contracture of the scar tissue near joints causes deformity and sometimes, particularly in young subjects, metaplastic bone forms in the granulation tissue — so-called MYOSITIS OSSIFICANS.

785

MUSCLE DAMAGE

SECONDARY MUSCLE DISORDERS (continued)

(b) Inflammation

In most inflammatory processes, including the common pyogenic infections, the intermuscular fascial planes are involved and muscle damage is negligible and superficial, consisting of degeneration and necrosis of individual fibres.

Abscess formation may follow intramuscular injections.

Viral myositis:

A true myositis with focal necrosis of fibres, lymphocyte and macrophage infiltration can be caused by the *Coxsackie group* of viruses. The muscles of the upper thorax are particularly affected.

Parasitic myositis

In trichinosis, the parasitic larvae encyst in the interstitial tissues within muscles. The adjacent muscle fibres become necrotic; focal calcification is often a late sequel.

Repair of focal muscle damage

In cases of mild trauma and inflammation where there is only focal muscle fibre damage, and particularly when the endomysium remains intact, complete restoration to normal is effected by muscle cell regeneration.

2. THE MYOPATHIES

In this broad group of disorders, the abnormalities, which are essentially disturbances of muscle metabolism, are within the muscle fibres and are reflected in a limited, non-specific range of morphological changes.

Normal — Fibres

Myopathy
- Fibre thinner and rounded
- Splitting
- Cytoplasm homogeneous and eosinophilic
- Flocculation and vacuolation
- Nucleus often centrally placed

Loss of striations

MYOPATHIES

Normal

No fat

Endomysium very thin

MYOPATHIES

Endomysium thickened

Fat cells

Macrophages invading the endomysium of a necrotic fibre

In some disorders, the fat may mask the muscle atrophy and there may even be pseudohypertrophy.

Note: Inflammation is not a feature of most myopathies: there may be a mild inflammatory response to actual muscle necrosis.

A case of **Duchenne dystrophy:**
Prominent winging of scapulae and scoliosis due to muscle weakness
Pseudohypertrophy of calves due to fatty infiltration

In some disorders, occasional muscle fibres show hypertrophy alongside atrophic fibres, and regenerating fibres may also be seen. Since these basic changes vary in their incidence within muscles and in their rate of progress, a cross-section of affected muscle need not be expected to show them all at one time.

Biopsy of:

Moderately affected muscle

A group of normal fibres

Fat cells

Neuromuscle spindle

Fibres showing various degrees of atrophy

Late stage muscle

Almost complete replacement of muscle by fat; only a few atrophic fibres remain.

787

INHERITED MYOPATHIES

The myopathies will be considered further under two main headings:
The abnormality is (1) GENERALLY determined, or (2) ACQUIRED.

1. The INHERITED MYOPATHIES

Muscular dystrophies

In this group, the nature of the abnormality within the fibre is unknown. Various disorders are separated and identified by their particular type of inheritance, clinical differences including age of onset, rate of progression and particular groups of muscle affected.
    Three dystrophies are described:

1. **The Duchenne type** (pseudohypertrophic muscular dystrophy)
Inheritance — X-linked recessive. Affects boys exclusively (apart from a few cases recorded in Turner's syndrome).
    The muscle changes are present *in utero,* but usually the first clinical disability presenting as lower limb weakness appears in childhood; progress is relentless with involvement later of the shoulder muscles. Death often occurs in the teens due to bronchopneumonia or cardiac failure.
    The pathological mechanism includes lack of the protein, **dystrophin,** which is normally present at neuromuscular junctions.

2. *Facioscapulohumeral dystrophy*
Inheritance — autosomal dominant. Affects both male and female.
Age of onset variable — if in childhood, progress is often fairly rapid.
                        — if in adult life, progress may be very slow.
    Muscle changes begin in facial and shoulder muscles and are often assymetrial; lower limb muscles may be affected late in the disease.

3. The myotonic disorders in which voluntary muscle movement, particularly in the cold, is slower to initiate and lasts longer than normal, is exemplified by:

Myotonic dystrophy

Inheritance — autosomal dominant. Affects both male and female. Age of onset — usually in adult life.
    The facial and tongue muscles are affected first, followed by the distal limb muscles; progress is slow but inexorable.
    This dystrophy is usually associated with abnormalities in other systems, e.g. gonadal atrophy, cataracts, cardiac conduction defects, defective androgen production or abnormal insulin response may be present.
    The disease shows genetic linkage with the secretor ABH system so that its diagnosis *in utero* can be inferred from genotyping using the presence of ABH antigen in amniotic fluid.

INHERITED MYOPATHIES

The inherited myopathies (continued)

Specific metabolic defects

An enlarging group of genetic myopathies with specific biochemical or morphological abnormalities is emerging due to the application of modern biochemical, histochemical and morphological (e.g. EM) techniques.

In some, the specific inborn error of metabolism is generalised and includes muscle; in others it is confined to the muscle fibre. Some examples will be given under broad headings:

(1) **Glycogen storage**	(2) **Lipid metabolism**	(3) **Periodic paralyses**
Type 2 — deficiency of (Pompe) acid maltase Type 5 — muscle (McArdle) phosphorylase Type 7 — phosphofructo-kinase (PEK)	Defect in free fatty acid transport into and utilisation within fibre. (a) carnitine palmityl transferase (CPT) (b) and muscle carnitine deficiency	Associated with hypo- and hyperkalaemia — defect in muscle cell not yet known

(4) Morphological abnormalities
  (a) *Mitochondrial*   (b) *Others*

(a)	(b)	

Large or increased numbers of mitochondria — abnormal oxidative processes	(i) Central core myopathy
	  Central area is abnormal
	
	(ii) Rod body myopathy
	  (nemaline) Rods of tropomysin under sarcolemma
		(iii) Centronuclear myopathy
		  Nucleus in middle of cell
		
		(iv) Disproportion of fibre types I and II

These various myopathies exhibit a wide range in respect of age of onset, clinical presentation and prognosis.

A further rare but interesting genetic abnormality of muscle of unknown aetiology is malignant hyperpyrexia. In this condition the administration of general anaesthetic precipitates acute muscle damage. Clinically, there is very high fever, muscle stiffness, cyanosis and acidosis very often resulting in death.

789

ACQUIRED MYOPATHIES

2. The ACQUIRED MYOPATHIES

Cachectic myopathy

In any wasting disease, loss of muscle with weakness is seen.

Primary condition

| Chronic infection
Malabsorption
Cancer
Endocrine disorder
Extreme old age | → Generalised
CATABOLISM
↓
The protein of muscle
is particularly affected → | Loss of muscle bulk;
fibres smaller with
nuclei closer together;
muscle fibre loss —
predominantly type II. |

Endocrine, toxic and nutritional myopathies

(a) Myopathy is seen in acromegaly, hyperthyroidism, hypothyroidism, hyperaldosteronism (due to hypokalaemia), hyperparathyroidism and in corticosteroid excess. (b) In alcohol and a variety of drugs in addition to corticosteroids, e.g. chloroquine, vincristine; and in vitamin D deficiency.

Polymyositis

This important condition links the myopathies with the inflammatory disorders of muscle. There is very strong evidence that it is an *autoimmune* disorder in which lymphocytes sensitised to muscle constituents cause destruction of muscle fibres, mimicking myopathy.

The onset is in middle life with a preponderance in women. Progress is variable; deterioration may be rapid or very slow, remissions are not uncommon and recovery is possible.

In a proportion of cases when the disorder also affects the skin, the term **dermatomyositis** is applied.

Aetiology

In 2/3 cases, the disorder is 'idiopathic', in 1/3 cases there is an associated
disease which falls into one of two main groups:
1. *Cancer* — the tumour may be clinically latent at
   the time of the presentation of the myositis.
2. *Generalised collagen or vascular disease* e.g.
   systemic lupus erythematosis, polyarteritis,
   rheumatoid arthritis.

Pathology

A mixture of chronic inflammatory
infiltrate and muscle fibre damage
ranging from necrosis to atrophy.

MYOPATHY DIAGNOSIS

In clinical practice, although in only a few conditions is curative therapy available, accurate diagnosis of cases of muscular weakness and atrophy is important since there is considerable variation in prognosis and management of these diverse disorders.

A diagnosis is usually reached from a synthesis of the information obtained from investigations under three main headings:

1. **General clinical considerations are fundamental.** Of particular importance are *family history, age of onset, distribution of muscle weakness* and *rate of progress.* To these are added clinical neurological assessment.

2. **Special investigation of neuromuscular electrical activity.** The rate of motor and sensory nerve conduction can be measured electrically.

   The ELECTROMYOGRAM records the activity of groups of muscle fibres and even of individual fibres (usually fine needle electrodes). The broad basic pathological changes already described are reflected in variations of the electrical potential within the muscle during various types of activity.

   These methods are particularly useful in distinguishing primary myopathies, including myotonias, from denervation atrophy.

3. **Laboratory tests**
   (a) *MUSCLE BIOPSY.* The motor unit area of a moderately weak muscle is chosen (end-stage muscle) should not be taken). Special precautions must be taken to minimise artefacts. Routine histological examination will usually distinguish the broad groups of disorders and identify the occasional rare myopathy with specific morphological features.

   Histochemical and EM examination and biochemical analysis may identify specific disorders.

   (b) *SERUM ENZYMES.* In the myopathies where actual muscle fibre destruction is proceeding, increased levels of creatine kinase (CK) and aldolase (ALS) are found.

791

POST-VIRAL FATIGUE SYNDROME

This syndrome has recently come to prominence due to an increased prevalence, both in sporadic cases and in small epidemics. For many years, post-viral depression (e.g. after influenza) and fatigue (e.g. after glandular fever) have been recognised and are self-limiting usually after only a few weeks; the pathological mechanisms remain obscure.

The syndrome now so prevalent is associated particularly with **enterovirus infection** (e.g. Cocksaxic viruses) and there may be severe functional deficits which are often long-lasting (years). Alternative names for the syndrome are **myalgic encephalomyelitis (ME)** or **chronic fatigue syndrome** (U.S.A.).

The clinical signs and symptoms are protean, but the major complaint is extreme fatigue after minimal exercise. For many years the condition was considered to be psychologically induced and was labelled a form of hysteria.

It is now clear that there is a firm organic basis, but the mechanisms are not yet established with certainty.

The flow diagram illustrates possible mechanisms:

BONE

A bone shows two gross anatomical forms in varying proportions, depending on the particular type of supportive function required of it.

1. COMPACT BONE,

seen well in long bone shaft, contributes rigidity and forms the dense outer shell (cortex).

The basic units of compact bone are Haversian systems (osteons) arranged in vertical columns.

Periosteum

Thin layers of cancellous trabeculae

Cement lines between osteons

Medullary cavity

T.S.

2. CANCELLOUS BONE

(along with marrow) occupies the medullary cavities. This arrangement as exemplified in a vertebral body contributes some compressibility and pliability.

The basic unit of cancellous bone is the trabecula, arranged less regularly but not randomly.

In both types of bone, there is a basic **lamellar** structure.

A single Haversian system showing central canal with capillaries, concentric laminae and osteocytes in lacunae.

A single trabecula showing:

Capillaries in marrow tissue

parallel lamellae, osteocytes in lacunae;

occasional osteoblasts on surface.

Bone GROWTH

In **endochondrial ossification,** seen at the metaphyseal ends of long bones, the cartilage dies and is invaded by osteoblasts which lay down bone to replace it.

In **membranous ossification,** seen in certain flat bones, the osteoblasts appear in an immature connective tissue matrix.

In pathological processes where new bone is formed, both methods of deposition are encountered.

BONE

Bone DEPOSITION

Rows of plump osteoblasts laying down lamellar collagen matrix. They are incorporated into the bone and housed in small lacunae as *osteocytes*.

Haversian system

Note the newly formed non-calcified *osteoid* in the centre of the osteon and on the surface of the trabecula. Normally calcification very quickly follows.

Note: During osteoblastic activity, **alkaline phosphatase** is liberated into the local tissue fluids and thence to the blood. In bone disorders, a raised serum alkaline phosphatase indicates increased osteoblastic activity.

Bone RESORPTION

Osteoclasts — multinucleated phagocytes removing bone. The indentations formed are called Howslip's lacunae.

Note that all the constituents of the bone including calcium are removed. This process is called **OSTEOCLASIS.**

The *osteocytes* lying in the bone lacunae have long branching processes which permeate fine channels in the bone. Their function is to control and maintain the integrity of the bone matrix, including the crystalline calcium content. One activity is to release calcium into the blood without disruption of the matrix. This process is called **OSTEOLYSIS.**

In **bone NECROSIS** the osteocytes are dead and the lacunae empty. The integrity of the matrix cannot be maintained, and although the lamellar structure may be seen for a considerable time, the staining properties of living bone are lost.

BONE

WOVEN BONE (non-lamellar), a primitive form laid down in fetal development.

Irregular trabeculae in primitive matrix — — — — —

Osteoblasts

Interwoven collagen

In adult life, this type is seen in bone regeneration and tumours. It may be later replaced by lamellar bone.

BONE and CALCIUM

(a) Calcification of bone

Exactly how precipitation of calcium phosphate occurs in osteoid is not known.

In a solution containing Ca^{++} and PO_4 , when the product of Ca^{++} and PO_4 exceeds a critical level, precipitation occurs. Where plasma calcium is low, usually due to inadequate absorption, bone calcification is defective and the diseases rickets and osteomalacia result (see p.821).

(b) Bone and calcium haemostasis

The bony skeleton acts as a reservoir for calcium and responds to the need to maintain plasma levels within a fairly narrow range (9.2 – 10.4 mg/dl or 2.3 – 2.6 mmol/l — these figures are for total plasma calcium and are used in clinical practice). This response is controlled mainly by a direct action of parathormone on bone as shown below.

(i) Response to low blood calcium

Low blood Ca^{++}

Direct stimulation of parathyroids

Parathormone

Restoration of blood Ca^{++}

BONE — Direct action induces osteolysis and osteoclasis

Ca^{++}

In parathyroid hyperplasia or neoplasia, this process occurs in excess, causing hypercalcaemia and pathological bone resorption.

(ii) When the blood calcium is high, parathormone is not secreted and bone resorption is in abeyance.

Calcitonin antagonises the action of parathormone, but its role in health and disease has not yet been fully assessed.

795

OSTEOPOROSIS

OSTEOPOROSIS (bone atrophy) is defined as a reduction in the amount of bone tissue; the tissue remaining is normally calcified.

In *normal* bones the dynamic processes of deposition and resorption are in balance.

In *osteoporosis* the balance is upset by

(1) diminished deposition
(2) increased resorption
(3) both 1 and 2 together

This imbalance may be continuous with progressive loss of bone substance, or sometimes the balance is temporarily or permanently restored with arrest of the process.

The bone loss is most obvious in cancellous bone with rapid turnover, but the changes eventually are recognisable even in the cortical haversian systems.

The following changes in vertebral bodies are illustrative.

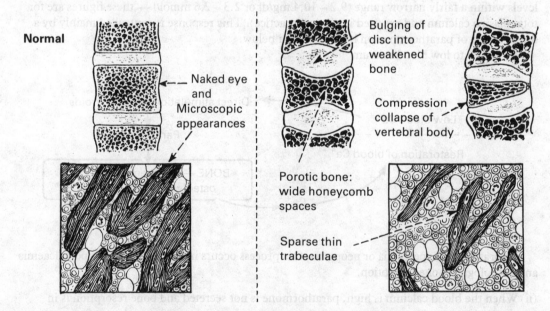

Normal

Naked eye and Microscopic appearances

Bulging of disc into weakened bone

Compression collapse of vertebral body

Porotic bone: wide honeycomb spaces

Sparse thin trabeculae

Note: The atrophied trabeculae have a normal calcium content, but because the total trabecular mass is reduced, the total bone calcium is also reduced.

OSTEOPOROSIS

Osteoporosis may be localised or general.

Localised osteoporosis is commonly due to disuse and is seen as a complication of other disorders, e.g. local IMMOBILISATION following fracture; limb paralysis and adjacent to severe joint disease with limitation of movement.

This process can be acute with active osteoclasis, but when function is resumed, normal bone structure is often restored.

General osteoporosis. Renal calculus is an important complication.

General IMMOBILISATION, particularly if prolonged, leads to —

Mechanism:

General $\rightarrow$ General $\rightarrow$ Ca^{++} mobilised $\rightarrow$ Hypercalcaemia $\rightarrow$ Hypercalcuria $\rightarrow$ Renal
immobilisation osteoporosis from bones calculus

IDIOPATHIC GENERALISED OSTEOPOROSIS

This is the most common disorder of bone. From middle age onwards there is progressive atrophy of bone with changes similar to those seen in osteoporosis, and some consider that generalised osteoporosis is an accelerated form of ageing atrophy. The dividing line between the conditions is ill-defined. Although the disease is generalised, weakness at particular sites leads to important complications:

1. Compression fracture (collapse) of vertebral bodies (usually preceded by gradual loss of height and kyphosis); often associated with sudden pain on weight lifting

2. Fracture of neck of femur or other long bones

3. In the elderly, during manual cardiac massage, fracture of the ribs or sternum may be sustained.

Note: In this type of osteoporosis, the routine serum biochemical tests — particularly the calcium levels — are within the normal range.

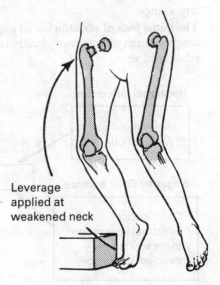

Leverage
applied at
weakened neck

797

OSTEOPOROSIS

Aetiology and mechanisms

Although the majority of cases are idiopathic, there are some pointers to indicate a multifactorial aetiology.

1. **Hormonal influences**
    (a) Incidence: female>male.
    Progressive after the menopause;
    rate of bone loss is greater in
    female than in male.
    (b) A severe type of osteoporosis is
    seen in Cushing's syndrome
    (glucocorticoid excess) and complicating
    prolonged steroid therapy.
    This suggests that the balance between anabolic steroids (androgens and oestrogens) and antianabolic steroids (cortisol, etc.) is important.
    (b) Other hormones have an influence — untreated thyrotoxicosis may be complicated by osteoporosis, and parathyroid function has already been dealt with.
    It is possible that disturbances of various hormones influence the cellular activities of bone and upset the balance of deposition and resorption.

2. **Calcium haemostasis**
    Although there is no evidence that calcium metabolism at the bone trabecular level is abnormal, over the years there is a net total calcium loss and it is suggested that a mildly deficient calcium absorption may contribute. In these circumstances, the action of parathormone assumes importance.

3. **The initial bulk of skeleton** has an important theoretical bearing on whether osteoporosis will be severe enough to cause complications in old age. The following diagram illustrates the possible relationships:

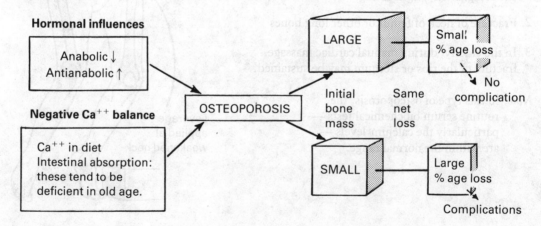

It is important in the treatment of osteoporosis that mobility and activity be maintained. The superimposed effects of disuse atrophy can be very serious.

OSTEOMALACIA AND RICKETS

Osteomalacia and rickets are disorders of bone in which the essential defect is failure of calcification in newly formed osteoid, caused by vitamin D deficiency.

Osteomalacia occurs in adult life and affects the osteoid which is being continually laid down in the normal remodelling bone.

Rickets affects the growing child, and serious additional disturbances are seen at the growing ends of long bones. Clinically there is pain, weakness of bones with a tendency to distortion and even fracture. Looser's zones, seen in X-ray, are linear partial fractures of long bones which have failed to calcify.

The mechanisms by which vitamin D deficiency prevents calcification are complex and not completely elucidated. The following simplified diagram indicates the important sites of activity.

Lack of vitamin D due to poor diet – no sunlight, – malabsorption D_2 D_3 → Via LIVER → KIDNEYS → Lack of active metabolite 1,25 dihydroxy-cholecalciferol (1,25 DHCC)

Disturbance of Ca and P balance in serum and extracellular fluid

(1) **Deficient** intestinal **absorption of Ca** (serum Ca not always low)
(2) and of P: also increased renal clearance of P **(serum P always LOW)**

Ca x P low

Action on newly deposited bone.

(1) **Osteoblasts** form defective matrix; osteoblasts often increased in number
(2) **Oateoclasts** prevented from responding to parathormone

Tends to increase renal production of 1,25 DHCC

Parathyroid hyperplasia

In some cases causes serious osteoclasis

Failure of calcification

Bone trabecula of *normal* size

Thick osteoid layer deposited by increased osteoblastic activity

Calcified bone stained black by Von Kossa's method

Serum alkaline phosphatase raised

Note:
1. In many cases the serum calcium may not be low.
2. Parathyroid activity may cause bone resorption.

OSTEOMALACIA AND RICKETS

In **rickets** there are important changes at the growing ends of long bones.

Normal **Rickets**

This results in stunting of growth and bowing of the lower limbs.
In female's permanent deformities of the pelvis can cause serious difficulty during childbirth

Regularly arranged columns of cartilage cells being replaced by columns of well calcified bone

Thickened irregular cartilage — poorly calcified, scanty bone formation

Since osteomalacia can be treated by vitamin D, it is important to distinguish it from osteoporosis: bone biopsy and biochemical tests are useful.

	Osteomalacia	Osteoporosis
Biopsy — appearance of trabeculae	Size — normal Thick uncalcified osteoid seams	Thin and small Normal calcification
Osteoblasts	Often increased	Normal numbers
Serum biochemistry Alkaline phosphatase	Raised	Normal
Phosphate	Low	Normal
Calcium	May be low	Normal

In cases of malabsorption occurring after middle age, in women particularly, osteomalacia and osteoporosis occur together.

Renal osteodystrophy (renal rickets)

In any renal disease associated with uraemia, abnormalities of bone occur. They are the result of abnormal calcium/phosphate balance, causing an osteomalacia-like disorder and secondary hyperparathyroidism causing osteoclasis. Additional factors may be failure of the diseased kidney to form 1,25 DHCC, the active metabolite of vitamin D, and urinary loss of phosphate due to tubular abnormalities.

BONE — MISCELLANEOUS

HYPERPARATHYROIDISM

In about 20% of cases of primary hyperparathyroidism, due either to adenoma or idiopathic hyperplasia, bone changes are marked (see also p.840).

The essential change is increased bone resorption due to greatly increased osteoclastic activity; usually osteoblastic activity is also increased but cannot cope with the resorption.

Numerous osteoclasts attacking trabeculae

Osteoblasts on opposite surface

Giant cells (osteoclasts) and spindle cells occupying the marrow tissues

These changes, although generalised, may be locally severe causing cystic spaces — the fully developed disorder is called **osteitis fibrosa cystica.** If haemorrhage occurs, giant cell tumour of bone may be mimicked.

The biochemical changes are (1) RAISED blood CALCIUM — due to mobilisation from bones and increased activity of 1,25 DHCC and (2) RAISED alkaline PHOSPHATASE due to increased osteoblast activity.

HYPERTROPHY OF BONE

In **acromegaly** the enlargement of the jaws, hands and feet is due to subperiosteal osteoblastic proliferation and the re-establishment of endochondrial bone formation under the influence of pituitary growth hormone.

Hypertrophic osteoarthropathy (including finger clubbing) affects the digits, distal ends of long bones and the distal joints.

Oedema and increase of vascular connective tissues under nail bed

Periosteal new bone formation

The mechanism is unknown, but the condition is associated with chronic lung disease, cyanotic heart disease and chronic intestinal inflammatory conditions.

Its importance is as an indicator of serious disease elsewhere, and it is of interest that if the primary disease can be cured, the osteoarthropathy may resolve.

BONE — MISCELLANEOUS

Fibrous dysplasia of bone

This disorder of unknown
aetiology may affect a single (monostotic)
or several bones (polyostotic). The lesion is a
well demarcated fibrous tissue containing small
abnormal bone trabeculae. The normal bone is
gradually replaced; small cysts may be present.
Complications
Fracture or deformity of the weakened bone.

Well
circumscribed
lesion — partly cystic

Beaked
trabeculae

Paget's disease of bone (Osteitis deformans)

This disease of unknown aetiology usually presents after the age of 50 years and affects males
predominantly. It is fairly common (3% of autopsies), but only in its more severe forms are there
clinical symptoms. The disorder is focal but tends to spread slowly but progressively. The bones
particularly affected are the pelvis, lower vertebrae, skull and lower limbs.

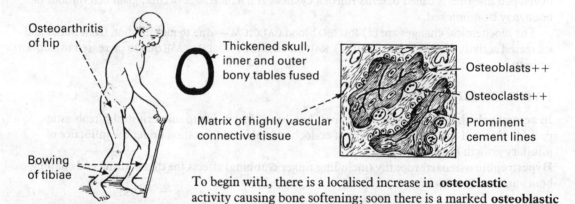

Osteoarthritis
of hip

Thickened skull,
inner and outer
bony tables fused

Matrix of highly vascular
connective tissue

Bowing
of tibiae

Osteoblasts++

Osteoclasts++

Prominent
cement lines

To begin with, there is a localised increase in **osteoclastic**
activity causing bone softening; soon there is a marked **osteoblastic**
reaction with bone resorption and deposition proceeding

chaotically, so that a mosaic of defective irregularly calcified bone trabeculae is
formed. The bone may be thickened, but its structure is defective and weak.
Biochemical changes reflect the cellular activity at trabecular level:
Alkaline phosphatase ↑ (osteoblastic); *urinary hydroxyproline* ↑ (collagen destruction).

The important **complications** are:

1. **Fracture** of weakened bones (including partial long bone fracture and vertebral compression).
2. **Osteoarthritis** of joints due to abnormal stresses caused by bony deformity.
3. An increased risk (×30) of the development of **bone sarcoma.**
4. The increased circulatory load through the vascular stroma may cause high output cardiac
   failure.

   Calcitonin, the physiological antagonist of parathormone, offers effective therapy in many
cases.

BONE — MISCELLANEOUS

Avascular bone necrosis

(a) The usual processes involved in fracture healing have been dealt with (p.88). Due to details of vascular anatomy at particular sites, fractures may be complicated by severance of the blood supply to one of the bone fragments. This results in a high incidence of **avascular (aseptic) bone necrosis.** Fractures of the femoral neck and scaphoid bone are good examples.

(b) In other cases of aseptic bone necrosis, trauma is not obviously an aetiological factor. In some, but not all of a miscellany of conditions, (which includes working at increased atmospheric pressure (Caisson disease), hyperlipidaemia, Gaucher's disease, gout, sickle cell anaemia and prolonged corticosteroid therapy), local ischaemia may be due to sludging of blood in end arteries to bone.

Bone necrosis of this type has important effects when it occurs at an articular surface: serious degenerative arthritis may ensue.

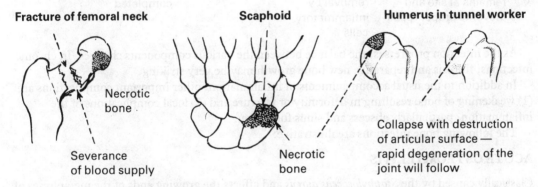

Fracture of femoral neck   **Scaphoid**   **Humerus in tunnel worker**

Necrotic bone

Severance of blood supply

Necrotic bone

Collapse with destruction of articular surface — rapid degeneration of the joint will follow

Note: These areas of necrotic bone may be relatively radiodense due to disuse osteoporosis of the adjacent living bone.

(c) In children and adolescents osteonecrosis occurs at several epiphyseal sites for no known cause (repeated minor trauma may be operative in some cases). The general name for this condition is osteochondritis juvenalis, and various eponymous terms are applied depending on the site affected. The commonest is Perthes' disease in which necrosis of one or both femoral heads occurs in children aged 4 – 10 years: (male : female =5:1)

Subperiosteal haematoma

In scurvy, the lack of vitamin C is the cause of abnormal collagen synthesis and there is a bleeding tendency due to capillary fragility.

In very young children, large haematomas may form under the periosteum in response to relatively minor trauma. The osteoblasts on the undersurface proceed to form irregular bone and considerable time is required for remodelling to occur. Similar haematomas with ossification may be seen on radiographs of the bones of 'battered babies'.

INFECTIONS OF BONE

The following basic pathological processes occur in all bone infections.

1. Destruction of bone due to necrosis. **2. Reactive and reparative processes.**

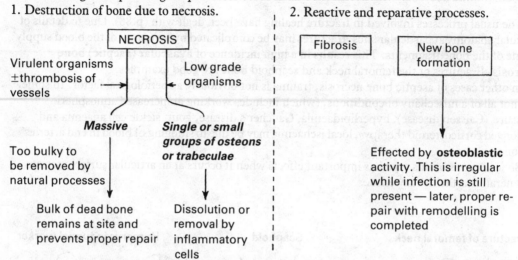

As the infection progresses, the balance between the various components changes. In chronic infections, fibrosis and reparative new bone growth may be very striking.

In addition to the usual accompaniments of inflammation, other important complications are: (1) weakening of bone resulting in deformity or fracture and (2) local complications of the inflammation, particularly abscess and sinus formation.

The following bone infections are illustrative:

ACUTE OSTEOMYELITIS

Classically caused by the *Staphylococcus aureus* and affects the growing ends of the metaphyses of long bones in children. Nowadays the incidence has been greatly reduced by the use of antibiotics. The organisms are blood borne and settle in the cancellous bone of the metaphysis. The effects are dramatic and rapidly progressive.

INFECTIONS OF BONE

Acute Osteomyelitis (continued)

Unless treatment is started promptly, the expanding inflammatory process within the rigid bone is seriously complicated.

New bone beginning to be laid down by raised periosteum

Extensive bone NECROSIS due to local toxicity and vascular thrombosis

Penetration into soft tissues and through skin

End result

Sequestrum of dead bone

Involucrum of new irregularly formed bone

Discharging sinus

The presence of necrotic bone ensures that the inflammation and sinus discharge continue. With large sequestra, the usual natural methods of removal of dead tissue are inadequate so that surgical treatment is necessary.

At a late chronic stage, in addition to the local disability and disturbance of bone growth, **AMYLOID** disease may supervene.

Other pyogenic bacteria can cause osteitis — the salmonella group (esp.*S.typhi*) and brucella, the latter often causing a low grade osteitis of the spine.

With inadequate antibiotic treatment, acute inflammatory processes may be converted into low grade osteitis. Staphylococcal infection of the spine may present in adults in this way.

TUBERCULOSIS

The incidence of bone and joint infection parallels the incidence of the more common pulmonary and intestinal infections. It is therefore very low in developed countries but still significant elsewhere.

The spine and growing ends of long bones including the epiphyses are commonly affected by blood borne spread and, because of the proximity of joints, tuberculous arthritis is a frequent concomitant.

The basic pathological process is destruction of bone and replacement with tuberculous granulation tissue. Caseous necrosis is common and tracking and spread into adjacent tissues, particularly in relation to spinal tuberculosis, leads to cold abscess formation.

Although the progress is much less rapid than in acute osteomyelitis, without adequate treatment serious damage to bones and joints occurs.

DEVELOPMENTAL ABNORMALITIES

Local abnormalities are fairly common and include cleft palate, spina bifida and many structural variations of limb development. In the majority the aetiology is uncertain: the presence of teratogens (e.g. thalidomide) is suspected in many and, in a few, genetic inheritance has been established.

Generalised abnormalities are rare and usually inherited.

1. **ACHONDROPLASIA** causes a particularly striking dwarfism.

Short, deformed limbs cause a waddling gait. The bones at the skull base are underdeveloped.

The basic abnormality is defective, irregular development of cartilage cells, particularly at the growing metaphyseal plate. This results in stunted long bones.

2. In **OSTEOGENESIS IMPERFECTA,** if there is survival beyond infancy, the thin brittle bones fracture easily and a history of multiple fractures with minimal cause is the usual presentation.

The basic defect is in the osteoblasts which fail to synthesise lamellar collagen properly.

A long bone showing three fractures.

Old, with deformity

More recent, with exuberant callus

Recent, with displacement

Associated conditions due to the same defect are:
(a) very thin sclerae which appear blue
(b) abnormal tooth development due to defective denture formation.

3. **OSTEOPETROSIS** (Marble bone disease of Albers-Schönberg) is a disorder in which failure of conversion of calcified cartilage to bone and failure of bone remodelling leads to increased density of the skeleton.

Complications are: (a) anaemia due to marrow replacement
       (b) fractures
       (c) cranial nerve compression.

CYSTIC LESIONS IN BONE

True, simple cysts in bone are rare. They have a well
defined collagenous capsule and occur in the proximal
humeral and femoral metaphyses in children. As they expand,
the risk of fracture increases and this is the most usual
presenting sign.

Contains
clear watery
fluid

Capsule

There is no
distortion
of bone
shape

In contrast, cyst-like spaces occur in many bone disorders
and even fairly solid non-calcified lesions may appear
cystic on radiological examination. Examples of such disorders
are cystic degeneration adjacent to osteoarthritic
joints, giant cell tumour of bone, aneurysmal bone cyst,
hyperparathyroidism, histiocytosis X, localised developmental
defects involving fibrous tissue or cartilage and, most
commonly, metastatic tumour in bone. Because of the very different prognostic
implications, in clinical practice accurate histological diagnosis is essential.

Eosinophilic granuloma (at the benign end of
the spectrum of histiocytosis X,
see p.607) usually presents as single osteolytic
radiolucent lesions of bone in children. The
effects may be serious if skull bones are destroyed,
otherwise resolution is to be expected.
The histological appearances are typical.

Eosinophils

Foamy
histiocytes
containing
lipid, in a
vascular
connective
tissue stroma

Multinucleate giant cells

TUMOURS IN BONE

Simple tumours present as proliferations of a variety of tissues, varying from rounded excrescences
of hard bone (simple exostoses and osteomas) through multiple irregular nodules of cartilage
(endochondromas) to areas of replacement of bone by fibrous or myxomatous tissue. In the field
of simple bone tumours, the borderland between true neoplasia and developmental defect is ill-
defined.

The importance of simple bone tumours is that:

1. They may cause cosmetic and slight functional defects.
2. Pathological fracture may occur.
3. In some conditions (e.g. multiple enchondromatosis and giant cell tumour), there is a tendency
   to malignant transformation.

807

TUMOURS IN BONE

Osteoid osteoma

Although rare, this is worthy of particular mention since it has a striking classical presentation and a specific pathology.

Clinical: Classically, an adolescent complains of well localised, increasingly severe pain in a lower limb long bone.

Pathological: The essential lesion is a small focus of newly formed irregular trabeculae of osteoid or poorly calcified woven bone in a highly vascular stroma.

Marked osteoblastic activity ------

Highly vascular stroma ------

Active remodelling by osteoclasts; lesion rarely exceeds 1cm diameter

Radiologically a very small radiolucent area is surrounded by densely calcified bone

Note reaction in surrounding bone; sclerosis of adjacent cortex and periosteal bone thickening.

Giant cell tumour (osteoclastoma)

This is not a common tumour but presents characteristic histological appearances. The tumour arises in adult life (age 20 – 40 years), usually at the end of a long bone — especially adjacent to the knee. The basic pathological process is essentially destructive of bone so that the cortex, gradually expanded by the tumour, becomes egg-shell thin and may be ruptured. Pathological fracture is common.

Lower end of femur showing expansion of cortex by partly cystic, partly solid haemorrhagic tumour

Numerous osteoclast-like giant cells in a spindle cell vascular stroma

Behaviour: 50% of tumours are *benign* and are cured by thorough removal, 30% recur and 20% are beginning or after recurrence — they metastasise to the lungs.

In general terms, a tumour showing cellular pleomorphism and abnormal mitotic activity can be expected to behave as a sarcoma, but unfortunately behaviour cannot always be certainly assessed from histological appearances.

TUMOURS IN BONE

MALIGNANT TUMOURS

Primary malignant tumours of bone are not common, but they assume importance because some arise in young people and are highly malignant and in a few, specific pre-existing bone disorders are known precursors, e.g. Paget's disease, multiple enchondromatosis.

Osteosarcoma (Osteogenic sarcoma)
This highly malignant tumour is the commonest primary malignant tumour of bone (excluding myelomatosis). It affects two distinct age groups and there is a preponderance of males over females.

Young age group — majority of cases (10-25 years)
The tumour usually arises near the end of a limb long bone (particularly around the knee.

Elderly subjects (over 60 yrs.)
In 50% of this group, Paget's disease is associated. Vertebrae, pelvis and skull are often affected, and tumours may be multicentric in origin.

The classical tumour in a young man will be described: tumour growth begins in the medullary cavity and is latent. Clinical signs present relatively late, i.e. when the cortex has been destroyed and penetrated.

Tumour begins here: spread through cortex has occurred

Periosteum stripped from bone

Spicules of reactive bone forming

The clinical signs are pain, swelling and redness of the lower thigh

The radiological counterpart is a patchily radiolucent tumour

Sun-ray appearance due to new bone spicules

Codman's triangle (new bone forming where periosteum is being stripped)

NB at this stage lung metastases may be present.

The tumour arises from primitive cells which retain to a varying extent the ability to form bone. Histologically, varying amounts of osteoid, irregularly woven bone and sometimes islands of primitive cartilage are seen in a vascular sarcomatous matrix of which the cells are pleomorphic.

TUMOURS IN BONE

Chondrosarcoma
This shows a much slower growth pattern and affects the age group 40 – 70 years. Multiple enchondromatosis pre-exists in a number of cases. The tumours arise particularly in the spine and pelvis and consist of primitive cartilage. Progressive local destruction followed by metastasis to the lung is usual.

Ewing's tumour
This is a rare malignant tumour of unknown histogenesis arising in long bones of young subjects. The tumour cells are fairly uniform with small dark nuclei resembling large lymphoid cells.

Lymphoid tumours
Lymphoid tumours, including myelomatosis (see p.605), arise in bone, causing osteolysis.

SECONDARY TUMOURS IN BONE

This is the most common type of tumour in bone. Metastases are usually multiple: occasionally latent renal and thyroid cancers present as single bony metastases with pathological fracture. Tumours which show a predilection for spread to bone are carcinoma of the PROSTATE, BREAST and LUNG particularly. The incidence of bone secondaries ESPECIALLY IN THE SPINE is very high when these tumours become widespread.

The effects of metastatic growth are essentially osteolytic with extensive destruction of bone. In a minority of cases, osteoblastic activity is stimulated by the presence of the tumour so that dense reactive bone is formed. Osteosclerotic secondaries of this type are seen particularly in cancers of the PROSTATE and BREAST.

JOINTS

The diagram illustrates the important components of a **diarthrotic joint.**

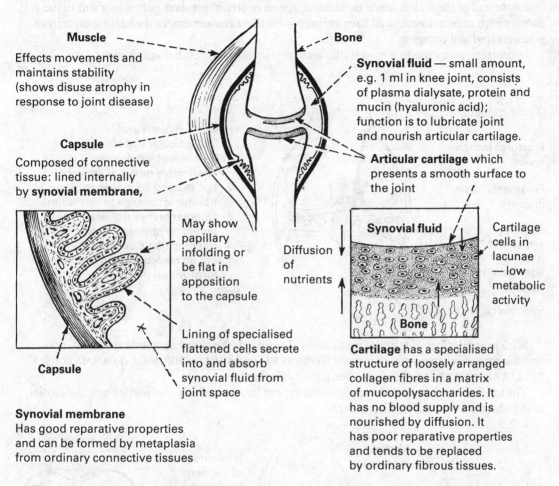

Muscle

Effects movements and maintains stability (shows disuse atrophy in response to joint disease)

Bone

Synovial fluid — small amount, e.g. 1 ml in knee joint, consists of plasma dialysate, protein and mucin (hyaluronic acid); function is to lubricate joint and nourish articular cartilage.

Capsule

Composed of connective tissue: lined internally by **synovial membrane,**

Articular cartilage which presents a smooth surface to the joint

May show papillary infolding or be flat in apposition to the capsule

Diffusion of nutrients

Synovial fluid

Cartilage cells in lacunae — low metabolic activity

Bone

Capsule

Lining of specialised flattened cells secrete into and absorb synovial fluid from joint space

Cartilage has a specialised structure of loosely arranged collagen fibres in a matrix of mucopolysaccharides. It has no blood supply and is nourished by diffusion. It has poor reparative properties and tends to be replaced by ordinary fibrous tissues.

Synovial membrane
Has good reparative properties and can be formed by metaplasia from ordinary connective tissues

The two most common joint diseases illustrate how individual components of a joint may be initially affected:

| **Rheumatoid Arthritis** essentially an inflammation of **synovial membrane** | **Osteoarthritis** essentially a degeneration of **articular cartilage** |

As the diseases progress, other secondary effects are added and may obscure the basic pathology.

JOINTS

Trauma is very variable in its severity and effects.

At one end of the scale a single incident of 'sprain or strain' involves only minor soft tissue damage with minimal associated haemorrhage — in these circumstances the healing capacity of joints is rapid and complete.

In contrast, many modern road traffic accidents involve serious damage to joints.

These include:

Fractures into join space

Fragments loose in joint

Capsular and ligamentous tears

Haemorrhage into joint

Possible sequels are:
1. The articular surface is permanently deformed (ineffective repair of cartilage).
2. Loose body continues to cause traumatic damage to synovium.
3. Ligaments may not heal or are united by poor scar tissue.
4. Haemorrhagic exudate may not be resorbed — adhesions form within the joint.

With lesser degrees of trauma, particularly if repeated, the synovial membrane shows non-specific reactive changes which include **HYPERAEMIA** and a **MILD CHRONIC INFLAMMATORY CELLULAR INFILTRATE**. There is often a joint **effusion.**

The knee joint is susceptible to a particular type of injury in which one (particularly the medial) of the fibrocartilagenous menisci is torn.

Medial meniscus

Movement of sudden flexion and rotation — cartilage caught between femur and tibia.

Linear tear

Repair of the tear is by poor scar tissue; recurrence with locking of the joint and effusion is common.

Apart from damage directly attributable to trauma, the most important sequel is that the scene is set within the joint for the more rapid development of **DEGENERATIVE DISEASE**.

JOINTS

OSTEOARTHRITIS (OA)

This is the commonest disorder of joints and, by causing pain and stiffness, is the commonest cause of chronic disability after middle age. The basic pathological progress is degenerative and is similar to that seen in lesser degree in simple ageing. The suffix 'itis' is really inappropriate since any inflammatory changes are secondary.

The disorder is divided into two main groups:

1. In **secondary OA** there is a clear association with some predisposing condition which may be virtually any abnormality of a joint. Of particular importance are
   (a) alterations to the joint mechanics (e.g. abnormal alignments and angulations); a particularly severe form (Charcot's joint) is seen when the nerve supply to a joint and its adjacent muscles is defective.
   (b) abnormality of the articular surfaces (e.g. following injury).
   (c) abnormal stresses on the joint (e.g. the increased weight-bearing demanded by obesity; association with particular occupations and sports).

2. In **primary OA,** no obvious predisposing cause is evident; there is a presumptive abnormality of chondrocyte metabolism but its essential nature remains obscure. A familial pattern is apparent in some cases.
   In both types of osteoarthritis the basic pathological processes are the same.

Normal

Surface loss

Cartilage

Replacement by chondrocytes

Bone

The integrity of the articular cartilagenous surface represents a fine balance between 'wear and tear' losses and replacement by chondrocytes of the specialised matrix.

The earliest change in ageing and OA is in the chemical composition of the matrix which becomes softer. This is followed by progressive characteristic morphological changes.

At site of pressure

Early

Flaking and fibrillation of surface

Areas of cystic degeneration

Later

Loss of cartilage; exposure of bone — becomes hard and polished (eburnated)

JOINTS

OSTEOARTHRITIS (continued)

At edge of joint

Bone forming from cartilage

Outgrowth of irregular bone (osteophyte) forming a lip round the joint margin

Osteophytes may contribute to limitation of movement

Cystic degeneration of bone

Extensive loss of cartilage with exposed eburnated bone

The synovial membrane may show mild, non-specific inflammation and effusion may occur but these changes are secondary.

Distribution: secondary OA often affects a single predisposed joint.

In primary OA, the larger weight bearing joints and the spine in particular are susceptible, but in addition, especially in women, the terminal phalanges immediately adjacent to the interphalangeal joint bear osteophytic outgrowths (Heberden's nodes). Similar lesions (at the proximal interphalangeal joints — Bouchard's nodes) superficially mimic the deformities of rheumatoid arthritis; they are, however, not associated with severe disability and muscle wasting in negligible.

Cervical spondylosis. When osteophytes form around the various intervertebral joints, particularly in the cervical spine, neurological complications ranging from compression of individual nerves to actual spinal cord damage are seen.
Note: OA is a local degenerative disease; there is no associated systemic illness.

Gout. The arthritis of gout begins as an acute inflammatory process affecting usually a great toe; with repeated attacks, degenerative arthritis supervenes.
Aetiology: the disease is a disorder of purine metabolism. There is hyperuricaemia (serum uric acid>7 mg/dl). Periodically, urate crystals are deposited within the affected joint, at first in the articular cartilage, but later both in the adjacent bone and soft tissues. An acute inflammatory reaction is evoked.

Pseudo-gout. In this condition, crystals of calcium pyrophosphate are deposited in the joint, evoking a similar inflammatory reaction. Larger joints such as the knee tend to be affected; chronic degenerative arthritis supervenes.

RHEUMATOID ARTHRITIS

Rheumatoid arthritis (RA) is a fairly common systemic disease (1 – 3% of population in Europe). The main target tissue is the synovial membrane of joints (polyarthritis). The typical clinical course is insidious in its onset and progression. In a minority of cases, the onset is acute and the progress rapid. Frequently there are remissions and exacerbations.

Incidence: female>male
　　　　　2 – 3 : 1

Age of onset: usually 35 – 55 years, but also in childhood — usually severe.

Typically, the joints of the hands and feet and the knee joints are affected; less commonly there is involvement of the cervical spine and temporomandibular joints.
Pathology: The essential condition is an active chronic inflammation of the synovial membrane.

Early

Swollen inflamed synovium

Fluid contains fibrin and polymorphs

— Fibrinous exudate

Intense infiltration with lymphocytes and plasma cells

Signs of inflammation with *swelling* over *joints*

A raised ESR and normochromic anaemia are evidence of the systemic illness.

Intermediate

Laxity of capsule and soft tissue — inflammation in periarticular tissues

Destruction of cartilage by enzymatic action and granulation tissue spreading over the articular surface (pannus)

Joints swollen + marked muscle wasting (interosseous and thenar muscles)

Late

Inflammation usually less marked — fibrous adhesions across joint – may be irregular bony union

Severely distorted joint

Permanent deformity due to contracture and often subluxation

RHEUMATOID ARTHRITIS

The **aetiology and mechanisms** responsible for the disorder remain unknown. A popular current hypothesis is:

The local condition is aggravated by affection of other synovial tissues — particularly tendon sheaths and bursae.

The systemic nature of the disease is illustrated by inflammatory processes affecting the connective tissues at other sites.

1. **Rheumatoid nodules** occur under the skin at pressure points, particularly in the forearms and elbow joints in 1/5 of cases. They range in size up to a few centimetres in diameter. The histological appearance is striking.

Nodule under skin of elbow.

Central area of well demarcated fibrinoid necrosis

Pallisade of fibroblasts

Well collagenised granulation tissue

2. The lung may be diffusely affected or, in some cases, lesions similar to rheumatoid nodules are seen. In coal miners, the mixture of coal dust and collagen gives characteristic radiological and pathological appearances — Caplan's nodules (see p.345).
3. Necrotising arteritis is a serious concomitant in a few cases.
4. A mild interstitial myocarditis, polymyositis or neuritis may be seen in some cases.
5. Lymphoid and splenic reactive enlargements (Still's disease).

Complications:

1. Amyloid disease.
2. Splenomegaly causing hypersplenism — so-called Felty's syndrome.

POLYARTHRITIS

Ankylosing spondylitis (AS) is an arthritis affecting particularly the sacroiliac, costovertebral and vertebral joints.

Incidence: .05 per cent of population
male>female; 8:1

Age of onset: Young adults progressive into middle age. Rheumatoid factor negative

The disorder is, like RA, an active chronic arthritis, but differs in that it proceeds inexorably to calcific and osseous ankylosis, so that no movement of the affected joints is possible.

Bony union on the periphery of the intervertebral discs gives the characteristic radiological appearance — bamboo spine.

The aetiology and mechanisms of the disorder is not known — a few cases are associated with Reiter's syndrome or chronic inflammatory bowel disease.

Psoriatic arthritis is very similar to RA, but rheumatoid factor is absent.

Reiter's syndrome (polyarthritis, urethritis and conjunctivitis) has similar chronic inflammatory joint disease, but rheumatoid factor is negative. There is strong evidence that a chlamydial infection is primary, but the detailed mechanisms remain obscure.

HLA association (see introduction). It is of great interest in that ankylosing spondylitis, psoriatic patients with arthritis and Reiter's syndrome all have a close association with HLA-B27 (90% in AS). This suggests that a genetic susceptibility is an important factor predisposing to the arthritis.

No such association with HLA-B27 is evident with RA, which however shows an association (60%) with HLA-DRW4.

Arthritis in acute rheumatic fever
During this stage, arthritis of the knee, ankle and wrist joints is common. The synovial tissues are inflamed and there is an inflammatory cellular infiltrate : the joint fluid contains polymorphs but is sterile. The arthritis is usually self-limiting and without sequelae, in contrast to the cardiac valvular lesions.

817

OSTEO — AND RHEUMATOID ARTHRITIS — COMPARISON

	OSTEOARTHRITIS	RHEUMATOID ARTHRITIS
Type of disorder	Degenerative	Inflammatory
Site of initial damage	Articular cartilage	Synovial membrane
Age	Late middle age +	3rd decade (any age)

Joints affected	Large weight bearing
	    often single,
	    pre-existing local
	    factors in some cases
		Small
		    of hands and feet,
		    multiple

Systemic disease	None ESR – normal Rheumatoid factor — absent	++ ESR ↑ Rheumatoid factor positive Secondary anaemia

INFECTIONS OF JOINTS

1. **Acute infective arthritis**

    (a) Primary pyogenic haematogenous infection is rare nowadays. It remains, however, a serious complication in joints already damaged. The essential changes are:

    (b) Arthritis complicating **gonorrhoea** and **brucellosis.**

    In both of these conditions, a polyarthritis may occur in the acute phase and, in a small number, continues as a low grade arthritis. The spine particularly is affected in brucellosis.

2. **Tuberculous arthritis**

    In Western countries the incidence is low: a few cases arise complicating reactivated pulmonary tuberculosis in the elderly. If untreated, there is a low grade chronic inflammation with effusion and progressive destruction of tissues.

    The diagnosis requires culture of joint fluid and/or biopsy when the typical histology of tuberculosis is seen.

PROLIFERATIONS AND TUMOURS OF SYNOVIAL TISSUES

Pigmented villonodular synovitis (PVNS)
This may affect any synovial tissue, but the knee and hip joints are most commonly affected. There is a strong male predominance (age 20 – 50). The synovial membrane shows a striking proliferation either in the form of brown pigmented large villi or rounded nodules.

Proliferating synovial cells on surface

Underlying tissue: Macrophages with iron^{++}, fat^{+} Giant cells

Villous and nodular growth

The exact nature of the lesion is not certain. It may be reactive or neoplastic **but it certainly never metastasises.**

The so-called benign giant cell tumour of tendon sheath is now considered to be a solitary variant of PVNS.

Synovial sarcoma (malignant synovioma)
This is a rare but highly malignant tumour arising adjacent to a joint (usually the knee or ankle) in young adults. The histological distinction from other sarcomas requires the demonstration of synovial spaces in the tumour.

Pseudo epithelial synovial clefts

Pleomorphic spindle cells

LOOSE BODIES IN JOINTS

Loose bodies are usually found in diseased or damaged joints and their presence tends to aggravate any existing disease. Clinically, there is often recurrent 'locking' of the joint.

Traumatic:
Fragments derived from fractures: tearing of cartilage and synovium

Degenerative:
Melon seed bodies
Fragments of osteophytes } Products of arthritis

Synovial chondromatosis — numerous polypoidal projections of cartilage (aetiology unknown)

PARA-ARTICULAR TISSUES — MISCELLANEOUS

Bursae
These are synovial-lined spaces usually overlying bony prominences and often connected with adjacent joint spaces. They are subject to traumatic and inflammatory disorders as have been described in joints.

Ganglion
This is a swelling which forms in relation to joint synovium or more usually, tendon sheath. The essential lesion is a myxomatous degeneration of the sheath substance; it is not lined by synovium. Ganglia are classically seen around the wrist.

This type of myxomatous cystic degeneration may occur at other less prominent sites, e.g. within the cartilagenous menisci of the knee.

Dupuytren's Contracture. See page 166.

CONNECTIVE TISSUE DISEASES

Some four decades ago, the idea that the collagen component of the connective tissues throughout the body were subject to specific disorders gave rise to the concept of diffuse collagen diseases. Since, in fact, damage to collagen is not usually the primary event, the name was changed to the CONNECTIVE TISSUE DISEASES.

The group includes the 'rheumatic' diseases — rheumatoid arthritis (RA), ankylosing spondylitis (AS) and rheumatic fever; systemic lupus erythematosis (SLE); scleroderma; polyarteritis nodosa (PAN) and dermatomyositis.

Some of these disorders have already been described (RA p.815; AS p.817: rheumatic fever p.270; PAN p.223; dermatomyositis p.790).

CONNECTIVE TISSUE DISEASES

Systemic lupus erythematosis (SLE)
This is a rare disease predominantly affecting young women. The clinical progress varies from acute and rapid to insidious and slow. Most frequently the skin, kidneys, serous membranes and endocardium are damaged and, in a few cases, the central nervous system. The essential lesion is a vasculitis affecting arterioles, capillaries and venules with fibrinoid necrosis and a variable inflammatory cellular infiltrate. In the kidney, the lesion is a glomerulitis (see p.634).

The formation of various autoimmune antibodies is the basic abnormality. Various cell constituents including nuclear DNA are destroyed. Lymphocytotoxic antibodies, by destroying T lymphocytes, further disturb the balances within the immune system, e.g. loss of self recognition and tolerance, and allow unsuppressed B cell proliferation.

Progressive systemic sclerosis
This is a rare, slowly progressive disease in which there is gradual fibrosis of various organs including the skin (face and hands), gastrointestinal tract, heart and lungs. Raynaud's disease is a common concomitant. The basic abnormality is in the small blood vessels, which show sclerosis with intimal thickening. The change is associated with fibrosis of the surrounding tissues by a mechanism as yet undetermined. The evidence for an autoimmune basis is less clear in systemic sclerosis than in the other disorders in this group.

From the descriptions of these various disorders it will be seen that the basic mechanisms are essentially inflammatory and are mediated by autoimmune processes. The inflammatory damage is very variable in its severity, its site of predilection and even in its local effects. Multiple factors, of which inherited susceptibility and resistance are important, are involved. The following diagram illustrates the basic mechanisms:

GLAND

CHAPTER 16

ENDOCRINE SYSTEM

PITUITARY GLAND

The endocrine organs form a control system related to the function and metabolism of the organs and peripheral tissues. In this, the pituitary plays a central role.

Anterior pituitary (Adenohypophysis)

Adeno-
hypophysis

Neuro-
hypophysis

ADH
oxytocin

The blood supply to the anterior pituitary is via a portal system which involves the hypothalamus as well as the pituitary, i.e. the direct arterial supply to the pituitary is small.

Histology: Three types of cell are recognised.

Non-granulated
Chromophobes
(50%)

Cells which have
discharged secretion

Basophils
(12%)

Eosinophils (35%)

Thyrotrophin(TSH)

Adrenocorticotrophic
hormone
(ACTH)

Gonadotrophins
(FSH and LH)

Prolactin

Growth hormone
(somatotrophin)

Control of endocrine function

A two tier system operates controlling the function of the pituitary and the other endocrines.

1. **Peripheral control.** This can be illustrated by thyroid function.
   The blood level of the peripheral hormone controls the pituitary secretion of the stimulating hormone.

Stimulates
anterior
pituitary

Secretion
of TSH

Depression
of pituitary
secretion

Fall in
blood thyroid
hormone

Secretion
of thyroid
hormone

Demand for
thyroid
hormone

Tissues

PITUITARY GLAND

Control of endocrine function (continued)

2. **Central control.** In the hypothalamus (median eminence), peptide substances are produced which are transmitted to the anterior pituitary via the portal system of vessels. These peptides act as permissive hormones, allowing release or inhibition of pituitary hormone secretion. Releasing substances have been identified for TSH, LH/FSH, and GH. An inhibiting substance, somatostatin, has been discovered. It inhibits not only growth hormone secretion, but also secretion of insulin, glucagon and prolactin. It is thought there is a release-inhibition mechanism for each pituitary hormone. The action of the hypothalamic centres is controlled directly or indirectly (it is not always clear which) by the concentration of hormones in the blood.

Action of anterior pituitary hormones

Growth hormone
1. Stimulates growth.
2. Acts with insulin and thyroid hormone in controlling protein, fat and carbohydrate metabolism. Promotes nitrogen retention and stimulates protein synthesis.

Prolactin
Helps to initiate and maintain lactation.

Gonadotrophins

1. FSH — Promotes growth of follicles in ovary
— Promotes spermatogenesis

2. LH — Induces ovulation
— Stimulates testosterone production by testes

Thyroid-stimulating hormone
Induces secretion of thyroid hormones and can cause hyperplasia of thyroid epithelium.

Adrenocorticotrophic hormone
Stimulates secretion of glucocorticoids by the adrenal cortex.

PITUITARY GLAND

Inflammations of the pituitary gland

Apart from involvement in acute meningitis inflammation, acute or chronic, is uncommon. Tuberculosis, syphilis and sarcoidosis have been reported.

Lesions of the anterior pituitary generally result in hypofunction or hyperfunction.

ADENOHYPOPHYSEAL HYPOFUNCTION

This produces characterisitic syndromes:

IN CHILDHOOD
Normal child
aged 13 yrs

(a) **Lorain-Levi syndrome (Pituitary dwarfism)**
Growth hormone secretion is
deficient. There may also be
deficiencies of other pituitary
hormones. Attacks of hypoglycaemia
occur. Gonadotrophins
are usually lacking and
puberty does not occur.
In ⅔ of cases, no cause can
be found. The condition may
be familial and in these circumstances
the only deficiency may
be of growth hormone. A pituitary
tumour or craniopharyngioma
is the cause in other cases.

- Skeletal growth diminished
- Retarded sexual development.
- Normal intelligence

(13 yrs)

(b) **Frohlich's syndrome**
Stunting of growth.
Obesity: feminine distribution of fat.
Arrested sexual development
Mentally subnormal.
Decreased production of growth and
other pituitary hormones.
The cause is a lesion affecting the
hypothalamus or anterior pituitary or both.
Sometimes it is a tumour *e.g.* craniopharyngioma,
chromophobe adenoma, glioma or meningioma.
A similar condition is found in adults and in
some cases a chromophobe adenoma is present.

(13 yrs)

PITUITARY GLAND

ADENOHYPOPHYSEAL HYPOFUNCTION (CONTINUED)

IN ADULTS

Simmond's disease (Sheehan's syndrome)

This occurs in women and is due to ischaemic necrosis of the pituitary following post-partum haemorrhage. The normally low pressure in the pituitary portal vascular supply increases the susceptibility of the gland. The results vary with the extent of necrosis and may include the following:

Lack of TSH — low BMR, features of hypothyroidism, sensitivity to cold, coarsening and loss of hair

Lack of prolactin — failure of lactation, and later breast atrophy

Lack of ACTH — deficiency of glucocorticoids — weakness, low BP, hypoglycaemia

Lack of gonadotrophins — amenorrhoea, sterility, loss of libido

Erythema ab igne

Loss of pubic hair

Where the necrosis is extensive, death may occur due to the complete loss of control of metabolism. With lesser degrees, lack of one or other of the pituitary hormones may be the dominating feature. In time, the peripheral endocrine organs — thyroid, adrenals, ovaries — show atrophy.

ADENOHYPOPHYSEAL HYPERFUNCTION

In most cases, this is the result of tumour formation in the pituitary.

Giantism and acromegaly

These are both the result of excess production of growth hormone by an eosinophil adenoma. Giantism arises in children before the epiphyses have fused; acromegaly arises in adult life.

Giantism

The excess growth hormone induces skeletal growth, the bones retaining their normal shape and relative proportions. Fusion of epiphyses is delayed, but eventually occurs and the features of acromegaly appear. As in acromegaly, there is initially increase in pituitary secretions and there may be sexual precocity.

827

PITUITARY GLAND

Acromegaly

The soft tissues increase in thickness. This is followed by periosteal ossification causing thickening of bones.

Clinical signs

Features coarsened: nose enlarged.
Prognathic (projecting jaw).
Irregular bone formation — interferes with joint
    function — leads to osteoarthritis.
Limbs enlarged.

Pain due to nerve compression is common.
Initially, secretion of other pituitary hormones is increased leading to increased strength and increased libido. Glucose tolerance is diminished. Diabetes occurs in 10% Later, tumour destroys other parts of the pituitary causing weakness, muscle wasting and increased glucose tolerance. High blood pressure with cardiac hypertrophy and extensive atheroma is common, and the patient may die in cardiac failure.

In both giantism and acromegaly, the tumour may compress surrounding structures, *e.g.* optic nerves, leading to hemianopia; or the hypothalamus leading to diabetes insipidus.

Prolactinoma. Small adenomas, often of chromophobe cells, may secrete prolactin and cause infertility in the female (see p.698).

POSTERIOR PITUITARY (**NEUROHYPOPHYSIS**)

This is composed of neural tissue and serves as a store for two hormones produced in the hypothalamus.

1. **Vasopressin (antidiuretic hormone, ADH)**

   By altering the permeability of renal collecting tubules and concentrating the urine, vasopressin helps to control water balance. Diabetes insipidus is the condition which results when it is deficient. Absence of the concentrating mechanism results in the loss of large quantities of fluid. Abnormal thirst and polydypsia result. The condition results from damage (injury, tumour or encephalitis) to the hypothalamus.

2. **Oxytocin**

   This hormone causes contraction of smooth muscle and is often used to aid uterine contraction in labour. It also causes expulsion of milk during lactation.

THYROID GLAND

Normal bilobed gland weighs approximately 25g

Colloid storing thyroid hormones

Parafollicular cells (source of calcitonin)

Follicles lined by cuboidal epithelium

Rich capillary network

The thyroid gland is under the control of the pituitary thyroid-stimulating hormone (TSH).

Iodide in diet Bowel

Absorption facilitated by TSH

Iodine + Tyrosine

Monoiodo- and diiodo-tyrosine

(Triiodothyronine)
T_3

T_4
(Thyroxine)

Secretion stimulated by TSH

Blood

The secretion of TSH is determined by the level of T_3 and T_4 in the blood.

THYROID HYPOFUNCTION

Insufficient thyroid hormone is produced, resulting in myxoedema in adults and cretinism in children.

Adults — MYXOEDEMA

Clinical signs

- Basal metabolic rate reduced.
- Body temperature falls. *cold intolerant*
- Lethargy and apathy.
- Appetite reduced.
- Constipation.
- Respiratory and heart rates reduced.
- Diminished libido.
- Lack of ovulation.
- Skin thickened, non-pitting oedema due to increase in mucoprotein ground substance.
- Hair brittle, dry and falls out.
- Blood cholesterol is raised.
- TSH secretion is increased.
- T_3 and T_4 blood levels low.

THYROID GLAND

Myxoedema (continued)
Causes

1. Autoimmune thyroiditis
   (a) Atrophic form — so-called
   primary myxoedema — the
   commonest cause of hypothyroidism
   (b) Goitrous form —
   Hashimoto's disease.
2. Severe iodine deficiency.

3. Dyshormonogenesis — inborn errors
   in the formation of thyroid hormones.
4. Anti-thyroid drugs.
5. Excessive surgical resection of thyroid gland.
6. Treatment with radioiodine.
7. Hypopituitarism ⟶ reduced TSH.

Pathological changes in primary myxoedema

The thyroid is
shrunken, white
and firm

Cells in follicles large
with bizarre nuclei and
granular pink cytoplasm
(Askanazy cells)

Isolated islands
of small
follicles
embedded in
fibrous tissue

Lymphocytes
+ plasma cells

Lack of colloid

Children — CRETINISM

Infants normal at birth, but abnormality appears within weeks.

Clinical Signs
Protruding tongue

Dwarf with short limbs
Coarse dry skin
Lack of hair and teeth
Mental deficiency

Pot belly — often umbilical hernia

Changes are irreversible unless treatment is given
early.
Two forms are recognised:

(1) endemic and (2) sporadic cretinism.

THYROID GLAND

Endemic cretinism

This occurs in districts where goitre is common due to iodine deficiency. It rarely appears until the 3rd generation of a goitrous family and the mother almost always has a goitre.

The infantile thyroid is usually enlarged and nodular. Histologically, there are hyperplastic foci containing colloid which compress and cause atrophy of the intervening tissue. In some instances the whole gland is atrophic.

Sporadic cretinism

This is due to congenital hypoplasia or absence of the thyroid. The cause is unknown. Deaf mutism is often present.

Dyshormonogenesis

In this condition, cretinism is due to a congenital familial recessive enzyme defect leading to inability to complete the formation of thyroid hormone. The thyroid gland is enlarged and shows epithelial hyperplasia. TSH is increased.

THYROID HYPERFUNCTION

Excessive quantities of circulating thyroid hormone (T_3 and T_4) cause thyrotoxicosis.

Clinical signs
- Exophthalmos — not always present.
- Prominent thyroid.
- *BMR increased.*
- Skin warm and sweaty : heat intolerance.
- Weakness, hyperkinesia and emotional instability.
- Loss of weight.
- Glucose tolerance diminished, glycosuria.
- Rapid Pulse.
- Cardiac arrhythmia and failure in older patients.
- TSH low.

Three types of thyroid lesion can give rise to thyrotoxicosis.

1. Graves disease (exopthalmic goitre).
2. Toxic adenoma.
3. Toxic nodular goitre.

THYROID GLAND

Graves' disease (exophthalmic goitre)

Gland is diffusely enlarged; pale pink in colour

Gland is hyperplastic; numerous closely packed acini of various sizes

Sometimes intra-acinar papilliform growths

Colloid absent

Cells columnar

In some cases there are foci of thyroiditis with lymphocytes and plasma cells.

Other changes: 1. Thymus is enlarged with increase of lymphocytes. This may be an immune response.
2. Patches of myxoedema — usually on pre-tibial aspect of legs.
3. Exophthalmos, due to fatty infiltration of eye muscles.

Aetiology 1. Usually occurs in females
2. More common in families showing high incidence of autoimmune disease, e.g. thyroiditis, pernicious anaemia.
3. The stimulation of the thyroid is due to an autoantibody (long-acting thyroid stimulator, LATS) which reacts with and activates the surface receptor for TSH on thyroid epithelium. Cyclic AMP is formed and this stimulates hyperplasia of the epithelium and increased formation of thyroid hormone. With the increase in hormone, the blood TSH falls.

Toxic adenoma

Most adenomas are non-active; only a small proportion (1%) give rise to toxic symptoms.

There is usually only one large adenoma present. The histological features are the same as in Graves' disease. Increased production of thyroid hormone by the adenoma, which is autonomous, causes a fall in TSH, and the remainder of the thyroid is inactive.

Toxic nodular goitre

This develops in some cases of non-toxic nodular goitre. Nodules of hyperplasia are interspersed with inactive tissue. The condition is more common over the age of 50. Exophthalmos is absent. Cardiac arrhythmias and failure are common.

THYROID GLAND

Non-toxic goitre

This is a simple enlargement of the thyroid gland, not associated with increased secretion of thyroid hormone.

Two morphological forms are found: (1) parenchymatous and (2) colloid.

1. *Parenchymatous goitre.* The gland is enlarged and pale pink. Two phases can be recognised:

(a) **Diffuse hyperplasia:** The gland consists mainly of small closely packed acini lined by columnar epithelium and containing a small amount of poorly stained colloid. Occasional intra-acinar papilliform epithelial projections may be seen.

(b) **Nodular hyperplasia:** This is a later stage. Areas of marked hyperplasia cause atrophy of intervening parenchyma. It appears to be related to continuing severity of iodine deficiency.

2. *Colloid goitre.* The enlarged gland is translucent and brown due to the large amount of stored colloid.

This is common in women and appears at puberty or during pregnancy.

There are usually no symptoms, but pressure symptoms develop if the thyroid is retrosternal, e.g. pressure on trachea causing stridor, pressure on recurrent laryngeal nerve → hoarseness.

Vesicles large and full of dense colloid

Small cysts common

Epithelium flattened

Aetiology. Goitre is endemic in certain areas of the world, mountainous regions remote from the sea — Switzerland, Himalayas, Andes, etc. There is a lack of iodine in the soil, hence in the food. Sporadic goitre may be induced by other factors.

(1) Lack of iodine in food

(2) Inhibited by drugs

Iodide

(2) Inhibited by excess iodine

Iodine + Tyrosine

Monoiodo-tyrosine

Diiodo-tyrosine

(3) Inhibited by inherited congenital lack of enzymes

Thyroid gland

T_3

T_4

Mechanism of goitre production

Lack of iodine → Deficient production of thyroid hormone → TSH secretion → Enlargement of thyroid to Extract maximum amount of iodine from blood

Where the lack of iodine is severe, proliferation is marked (parenchymatous goitre). In colloid goitre, the process is milder.

833

THYROID GLAND

AUTO-IMMUNE THYROIDITIS

This type of disease is associated with the appearance of thyroid antibodies in the blood and inflammatory changes with lymphocyte and plasma cell reaction in the thyroid gland. The degree of pathological change and the clinical effects tend to form a spectrum, but three conditions can be defined.

1. **Hashimoto's thyroiditis (lymphadenoid goitre)**

    This is the most distinctive type of autoimmune thyroid disease, and the changes are widespread. *may progress to lymphoma (malignant)*

Round cell infiltrate

Germinal follicle

Many small acini

Acini lined by pink cell (Askanazy or Hürthle cells)

Lymphocytes and plasma cells

Nuclei often large and irregular

Clinical effects: While the patients may be euthyroid, it is obvious that the balance is precarious. In 50%, the patient, usually a middle-aged female, develops hypothyroidism. Any attempt to reduce the size of the goitre by surgery inevitably causes hypothyroidism.

The uptake of iodine is reduced and the combination with tyrosine is abnormal. Abnormal thyroid hormone is produced. Antibodies to thyroglobulin and to cytoplasmic microsomes of thyroid epithelium are usually present in high concentration.

2. **Primary Myxoedema.**
Antibodies to thyroid hormones and epithelium are found in this disease (p.829) also, but the plasma concentration is lower than in Hashimoto's disease.

3. **Focal thyroiditis**
This form of autoimmune disease is usually asymptomatic, but again the balance is disturbed and surgical interference may precipitate hypothyroidism. The concentration of antibodies in the plasma is always low. The thyroid in Graves' disease often shows a form of focal thyroiditis and this may account for the occasional occurrence of hypothyroidism as a late complication in that disease.

Patients with autoimmune thyroiditis are apt to have other organ-specific antibodies, e.g. gastric, adrenal etc., and pernicious anaemia and adrenal insufficiency may occur.

THYROID GLAND

Auto-immune thyroiditis (continued)

Aetiology 1. These conditions are usually found in females.
2. Sometimes autoimmune disease develops in siblings of the patient or near relatives, suggesting an inherited predisposition.
3. The exact cause is unknown, but the fact that various forms of organ-specific autoimmune disease may occur in the same patient might indicate a basic disorder in the immune system.

TUMOURS OF THE THYROID

Adenoma of the thyroid

This is a fairly common condition. The tumours are usually multiple but well encapsulated by fibrous tissue. It is difficult in some cases to distinguish between adenomas and nodular goitre. Their structure varies. Some are 'colloid adenomas', some are solid and consist of closely packed small acini. The latter may induce symptoms of hyperthyroidism.

Carcinoma of the thyroid

This is an uncommon condition, but the incidence is not truly known because of the difficulty in diagnosis, even on histological examination.

Two main forms are recognised:

1. *Papillary cystadenocarcinoma.* This is the commonest form. It is a well-differentiated tumour consisting of small cysts filled by papillary ingrowths. The epithelium covering the papillae is remarkably uniform and shows few mitoses, but the tumour is unencapsulated and spreads to the local lymph nodes. Distant metastases are unusual.
2. *Follicular adenocarcinoma.* This is an encapsulated tumour which may resemble solitary adenomas. Microscopically, mitotic activity and pleomorphism indicate malignancy. This type invades blood vessels and metastases to lungs and bones are common.

Anaplastic tumours also occur. — *even worse*

Thyroid carcinoma causes symptoms mainly by compressing structures in the neck — trachea, recurrent laryngeal nerve etc.

Medullary carcinoma

This is a rare tumour arising from the calcitonin-producing cells of the thyroid. Blood calcitonin is high. In addition, there may be production of other hormones resulting in a carcinoid or Cushing's syndrome. There is a familial form in which there are multiple tumours of a number of endocrine organs.

ENDOCRINE PANCREAS

The islets of Langerhans form 1 – 2 per cent of the pancreatic tissue. Three types of cell make up the islets. The majority are ß cells.

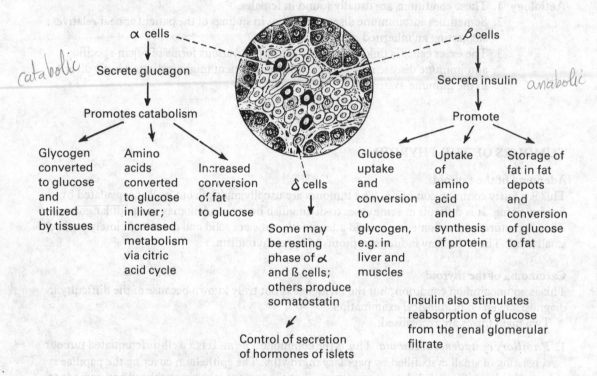

catabolic

α cells

Secrete glucagon

↓

Promotes catabolism

- Glycogen converted to glucose and utilized by tissues
- Amino acids converted to glucose in liver; increased metabolism via citric acid cycle
- Increased conversion of fat to glucose

δ cells

↓

Some may be resting phase of α and ß cells; others produce somatostatin

↙

Control of secretion of hormones of islets

anabolic

β cells

Secrete insulin

↓

Promote

- Glucose uptake and conversion to glycogen, e.g. in liver and muscles
- Uptake of amino acid and synthesis of protein
- Storage of fat in fat depots and conversion of glucose to fat

Insulin also stimulates reabsorption of glucose from the renal glomerular filtrate

Insulin and glucagon have virtually opposite actions. The action of insulin is also opposed by growth hormone and glucocorticoids.

DIABETES MELLITUS

This condition is due to a lack of insulin activity. Commonly this is the result of diminished production of insulin, but sometimes there appears to be some interference with its function. The condition is a disease complex of mixed aetiology and the manifestations are the result of biochemical abnormalities induced by an inability to control carbohydrate metabolism.

ENDOCRINE PANCREAS

BIOCHEMICAL CHANGES AND CLINICAL EFFECTS

The main results of insulin lack are:

1. **Inability to control carbohydrate metabolism,** causing:

2. **Increased fat catabolism**
   Leads to:

   Excess production of acetyl CoA

   Conversion to ketone bodies (acetone + ß hydroxybutyric acid)

   Ketosis ⟶ Acidosis ⟶ Acid excreted in combination
   with Na$^+$ and K$^+$

   Further electrolyte depletion

3. Increased catabolism of amino acids prevents proper protein synthesis and this, together with (1) and (2) above, leads to loss of weight despite polyphagia.

TYPES OF DIABETES

Primary forms

**Insulin-dependent diabetes
(juvenile or early onset diabetes)**
This form is due to actual
destruction of ß cells in the
islets of Langerhans.

ß cells are
progressively
destroyed

α cells persist

δ cells may
increase

Fibrosis and
sometimes
amyloid
deposition occurs

Lymphocytic reaction
may be present

ENDOCRINE PANCREAS

Types of Diabetes (continued)

Insulin-Dependent Diabetes (*continued*)

The onset is acute and the peak of incidence is around 13 years. Three factors appear to be of importance in the aetiology.

1. There is a familial incidence and affected individuals appear to have a defect in chromosome 6 and possess particular HLA antigens.
2. The onset of the condition is commonest in autumn and winter.
3. Cell-mediated immunity against islet antigens and humoral antibodies are present in at least 50% of cases at onset.
   This has given rise to a theory of pathogenesis.

Other forms of autoantibody, e.g. gastric, thyroid, adrenal, have been demonstrated.

Both sexes are affected and the condition is commoner in lower socio-economic groups. In a small group of children, a milder form, usually not requiring insulin, is inherited as an autosomal dominant.

Non Insulin-Dependent Diabetes (Maturity of Late onset Diabetes)

This is the commonest form of diabetes. It is more frequent in females and the incidence increases with age, peaking at 70 in males and at 80 in females. The islet tissue is virtually normal or only slightly reduced in amount. ß cells appear healthy. Blood insulin values vary — frequently moderately reduced, sometimes high. The cause is unknown. There is no association with autoimmune diseases and antibodies to islet tissue are almost never present. No relationship to the HLA system has been demonstrated. Its occurrence in identical twins however indicates some genetic disorder. Most patients are obese and it has been suggested that they lack cell receptors for insulin. Symptoms are usually mild and the patient often presents with vascular complications. Diet and hypoglycaemic drugs usually control the blood sugar.

Gestational Diabetes

This is associated with glycosuria during pregnancy and the birth of overweight babies. Control of the maternal blood sugar reduces birth weight to normal. Permanent diabetes is apt to develop at a later date.

ENDOCRINE PANCREAS

Types of Diabetes (continued)
Secondary forms

Diabetes may complicate:
1. A number of endocrine diseases (acromegaly, Cushing's syndrome, Conn's syndrome)
2. Metabolic diseases (haemochromatosis, pancreatic calcification, hypocalcaemia)
3. Drug therapy (steroids, thiazide diuretics)
4. Pancreatic inflammation, etc., (chronic pancreatitis, mumps, cystic fibrosis).

COMPLICATIONS OF DIABETES

1. **Diabetic Coma.** Three forms of coma occur:

    (a) **Keto-acidotic coma.** This is the type which is common in insulin-dependent diabetes. Hyperosmolarity, hypovolaemia, acidosis and loss of electrolytes if unchecked lead to coma.
    (b) **Hyperosmolar non-ketotic coma.** This develops slowly in mild diabetes. Hyperglycaemia builds up (blood glucose > 55.6 mmol/l) and produces profound dehydration. The cause is unknown.
    (c) **Lactic acidosis coma.** This is uncommon, although increase in lactic acid is frequent in diabetes.

2. **Hypoglycaemic coma.** This occurs when insulin intake is excessive for the amount of food consumed.

3. **Cardiovascular lesions**

    (a) Atheroma develops at an earlier age and with increased severity. Coronary thrombosis is not uncommon.
    (b) Monckeberg's sclerosis shows an increased incidence.
    (c) Microangiopathy causing occlusion of arterioles and capillaries. These vascular lesions are responsible for many of the clinical lesions e.g. cardiac failure (the commonest cause of death in diabetes) retinopathy, neuropathy, gangrene of limbs, Kimmelstiel-Wilson lesions in the kidney.

4. **Renal failure.** This is the other common cause of death. It may be due to glomerulosclerosis, but pyelonephritis and renal papillary necrosis are other causes.

5. **Infections.** There is an increased susceptibility to sepsis and fungal infections. Tuberculosis is also common.

ENDOCRINE PANCREAS

HYPERFUNCTION

This is the result of tumours of the islet cell tissue (adenoma or carcinoma). These tumours are apudomas (amine precursor uptake and decarboxylation). In common with similar tumours found in the pituitary, thyroid, gastrointestinal tract and bronchi, they are able to form peptide hormones. Frequently tumours may arise simultaneously in various sites in the body. In the cases of the pancreas, 10% are malignant. The clinical effects vary with the hormone producted:

1. Insulin-secreting tumours arising from ß cells produce attacks of hypoglycaemia.
2. Gastrin-secreting tumours cause multiple peptic ulcers (Zollinger-Ellison syndrome).
3. Glucagonoma inducing a diabetic condition.
4. Inappropriate hormone secretion, e.g. carcinoid syndrome, Cushing's syndrome, etc.

PARATHYROID GLANDS

The parathyroids are four small glands lying posterior to the thyroid gland.

Site of these glands is very variable

Thyroid (posterior view)

Three types of cell are found:
1. Water clear principal cells — actively secreting parathormone.
2. Darker principal cells — representing a resting phase
3. Oxyphil cells — function unknown

Action of parathormone

With vitamin D it regulates absorption of calcium and phosphorus according to blood levels

Controls reabsorption of calcium and excretion of phosphate

Controls mobilisation of calcium and phosphorus from bone

Kidney

Gut

Maintains relative concentrations of calcium and phosphorus in the blood and helps control acid/base balance

Bone

PARATHYROID GLANDS

HYPERFUNCTION (see p.801)

Two forms exist:

↗8010

Primary

This is due to hyperplasia, <u>adenoma</u> or carcinoma of the principal cells. Excess parathormone may also be produced by carcinoma of the bronchus or kidney.

The blood calcium is raised, much of it mobilised from the bones. The effects are:

1. Formation of renal calculi leading to renal failure
2. Osteitis fibrosa cystica
3. General muscle weakness
4. Metastatic calcification.

Secondary

This is a reaction to hypocalcaemia produced by chronic renal failure and malabsorption syndromes. Parathyroid hyperplasia may proceed to adenoma formation. Various syndromes are associated with this condition, e.g. renal rickets. *Vit D deficiency*

HYPOPARATHYROIDISM

This occurs in three circumstances:

1. Accidental surgical removal of the parathyroids during thyroidectomy
2. Autoimmune disease
3. Congenital deficiency.

↑ bone density

hair less
brittle nails
cataracts

ADRENAL GLAND

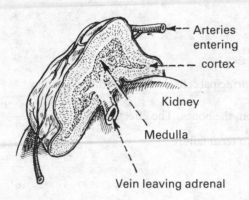

- Arteries entering
- cortex
- Kidney
- Medulla
- Vein leaving adrenal

- Zona glomerulosa (source of mineralocorticoids)
- Zona fasciculata
- Zona reticularis (Source of glucocorticoids)
- Medulla (Source of catecholamines)

Mineralocorticoids

The main one is aldosterone.
It is involved with the renin-angiotensin system and ADH in the maintenance of blood volume. The mechanism is as follows:

Fall in renal output of NaCl   Fall in renal perfusion
↓
Stimulation of juxtaglomerular system
↓
Renin secretion
↓
Angiotensin formed in blood
↓
Aldosterone secretion
↓
Increase in renal absorption of sodium and chloride   Increased tubular secretion of K^+
↓
Blood osmolarity rises
↓
ADH secretion stimulated
↓
Retention of fluid
↓
Blood osmolarity returns to normal

Glucocorticoids cortisol

Their actions are:

- Anti-inflammatory action
- Prevents migration and activity of polymorphs and macrophages
- Increased gluconeogenesis from protein
- Deposit of subcutaneous fat in trunk and face
- Suppress secretion of growth hormone

↓
- Increased protein catabolism
- Blood sugar increases
- Cytotoxic effect on lymphocytes

↓
- Diminished protein synthesis
- Glycogen deposition in liver
- Suppression of immunological response

ADRENAL GLAND

Control Mechanism

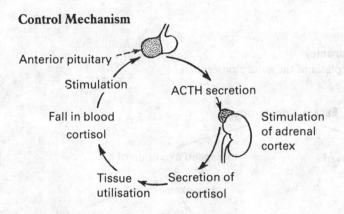

Anterior pituitary

Stimulation

ACTH secretion

Fall in blood cortisol

Stimulation of adrenal cortex

Tissue utilisation

Secretion of cortisol

There is also a centre in the hypothalamus which formulates a releasing hormone controlling the secretion of ACTH.

Sex hormones — androgens and oestrogens — are also produced in small quantities.

HYPERACTIVITY

This manifests itself in three ways:

1. **Cushing's syndrome (hypersecretion of cortisol)**

   This condition is commonest in women, but occurs also in men and children.

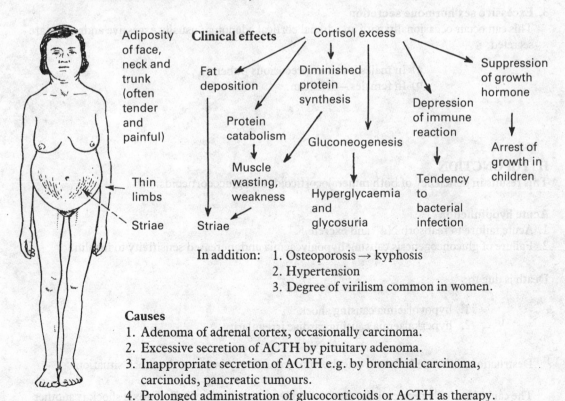

Adiposity of face, neck and trunk (often tender and painful)

Thin limbs

Striae

Clinical effects

Cortisol excess

Fat deposition

Diminished protein synthesis

Protein catabolism

Gluconeogenesis

Muscle wasting, weakness

Striae

Hyperglycaemia and glycosuria

Suppression of growth hormone

Depression of immune reaction

Arrest of growth in children

Tendency to bacterial infection

In addition:
1. Osteoporosis → kyphosis
2. Hypertension
3. Degree of virilism common in women.

Causes

1. Adenoma of adrenal cortex, occasionally carcinoma.
2. Excessive secretion of ACTH by pituitary adenoma.
3. Inappropriate secretion of ACTH e.g. by bronchial carcinoma, carcinoids, pancreatic tumours.
4. Prolonged administration of glucocorticoids or ACTH as therapy.

ADRENAL GLAND

Hyperactivity (continued)

2. Hyperaldosteronism (Conn's syndrome)
This is due to an adenoma or hyperplasia of the zona glomerulosa. ↑ aldosterone

Effects

Excess aldosterone

Increased reabsorption of
NaCl from renal tubule

↓

Sodium and
water retention

↓

Hypertension

Increased excretion of K⁺

↓

Hypokalaemia

↓   ↘

Possible cardiac   Alkalosis
irregularity
                         Tetany
                         Cramps

3. Excessive sex hormone secretion
This can occur occasionally with an adrenal cortical adenoma; usually excessive androgens are secreted.

      (a) In males it causes precocious puberty.
      (b) In females — virilism.

HYPOFUNCTION
This results in deficiency of both mineralocorticoids and glucocorticoids.

Acute hypofunction
1. Acute failure to reabsorb Na⁺ and excrete K⁺.
2. Failure of gluconeogenesis causing hypoglycaemia and increased sensitivity to insulin.

Death is due to:

      1. hypovolaemia causing shock
      2. hyperkalaemia causing cardiac irregularity.

Destruction of the medulla and catecholamine deficiency increase the shock situation.

The cause is usually septicaemia, especially due to meningococci. Endotoxic shock is another cause. These conditions result in necrosis of the cortex and gross haemorrhage in the medulla.

ADRENAL GLAND

Chronic Hypofunction

Inadequate production of MINERALOCORTICOIDS ↓AOH *aldosterone*

Waterhouse-Friderichsen syndrome → vascular collapse & shock due to acute hemorrhage of adrenal → meningitis

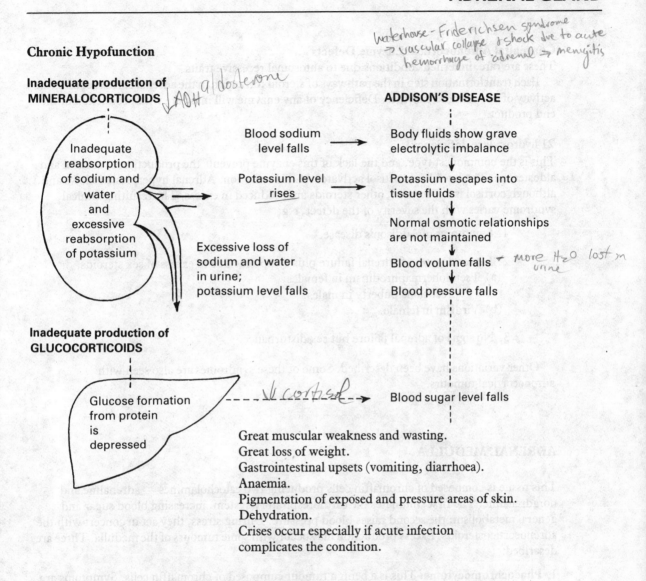

ADDISON'S DISEASE

Inadequate reabsorption of sodium and water and excessive reabsorption of potassium

Blood sodium level falls → Body fluids show grave electrolytic imbalance

Potassium level rises → Potassium escapes into tissue fluids

Normal osmotic relationships are not maintained

Excessive loss of sodium and water in urine; potassium level falls

Blood volume falls ← *more H₂O lost in urine*

Blood pressure falls

Inadequate production of GLUCOCORTICOIDS

Glucose formation from protein is depressed -----↓ *cortisol* → Blood sugar level falls

Great muscular weakness and wasting.
Great loss of weight.
Gastrointestinal upsets (vomiting, diarrhoea).
Anaemia.
Pigmentation of exposed and pressure areas of skin.
Dehydration.
Crises occur especially if acute infection complicates the condition.

Administration of adrenal hormones restores individual to normal.

Causes

1. Tuberculous destruction of adrenals.
2. 'Idiopathic' Addison's disease. This is now known to be due to an autoimmune reaction in at least 50% of cases.

Other autoimmune diseases affecting other endocrine glands are commonly associated with this form of Addison's disease.

ADRENAL GLAND

Congenital Adrenocortical Enzyme Defects

These are rare, inherited conditions due to autosomal recessive traits.

Each transformation step in the pathways of steroid formation in the adrenal cortex requires the activity of one or more enzymes. Deficiency of any enzyme will interfere with production of the end product.

21 hydroxylase deficiency

This is the commonest type, and the lack of this enzyme prevents the production of cortisol and aldosterone. The low blood cortisol activates ACTH secretion. Adrenal hyperplasia follows and, although cortisol is not formed, other steroids are produced in excess. The resulting clinical syndrome varies with the severity of the defect, e.g:

1. Symptoms of Addison's disease.

2. Lesser degrees of adrenal failure plus symptoms due to excess of sex steroids.
   (a) Pseudohermaphroditism in females;
       precocious puberty in males.
   (b) Virilism in female.

3. No signs of adrenal failure but sex disturbance.

Other variations have been described. Some of these syndromes are also seen with adrenocortical tumours.

ADRENAL MEDULLA

This tissue is composed of chromaffin cells producing two catecholamines — adrenaline and noradrenaline. The first stimulates the cardiorespiratory system, increasing blood sugar and general metabolism; the second raises blood pressure. During stress, they act in concert with the adrenocorticosteroids. Excess production may occur with some tumours of the medulla. Three are described:

1. **Phaeochromocytoma.** This is a benign tumour composed of chromaffin cells. Symptoms are due to paroxysmal overproduction of the amines with hypertension, raised metabolic rate and blood sugar. Arteriosclerosis develops rapidly and cerebral haemorrhage may occur.

2. **Ganglioneuroma:** a benign tumour, composed of well-differentiated ganglion cells (see p.771).

3. **Neuroblastoma:** a very malignant tumour of primitive nerve cells. Catecholamines are occasionally produced by the neurogenic tumours (see p.771)

INDEX

ABO blood groups, 533, 567, 568
Abortion, endometritis following, 667
Abscess (see also various tissues), 38
  amoebic, 473
  cold, 60, 805
  pyaemic, 52, 53
Achalasia of oesophagus, 376
Achlorhydria, in anaemia, 516, 520
  in chronic gastritis, 383
  in gastric carcinoma, 393
Achondroplasia, 806
Acidosis in diabetes 837
  in renal failure, 654
  in renal tubular, 640
Acoustic Schwannoma, 774
Acromegaly, 828
  bone in, 801
ACTH (see also Adrenocorticotrophic
  hormone), 824
Actinomycosis, 64
Active immunisation, 118
Acute bacterial endocardtis, 279
Acute inflammatory reaction, 30-36
Addisonian anaemia, 518-521
Addison's disease, 845
  pigmentation in, 845
Adeno-acanthoma of endometrium,
  670
Adenocarcinoma, 184
Adenoids, 290
Adenoma (see also various organs), 171
Adenomyoma of uterus, 674
Adenomyosis of uterus, 674
Adenosine diphosphate release
  platelets, 556
Adenosis of breast, 692
  sclerosing, 692
Adrenal glands, 842
  Addison's disease, 845
  auto-antibodies to, 845
  congenital anomalies, 846
  Cushing's syndrome and, 843
  hormones of, 842
  hyperfunction, 843

hypofunction, 844
  medulla, 846
  shock and, 152
  tuberculosis, 845
  tumours, 843, 844, 846
  virilism, 844
Adrenaline,
  production by tumours, 846
Adrenocortical hormones (see also
  Aldosterone etc.), 842
Adrenocorticotrophic hormone,
  secretion by tumours, 843
Adult Respiratory
Distress Syndrome (ARDS) 316
Afibrinogenaemia, 565
Aflatoxin, effects on liver, 477
Age, cancer and, 200
Ageing, 14
Agglutination reactions, 103
Agranulocytic angina, 550
Agranulocytosis, 550
AIDS, 113
Air embolism, 128
Albers-Schonberg disease, 806
Alcohol, chronic pancreatitis and, 495
  effects on liver, 455
Alcoholic cirrhosis, 461
  hepatitis, 455
  hyaline, 455
  Aldosterone
  Conn's syndrome and, 844
  primary hyperaldosteronism, 844
  renin and, 842
Aleukaemic leukaemia, 589
Alimentary tract, 366 et seq.
  lymphomas, 411
Alkaline phosphatase,
  in osteoblastic activity, 794, 802
Alkalosis, in Conn's syndrome, 844
  in intestinal obstruction, 428
  tetany and, 844
  vomiting and, 428
Allergic encephalomyelitis,
  experimental, 745

Allergy, 109
Alzheimer neurofibrillary
  degeneration, 732
Alzheimer's disease, 732
Amaurotic familial idiocy, 750
Amino-aciduria, in Fanconi's
  syndrome, 642
  in liver disease, 469
Amniotic fluid embolism, 128
Amoebiasis,
  hepatic, 473
  intestinal, 417
Amoebic dysentery, 417
Amylase levels in acute pancreatitis,
491
Amyloid degeneration, 15-18
  classification, 18
  distribution in tissues, 16
  etiology, 17
  in myelomatosis, 606
  nature of, 15
  nephrotic syndrome and, 638
  staining of amyloid, 15
Amyotrophic lateral sclerosis, 759
Anaemia
  Addisonian, 518-521
  aplastic, 512
  in chronic disease, 543
  classification, 511
  definition, 509
  dyshaemopoietic, 511, 512
  effects, 509, 526, 527
  folic acid deficiency, 522
  haemolytic, 23, 525-542
  hypersplenism, 542, 582
  hypochromic microcytic, 513, 545
  hypoplastic, 512, 557
  in malignant disease, 543
  iron deficiency, 513-516
  leuco-erythroblastic, 544
  macrocytic, 544
  megaloblastic, 517-522
  normocytic, 543
  pernicious, 518-521

Anaemia (Contd)
post-haemorrhagic, 523, 524
refractory, 544
sideroblastic, 544
splenic, 582
in uraemia, 543
Analgesic abuse, kidney in, 638
Anaphylactic immune reaction,
109, 110
in hay fever, 110
in asthma, 110
Anaphylactic shock, 110
Anaphylactoid purpura, 566
kidney in, 634
Anaphylatoxins, 104
Anaplasia, definition of, 165
Anencephaly, 768
Aneurysmal bone cyst, 807
Aneurysms,
berry, 228, 725
cardiac, 263
causes, 226
cerebral, 725
cirsoid, 228
micro, 228
mycotic, 229
types, 227
Angina, agranulocytic, 550
pectoris, 254, 265
Vincent's, 370
Angiofibroma, juvenile, of nose, 294
Angioleiomyoma, 241
Angioma, 190
cavernous, 190
sclerosing, 242
Angioneurotic oedema, 142
Angiotensin
in hypertension, 218
Aniline dyes,
bladder cancer and, 663
Anisocytosis of red cells, 503
Ankylosing spondylitis, 817
Anoxaemia (see Hypoxaemia) 136
Anthracosis, 342
focal dust emphysema in, 342
progressive massive fibrosis in, 343
Antibodies (see also
Immunoglobulins)
agglutinating, 103
antigen-combining sites of, 96
anti-tumour, 205
auto-, 115-117
cross-reactions, 96
cytotoxic, 110

opsonic effect of, 103
precipitating, 103
specificity of, 95
Antibody production, 98
cells involved in, 98
plasma cells and, 98
primary response, 95
secondary response, 95
thymic-dependent, 97
thymic-independent, 97
Anticoagulants
endogenous, 560, 562
therapy, 563
Antidiuretic hormone, 828
Antifreeze poisoning, 639
Antigen-antibody complexes,
pathogenic effects of, 109-111
Antigen-antibody reactions, 95
Antigens, 96
determinant sites of, 96
tumour, 205
valency, 96
Antinuclear factors, 116, 821
Anti-oncogens, 198
Antiserum, 118
Antitoxic reactions, 103
Aorta,
aneurysm, 227
atheroma, 210
medial necrosis, 222
rupture of, 227
syphilis, 227
Aortic valve, calcific stenosis of, 277
chronic rheumatic disease of, 277,
278
incompetence, 278
in rheumatic fever, 274, 278
stenosis, 277
in syphilis, 278
Aortitis, syphilitic, 62
Aphthous stomatitis, 366
Aplastic anaemia, 512
classification, 557
drug-induced, 557
Apoplectic cyst, 723, 724
Apoptosis, 7
Appendicitis
acute, 42, 412
chronic, 415
gangrenous, 413
perforating, 413
Appendix,
abscess, 414
actinomycosis, 471

appendicitis, 412-415
carcinoid of, 410
concretions in. 413
mucocele, 415
obstruction, 413
Apudomas, 411
Aqueduct of Sylvius atresia, 766
Argentaffin cells, carcinoid and, 409
Arnold-Chiari malformation, 766
Arrhenoblastoma, 689
Arteries, 208-231
age effects of, 134, 216
aneurysms, 226-229
arteriosclerosis, 216
arteritis, 208, 223-225
atheroma, 134, 208-215
calcification, 216, 222
endarteritis obliterans, 221
Erdheim's medial degeneration, 235
fibrosis, 208, 216
hyaline change, 216, 221
hypertension changes in, 217, 221
medial calcification, 216, 222
Monckebergs' sclerosis, 222
narrowing, effects of, 210
occlusion, effects of, 210
polyarteritis nodosa, 208, 223
Raynaud's disease and
phenomenon (syndrome),
230, 231
in syphilis, 62
thrombosis, 120 et seq.
Arterioles,
arteriolosclerosis, 216
in benign hypertension, 221
in diabetes, 839
fibrinoid necrosis, 221
hyaline change, 221
in malignant hypertension, 221
Arteriosclerosis, 217
diabetes. 839
Arteriolosclerosis, 216
in hypertension, 221
senile, 216
Arteritis, 223-225
Buerger's disease, 224
in connective tissue diseases, 223
etiology, 224
giant cell, 225
polyarteritis nodosa, 223
syphilitic, 62
Takayashu's 225
temporal, 225
tuberculous, 734

Arteritis (Contd)
  in Wegener's granulomatosis, 223
Arthritis, 811-818
  acute infective, 818
  in ankylosing spondylitis, 817
  in brucellosis, 818
  gonococcal, 818
  in gout, 814
  neuropathic, 813
  osteoarthritis, 813, 814, 818
  in pseudo-gout, 814
  psoriatic, 812
  in Reiter's syndrome, 817
  rheumatic, 820
  rheumatoid, 815, 816, 818
  suppurative, 818
  tuberculous, 818
Arthus type of hypersensitivity, 111
Asbestosis, 346, 347
  mesothelioma and, 363
Aschoff body, 272
Ascites,
  chylous, 240
  in cirrhosis, 139, 460, 466
  in liver failure, 467
Askanazy cells 830
Aspergillosis, 348
Aspergillus flavus, aflatoxin and, 477
Aspirin,
  gastric haemorrhage and, 381
  peptic ulcer and, 388
Asthma,
  bronchial, 110
  cardiac, 251
Astrocytes, 713
Astrocytoma, 770
Ataxia, cerebellar, 761
  Friedreich's, 761
Atelectasis of lung, 314
Atheroma, 209-215
  changes in, 209, 210
  complications, 210
  etiology, 214, 215
  mechanisms, 211-213
  thrombosis in, 210
Atheromatous aneurysm, 210, 227, 229
Atopy, 109
Atrial fibrillation, 276
Atrophy, 13
  brown, 269
Auditory nerve,
  Schwannoma of, 774
Auer rods, 590
Auto-antibodies, 116

to adrenal, 845
colonic epithelium, 419
gastric mucosa, 383, 520
glomerular basement membrane, 62?
heart muscle, 276
intrinsic factor, 520
liver, 463
mitochondria, 116
nervous tissue, 747
nuclei, 116
platelets, 566
red cells, 537
smooth muscle, 116
skeletal muscle, 790
thyroid gland, 116, 830
Auto-antigens, tolerance to, 108
Auto-immune diseases (see also
    various organs and tissues),
    115-117
  auto-antibodies, 116, 117
Auto-immune haemolytic anaemia, 537
Autolysis, 6

Bacillary dysentery, 416
Bacteraemia, 52
Bacterial endocarditis, 279, 280
  infections, 48-64
Bacterial shock, 145, 156
Bacteriuria,
  asymptomatic, 645
  in pyelonephritis, 645
Bagassosis, 348
Bamboo spine, 817
Basal-cell carcinoma, 183
Battered baby syndrome, 803
Bell's palsy, 764
Bence-Jones protein, 606
Benign tumours, general features, 163
  of connective tissue, 166-169
  of epithelium, 170-173
Benzidine, bladder cancer and, 663
Benzpyrene, 194
Berry aneurysm, 228, 725
Bile changes in composition of, 480
  'white', 486
Bile ducts,
  calculi in, 484
  carcinoma 487
  infection, 486
  obstruction, 22, 486
  in primary biliary cirrhosis, 463
  proliferation in cirrhosis, 464

tumours, 487
Bile pigment,
  formation of, 21, 527
  in jaundice, 22
  metabolism, 21
  stones, 484
Bile salts, in cholecystitis, 480
Biliary,
  abscesses, 471
  cirrhosis, primary, 463
  cirrhosis, secondary (obstructive),
    464
  colic, 486
  pigmentation, 22
Bilirubin formation, 21, 527
  glucuronide, 21
  metabolism, 527
Bird-fancier's lung, 348
Bittner milk factor, 197
Blackwater fever, 541
Bladder (see also Urinary bladder),
  660
Bleeding time, in haemophilia, 564
  in idiopathic thrombocytopenic
      purpura, 566
Blood,
  absolute values, 502, 503
  clotting factors, 561
  coagulation, 560, 561
  cross-matching, 567-570
  fibrinolytic system, 562
  groups, 567, 568
  volume, 136, 151
Blood groups,
  gastric carcinoma and, 393
Blood pressure in shock, 146
Blood transfusion, 567-570
  haemolytic reactions, 533-534
  serum hepatitis and, 570
Bone, 793-810
  achondroplasia, 806
  in acromegaly, 801
  in Albers-Schönberg disease, 806
  atrophy, 796
  avascular necrosis, 803
  calcification, 795
  compact, 793
  in battered baby syndrome, 803
  in Cushing's syndrome, 798
  cysts of, 807
  eosinophil granuloma, 807
  in fibrous dysplasia, 802
  formation, 795
  fracture healing, 88-91

Bone (*Contd*)
  in Hand-Schuller-Christian disease, 607
  haversian system, 794
  in hyperparathyroidism, 801
  in hypertrophic osteoarthropathy, 801
  involucrum, 805
  lamellar, 793
  in malabsorption syndrome, 408
  metaplastic, 785
  in myelomatosis, 605
  normal structure, 793-795
  in osteitis deformans, 802
  osteochondritis juvenilis, 803
  osteogenesis imperfecta, 806
  osteomalacia, 799, 800
  osteomyelitis, 804, 805
  osteopetrosis, 806
  osteoporosis, 796-798
  in Paget's disease, 802
  parathormone, 795, 841
  pyogenic infections, 804
  in renal tubular disease, 800, 841
  resorption, 796
  rickets, 799
  in scurvy, 803
  sequestrum 805
  subperiosteal haematoma, 803
  tuberculosis, 805
  tumours, primary, 807-810
    secondary, 697, 704, 810
  in uraemia, 800
  in vitamin C deficiency, 803
  in vitamin D deficiency, 799, 800
  woven, 795
Bone marrow,
  aplasia, 557
  erythropoiesis in, 524
  in haemolytic anaemia, 528
  haemopoiesis in, 500
  hyperplasia, 512, 546, 547
  in iron deficiency anaemia, 512
  leucopoiesis in, 548, 549
  in leukaemia, 586-594
  in lymphocytic leukaemia, 592
  in megaloblastic anaemia, 520·
  in myelomatosis, 605
  in myeloproliferative disorders, 557
  platelet production in, 556
Bouchard's nodes, 814
Boundary Zones, 153, 722
Brain (see also Nervous system)
  abscess, 733-735

ageing, 731
Alzheimer's disease, 732
in amoebiasis, 744
aneurysms, 725, 726
applied anatomy, 710
atheroma, 721
atrophy, 722, 731
cerebral haemorrhage, 724, 725
cerebrospinal fluid, 778
chorea, 754
circulatory disturbances, 161, 719
concussion, 728
congenital abnormalities, 768
coning, 717
demyelinating diseases, 745-747
distortions and dislocations, 717
encephalitis, 741, 742, 745
encephalomyelitis, 745
encephalopathy, 748
expanding lesions, intracranial, 716
extrapyramidal disorders, 753, 754
in general paralysis of the insane, 63
gliosis, 713
haemorrhage, intracranial, 724-727
  extradural, 729
  intracerebral, 724-747
  subarachnoid, 725
  subdural, 729
  traumatic, 727, 728
in head injury, 727
herniation, 717
in Huntington's chorea, 754
hydatid cyst, 744
hydrocephalus, 765-767
in hypertension, 726
in hypoglycaemia, 752
infarction, 130, 153, 721-723
inflammation, 733-735
kernicterus, 535
in liver failure, 468
in malaria, 742
meninges, 710,711
meningitis, 733-736
neuroglia, 713
neurones, 712
nuclear jaundice, 535
oedema, 715
in phenylketonuria, 750
senile dementia, 732
Tay-Sach's disease, 750
syphilis, 63
thrombosis, 721
in toxoplasmosis, 743
trauma, 727, 728

in trypanosomiasis, 744
tuberculosis, 736
tumours,
  primary 769-773
  secondary, 775
vascular malformations, 772
virus infections, 737-742
Breast (see also Nipple), 692
  abscess, 692
  adenosis, 693
  carcinoma, 696-697
  in mice, 197
  cystadenoma, papillary, 694
  cystic disease, 693
  duct ectasia, 692
  epitheliosis, 693
  fibroadenoma, 173, 693
  giant intracanalicular, 694
  intraduct carcinoma, 695
  intraduct papilloma, 694
  mastitis, 692
  mastopathy, cystic, 693
  Paget's disease of nipple, 695
  papilloma, 694
  sarcoma, 694
  sclerosing adenosis, 693
  tumours, primary, 693-697
Brenner tumour, 691
Bronchi and bronchioles, 299 et seq.
  adenoma, 352
  in asthma, 302
  bronchiectasis, 304-307
  bronchiolitis, 299 et seq.
  bronchitis, 299
  carcinoma, 353-360
  obstruction, 306, 317, 331
  virus infection, 299
Bronchiectasis, 304-307
Bronchitis, 299
Bronchopneumonia (see also
    Pneumonia), 319-321
  aspiration, 328
  influenzal, 325
  simple nom-suppurative, 319
  suppurative, 321
  tuberculous, 337
Bronzed diabetes, 24
Brown atrophy, 25, 269
Brown-Kelly-Paterson syndrome, 516
Brucellosis, 818
Buerger's disease, 224
Bulbar paralysis, progressive, 759
Burkitt's lymphoma, 197, 198, 608
Burns, 155

Burns (contd)
  renal failure and, 639
  shock in, 155
Burr cells, 503
Bursa of Fabricius, 97
Bursae, 820
Byssinosis, 348

Caecum
  'hyperplastic tuberculosis'
    of, 402
Caeruloplasmin, 751
Calcification,
  of bone, 795
  pathological, 19
Calcitonin, 795, 802
Calcium carbonate stones
  biliary, 484
  pancreatic, 495
Calculi, biliary (gallstones), 484
  renal, 661
  salivary, 371
  urinary, 661
  vesical, 662
Callus, 88, 89
Campylobacter pylori, 388, 389
Candidiasis, 71, 330
  of oesophagus, 375
  of oral mucosa, 366
Capillaries, in inflammation, 31
  sphincter control of, 31
  thrombosis, 125
Capillary angioma, 190
Carbon tetrachloride,
  effects on kidney, 639
  effects on liver, 444
Carcino-embryonic antigen, 426
Carcinogenic agents,
  chemical, 194, 195, 360
  hormones, 199
  initiating factors, 195, 202
  promoting factors, 199, 203
  radiation, 196
  trauma, 200
  viruses, 197, 198
Carcinoid syndrome, 410, 411
  valvular lesions in, 411
Carcinoid tumour, bronchial, 352
  intestinal, 410
Carcinoma (see also various organs)
  definition, 175
  metastases, distribution of,

176 et seq.
  myopathy and, 790
  predisposing conditions, 199, 200
  spread of, 176, et seq.
  varieties of 182-184
Carcinoma-in-situ, 174
  of cervix, 676, 677
Cardiac (see also Heart)
  aneurysm, 263
  arrhythmias, 261
  asthma, 251
  fibrosis, 254, 264
  musculature, 252
  output, 253
  tamponade, 284
Cardiogenic shock, 145, 149
Cardiomyopathy, 268
Carditis, rheumatic, 270-273
Carotid body tumour, 241
Cartilage, in stroma of tumours,
  tumours of, 372
Caseation, 5, 58
Casts, urinary, 618
Catarrhal inflammation, 41
Catecholamines, 146, 846
Cats, virus leukaemia of, 197
Cat-scratch fever, 574
Cavernous angioma, 190
Cells,
  damage, 2-12, 28
  death, 2
  giant, 43, 69
  labile, 81
  permanent, 81
  stable, 81
Cellulitis, 46
Cerebrospinal fluid, 765, 778
  abnormalities, 778
  circulation, 765
  normal, 778
  pressure raised, 765
Cervix uteri,
  carcinoma, 678
  carcinoma-in-situ, 677
  congenital erosion, 675
  cytology, 680
  endocervicitis, 676
  epidermidisation, 676
  erosions, 675
Chains (lg), 99
Chalone, 82
Chancre, syphilitic, 366
Cheilosis, 516
Chemical carcinogens, 194, 195

Chemodectoma, 241
Chemotaxis, 34
  complement and, 104
Chimney sweep's cancer, 706
Chloasma, 20
Chloroform, effects on liver, 443
Cholangiocarcinoma, 475
Cholangitis, 471
  gallstones and, 486
Cholecystitis, 480
  composition of bile in, 480
Cholelithiasis, 483, 484
Cholera, 400
Cholestasis, cirrhosis and, 463
  drug-induced, 465
  extrahepatic, 464
  intrahepatic, 463
  obstructive jaundice and, 463
Cholesterol (see also
    Hypercholesterolaemia)
  in atheroma, 212
  in gallbladder, 482
  gallstones, 484
Cholesterosis of gallbladder, 482
Chondroma, 168
Chondromatosis, synovial, 819
Chondrosarcoma, 810
Chorea, 754
Choriocarcinoma, 672
  hormonal changes of, 672
  in teratoma, 707
Chorionic gonadotrophins, 672
Christmas disease, 561, 564
Chromaffin cells, 846
Chromosomal abnormalities,
  in chronic myeloid leukaemia, 591
  in Klinefelter's syndrome, 698
  in Turner's syndrome, 698
Chronic granulomatous disease, 551,
  552
Chronic inflammation, 39, 43
Chronic venous congestion, 135
Chylous ascites, 240
Cigarettes, bronchial carcinoma and,
  360
  chronic bronchitis and, 301
  co-carcinogenic action of, 360
  peptic ulcer and, 388
Circumcision
  cervical carcinoma
    and, 680
  penile carcinoma and, 705
Cirrhosis of liver, 457
  active chronic hepatitis and, 452

Cirrhosis of liver (*Contd*)
alcoholic, 461
auto-antibodies and, 459, 462, 463
biliary, primary, 463
secondary (obstructive), 464
carcinoma and, 460
cardiac, 465
in childhood, 461
cryptogenic, 465
dietary iron and, 24, 465
effects of, 459
etiology, 461 et seq.
in haemochromatosis, 465
macronodular, 457
malnutrition and, 461
micronodular, 457
obstructive biliary, 464
pigment, 465
post-hepatitic, 462
post-necrotic, 444
types of, 457
virus hepatitis and, 462
in Wilson's disease, 465
Cirsoid aneurysm, 228
Clear-cell renal carcinoma, 657
Clones in malignancy, 201
Clonorchis sinensis and
cholangiocarcinoma, 477
Clostridial infections, 56, 57
Cloudy swelling, 8
Clubbing of fingers, 307, 801
Coagulation of blood, 560
deficiency diseases, 561-565
Coagulative necrosis, 3
Coal miners,
anthracosis in, 342, 343
focal dust emphysema in, 342
progressive massive pulmonary
fibrosis in, 343
Co-carcinogens, 199, 200
Codman's triangle, 809
Coeliac disease, 406
Cold abscess, 60
Cold haemagglutinin disease, 538
Colitis (see also Dysentery),
in regional enteritis, 403
ulcerative, 418
uraemic, 654
Collagen diseases, see Connective
tissue diseases, 820, 821
Collagen, formation of, 80
Collateral circulation, 129
Colliquative necrosis, 4
Colloid casts, 618

Colostrum, Ig in, 100
Coma,
diabetic, 776, 839
hepatic, 468
hypoglycaemic, 839
uraemic, 635
Comedo-carcinoma of breast, 695
Common bile duct, obstruction of, 486
Compensatory hypertrophy, 160
Complement, 103, 104
in acute glomerulonephritis, 623
Concussion, 728
Congestive splenomegaly, 580
Connective tissue diseases, 820, 821
Raynaud's phenomenon in, 231
tumours 166-169, 185-188
Conn's syndrome, 844
Constrictive pericarditis, 284
Contact inhibition, 81, 82
Contraceptive pill, 668
Contre-coup lesion, 728
Coronary arterial atheroma, 255-257
Coronary artery obstruction, effects
of, 254-256
Corrosive chemicals, effects of, 375
Coryza, acute, 290
Councilman body, 445
Coxsackie virus infections, 786
Craniopharyngioma, 773, 826
Creatinine clearance, 619
excretion, 619
Cretinism, 830
Crohn's disease, 403
Crush syndrome, 785
Cryoglobulinaemia, 604
Cryptococcosis, 742
Curling's ulcer, 152
Cushing's syndrome, 843
Cyanocobalamin, see vitamin B_{12}
Cyanosis, 136
Cystadenocarcinoma, 688
Cystadenoma, 172
multilocular of ovary, 172, 687
serous of ovary, 172, 686
Cystic disease of breast, 694
duct obstruction, 692
hygroma, 243
Cystitis, 660
Cytology, exfoliative, 680
cervical and vaginal, 680
nipple discharge, 694
Cytotoxic antibody, hypersensitivity
and, 110

Degenerations, definition, 26
Delayed hypersensitivity reactions,
109, 111
cells concerned in, 106
Dementia,
pre-senile, 732
senile, 732
Dermatomyositis, 790
Dermatopathic lymphadenopathy, 577
Dermoid cysts,
of nervous system, 773
of ovary, 189, 190
Desensitisation in allergy, 108
Diabetes, bronzed, 24
insipidus, 828
Diabetes mellitus, 836
kidney in, 637
peripheral neuropathy in, 764, 839
types of, 837-839
Diffuse lymphoma, 600-602
Diphtheria, 42, 292, 370
heart in, 267
larynx in, 292
neuropathy in, 764
prophylaxis, 118
Dissecting aneurysm, 228
Disseminated intravascular
coagulation, 148
Disuse atrophy, 13
Diuresis, osmotic, 837
Diverticula
intestinal, 427
B_{12} deficiency and, 427
Meckel's 389
oesophageal, 376
Diverticulitis, 427
Donovan bodies, 681
Ductus arteriosus, patent, 285
Duodenum (see also Intestine)
Curling's ulcer of, 152
peptic ulcer of, 386
Dupuytren's contracture, 166, 820
Dwarfism, achondroplastic, 806
in cretinism, 830
pituitary, 826
renal, 841
Dysentery,
amoebic, 417
bacillary, 416
Dysgerminoma, 690
Dyshaemopoietic anaemias, 511, 512
Dysplasia, 161, 174
Dysphagia, 516
Dystrophia adiposo-genitalis, 826

Dystrophic calcification, 19
Dystrophy, muscular, 788

Ectopic ACTH syndrome, 835, 840
Ectopic pregnancy, 684
Electrocardiography, 266
Electrolytes,
　in Addison's disease, 845
　in Conn's syndrome, 844
　in renal failure, 654
Elephantiasis, 240
Embolism, 128
　air, 128
　amniotic, 128
　fat, 90, 128
　parenchymal cell, 128
　pulmonary, 128, 132
　tumour, 128, 176-180
Emigration of leucocytes,
　in inflammation, 33,34
Emphysema,
　acute vesicular, 309
　atrophic (senile), 313
　centrilobular, 310
　classification, 308
　focal dust, 313
　interstitial, 313
　panacinar (panlobular), 309
Empyema, 46
　pleural, 362
Encephalitis, 733
　acute necrotising, 740
　lethargica, 741
　herpes simplex, 740
　measles, 741
　rabies, 741
　subacute sclerosing, 741
　toxoplasmosis, 743
　virus, 738
　zoster, 740
Encephalocele, 768
Encephaloid carcinoma, 696
Encephalomyelitis,
　acute disseminated, 745
　acute haemorrhagic, 745
　experimental allergic, 745
　post-infectious, 745
　post vaccinial 745
Encephalopathy, 748
　hepatic, 468, 749
　hypertensive, 726
　Wernicke's 748

Enchondroma, 168
Enchondromatosis, multiple, 168
End-arteries, 130
Endarteritis, 43
Endocarditis, acute bacterial, 124, 279
　rheumatic, 124, 272, 274
　subacute bacterial, 279
Endocrine glands, 824
Endogenous pigments, 20 et seq.
Endometriosis, 674
Endometritis, 667
Endometrium,
　adeno-acanthoma, 670
　adenomatous hyperplasia, 669
　carcinoma, 670
　cyclical changes in, 665, 666
　cystic hyperplasia, 668, 669
　endometritis, 667
　and oral contraceptives, 668
　polyps, 670
　stromal sarcoma, 671
　tuberculosis, 668
Endotoxic shock, 156
Endotoxins, 51, 156
End-stage kidney, 653
Enteric fever (see also Typhoid), 396
Enteritis, 395
Enterocolitis, 399
Eosinophil granuloma of bone, 807
　leucocytes, 553
　leucocytosis, 553
Epidermidisation of cervix, 676
Epididymitis, gonococcal, 700
　tuberculous, 701
Epilepsy, 777
Epithelial crescents, 621
　mucin, 26
　tumours
　　benign, 170
　　malignant, 175
Epithelioid cells, 58
Epitheliosis of breast, 693
Epithelium, repair of, 76
Epstein-Barr virus, 68, 148, 608
Epulis, 368
Erdheim's medial degeneration, 222
Erosions, cervical, 675
　gastric, 381
Erythroplasia of Queyrat, 705
Erythropoiesis, control of, 501
　essential factors in, 501
　megaloblastic, 507
　noromoblastic, 507
Erythropoietin, 501

in secondary polycythaemia, 546
Essential hypertension, 219
　kidney in, 649
Estrogens and cancer, 671, 697
Ethylene glycol poisoning, 639
Ewing's tumour of bone, 810
Exogenous pigments, 25
Exophthalmos, 831
Exostosis, 178, 807
Exotoxins, 51
Extradural haematoma, 729
Extramedullary haemopoiesis, 559
Extrapyramidal disorders, 753, 754
Eye in diabetes, 839
　retinoblastoma, 771

Fabricius, bursa of, 97
Facio-scapulo-humeral muscular
　dystrophy, 788
Fallopian tube,
　in ectopic pregnancy, 684
　haematosalpinx, 684
　hydrosalpinx, 683
　pyosalpinx, 683
　salpingitis, 683
　tuberculosis, 683
　tumours, 683
Fallot's tetralogy, 285
Fanconi's syndrome, 642
Farmer's lung, 348
Fat, abnormal storage, 9
　embolism, 90, 128
　necrosis, 491
　in pancreatitis, 491
Fatty change, 9, 10, 11
Fc fragment of immunoglobulins, 99
Feminisation, testicular, 698
Ferritin, 514
Fetal haemoglobin, 531
Fever, 72
　blackwater, 541
　glandular, 68, 573
　typhoid, 396-398
　uveo-parotid, 371
Fibrin formation, 560
Fibrinogen, conversion to fibrin
　deficiency, 560
Fibrinoid necrosis of arterioles, 221
Fibrinolysis, 126, 562, 563
Fibro-adenoma of breast, 173, 693
　giant intracanalicular, 694
Fibroblasts, 80

Fibrocystic disease of pancreas, 496
'Fibroid', uterine, 169, 673
Fibroma, 166
Fibromatosis, 166
Fibrosarcoma, 186
Fibrosis, 39, 40, 80
    cardiac, 254
Fibrous dysplasia of bone, 802
Filariasis, 240
Fistula, 46
Fluid balance, disturbances of,
    140 et seq.
Folic acid, 522
    action of, 517
    in malabsorption syndrome, 408
Follicle-stimulating hormone (FSH),
    666
Follicular lymphoma, 618, 620
Food poisoning, 400
Foramen ovale, persistent, 285
Fracture,
    complications, 90
    factors influencing, 91
    healing, 88
    pathological, 90
Friedreich's ataxia, 761
Fröhlich's syndrome, 826
Fungal infections in diabetes, 839
    of lung, 330
    of mouth, 366
    of oesophagus, 375
    opportunistic, 71
    of vulva, 681

Galactosaemia, 465
Gallbladder, 479
    cholecystitis, 480
    cholesterosis, 482
    gallstones, 483
    mucocele of 481, 486
    'strawberry', 482
    in typhoid fever, 396
Gallstone ileus, 486
Gallstones
    calcium carbonate, 484
    carcinoma and, 486
    cholesterol, 484
    effects of, 486
    in haemolytic anaemia, 484
    inflammatory, 485
    metabolic, 485
    mixed (laminated), 485

pigment, 484
Gammaglobulins, see
    immunoglobulins, 99-101
Ganglion, 820
Ganglioneuroma, 771
Gangrene, 4, 56
    in diabetics, 839
    dry, 56
    primary, 56
    wet, 56
Gas gangrene, 4, 56
Gastric atrophy, 383, 520
    mucosa, 382
        autoantibodies to, 383
        heterotopia, 389
        repair, 386
        ulcer, 384 et seq.
Gastrin-secreting tumours, 840
Gastritis,
    acute, 381
    atrophic, 382
    auto-immune, 383, 520
    chronic, 382
    iron deficiency and, 516
    pernicious anaemia and, 383, 520
    superficial, 382
    vitamin B_{12} deficiency and, 383, 520
Gastro-enteritis of infants, 395
Gaucher's disease, 27
General paralysis of the insane, 63
Germinal centres, lymphoid, 98
Ghon focus, 59, 332
Giant-cell, arteritis, 225
    epulis, 368
    tumour of bone, 187, 808
    tumour of tendon sheath, 819
Giant cells, 43
    virus-induced, 69
Giantism, pituitary, 827
Glandular fever, 68, 573
Glioblastoma multiforme, 770
Gliomas, 770
Gliosis, 713
Global infarct of heart, 258
Glomangioma, 241
Glomerulonephritis (see also
    Nephritis),
    acute diffuse proliferative, 621
    chronic, 635
    classification, 620
    complement and, 633
    focal, 626
    immunological features, 632
    membrano-proliferative, 631

membranous, 627
    minimal-change, 629
    oedema in, 622
    post-streptococcal, 621
    rapidly progressive, 624
Glomerulosclerosis, diabetic, 637
Glomus bodies, 241
Glomus jugulare tumour, 241
Glossitis, atrophic, 516
Glucocorticoid hormones,
    in Cushing's syndrome, 843
Glutamic-oxalacetic transaminase, 447
    -pyruvic transaminase, 447
Gluten enteropathy, 406
Glycogen storage disorders, 27, 465
Goitre,
    colloid, 833
    endemic, 833
    exophthalmic, 831
    iodide, 833
    iodine deficiency, 833
    non-toxic, 833
    parenchymatous, 833
    sporadic, 833
    toxic nodular, 831
Gonadotrophic hormones, 825
    production by tumours, 672, 707
Gonorrhoea,
    arthritis in, 818
    epididymitis in, 700
    prostatitis in, 55, 700
    salpingitis in, 55, 683
Goodpasture's syndrome, 625
Gout,
    joints in, 814
    kidney in, 642
Granular-cell myoblastoma,
    of tongue, 368
Granulation tissue, formation of, 39
    healing of wounds by, 76
Granuloma, 43
    eosinophil, 807
    infective, 43
    inguinale, 681
    talc, 43
    Wegener's, 223
Granulomatous disease,
    chronic, 552
    orchitis, 701
Granulosa-cell tumour, 689
Graves' disease, 117, 832
    immune mechanism in, 117, 832
Grawitz tumour, 657
Growth hormone, 824

Gumma, syphilitic, 62
Gynaecomastia, 697

Haemangio-endothelioma, 243
Haemangioma, 190
Haemangiosarcoma, 243
Haematocrit, 502
Haematosalpinx, 684
Haemochromatosis, 24
  liver in, 465
  pancreas in 24, 839
  skin pigmentation in, 24
Haemoglobin, abnormal forms, 532
  breakdown, 21
  concentration, 502
  MCH, 502
  MCHC, 502
  variations in level, 502
Haemoglobinopathies, 531, 532
Haemoglobinuria,
  in auto-immune haemolytic
    anaemia, 538
  in blackwater fever, 541
  cold, 538
  kidney in, 533, 641
  march, 540
  in transfusion reaction, 533
Haemolysis,
  kidney in, 528, 641
  in transfusion reactions, 533, 639
Haemolytic anaemia,
  auto-immune, 537
  bile pigment metabolism in, 22, 527
  blackwater fever, 541
  bone marrow, 528
  in burns, 542
  changes, 327, 528
  classification, 529
  causes of, 529
  drug-induced, 539
  general features, 525-542
  glucose-6-phosphate deficiency, 530
  haemoglobinopathies, 531, 532
  haptoglobins in, 528
  hereditary elliptocytosis, 529
  hereditary spherocytosis, 529
  hypersplenism in, 542
  malaria, 539, 541
  march haemoglobinuria, 540
  microangiopathic, 540
  of newborn, 534, 536
  paroxysmal nocturnal

  haemoglobinuria, 529
  pyruvate kinase, 530
  radioisotopes, use of, 526
  sickle-cell disease, 532
  thalassaemia, 532
Haemolytic antibodies, 533-538
  disease of newborn, 534
  jaundice, 527
  toxins and chemicals, 539
Haemolytic uraemic syndrome, 641
Haemopericardium, 284
Haemophilia, 564
Haemopoiesis, 500
Haemopoietic stem cells, 500 et seq
Haemorrhage (see also Purpura),
  acute renal failure following, 151
  petechial, 565, 566
  shock and, 145
Haemorrhagic diseases, 562-566
  erosions of stomach, 381
  inflammation, 42
  sarcoma (Kaposi), 243
  telangiectasis, hereditary, 242
  thrombocythaemia, 566
Haemorrhoids, 139, 232
Haemosiderin deposition, 23, 525
  et seq.
Haemostasis, 560
Haemothorax, 318
Hamartoma, definition, 190
Hamman-Rich syndrome, 349
Hand-Schüller-Christain disease, 607
Haptens, 96
Haptoglobins,
  in haemolytic anaemia, 528
Hashimoto's disease, 116
Hay fever, 110, 291
Headache, 776
Head injury,
  brain damage in, 728
  delayed complications, 729, 730
  extradural haemorrhage, 729
  fracture of skull in, 727
  subdural haematoma in, 729
Healing,
  chalones, 82
  collagen synthesis, 80
  complications, 79
  contraction, 78
  contact inhibition, 82
  factors influencing, 80
  fibrosis, 80
  by first intention, 76
  regenertion, 81, 82

  by second intention, 77
  special situations, 83-91
  vitamin C deficiency and, 80, 91
  wound healing, 76-79
Heart (see also Cardiac)
  adiposity, 269
  amyloidosis, 16
  aneurysm of, 263
  atrophy, 269
  block, 282
  cardiomyopathy, 268
  compensatory mechanisms, 246, 248
  congenital malformations, 285
  coronary artery disease, 254-257
  endocarditis, bacterials, 279, 280
  failure, 245-253
  fatty change, 10, 269
  hypertrophy, 248
  infarction, 131, 258-263
  ischaemia, chronic, 264
  myocarditis, 267
  pericardium, 283, 284
  rheumatic disease of, 270-273
  rupture of, 262
  septal defects, 285
  in shock, 149
  thrombosis in, 124, 261
  tumours, 284
  valvular diseases, 274-278
Heavy chains, 99
Heberden's nodes, 814
Heinz bodies, 505
Helicobacter pylori, 388, 389
Henoch-Schönlein purpura, 566
Hepatic
  encephalopathy, 470
  venous obstruction, 460
Hepatisation of lung, 322
Hepatitis,
  active chronic, 452
  alcoholic, 455
  amoebic, 473
  chronic, cirrhosis and, 462
  infective, 445
  transaminase levels in, 447
  virus, 445
Hepato-cellular failure, 467-470
  jaundice, 22
Hepato-lenticular degeneration, 465
Hepatoma, 475
Hermaphroditism, 698
Hernia, of brain, 716, 717
  hiatus, 375
  of intestine, 430

Herpes
  simplex, 67, 740
  zoster, 67, 740
Hiatus hernia, 375
Hirschsprung's disease, 434
Histamine
  in anaphylaxis, 110
  -fast achlorhydria, 520
  in inflammation, 36
Histiocytes, 607
'Histiocytosis X', 607
Hodgkin's disease, 595-598
  anaemia in, 598
  blood picture in, 597
  depression of 'T' cell function in, 598
  lymphocyte predominant, 597
  lymphocyte depleted, 597
  microscopic appearances, 597
  mixed cellularity, 597
  nodular sclerosing, 597
  spleen in, 596
  staging, 596
  variants, of, 597
'Honeycomb' lung, 350
Hormone-dependent tumours, 671, 697
Hormones
  carcinogenic effects on, 671
  production of, by tumours, 357
Horse-shoe kidney, 655
Hour-glass stomach, 386
Howell-Jolly bodies, 505, 519
Howslip's lacunae, 794
Hüntington's chorea, 754
Hurthle cells, 834
Hyaline degeneration, 26
  membrane disease, 315
Hyaluronidase, streptococcal, 54
Hydatid disease, 474, 744
Hydatidiform mole, 672
  penetrating, 672
Hydrocephalus, 765-767
  acquired, 766
  communicating, 765
  congenital, 766
  non-communicating, 765
  secondary, 767
Hydronephrosis, 658
Hydrophobia, 741
Hydropic swelling, 8
Hydrops foetalis, 535
Hydrosalpinx, 683
Hydrothorax, 333, 337, 361
5-Hydroxytryptamine, 410

Hygroma, cystic, 243
Hyperaemia,
  active, 30, 31
  inflammatory, 30, 31
Hyperaldosteronism, 844
Hyperbetalipoproteinaemia, 27
Hypercalcaemia,
  in bronchial carcinoma, 357
  in hyperparathyroidism, 841
  in hypervitaminosis D, 642
  in immobilisation, 797
  in myelomatosis, 605
Hypercholesterolaemia, 27
  in atheroma, 214
  essential familial, 27
  in myxoedema, 829
  in nephrotic syndrome, 628
Hypergammaglobulinaemia, 73
Hyperglycaemia, 837
Hyperlipidaemia,
  in nephrotic syndrome, 628
Hypernephroma, 657
Hyperparathyroidism, 841
  bone changes in, 801
  primary, 841
  secondary, 841
Hyperplasia, 160
Hyperplastic caecal tuberculosis, 402
  cystic disease of breast, 693
Hypersensitivity reactions, 109-111
  anaphylactic (type I), 110
  Arthus (type III), 111
  atopic (type I), 109
  auto-immune, 115
  cytotoxic (type II), 110
  delayed (type IV), 111
  immune-complex (type III), 111
  types of, 109 et seq.
Hypersplenism, 581
Hypertension, systemic,
  arteriolosclerosis in, 216, 221
  arteriosclerosis in, 216, 221
  benign, 220, 221
  brain in, 726
  classification 220
  in Conn's syndrome, 219, 844
  essential, 219
  etiology, 218
  heart in, 221, 247
  hyperaldosteronism in, 219, 844
  kidney in, 219, 221, 649
  malignant, 220, 221
  phaeochromocytoma and, 219, 846
  portal, 460

  primary, 219
  pulmonary, 234, 251, 312
  renal, 652
  secondary, 219
  vascular changes in, 221
Hypertensive encephalopathy, 726
Hyperthyroidism, 832
Hypertrophic, pulmonary
  osteoarthropathy, 801
Hypertrophy, 160
Hyperuricaemia, 814
Hypervitaminosis D, 642
Hypoaldosteronism, 845
Hypocalcaemia, parathyroid
  deficiency and, 841
  in renal failure, 800
  in rickets, 799
Hypochromic microcytic anaemia, 545
Hypoglycaemia, 839
Hypoparathyroidism, 841
Hypophysis (see also Pituitary), 824
Hypoplastic anaemia (see Aplastic
  anaemia)
Hyposplenism, 583
Hypotension
  in Addison's disease, 845
  in myocardial infarction, 145
  in shock, 148
  in vaso-vagal attack, 154
Hypothyroidism, 829
Hypovolaemia, 145
Hypovolaemic shock, 145
Hypoxia, 136
  cerebral, 719, 720

Icterus gravis neonatorum, 534, 535
Ileitis, regional, 403
Ileus, 434
  biochemical changes, 434
  gallstone, 486
  paralytic, 434
Immediate type hypersensitivity, 109
Immobilisation osteoporosis, 797
Immune-complex nephritis, 634
Immune-complex reactions, 111
Immune reactions, 102-104
Immune response, 94-98
  cell co-operation in 94
  cell mediated, 98, 106
  cellular basis of, 97, 98
  humoral, 98
  in infections, 94

Immune response (Contd)
  primary, 95
  secondary, 95
  specifically responsive cells in, 98
  thymic-dependent, 97
Immune serum, 118
Immunisation, active, 118
  passive, 118
Immunity, 94-118
  applications, 118
  memory and recognition, 95, 98
  non-specific associated
    mechanisms, 94
Immunoglobulin, A(IgA), 101
Immunoglobulin, D(IgD), 101
Immunoglobulin, E(IgE), 101
Immunoglobulin, G(IgG), 100
Immunoglobulin, M(IgM), 100
Immunoglobulins, 99-101
  Fab fragment of, 99
  Fc fragment of, 99
  heavy chains of, 99
  light chains of, 99
  myeloma, 604
  in myelomatosis, 605
Immunological tolerance, 108
Immunopathology, 109 et seq.
Inclusion bodies, 69
Infantile paralysis (see Poliomyelitis)
Infantilism, pituitary, 826
Infarction, 130-133
  cardiac, 256-263
  effects of, 130, 261-263
  enzyme changes, 266
  global, 258
  septic, 52, 53
Infection,
  acute bacterial, 54-57
  chronic, 58-64
  defence mechanisms in, 49, 50
  definition of, 48
  effects of, 72, 73
  ESR, 73
  factors influencing, 49, 50
  failure of defence mechanisms, 50
  fever in, 72
  immune response in, 50, 51
  mechanism of production, 51 et seq.
  metabolic effects, 73
  'opportunistic', 71
  plasma proteins, 73
  pyogenic, 54, 55
  routes of entry, 48
  virus, 65-70

Infectious mononucleosis, 68, 573
Infective endocarditis, 279, 280
Infective hepatitis, 445
Infertility, 698
Inflammation, 30-46
  abscess, 38
  acute, 30-32
  blood flow, changes in, 31
  catarrhal, 41
  causes, 30
  chemotaxis in, 34
  chemical factors, 36
  chronic, 43 et seq.
  emigration of polymorphs in, 33
  exudation in, 32, 41
  granuloma, 43
  margination of polymorphs in, 33
  microcirculatory changes in, 31
  oedema in, 32, 142
  organisation, 40
  phagocytosis in, 34, 35
  resolution of, 37
  sequels of, 37-40
  signs of, 30
  suppuration, 38, 42
  ulceration, 44
  vascular hyperaemia in, 30, 31
  vascular permeability in, 32
Inflammatory oedema, 32, 142
Influenza, 325
Insect bite, 111
Insulin, antibodies to, 838
  diabetes and, 838
Insulin-secreting tumours, 840
Interferon, 70
Interstitial-cell tumour of testis, 707
Interstitial fluid, control of changes
    in, 140
  myocarditis, 267
  nephritis, 643
  salpingitis, 683
Intervertebral disc, prolapse of, 755
Intestine (see also Appendix,
    Caecum, Rectum)
  amoebiasis, 417
  amyloidosis, 16
  appendicitis, 412 et seq.
  auto-antibodies to, 406
  bacillary dysentery, 416
  carcinoid, 409-411
  carcinoma, 409, 424-426
  cholera, 400
Crohn's disease, 400, 403, 404, 420
  diverticula, 427

  duodenal ulcer, 388, 389
  dysentery, 416
  enteritis, 395
  enterocolitis, 399
  in food poisoning, 400
  gastro-enteritis of infancy, 400
  gluten-enteropathy, 406
  hernia, 430
  Hirschsprung's disease, 434
  ileus, 434
  infarction, 133
  intussusception, 432
  lymphoid polyposis, 423
  lymphoma, 411, 608
  malabsorption syndrome, 405-408
  Meckel's diverticulum, 384
  obstruction, 428 et seq.
  paratyphoid fever, 398
  peptic ulceration of, 384-389
  Peutz-Jeghers syndrome, 367, 409
  polypi, 409, 421
  polypoid adenoma, 421
  polyposis coli, 423
  proctitis, 420
  pseudopolyposis, 423
  regional enteritis, 403
  stercoral ulcer, 429
  strangulation, 431
  tropical sprue, 406
  tuberculosis, 401
  tumours of large intestine, 421
  tumours of small intestine, 409
  typhoid fever, 396-398
  ulcerative colitis, 418
  in uraemia, 654
  villous papilloma, 422
  volvulus, 433
  Whipple's disease, 406
Intracranial pressure increased,
    716-718
Intraduct carcinoma of breast, 695
Intrinsic factor, 518
  auto-antibodies to, 520
Intussusception, 432
Involucrum, 805
Iodine deficiency, 833
  metabolism, 829
Ionising radiations, 196
Iron balance, 515
  metabolism, 514
Iron-binding capacity in iron
    deficiency, 513
Iron-deficiency anemia, 513-516
  associated changes, 516

Ischaemia,
 cerebral, 719 et seq.
 local, 129 et seq.
Ischaemic heart disease, 245, 254
 et seq.
Islet cell tumours, 840
Iso-antibodies, 533
 antigens, 533

Jaundice
 cholestatic, 463
 haemolytic (acholuric), 527
 obstructive, 486
Joints
 arthritis, 811-818
 Charcot's, 813
 effusion, 812
 loose bodies in, 819
 neuropathic, 813
 normal structure, 811
 in osteoarthritis, 813, 814, 818
 pigmented villondular synovitis, 819
 in rheumatoid arthritis, 815, 816,
  818
 synovial chondromatosis, 819
 synovial sarcoma, 819
Juxtaglomerular apparatus, 218

Kallikrein, 36
Kaposi's haemorrhagic sarcoma, 243
Kappa chain, 99
Karyolysis, 3
Karyorrhexis, 3
Kayser-Fliescher ring, 751
Keloid, 79, 166
Kernicterus, 535
Kernohan's notch, 717
Ketonuria in diabetes, 837
Ketosis in diabetes, 837
Kidney
 abortion and, 636
 acute tubular necrosis, 636, 639
 agenesia of, 655
 amyloidosis of, 16, 638
 in analgesic abuse, 638
 in anaphylactoid purpura, 634
 in arteriosclerosis, 221, 649
 in benign essential hypertension, 649
 chemicals, nephrotoxic and, 639
 congenital abnormalities, 655

cortical necrosis, 641
in 'crush syndrome', 785
in diabetes mellitus, 637
in drug hypersensitivity, 638
in eclampsia, 636
end-stage, 653
failure, see Renal, 653
fatty change, 10
functions, 612-619
glomerulonephritis, 620
in Goodpasture's syndrome, 625
in gout, 642
granular contracted, 635
haemolytic uraemic syndrome, 641
horseshoe, 655
hypertensive changes, 651
in hyperuraemia, 642
hypoplasia, 655
infarction of, 130
juxtaglomerular apparatus, 218
lipoid nephrosis, 628
lower nephron nephrosis, 639
in malignant hypertension, 651
in massive hepatic necrosis, 469
in microangiopathic polyarteritis,
 634
in myeloma, 606
nephritis, 620
nephrocalcinosis, 642
nephrotic syndrome, 627
nephrotoxic chemicals and, 639
papillary necrosis, 638, 644
in periarteritis nodosa, 223, 634
polycystic disease, 656
in pregnancy, 636
pyelonephritis, 644
in shock, 151, 639
in subacute bacterial endocarditis,
 280
in systemic lupus erythematosus, 634
'transfusion', 533, 639
tuberculosis, 648
tumours of, 657, 658
ultrastructure of, 613
Kimmelstiel-Wilson lesion, 637
Kinins, in inflammation, 36
Klinefelter's syndrome, 698
Koilonychia, 516
Krukenberg tumour, 392
Kulschitsky cells, carcinoid and, 409
Kuru, 68, 742

Labile cells, 81
Lacrimal gland in Sjögren's
 syndrome, 371
Lactogenic hormone, 825
Landry-Guillain-Barré syndrome, 763
Langhans' giant cells, 43
Larynx
 in angioneurotic oedema, 142
 diphtheria, 292
 inflammation, 292
 oedema glottidis, 292
 singers' node (fibroma), 294
 syphilis, 292, 293
 tuberculosis, 306
 tumours, 294
 in typhoid fever, 292
LATS, 832
Lead poisoning,
 neuropathy in, 764
 punctate basophilia in, 505
Leather-bottle stomach, 391
Left ventricular failure, 250-253
 hypertrophy, 247
Legionnaire's disease, 327
Leiomyoma, 169, 673
Leiomyosarcoma, 188
Leprosy, 64
Leptospirosis, 472
Letterer-Siwe disease, 607
Leucocytes, 548 et seq.
Leucocytosis, 549
Leuco-erythroblastic anaemia, 544
Leucopenia, 501, 550, 554
Leukaemia, 586-594
 acute, 589
 aleukaemic, 586
 bone marrow in, 604, 607
 chronic lymphocytic, 592, 593
 chronic myeloid, 591
 cytochemical tests in, 589
 lymph nodes in, 592
 monocytic, 589
 Philadelphia chromosome in, 591
 spleen in, 591, 592
 virus, in animals, 197
Leukaemoid reactions, 594
Leukodystrophy, 750
Leukoencephalitis, acute
 haemorrhagic, 745
Leukoplakia, 367, 682
Leydig-cell tumour, 707
Light chains, 99
Lipid
 abnormal accumulation of, 27

Lipid *(Contd)*
  in atheroma, 212
  storage diseases, 27
Lipofuscin, 25
Lipoma, 167
Lipo-melanic reticulosis, 577
Lipoproteins,
  disturbed metabolism, 27
  high density, 214
  very low density, 214
Liposarcoma, 188
Lips (see also Oral cavity), 366
Liver
  actinomycosis, 471
  acute yellow atrophy, 444, 447
  aflatoxin, effect on, 477
  alcohol and, 453-456
  amoebiasis, 473
  anatomy and physiology, 440-442
  auto-antibodies and, 463
  bacterial infections of, 471, 472
  in biliary obstruction, 463, 464
  cells,
    alcoholic hyaline, 455
    ballooning, 445, 455
    Councilman lesion, 445
    hyaline change, 455, 456
  cholestasis, 463
  chronic venous congestion, 138
  cirrhosis, 457 et seq.
  clotting defects and, 467, 469
  encephalopathy, hepatic, 468, 470
  endocrine disturbances and, 469
  failure, 467 et seq.
  fatty change, 10
  fluke, cholangiocarcinoma and, 474
  function, disturbances of, 442
    tests of, 442
  in haemochromatosis, 465
  healing, 84
  hepatitis, 445-451
  in hepato-lenticular degeneration, 465
  hydatid disease, 474
  injury, causes of, 444
  in kala-azar, 473
  in leptospirosis, 472
  in malaria, 473
  in malnutrition, 9
  metastatic tumours, 478
  multiple nodular hyperplasia, 444
  necrosis, 443
    centrilobular, 443
    focal, 445

massive, 444
mid-zonal, 443
peripheral zonal, 443
post-necrotic scarring, 444
pyogenic infections of, 414, 471
repair and regeneration, 446
schistosomiasis, 473
syphilis, 472
tropical abscess, 473
tuberculosis, 471
tumours, 475, 476
virus disease, 445 et seq.
Lobar pneumonia, 322-324
Local oedema, 142
Long-acting thyroid stimulator, 832
Loose bodies in joints, 819
Looser's zones, 799
Lorain-Levi syndrome, 826
Lower motor neurone disease, 757-760
Lower nephron nephrosis, 639
Lung
  anatomy, 295, 296
  asthma, bronchial, 302, 303
  atelectasia, 314
  in bagassosis, 348
  bird-fancier's, 348
  bronchiectasis, 304-307
  bronchitis, 299-301
  bronchopneumonia, 319
  in byssinosis, 348
  chronic venous congestion, 137
  emphysema, 308 et seq.
  empyema, 364
  extrinsic allergic alveolitis, 348
  farmer's, 348
  in fibrocystic disease of pancreas, 306
  fibrosis, 349
  fungal infections, 348
  Ghon focus, 59
  in Hamman-Rich syndrome, 349
  'honeycomb', 350
  hyaline membrane disease, 316
  hypostatic congestion, 321
  infarction, 132
  in influenza, 325
  in left ventricular failure, 251
  in measles, 326
  metallic dusts and, 349
  'mushroom pickers', 348
  oedema of, 143
  'opportunistic' infections of, 330
  in ornithosis, 326
  in paraquat poisoning, 351
  pneumoconiosis, 341 et seq.

pneumonia, 319 et seq.
progressive massive fibrosis, 343
in psittacosis, 326
pyaemic abscesses, 331
in shock, 149
suppuration, 321, 328, 330, 331
tuberculosis, 59, 60, 332
tumours, 352 et seq.
in uraemia, 654
virus infections of, 325, 326
Lupus erythematosus,
  systemic, 116, 821
Lymph nodes, 571-577
  acute lymphadenitis, 573
  in cat-scratch fever, 574
  chronic enlargements of, 592-594
  dermatopathic lymphadenopathy, 577
  glandular fever, 573
  in 'histiocytosis X', 607
  Hodgkin's disease, 595-598
  in immune responses, 98
  in infectious mononucleosis, 573
  in leukaemia, 592
  in lipid storage disease, 27
  lipo-melanic reticulosis, 577
  in lymphogranuloma venereum, 574
  in malignant lymphoma, 595-609
  measles, 574
  normal structure of, 571
  pigmentary infiltrations, 577
  reactive hyperplasia, 572
  in sarcoidosis, 575
    thymic dependent areas of, 98
  toxoplasmosis, 576
  tuberculosis, 575
  tumours
    primary, 577
    secondary, 576
  in typhoid fever, 396
  in Waldenstrom's
    macroglobulinaemia, 604
Lymphadenitis, 573, 575
Lymphangiectasis, 243
Lymphangiosarcoma, 243
Lymphangitis, 238
Lymphatic obstruction, 239, 240
Lymphatics, diseases of, 238-240
Lymphocytes, 97, 554
  'B' cells, 97
  in inflammation, 39
  surface markers, 97
  'T' cells, 97
  thymic origin of, 97

Lymphocytes (*Contd*)
  transformation, 98
Lymphocytic leukaemia, 592
Lymphoedema, 239
Lympho-epithelioma, 294, 370
Lymphogranuloma venereum, 574
Lymphoid tissues
  dendritic cells of, 571
  diseases of, 571-577
  germinal centres in, 98
  paracortex, 98
  spleen, 578-583
  tumours, 595 et seq.
Lymphokines, 106
Lymphoma, 586, 595-609
  alimentary tract, 411, 421
  Burkitt's, 608
  cell types, 601
  classifications, 599-602
  complications, 603
  diagnosis, 609
  diffuse, 600
  follicular, 600
  Hodgkin's disease, 595-598
  lymphoplasmacytic, 604
  macrophage, 607
  non-Hodgkin, 599-609
  plasma cell, 605, 606
  staging, 596
Lymphopenia, 554
Lymphoplasmacytic tumours, 604
Lympho-reticular tissues, 571-609
  neoplasia, 586-609
Lysosomal enzymes, 36
Lysozymes, 49

Macrocytic anaemia, 545
  pernicious anaemia, 519-521
  other forms of, 545
Macroglobulin, 100
Macrophages,
  inhibition of migration of, 107
  role in immune responses, 103, 105
  tumours, 607
Malabsorption syndrome, 405-408
  anaemia in, 408, 522
  bone changes in, 408
  coagulation defect in 565
  spleen in, 406
Malaria, 539, 541, 542
  Burkitt's tumour and, 608
  liver in, 541

pigment in, 25
Malignant hypertension, 220, 221
  kidneys in, 651, 652
Malignant melanoma, 193
Malignant tumours
  epithelial, 175-184
  non-epithelial, 185-188
Mallory bodies, 455
Mammary duct ectasia, 692
Marble bone disease, 806
March haemoglobinuria, 540
Marfan's syndrome, 222
Mast cells in anaphylaxis, 109
Mastitis, 692
Mastopathy, cystic, 693
McArdle's syndrome, 789
Mean corpuscular haemoglobin
    (MCH), 503
  haemoglobin concentration
    (MCHC), 502
  in hypochromic microcytic
    anaemia, 513
  in pernicious anaemia, 519
  volume (MCV), 503
  in hypochromic microcytic
    anaemia, 513
  in pernicious anaemia, 519
Measles, encephalitis and, 741
  giant-cell pneumonia in, 326
  lymphoid tissues in, 574
Meckel's diverticulum, 384
Medial calcification of arteries, 222
Medullary carcinoma of thyroid, 835
Medulloblastoma, 771
Megaloblastic anaemia, 517-522
Megaloblasts, 507
Meig's syndrome, 691
Melanin pigment, 20
Melanocyte stimulating hormone, 20
Melanocytes, 20
  tumours of, 191-193
Melanoma, 193
  malignant, 193
Melanophores, 20
Melon seed bodies, 819
Memory cells, 98
Meninges, 710, 711
  meningioma, 772
  meningitis, 733, 734
  meningocele, 768
Meningioma, 772
Meningitis, 733, 734
  aseptic, 738
  meningococcal, 55

pyogenic, 733
  tuberculous, 735
  virus, 738
Meningocele, 768
Meningomyelocele, 768
Meniscus, tear of, 812
Mesangial cells, 613
Mesaortitis, syphilitic, 62
Mesothelioma, malignant, 347
Metabolism, inborn errors, 27
Metamyelocytes, 548
Metaplasia, 161, 174
  in stroma of tumours, 189
Metastasis of tumours, 176 et seq.
Metastatic calcification, 19
Mice, breast cancer in, 197
Micro-aneurysms, cerebral, 228
Micro-angiopathic haemolytic
    anaemia, 540
Microcytic anaemia, 513, 545
Microglia, 713
Miliary tuberculosis, 59, 339
Milk factor of Bittner, 197
Mineralocorticoid hormones, 842
Mitral valve incompetence, 275
  stenosis, 274
Mixed tumours, 189
  of parotid gland, 189, 372
Monckeberg's sclerosis, 222
Moniliasis and candidiasis, 71
Monoclonal proliferation, 202, 593,
  604
Monocytes, 555
  change to macrophages, 555
Monocytic leukaemia, 589
Monocytosis, causes of, 555
Mononuclear phagocyte system, 105
Monospot test, 574
Motor neurone disease, 757-759
Mouth, 366
Mucocele, of appendix, 415
  of gallbladder, 481
Mucoid carcinoma, 425
  degeneration, 26
Mucoviscidosis, 496
Multiple, enchondromatosis, 168
  endocrine adenoma syndrome, 840
  myeloma (see Myelomatosis), 605,
    606
  sclerosis, 746, 747
Mumps, 371
  orchitis, 701
Mural thrombus, 261
Muscle healing, 85

Muscle, smooth
  auto-antibodies to, 116
  tumours of, 169
Muscle, skeletal, 780-792
  applied anatomy, 780-784
  atrophy, 781-784
  auto-antibodies to, 790
  biopsy, 791
  dystrophy, 787, 788
  hypertrophy, 784
  infective myositis, 786
  innervation, 781, 782
  ischaemic necrosis, 785
  muscular dystrophy, 788
  metabolic defects, 789
  motor end-plate, 784
  in myasthenia gravis, 784
  myopathy, 786-792
  myositis ossificans, 785
  in neural atrophy, 782
  normal structure, 780, 781
  in periodic paralysis, 789
  polymyositis, 790
  repair, 785
  in rheumatoid arthritis, 790
  serum enzymes, 791
  spindles, 783
  types, 781
Muscular dystrophy, 788
Mushroom picker's lung, 348
Mutation,
  cancer and, 197, 202
  radiation-induced, 197
Myalgic-encephalomyelitis (ME), 792
Myasthenia gravis, 117, 784
  thymus in, 585
Mycotic aneurysm, 229
Myeloblasts, 548, 589
Myelocytes, 548
Myelofibrosis, 558
Myeloid leukaemia, 587, 589, 591
Myeloid metaplasia, 559
Myeloma cells, 605
  protein, 606
Myelomatosis, 605, 606
  amyloid in, 606
  hypercalcaemia in, 605
  immunoglobulins in, 606
  renal changes in, 606
  skeletal changes in, 605, 810
Myeloproliferative disorders, 557
Myocardial infarction, 254 et seq.
Myocarditis, 267
Myoglobinuria, kidney in, 785

Myomalacia cordis, 262
Myopathy, 786-791
Myositis, 786
  ossificans, 785
Myotonic dystrophy, 788
Myxoedema, 829
  pretibial, 832
Myxoma, 167

Naegeli type of leukaemia, 589
Naevus,
  junctional, 192
  pigmented, 192
  spider, 242
Necrobiosis, 7
Necrosis, 2-6
Negri bodies, 69
Nephritis (see also
    Glomerulonephritis)
  immune-complex, 621 et seq.
  interstitial, 638
Nephroblastoma, 658
Nephrocalcinosis, cell injury in, 642
  in hyperparathyroidism, 642
  in hypervitaminosis D, 642
  in renal tubular acidosis, 642
Nephrosis, lipoid, 629
  lower nephron, 639-640
Nephrotic syndrome,
  in amyloidosis, 638
  in diabetes mellitus, 637
  in focal glomerulosclerosis, 630
  in membranous glomerulonephritis,
    627, 628
  in minimal-change
    glomerulonephritis, 629
  oedema in, 628
  in systemic lupus erythematosus, 634
Nerve cells, see Neurones, 712
Nerves, peripheral, 761-764
  healing, 85-87
  neuritis, 763
  neurofibromatosis, 773, 774
  neuropathy, 761-764
  tumours of, 773
Nervous system, 710-778
  anatomy and physiology, 710, 711
  cerebrospinal fluid, 710, 711, 768
  congenital abnormalities, 766, 768
  demyelinating diseases, 745-747
lipidoses, 27
  meninges, 710, 711

metabolic defects, 748-752
  neuroglia, 713
  neurones, 712
  repair, 85-87
  spinal cord, 755
  tumours, 769-775
Neurilemmoma, 773, 774
Neuritis (see also Neuropathy),
    interstitial, 763
Neuroblastoma, 771, 846
Neuro-ectodermal tumours, 769
Neurofibroma, 773
Neurofibromatosis, 774
Neurofibrosarcoma, 774
Neuroglia, 711, 713
Neuroma, traumatic, 87
Neurons, 712
  chromatolysis, 712
  degenerations, 712
    Wallerian, 86
  tumours of, 770, 771
Neuropathic arthritis, 813
  muscle atrophy, 782
Neuropathies, 762-764
  carcinomatous, 762
  definition, 761
  parenchymatous, 761
  Schwann cell dysfunction, 762
  segmental, 762, 764
  vascular, 763
  in vitamin deficiencies, 762
Neuronophagia, 739
Neutropenia, 550
Neutrophil leucocytes, 550
  in Arthus reaction, 111
  in chronic granulomatous disease,
    551, 552
  functional defects of, 551
  in inflammation, 33 et seq.
  phagocytosis by, 34, 551
  production of, 548
  in suppuration, 38
Neutrophil leucocytosis, 549
  leucopenia, 550
Niemann-Pick's disease, 27
Nipple, areolar infection, 692
  discharge, 694
  Paget's disease of, 695
  papilloma, 694
Nodes,
  Bouchard's, 814
  Heberden's, 814
Noradrenaline,
  production by tumours, 846

Normoblasts, 507
Normocytic anaemia, 545
Nose,
    polypi, 290
    rhinitis, 288-291
    tumours, 294
Nuclear jaundice (see Kernicterus), 535
Nucleus, folic acid and, 517
    radiation changes, 197
    vitamin B_{12} and, 517
Nutmeg liver, 138
Nutritional oedema, 144

Oat cell carcinoma, 359
Obesity, 11
    Fröhlich's syndrome and, 826
    gallstones in, 485
    heart in, 269
    late-onset diabetes and, 838
    osteoarthritis and, 813
Obstructive jaundice, 486
Ocular melanoma, 193
Oedema, 141
    of brain, 715
    generalised, 144
    glottidis, 292
    inflammatory, 32, 142
    local, 141
    pulmonary, 143
Oesophagus, 375
    achalasia, 376
    atresia, 377
    in Chagas's disease, 376
    diverticular, 376
    haemorrhage, 139
    hiatus hernia, 375
    inflammatory lesions, 375
    obstruction, 376
    'opportunistic' infections, 71, 375
    peptic oesophagitis, 375
    spontaneous rupture, 377
    tumours, 378
    varices, 139, 232, 377
Oestrogens and cancer, 199, 671, 689
Oligodendroglia, 713
Oligospermia, 698
Oncogenes, 198
Oöphoritis, 685
'Opportunistic' infections, 71, 375
    of lung, 330
    of oesophagus, 375

Opsonins, 103
Oral cavity,
    in Addison's disease, 367
    epulis, 368
    granular-cell myoblastoma, 368
    in iron deficiency, 516
    in lead poisoning, 367
    'leukoplakia', 367
    parabuccal mixed tumours, 372
    in pernicious anaemia, 521
    in Peutz-Jeghers syndrome, 367
    pigmentation, 367
    squamous carcinoma, 374
    syphilis, 366
    thrush, 366
    tumours, 367, 368
    in vitamin B deficiency, 366
Oral contraceptives, 668
Orchitis, 701
Organisation, 40, 127
Ornithosis, 326
Osmotic diuresis, 837
Osmotic fragility, 506
Osmotic pressure of plasma, 140
Osteitis deformans (Paget's disease of bone), 802
Osteitis fibrosa (see Hyperparathyroidism), 801
Osteoarthritis 813, 814, 818
Osteoblast, 794
Osteochondritis juvenilis, 803
Osteoclast, 794
Osteoclastoma, 187, 808
Osteodystrophy (renal), 800
Osteogenesis imperfecta, 806
Osteogenic sarcoma (see Osteosarcoma), 187, 809
Osteoid, 799
Osteoid osteoma, 808
Osteolysis, 794
Osteoma, 168, 807
Osteomalacia, 799, 800
Osteomyelitis
    pyogenic, 804
    tuberculous, 805
Osteopetrosis, 806
Osteophytes, 814
Osteoporosis, 796-798
Osteosarcoma, 187-809
Ovary,
    arrhenoblastoma, 689
    Brenner tumour 691
    carcinoma, 688 et seq.
    cystadenoma, multilocular, 172,

686, 687
    papillary serous, 172, 686
    dermoid cyst, 690
    dysgerminoma, 690
    endometriosis, 674
    fibroma, 691
    germ cell tumours, 690
    granulosa cell tumour, 689
    Krukenberg tumour, 691
    non-neoplastic cysts, 685
    oöphoritis, 685
    secondary tumours, 691
    teratoma, 690, 691
    thecoma, 689
    tubo-ovarian abscess, 685
    tumours, classification, 686
    in Turner's syndrome, 698
Oxalate stones. 661
Oxytocin 828

Paget's disease,
    of bone, 802
    of nipple, 695
Palmar fibromatosis, 166
Pancreas,
    acute haemorrhagic necrosis, 490
    calculi in, 495
    cysts, 494
    in diabetes, 836
    duct obstruction, 492
    exocrine, 488
    fat necrosis and, 491
    fibrocystic disease, 496
    islet-cell tumours, 840
    pancreatitis, 490
    in pluriglandular adenomatosis, 840
    in Zollinger-Ellison syndrome, 840
    tumours, 497
Pancreatic islets, 836
    tumours, 840
Pancreatitis,
    acute haemorrhagic, 490
    chronic, 494
Pancytopenia, 557-559
Pannus, 815
Papillary, cystadenoma, 172
    necrosis of kidney, 644
Papilloedema, 718
Papilloma, 170
Papovavirus and warts, 68
Pappenheimer bodies, 505
Parabuccal mixed tumours, 372

Paralytic ileus, 434
Paraquat poisoning, lung in, 351
Parathormone, 795
Parathyroid glands, 840
  adenomas, 841
  carcinoma, 841
  hyperparathyroidism, 841
  hypoparathyroidism, 841
  parathyroidectomy, effects of, 841
  tentany and 841
Paratyphoid, 398
Parietal-cell antibodies, 382, 520
Parkinsonism, 753, 754
Parotid gland
  cribriform cylindroma, 373
  mixed tumour, 189, 372
  suppuration, 371
  uveo-parotid fever, 371
Paroxysmal cold haemoglobinuria, 538
Passive immunisation, 118
Paul-Bunnell test, 574
Peau d'orange 240, 696
Pedicels, 613
Penis, condylomata acuminata, 705
  papilloma, 705
  Peyronie's disease of, 705
  Queyrat's erythroplasia of, 705
  squamous carcinoma, 705
  syphilitic chancre of, 61
Peptic ulcer, 384 et seq.
  carcinoma and, 387
  complications, 386, 387
  duodenal, 386, 387
  etiology, 388, 389
  gastric, 384-386
  of Meckel's diverticulum, 389
  oesophageal, 384
  perforation of, 384, 387
  types, 384, 385
Perforation of appendix, 413, 414
  of intestine, 398, 419, 429
  of stomach, 381, 384, 387
Periarteritis nodosa (see also
    Polyarteritis nodosa), 223
Pericarditis, 283, 284
  causes, 283
  in myocardial infarction, 263
  organisation of, 284
  rheumatic, 272
  uraemic, 283
Pericardium, 283
  effusion into, 283
  haemorrhage, 284
  pericarditis, 283

tumours, 284
Periodic paralysis, 789
Peritoneum,
  effusion into, 437
  peritonitis, 435
  tumours, 437
Peritonitis, 435
Permanent cells, 81
Pernicious anaemia, 518-521
  mucous membranes in, 521
  stomach in, 520
  subacute combined degeneration,
    521
  tongue in, 521
Perthes' disease of hip, 803
Petechial haemorrhages, 566
Peutz-Jeghers syndrome, 409
Peyronie's disease, 705
Phaeochromocytoma, 846
Phagocytosis, 34, 35
Phagosome, 34
Pharynx, 370
Phenylketonuria, 750, 751
Philadelphia chromosome, 591
Phlebitis, 232
  chronic, 234
Phlebothrombosis, 232
Phosphate stones, 661
Pigmentation
  in Addison's disease, 20
  anthracotic, 26
  biliary, 22
  endogenous, 20 et seq.
  exogenous, 25, 26
  haemosiderin, 23, 24
  lead, 26
  lipofuscin, 25
  malarial, 25
  melanin, 20
  in Peutz-Jeghers syndrome, 409
  silver, 26
  tattoo, 26
Pigmented naevus, 192
  villonodular synovitis, 819
Pituitary, 824
  in acromegaly, 828
  adenoma, 827
  anterior lobe, 824
  in Cushing's syndrome, 843
  in diabetes insipidus, 828
  dwarfism, 826
  in Fröhlich's syndrome, 826
  giantism, 827
  hyperfunction, 827

hypofunction, 826
  infantilism, 826
  in myxoedema, 829
  necrosis, 827
  posterior lobe, 828
  in pregnancy, 827
  in Sheehan's syndrome, 827
  in Simmond's disease, 827
  tumours, 826, 828, 843
Placenta, choriocarcinoma, 672
  hormones of, 672
  hydatidiform mole, 672
  penetrating mole, 672
Plasma cells 605, 606
  antibody production by 98, 606
  in inflammation, 39
  in multiple myeloma, 605
  origin of, 98
Plasmacytoma, 605
Plasmin, 562
Plasminogen, 562
Platelets, 556
  auto-antibodies to, 566
  function, 556
  origin, 556
  in thrombocytopenic purpura, 566
  in thrombosis, 120, 122
Pleura
  acute pleurisy, 361
  empyema, 362
  fibrosis, 361
  pneumothorax, 318, 337
  tuberculosis, 361
  tumours, 347
Pleural effusion, 252
Plummer-Vinson syndrome, 376
Pluriglandular adenomatosis, 840
Pneumoconiosis, 306, 341 et seq.
  anthracosis, 342, 343
  asbestosis, 346, 347
  siderosis, 137
  silicosis, 344, 345
Pneumocystis carinii, 330
Pneumonia, 319
  arthritis in, 345
  in aspergillosis, 330
  bronchopneumonia, 319
  in candidiasis, 330
  chemical, 351
  giant-cell, 326
  hypostatic, 321
  Legionnaire's disease, 327
  lipid, 329
  organisation of, 321

Pneumonia (*Contd*)
  in ornithosis, 326
  Pneumocystis carinii, 330
  primary atypical, 330
  in psittacosis, 326
  resolutionof, 324
  'rheumatic', 345
  tuberculous, 337
  in uraemia, 654
Pneumothorax, 318, 337
Podocytes, 613
Poikilocytosis of red cells, 503
Poliomyelitis, 739
Polyarteritis,
  nodosa, 223
  kidney in, 634
  microangiopathic, 540
  Wegener's granuloma and, 223
Polychromasia, 508
Polycystic disease of kidney, 656
Polycythaemia, 546, 547
  primary (vera), 546, 547
  secondary, 546, 547
Polymorphonuclear leucocytes, 548 et
  seq.
Polymyositis, 790
Polyneuritis (see also Neuropathy),
  762-764
Polyneuropathy (see Neuropathy), 762
Polyoma virus, neoplasia and, 197
Polyposis coli, 423
Polyuria in chronic renal failure, 653
  in diabetes insipidus, 828
  in diabetes mellitus, 837
Pompe's disease, 27
Porphyria, 764
Portal hypertension, 460
  pyaemia, 414
  venous obstruction, 139
Post-cricoid carcinoma, 378
Post-haemorrhagic anaemia, 523, 524
Post-necrotic scarring of liver, 444
Post-viral fatigue syndrome, 792
Potassium
  aldosterone and, 844
  in Conn's syndrome, 844
  paralysis and, 789
Precipitation reactions, 103
Pregnancy,
  abdominal, 684
  choriocarcinoma and, 672
  diabetes and, 838
  ectopic, 684
  hydatidiform mole and, 672

iso-immunisation in, 534
kidney disorders in, 636
macrocytic anaemia in, 522
penetrating mole and, 672
pyelonephritis in, 636
tubal, 684
Premalignant lesions, 367, 682
Pressure atrophy, 13
Proctitis in ulcerative colitis, 419
Progressive bulbar palsy, 759
  massive fibrosis of lung, 343
  systemic sclerosis, 821
Prolactin, 825
Promyelocytic leukaemia, 589
Prostaglandins, 36, 126
Prostate,
  carcinoma of, 704
  gonococcal infection, 700
  hyperplasia, 702
  latent carcinoma, 704
  prostatitis, 700
  tuberculosis, 701
Prothrombin, conversion to
  thrombin, 561
Pseudarthrosis, 91
Pseudo-
  -hypertrophic muscular dystrophy,
  788
  -membranous inflammation, 42
  -myxoma peritonei, 415
Psittacosis, 326
Puberty, precocious, 846
Pulmonary
  aspergillosis, 348
  candidiasis, 330
  collapse, 317
  embolism, 132
  hypertension, 312
  oedema, 143
  osteoarthropathy, 307
  tuberculosis, 332
    bronchopneumonia, 337
    in diabetics, 336
    effects of chemotherapy, 340
    localised metastatic, 339
    miliary, 339
    of pleura, 340
    primary, 332
    reinfection, 334
Pulmonary valve stenosis in
  carcinoid syndrome, 411
congenital, 285
Punctate basophilia, 505
Purpura

allergic, 566
  Henoch-Schönlein, 566
  thrombocytopenic, 566
Pus, 38
Pyaemia, 51, 52
Pyelitis, 643
Pyelonephritis
  acute, 643
  chronic, 646
  in diabetes, 637
  papillary necrosis in, 644
  in pregnancy, 636
  tuberculous, 648
Pyknosis, 3
Pylephlebitis, 414
Pyloric stenosis, congenital, 394
  peptic ulcer and, 386
  results of, 386, 394
Pyogenic bacteria, 54, 55
  infections, 54, 55
  membrane, 38
Pyogenic granuloma, 242
Pyometra, 678
Pyosalpinx, 683
  tuberculous, 683
Pyrexia, 72
Pyridoxine in sideroblastic anaemia,
  544
Pyrogens, 72

Q fever, 326
Queyrat's erythroplasia of penis, 705
Quinsy, 370

Rabies,
  vaccine, encephalomyelitis and, 745
Radiation,
  carcinogenic effects of, 196
  cell damage, 12
Raynaud's disease, 231
  phenomenon (syndrome), 230
Reagin, 101
Rectum,
  benign lymphoid polyposis, 423
  carcinoma, 424
  juvenile polyp, 423
  papilloma, 422
  tumours, 422 et seq.
Red cells
  absolute values, 502, 503

Red cells (Contd)
  auto-antibodies to 537
'balance sheet', 511, 515
  fragility, 506
  haemoglobin content, variations
    in, 502
  inclusions, 505
  life span of, 511, 526
  mean cell volume, 503
  number, variations in, 502
  packed cell colume, 502
  polychromasia, 508
  production of, 500
  shape and size, variations in, 503
  sickle cells, 504
  spherocytes, 504
  target cells, 504
Reed-Sternberg cells, 597
Refractory anaemia, 544
Regeneration, 81
Regional enteritis, 400, 403, 404
Reiter's syndrome, 660
Renal
  arteries, 612
    atheroma, 652
    stenosis, 652
  calculi, 661
    in hyperparathyroidism, 642
    in immobilisation, 797
  clearances, 619
  colic, 662
  dwarfism, 841
  failure, chronic, 653
    biochemical changes in, 654
    causes, 653
    clinical features, 653
    hypertension in, 653
    pathological changes, 653
    water excretion in, 653
  glycosuria, 837
  hypertension, 219, 652
  oedema, 144
  osteodystrophy, 800, 841
  pelvis, 658
  rickets, 800
  tubular acidosis, 640
  tubular necrosis, 639, 640
Renin
  in hypertension, 218
  in shock, 146
Repair (see Healing)
Reproductive system, female, 664
  male, 699
Resolution, 37, 324

Respiratory,
  distress syndrome of
    newborn, 315
  function, 297
  system, 288 et seq.
  viruses, 288
Reticulin formation, 80
Reticulocytes, 508
Retina, in diabetes, 839
  in malignant hypertension, 726
Retinoblastoma, 771
Retroplacental haemorrhage, kidney
    in, 641
Retroviruses, 65
Rhabdomyosarcoma, 188
Rhesus blood groups, 534
  in haemolytic disease of newborn,
    534
Rheumatic
  arthritis, 815
  fever, 270
  heart disease, 270-274
  nodules, 271
  Rheumatoid arthritis, 815, 816
    nodules, 816
    Sjögren's syndrome and, 371
Rhinitis, acute, 290
  allergic (atopic), 291
Rickets, 800
  non-dietary, 841
Rickettsial pneumonia, 326
Right ventricle,
  failure, 250, 251
  hypertrophy, 247
Rodent ulcer, 183
Rous sarcoma, 197
Rubber, bladder cancer and, 663
Rubella, cardiac anomalies in, 285
Rupture of heart, 262

Salivary glands, 371
  calculi in, 371
  in mumps, 371
  in Sjögren's syndrome, 371
Salmonellae, 396
Salpingitis, 683
Sarcoidosis
  lymph nodes in, 575
  uveo-parotid fever in, 371
Sarcoma
  definition, 185
  types, 186 et seq.

Sarcoma botryoides, 188
Satellitosis oligodendrocytic, 713
Scarring after would healing, 78
Schilling type of leukaemia, 589
Schistocytes, 503
Schistosomiasis of bladder, 663
  intestinal, 473
  of liver, 473
Schwannoma, 773, 774
Scirrhous carcinoma, 696
Scleroderma, 820
Sclerosing angioma of skin, 242
  adenosis of breast, 693
Scrotum, squamous carcinoma of, 706
Secondary hypertension, 219
  renal changes in, 652
Secretory piece, 101
Seminal vesicles, tuberculosis, 701
Seminoma, ovarian, 690
  testicular, 706
Senile arteriosclerosis, 216
  atrophy, 13
  dementia, 732
  emphysema, 313
Septal defects of heart, 285
Septic embolism, 52, 53
  spleen, 579
Septicaemia, 52, 54, 55
Sequestrum, bone, 805
Serotonin, 36, 410
Serum sickness, 118
Sex chromatin, 552
Sheehan's syndrome, 827
Shock, 145 et seq.
  bacterial, 145, 156
  in burns and scalds, 155
  causes, 145
  endotoxins, 156
  individual organs, 149-153
  mechanisms, 146, 147
  metabolism in, 148
  outcome, 157
  primary, 154
  types, 145
  vascular changes, 147
Shope papilloma, 197
Sickle-cell anaemia, 532
Sideroblastic anaemia, 544
Sideroblasts, 544
Siderosis, pulmonary, 137
Silica, cell injury and, 345
Silicosis, 344
Silver pigmentation, 26
Simmond's disease, 827

Singer's node (fibroma of larynx), 294
Sinus, 39, 46
Sinusitis, acute, 290
Sjögren's syndrome, 371
Skull fracture, effects of, 727-730
Sleeping sickness, 744
Slit pores, glomerular, 613
Slow virus infections, 68, 69, 742
Smegma, carcinogenic effect of, 680, 705
Sodium deficiency, 845
Softening, cerebral, 721-723
Soot, carcinogenic effect of, 706
Spherocytosis of red cells, 504, 529
Spider naevi, 242
Spina bifida, 768
Spinal cord, 756-761
    in amyotrophic lateral sclerosis, 759
    ascending degenerations, 756
    compression, 755
    congenital malformations, 768
    descending degenerations, 756
        in Friedreich's ataxia, 761
    motor neurons, lesions of, 758, 759
    in pernicious anaemia, 760
    in poliomyelitis, 739, 757
    in progressive bulbar palsy, 759
    in progressive muscular atrophy, 758
    in prolapsed intervertebral disc, 755
    subacute combined degeneration of, 760
    in syphilis, 63
    syringomyelia, 760
    in tabes dorsalis, 760
    transverse lesions, 755
    trauma of, 755
Spleen,
    atrophy 583
    in bacterial infections, 579
    chronic venous congestion, 580
    circulatory changes, 583
    enlargement, causes of, 579
    functions of, 578
    in Gaucher's diseases, 27, 581
    haemopoiesis in, 559
    in Hand-Schüller-Christian disease, 607
    in 'histiocytosis X' 607
    in Hodgkin's disease, 596
    hypersplenism, 582
    hyposplenism, 583
    infarcts of, 583
    in kala-azar, 579
    in lipid storage disorders, 581

    in malaria, 582
    in Niemann Pick disease, 581
    normal structure, 578
    septic, 579
Splenic anaemia, 582
Splenomegaly, 579 et seq.
    in bacterial infections, 579
    congestive, 580
    in haematological disorders, 582
    in lipid storage disorders, 581
    in protozoal infections, 541
Spondylosis, 814
Sprue, 406
Squamous carcinoma, 182
Stable cells, 81
'Staghorn' calculus, 662
Starvation, 9
Stercoral ulcers, 429
Sterility, male, causes of, 698
Still's disease, 816
Stokes-Adams attacks, 248
Stomach,
    achlorhydria, 383
    anatomy and physiology, 379, 380
    atrophic gastritis, 383
    auto-antibodies to, 383, 520
    carcinoma, 390
    dilatation, 394
    erosions, 381
    gastritis, 382
    gastroptosis, 394
    haemorrhage into, 387
    hour-glass, 386
    infections, 381
    leather bottle, 391
    leiomyosarcoma, 393
    linitis plastica, 391
    metaplasia, intestinal, 382
    peptic ulceration, 384 et seq.
    perforation, 387
    premalignant lesions, 387
    pyloric stenosis, 386
    tumours, 390-393
    ulcer, cancer, 387
Stomatitis, 366
Strangulation of gut, 134
'Strawberry' gall bladder, 482
    glomerulonephritis and, 621
    rheumatic fever and, 270
Struma ovarii, 691
Subacute bacterial endocarditis, 279
Subacute combined degeneration, 521, 760
Subacute sclerosing encephalitis, 741

Subarachnoid haemorrhage, 725
Subdural haemotoma, 729
Sub-phrenic abscess, 436
Suppuration, 38
Suprasellar cyst, 773
Surfactant, 316
Synovial chondromatosis, 819
    sarcoma, 819
Syphilis, 61-63
    neurological, 63
Syringomyelia, 760
Systemic lupus erythematosus, 821
    auto-antibodies and, 116, 821
    kidney in, 634

Tabes dorsalis, 6-3
Takayashu's disease, 225
Talc granuloma, 43
Tamponade, cardiac, 262, 284
Tar, carcinogenic effect of, 194
Tattooing, 26
Tay-Sach's disease, 750
Telangiectasis, 242
Temperature regulating mechanism, 72
Temporal arteritis, 225
Tendon sheath,
    giant-cell tumour of, 819
Tenosynovitis,
    pigmented villonodular, 819
Teratoma, 189, 190
    of brain, 773
    of ovary, 690
    of testis, 706
Testicular feminisation, 698
Testis,
    granulomatous orchitis, 702
    gumma, 702
    interstitial cell tumour, 707
    in Klinefelter's syndrome, 698
    lymphoma, 599
    orchitis, 701
    seminoma, 706
    syphilis, 702
    teratoma, 706
    tumours, 706
Tetanus, 57
    prophylaxis, 118
Tetany in hypoparathyroidism, 841
Tetany after parathyroidectomy, 841
Tetralogy of Fallot, 285
Thalassaemia, 532
Theca-cell tumour, 689

Theca-lutein cyst, 685
Thrombin, 561
Thrombo-angiitis obliterans, 224
Thrombocythaemia, 558
Thrombocytopenic purpura, 566
Thrombocytosis, 556
Thrombophlebitis, 178, 232-234
Thrombosis, 120-127
  coronary, arterial, 255
Thrombotic microangiopathy, 540
Thrush, 366, 375
Thymomas, 585
Thymus, 584, 585
  changes with age, 584
  hyperplasia, 585
  hypoplasia, 584
  in myasthenia gravis, 585
  normal function, 584
  tumours, 585
Thyroid gland, 829-835
  auto-immune thyroiditis, 116
Thyrotrophic hormone (TSH), 825
Tissue damage, 2, 3
Tolerance, immunological, 108
Tongue,
  glossitis, 366
  granular cell myoblastoma, 368
  squamous carcinoma, 369
  syphilis, 366
  tuberculosis, 366
Tonsilitis, 370
Toxic jaundice, 22
Toxins bacterial, 2, 51
  fatty change and, 9, 10
Toxoplasmosis, 576, 743
Trachea, 292
Transaminases,
  in liver disease, 447
  in myocardial infarction, 266
Transferrin, 24, 514
Transformation of small
  lymphocytes, 98, 106, 107
Transfusion, blood, 567-570
'Transfusion' kidney, 639
Trauma, acute renal failure in, 639
Treponema pallidum, 61
Tricuspid valve, incompetence, 278
Triple response of Lewis, 31
Tropical abscess of liver, 473
  sprue, 406
Trypanosomiasis, 744
Tubal pregnancy, 684
Tubercle, follicle, 43, 58
  immune reaction, 111

Tuberculoid leprosy, 64
Tuberculosis, 58-60
  Ghon focus, 59, 332
  lymph nodes in, 575
  pulmonary, 332-340
Tubo-ovarian abscess, 685
Tubular adenoma, 422
Tubular necrosis, renal, 151
Tubulorrhexis, renal, 639
Tumours, 162-206
  benign, 163
  classification, 163
  causation, 194-203
  connective tissue, 166
  criteria of malignancy, 165
  differentiation, 164
  epithelial varieties, 170 et seq.
  malignant, 175
  pre-malignant lesions, 174
  spread of, 176-181
  viruses and, 68, 197, 198
Turner's syndrome, 698
Typhoid, 396-398

Ulceration, 44, 45
Ulcerative colitis, 418
Upper motor neurone disease, 757-759
Uraemia, 635
Uraemic colitis, 654
  osteodystrophy, 654, 800
Urate stones, 661
Uretero-vesical reflux, 660
Ureters, 658, 659
Urethra,
  stricture, 700
  urethritis, 660, 699
Uric acid, 588, 814
Urinary bladder,
  calculi, 661, 662
  chemical carcinogens and, 663
  infections, 660
  malakoplakia, 660
  obstruction, 703
  schistosomiasis, 663
  tumours, 663
Urinary casts, 618
Urinary tract, 658-663
Urobilinogen, 527
Uterus, 667
  cervix uteri, 675
  choriocarcinoma, 672
  fibroid (leiomyoma), 169, 673

hydatidiform mole, 672
  tumours, 670-673
Uveo-parotid fever, 371

Vagina, 680
  inflammation, 680, 681
  tumours, 681, 682
Varices, oesophageal, 232, 377
Varicocele, 237
Varicose veins, 235-237
Vascular diseases, 208-243
Vasculitis, allergic, 224, 225
Vasopressin, 828
Vaso-vagal attack, 154
Veins, diseases of, 232-237
  in malignant disease, 234
  thrombophlebitis, 233
  thrombosis, 125, 232
  varicose, 235-237
Venous congestion, 134 et seq.
  general, 135-138
  local, 134
  oedema in, 136
Ventricular fibrillation, 281
Verruca vulgaris, 68
Vibrio cholerae, 400
Villous adenoma, 422
Vincent's angina, 370
Virilism, adrenal, 844, 846
Virulence of micro-organisms, 49
Virus infections, 65-70
  host/virus interaction, 69, 70
  immunity in, 70
  interferon production, 70
  latent, 67
  oncogenic, 68, 69
  slow, 68
Viruses,
  carcinogenic effects of, 197, 198
  cytopathic effects of, 2, 65, 69
  post-viral fatigue syndrome, 792
  respiratory, 288, 325
Vitamin B complex, 748
Vitamin B_{12} 518-521
  diverticulosis of small bowel and, 427
  subacute combined degeneration
    and, 521
Vitamin C deficiency,
  bones in, 803
  fracture healing in, 91
  wound healing in, 80
Vitamin D deficiency, 799, 800

Vitamin D deficiency (*Contd*)
   excess, 19
Vitamin K deficiency, 565
   haemorrhagic disease of newborn
     and, 565
Volvulus, 433
Von Gierke's disease, 27
Von Recklinghausen's
    neurofibromatosis, 774
Vulva, 681
   leukoplakia, 682
   tumours, 682

Waldenstrom's macroglobulinaemia,
   604
Wallerian degeneration, 86
Warthin-Finkeldey cells, 574
Warts, 68, 170
Waterhouse-Friderichsen syndrome,
   55
Wegener's granuloma, 223
Weil's disease, 472
Wernicke's encephalopathy, 748
Whipple's disease, 406'
White bile, 486
Wilm's tumour, 658
Wilson's diseae, 465-751
Wound healing, 76-79

Zenker's degneration, 398
Zollinger-Ellison syndrome, 840